young chas. MD

CLINICAL PEDIATRIC NEUROLOGY

A signs and symptoms approach

Gerald M. Fenichel, M.D.

Professor and Chairman
Department of Neurology
Vanderbilt University
School of Medicine
Nashville, Tennessee

1988
W. B. SAUNDERS COMPANY
Harcourt Brace Jovanovich, Inc.
Philadelphia   London   Toronto   Montreal   Sydney   Tokyo

W. B. SAUNDERS COMPANY
Harcourt Brace Jovanovich, Inc.

The Curtis Center
Independence Square West
Philadelphia, PA 19106

Library of Congress Cataloging-in-Publication Data

Fenichel, Gerald M.

Clinical pediatric neurology.

1. Pediatric neurology.   2. Nervous system—Diseases—
   Diagnosis.   I. Title. [DNLM: 1. Nervous System
   Diseases—diagnosis.   2. Nervous System Diseases—in
   infancy & childhood.   3. Neurologic Examination—in
   infancy & childhood. WS 340 F333c]

RJ486.F46 1988   618.92′8   87–26501
ISBN 0–7216–1896–0

Editor: Martin Wonsiewicz
Designer: Karen O'Keefe
Production Manager: Bob Butler
Manuscript Editor: Carol Robins
Illustration Coordinator: Peg Shaw
Indexer: Susan Thomas

Clinical Pediatric Neurology:
A Signs and Symptoms Approach   ISBN   0–7216–1896–0

Last digit is the print number: 9   8   7   6   5   4   3

*To Barbara—with love, on the occasion
of our thirtieth anniversary*

Preface

It is considerably easier to organize a textbook of child neurology by categories of diseases than by chief complaint. Unfortunately, patients present with complaints and not diseases. Complaints are the initial features of disease and therefore the starting point for diagnosis. From the chief complaint, a differential diagnosis is constructed and then tested to provide a single and, it is hoped, a correct final diagnosis.

Many disorders have the potential for what seems like an endless number of different presentations, e.g., migraine and epilepsy. Many symptoms are presenting features of what seems like an endless number of disorders, e.g., headache and dysphagia. This is the impediment to a text organized by chief complaint. In order to avoid constant repetition, the primary description of a disease has usually been assigned to a single chapter, although in some cases multiple entries have been made when variant forms of the same disease have different presentations, e.g., maple syrup urine disease. Tables are used generously in every chapter to provide differential diagnoses and to indicate the chapter containing the most complete description of a disease. The reader may sometimes have to flip back and forth between chapters, but this seems the best practical alternative.

This text is intended to provide practical information needed by physicians caring for children with neurologic disorders. With the text restricted in scope to diagnosis and therapy, no effort has been made to include basic science or pathologic considerations unless they are critical to understanding symptoms or therapy. References were selected because they were recent and easy to access, with literature summaries given preference over original reports. Eighteen major "presenting complaints" were chosen as chapter headings, and each chapter further refines that complaint by age at onset, course of illness, and other discriminating features.

Monographs have become a rarity in recent years because it is increasingly difficult for one person to be expert or interested in an entire specialty of medicine. This book, however, because of its orientation by presenting features, did not lend itself to using multiple authors, since the chapters are interrelated to a large extent. Consequently, it reflects my biases (learning disabilities were omitted) and some sections are written with more first-hand knowledge than others.

Several chapters were reviewed by true experts and I am grateful for their instruction: Dr. Michael H. Brooke, Dr. Robert B. Daroff, Dr. Owen B. Evans, Dr. Patrick J. M. Lavin, Dr. C. David Marsden, and Michael J. Painter, and Nole B. Tulipan. I am especially grateful to my pediatric neurology colleagues at Vanderbilt who were repeatedly pressed into service as reviewers: D. Anthony W. Kilroy and

Dr. Harry T. Whelan; to Dr. Zuo Chi-Hua who encouraged me to attempt this work when my courage faltered; and to Mrs. Lester Tilley, my secretary, research assistant, and friend.

I have learned a great deal writing this book, and I hope that it is as educational to others.

GERALD M. FENICHEL

Contents

1   Paroxysmal Disorders   1

2   Altered States of Consciousness   42

3   Headache   73

4   Increased Intracranial Pressure   89

5   Psychomotor Retardation and Regression   118

6   The Hypotonic Infant   147

7   Flaccid Limb Weakness in Childhood   170

8   Cramps, Muscle Stiffness, and Exercise Intolerance   199

9   Disturbances of Sensation   214

10   Ataxia   223

11   Hemiplegia   248

12   Paraplegia and Quadriplegia   263

13   Monoplegia   279

14   Movement Disorders   286

15 Disorders of Ocular Motility 302

16 Disorders of the Visual System 321

17 Lower Brainstem and Cranial Dysfunction 337

18 Disorders of Cranial Volume and Shape 359

Index 377

1 Paroxysmal Disorders

This chapter deals with disorders characterized by sudden and recurrent, but usually transitory, episodes of neurologic dysfunction. Paroxysmal disorders in children are frequently epileptic or migrainous in origin. Less common causes are syncope and other nonmigrainous vascular events, psychogenic disturbances, intermittent increased intracranial pressure, and metabolic disorders. Many "spells" remain unexplained even after intensive study. The differential diagnosis of paroxysmal disorders varies considerably from the newborn, to infancy, childhood, and adolescence and is best presented by age groups.

■ Paroxysmal Disorders of Newborns

Seizures are the major paroxysmal disorder of the newborn. The frequency of neonatal convulsions in one regional intensive care unit during the period 1976 to 1979 was approximately six per thousand live births (Bergman et al, 1983). This is comparable to the rate of five per thousand noted at several University Medical Centers twenty years previously (Holden et al, 1982). It is clear that seizures remain a common presenting symptom in the newborn. The challenge for the clinician is to differentiate seizure activity from normal neonatal movements and from pathologic movements due to other mechanisms (Table 1.1).

APPROACH TO DIAGNOSIS

Seizure Patterns

The clinical expression of seizures in the newborn, especially the premature, is poorly organized and difficult to distinguish from normal activity. Newborns with hydranencephaly or atelencephaly are capable of generating the full variety of neonatal seizure patterns. This supports the notion that seizures may arise from the brainstem as well as the hemispheres (Danner et al, 1985). Seizures arising in the brainstem may be confined there by the absence of myelinated pathways for propagation. For the same reason, seizures originating in one hemisphere are unlikely to spread beyond the contiguous cortex or to produce secondary bilateral synchrony.

Neonatal seizures are traditionally classified as (1) subtle, (2) multifocal clonic, (3) focal clonic, (4) tonic, and (5) myoclonic. This classification is useful, but does not do justice to the rich variety of patterns that are actually observed. Generalized tonic-clonic seizures do not occur (Kellaway and Hrachovy, 1983). Most newborns suspected of generalized tonic-clonic convulsions are *jittery* (see "Jitteriness" later on). Newborns paralyzed with pancuronium to assist mechanical ventilation pose a special problem in seizure identification. In this circumstance, physicians may be alerted to the possibility of seizures by the presence of rhythmic increases in systolic arterial blood pressure, heart rate, and oxygenation (Goldberg et al, 1982).

Subtle Seizures

Clinical Features. The term "subtle" encompasses several different patterns in which tonic or clonic movements of the limbs are lacking. Instead, behavioral changes or movements occur that cannot be distinguished from nonseizure activity. Subtle seizures are believed to be the most common neonatal seizure pattern, but this belief is probably based on faulty diagnosis.

1

Table 1.1 MOVEMENTS THAT RESEMBLE NEONATAL SEIZURES

Normal movement
Nonconvulsive apnea
Jitteriness
Benign nocturnal myoclonus
Pathologic myoclonus
Opisthotonos

Clinical observation alone is rarely accurate in discriminating subtle seizures from other kinds of movement.

Subtle seizure patterns are listed in Table 1.2. Of these, *apnea* poses the most vexing problem in differential diagnosis. Apneic spells are common in newborns, especially prematures, but should not be considered a seizure manifestation unless associated with tonic extension of the body or other subtle seizure patterns. Paroxysmal laughter has been reported as a seizure manifestation in two newborns and in both cases proved to be caused by congenital mass lesions of the posterior hypothalamus (Sher and Brown, 1976).

Diagnosis. The definitive identification of subtle seizures requires continuous electroencephalographic (EEG) monitoring. This can be accomplished by the use of 24-hour ambulatory cassettes that allow the acquisition of four or eight channels of data with the capability of marking the time of questionable events (Bridgers et al, 1986; Fenichel, 1987). When such monitoring is performed in newborns with subtle seizures, very few of the clinical episodes are associated with epileptiform activity. It seems unlikely that the abnormal activity was missed as a result of the small number of channels used. Epileptiform activity in the newborn is usually widespread, and epileptiform activity that is clinically asymptomatic is often detected (Fig. 1.1).

Subtle seizures are not associated with a specific etiology. Further diagnostic studies, treatment, and prognosis depend upon the underlying cause.

Multifocal Clonic Seizures

Clinical Features. Migratory jerking movements are noted first in one limb and then another; the face may be involved as well. The migration appears random and does not follow expected patterns of epileptic spread. Movements in one limb are sometimes prolonged, suggesting a focal rather than a multifocal seizure. The multifocal nature is detected later, when nursing notes are found to be contradictory concerning the side or the limb affected. Multifocal clonic seizures are a neonatal equivalent of generalized tonic-clonic seizures. They are ordinarily associated with severe, generalized cerebral disturbances such as hypoxic-ischemic encephalopathy.

Diagnosis. Multifocal epileptiform activity can usually be detected on a standard EEG. If epileptiform activity is not observed, a 24-hour monitor is recommended.

Focal Clonic Seizures

Clinical Features. These seizures are characterized by repeated, irregular jerking movements affecting one limb or both limbs on one side. The movements are irregular, are rarely sustained for long periods of time, and do not "march," as if spreading along the motor cortex. Focal clonic seizures occurring in a term newborn who is otherwise alert and responsive suggests a cerebral infarction or intracerebral hemorrhage (Fenichel et al, 1984). In newborns with states of decreased consciousness, focal clonic seizures may indicate a focal infarction superimposed upon a generalized encephalopathy (Clancy et al, 1985).

Diagnosis. During the seizure, a unilateral focus of high-amplitude sharp waves may be present adjacent to the Rolandic fissure. The discharge can spread to involve contiguous areas in the same hemisphere and can be associated with unilateral seizures of the limbs and adversive movements of the head and eyes. In the interictal period, the EEG usually demonstrates focal slowing or amplitude attenuation.

Newborns with focal clonic seizures should be evaluated by uncontrasted computerized tomography (CT) or ultrasound to determine the presence of intracerebral hemorrhage. If these studies are normal but the affected limbs seem paretic after the seizure has subsided, CT should be performed a week later to look for cerebral infarction. Ultrasound is not useful in detecting small cerebral infarctions.

Table 1.2 SUBTLE SEIZURE PATTERNS IN NEWBORNS

Apnea
Tonic deviation of the eyes
Repetitive fluttering of eyelids
Drooling, sucking, chewing
Swimming movements of the arms
Pedaling movements of the legs
Paroxysmal laughing

EKG

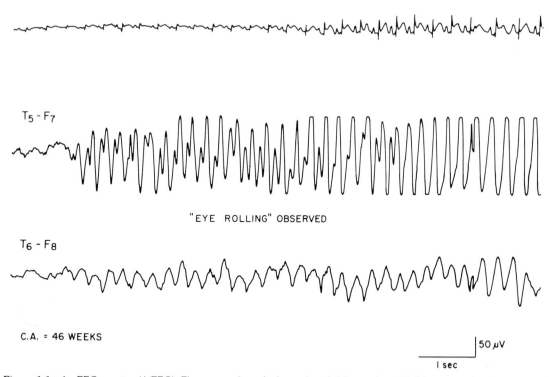

T5 - F7

"EYE ROLLING" OBSERVED

T6 - F8

C.A. = 46 WEEKS

50 μV

I sec

Figure 1.1 An EEG monitor (A/EEG). Electroconvulsive discharge from left hemisphere (T_5-F_7) associated with rolling back of the eyes.

Tonic Seizures

Clinical Features. These seizures are characterized by extension and stiffening of the body, usually associated with apnea and upward deviation of the eyes. Tonic posturing without the other features is rarely a seizure manifestation (Kellaway and Hrachovy, 1983). Tonic seizures are more common in prematures than term newborns and usually indicate structural brain damage rather than a metabolic disturbance.

Diagnosis. Tonic seizures in prematures are often symptomatic of intraventricular hemorrhage and are an indication for ultrasound study. Tonic posturing also occurs in newborns with forebrain damage, not as a seizure manifestation but as a disinhibition of brainstem reflexes. Prolonged disinhibition results in *decerebrate posturing*, an extension of the body and limbs associated with internal rotation of the arms, dilation of the pupils, and downward deviation of the eyes. This is often encountered as a terminal sign in prematures with intraventicular hemorrhage due to pressure on the upper brainstem (see Chapter 4).

Tonic seizures and decerebrate posturing must also be distinguished from *opisthotonos*, a prolonged arching of the back not necessarily associated with eye movements. Opisthotonos is probably caused by meningeal irritation and is seen in kernicterus, infantile Gaucher disease, and some aminoacidurias.

Myoclonic Seizures

Clinical Features. These seizures are characterized by brief repeated extension and flexion movements of the arms, the legs, or all limbs. They constitute an uncommon seizure pattern in the newborn but, when present, suggest severe, diffuse brain damage.

Diagnosis. There is no specific EEG pattern associated with myoclonic seizures in the newborn. Myoclonic jerks are often seen in babies born to drug-addicted mothers. It is not certain whether these movements are seizures, jitteriness, or myoclonus (discussed later).

Apnea

Clinical Features. An irregular respiratory pattern with intermittent pauses of three to six seconds, often followed by ten to fifteen seconds of hyperpnea, is regularly observed in prematures. The pauses are not associated with significant alterations in heart rate, blood pressure, body temperature, or skin color. This respiratory pattern, termed *periodic breathing*, is caused by immaturity of the brainstem respiratory centers. The incidence of periodic breathing correlates directly with the degree of prematurity. The rate of apnea is highest in active sleep and lowest in quiet sleep.

Apneic spells of ten to fifteen seconds are detectable at some time in almost all prematures and some term newborns. Apneic spells of ten to twenty seconds are usually associated with a 20 percent reduction in heart rate. Longer episodes of apnea are almost invariably associated with a 40 percent or greater reduction. The frequency of these apneic spells correlates with brainstem myelination. At forty weeks conceptional age, prematures continue to have a higher incidence of apnea than do term newborns (Albani et al, 1985). The incidence of apnea

sharply decreases in all infants at fifty-two weeks conceptional age.

Diagnosis. Apneic spells in otherwise normal-appearing newborns should be considered a sign of brainstem immaturity and not pathology. The brainstem auditory evoked response is useful in this regard. The interpeak latency of waves V-I is longer in prematures with apnea than in prematures without apnea at the same conceptional age. Apnea is common when the interpeak latency is greater than 6.0 ms and decreases in frequency as latencies less than 5.6 ms are attained (Henderson-Smart et al, 1983).

The sudden onset of apnea and states of decreased consciousness, especially in a premature, suggests an intracranial hemorrhage with brainstem compression. Immediate ultrasound is indicated.

An apneic spell is more likely to be a seizure manifestation when other seizure patterns are associated and bradycardia does not occur (Fig. 1.2) (Fenichel et al, 1980).

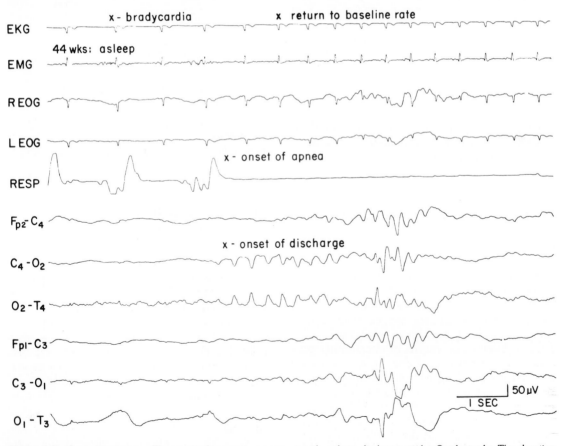

Figure 1.2 Convulsive apnea. The onset of apnea is concurrent with a theta discharge at the O_2 electrode. The duration of apnea exceeds the duration of discharge. (From Fenichel GM: Neonatal Neurology. Churchill Livingstone, New York, 1985.)

Benign Nocturnal Myoclonus

Clinical Features. Sudden jerking movements of the limbs during sleep occur in normal people of all ages (see Chapter 14). They appear primarily during the early stages of sleep as repeated flexion movements of the fingers, wrists, and elbows. When prolonged, they may be misdiagnosed as focal clonic or myoclonic seizures (Coulter and Allen, 1982).

Diagnosis. Nocturnal myoclonus can be distinguished from seizures and jitteriness because it occurs solely during sleep, it is not stimulus-activated, and the EEG is normal.

Treatment. Treatment is not required.

Jitteriness

Clinical Features. Jitteriness or tremulousness is an excessive response to stimulation. Touch, noise, and especially motion produce low-frequency, high-amplitude shaking of the limbs and jaw. It is commonly associated with a low threshold for the Moro reflex, but can occur in the absence of any apparent stimulation and be confused with myoclonic seizures.

Diagnosis. Jitteriness usually occurs in newborns with perinatal asphyxia, some of whom have seizures as well. It can be distinguished from seizures by EEG monitoring, by the absence of eye movements or alteration in respiratory pattern, and by the presence of stimulus-activation. Jitteriness is also encountered in newborns of addicted mothers and in newborns with metabolic disorders.

Treatment. Reduced stimulation decreases jitteriness. However, newborns of addicted mothers require sedation to facilitate feeding and to decrease energy expenditure.

DIFFERENTIAL DIAGNOSIS OF SEIZURES

Virtually any disorder of the newborn brain may result in a seizure. The time of onset of first seizure is very helpful in determining the cause (Table 1.3). Seizures occurring during the first twenty-four hours, and especially in the first twelve hours, are usually due to hypoxic-ischemic encephalopathy. Sepsis, meningitis, and subarachnoid hemorrhage are the causes next in frequency, followed by intrauterine infection and trauma. Direct drug effects, intraventricular hemorrhage at term, and pyridoxine dependency are relatively rare.

Table 1.3. DIFFERENTIAL DIAGNOSIS OF NEONATAL SEIZURES BY PEAK TIME OF ONSET

24 Hours
1. Bacterial meningitis and sepsis (see Chapter 4)
2. Direct drug effect
3. Hypoxic ischemic encephalopathy
4. Intrauterine infection (see Chapter 5)
5. Intraventricular hemorrhage at term (see Chapter 4)
6. Laceration of tentorium or falx
7. Pyridoxine dependency
8. Subarachnoid hemorrhage

24 to 72 Hours
1. Bacterial meningitis and sepsis (see Chapter 4)
2. Cerebral contusion with subdural hemorrhage
3. Cerebral dysgenesis (see Chapter 18)
4. Cerebral infarction (see Chapter 11)
5. Drug withdrawal
6. Glycine encephalopathy
7. Glycogen synthase deficiency
8. Hypoparathyroidism-hypocalcemia
9. Incontinentia pigmenti
10. Intracerebral hemorrhage (see Chapter 11)
11. Intraventricular hemorrhage in prematures (see Chapter 4)
12. Pyridoxine dependency
13. Subarachnoid hemorrhage
14. Tuberous sclerosis
15. Urea cycle disturbances

72 Hours to 1 Week
1. Benign familial neonatal convulsions
2. Cerebral dysgenesis (see Chapter 18)
3. Cerebral infarction (see Chapter 11)
4. Hypoparathyroidism
5. Intracerebral hemorrhage (see Chapter 11)
6. Kernicterus
7. Ketotic hyperglycinemias
8. Nutritional hypocalcemia
9. Tuberous sclerosis
10. Urea cycle disturbances

1 Week to 4 Weeks
1. Adrenoleukodystrophy, neonatal (see Chapter 6)
2. Cerebral dysgenesis (see Chapter 18)
3. Fructose dysmetabolism
4. Gaucher disease type II (see Chapter 5)
5. GM_1 gangliosidosis type I (see Chapter 5)
6. Herpes simplex encephalitis
7. Ketotic hyperglycinemias
8. Maple syrup urine disease, neonatal
9. Mitochondrial disorders
10. Tuberous sclerosis
11. Urea cycle disturbances

During the period from twenty-four to seventy-two hours, intraventricular hemorrhage is the most frequent cause of seizures in prematures, subarachnoid hemorrhage and cerebral contusion in large term newborns, and sepsis and meningitis at all gestational ages. Focal clonic seizures in term newborns suggest a cerebral infarction or an intracerebral hemorrhage. Seizures from cerebral dysgenesis may begin at this time and remain an important cause of seizures throughout infancy. All other conditions are relatively rare. Newborns with metabolic disorders other than hypoparathyroidism demonstrate lethargy and poor feeding before the onset of seizures.

After seventy-two hours, inborn errors of metabolism, especially aminoacidurias, become a more important consideration because protein and glucose feedings have been initiated. A battery of screening tests for metabolic disorders is outlined in Table 1.4. Herpes simplex infection is transmitted at the time of delivery and does not become symptomatic until the second half of the first week. Many conditions that cause seizures early can also cause seizures late: cerebral dysgenesis, cerebral infarction, and intra-

cerebral hemorrhage. In addition, seizures from kernicterus, neonatal adrenoleukodystrophy, and benign familial neonatal convulsions have their onset at this time.

Hypoxic-Ischemic Encephalopathy

Asphyxia at term is almost always an intra-uterine event, and hypoxia and ischemia occur together; the result is a hypoxic-ischemic encephalopathy (HIE). Acute total asphyxia usually leads to death from circulatory collapse. Affected fetuses are stillborn or die in the perinatal period. Occasional survivors are born comatose and have evidence of cranial nerve dysfunction. The usual mechanism of HIE in surviving term newborns is partial, prolonged asphyxia. In the monkey fetus, brain damage occurs when arterial oxygen is reduced by 90 percent and maintained at that reduced level for more than twenty-five minutes.

The fetal circulation accommodates to reductions in arterial oxygen by maximizing blood flow to the brain, and to a lesser extent the heart, at the expense of other organs. Heart rate and blood pressure remain undisturbed until arterial oxygen concentrations are reduced by 65 percent and then fall in a linear fashion with further reductions. The decline in heart rate and blood pressure can be maintained for several hours without producing encephalopathy if the arterial oxygen concentration is not reduced by more than 85 percent. This safety factor allows successful fetal monitoring.

Clinical experience indicates that the fetus may be subjected to considerable hypoxia without brain damage developing. The incidence of cerebral palsy among term newborns with a five-minute Apgar score of 0 to 3 is only 1 percent if the ten-minute score is 4 or higher (Nelson and Ellenberg, 1981). Any episode of hypoxia sufficiently severe to cause brain damage must also cause derangements in other organs (Fenichel, 1983). Newborns with mild to moderate HIE always have a history of irregularities in heart rate and usually pass meconium. Those with moderate to severe HIE may have lactic acidosis, elevated serum concentrations of hepatic enzymes, enterocolitis, renal failure, and fatal myocardial damage.

• HIE can be divided into three grades of severity by clinical symptoms: mild, moderate, and severe (Sarnat and Sarnat, 1976).

Clinical Features. Mild HIE is relatively common. Lethargy, without significant loss of consciousness, is noted immediately after birth. The

Table 1.4 SCREENING FOR INBORN ERRORS OF METABOLISM THAT CAUSE NEONATAL SEIZURES

Blood Glucose Low
1. Fructose-1,6-diphosphatase deficiency
2. Glycogen storage disease, type I
3. Maple syrup urine disease

Blood Calcium Low
1. Hypoparathyroidism
2. Maternal hyperparathyroidism

Blood Ammonia High
1. Argininosuccinic acidemia
2. Carbamylphosphate synthetase deficiency
3. Citrullinemia
4. Methylmalonic acidemia (may be normal)
5. Multiple carboxylase deficiency
6. Ornithine transcarbamylase deficiency
7. Propionic acidemia (may be normal)

Blood Lactate High
1. Fructose-1,6-diphosphatase deficiency
2. Glycogen storage disease, type I
3. Multiple carboxylase deficiency
4. Pyruvate cazboxylase deficiency
5. Pyruvate dehydrogenase complex disorders

Metabolic Acidosis
1. Fructose-1,6-diphosphatase deficiency
2. Glycogen storage disease, type I
3. Maple syrup urine disease
4. Methylmalonic acidemia
5. Multiple carboxylase deficiency
6. Propionic acidemia
7. Pyruvate carboxylase deficiency
8. Pyruvate dehydrogenase complex disorders

Urine Ferric Chloride or Dinitrophenylhydrazine
1. Maple syrup urine disease

No Rapid Screening Test
1. Adrenoleukodystrophy, neonatal form
2. Glycine encephalopathy
3. Glycogen synthase deficiency
4. Infantile GM_1 gangliosidosis, type I

characteristic features are jitteriness and sympathetic overactivity (tachycardia, dilation of pupils, and decreased bronchial and salivary secretions). Muscle tone is normal at rest, but mild head lag is demonstrated on the traction response. Tendon reflexes are normoreactive or hyperactive, and ankle clonus is usually elicited. The Moro reflex is complete, and repetitive extension and flexion movements are generated by a single stimulus. Seizures are not an expected feature, and their occurrence suggests concurrent hypoglycemia or the presence of a second condition.

Symptoms progressively diminish and disappear during the first week, with the exception that some degree of overresponsiveness may persist longer. Newborns with mild HIE probably recover completely; there is no evidence suggesting a cause-and-effect relationship with epilepsy or learning disabilities (Nelson and Broman, 1977).

Newborns with moderate HIE are lethargic or obtunded for at least the first twelve hours post partum and demonstrate jitteriness when aroused. The resting posture indicates hypotonia, and spontaneous movement of the limbs is lacking. Proximal weakness is present affecting the shoulder more than the pelvic girdle. In the period between forty-eight to seventy-two hours, some children begin to improve and then resemble newborns with mild HIE.

In others, there is continued obtundation or progressive stupor and coma. Seizures are an ominous sign and indicate a worsening prognosis.

Newborns with severe HIE are stuporous or comatose immediately after birth, and respiratory effort is insufficient to sustain life. Seizures begin within the first twelve hours. Hypotonia is severe, and tendon reflexes cannot be elicited. The Moro reflex and tonic neck reflex are absent as well. Sucking and swallowing are depressed or absent, but the pupillary and oculovestibular reflexes are present.

Some newborns experience a transitory improvement in state of consciousness between twelve and twenty-four hours post partum, but most remain comatose and have frequent seizures that progress to status epilepticus. The response to anticonvulsant drugs is usually incomplete. Generalized increased intracranial pressure develops between twenty-four and seventy-two hours. This is characterized clinically by coma, bulging of the fontanelle, loss of pupillary and oculovestibular reflexes, and respiratory arrest.

Death may occur at this time, or the child may remain stuporous for several weeks. The encephalopathy subsides after the third day, and survivors experience a decreasing frequency of seizures. Jitteriness is common as the child becomes arousable. Tone increases and the child becomes hypertonic in succeeding weeks.

The prognosis for newborns with moderate to severe HIE is poor. The mortality rate is 7 percent, and 34 percent will have neurologic impairment (Finer et al, 1981).

Diagnosis. An EEG is very helpful in determining the severity and prognosis of HIE (Holmes et al, 1982; Watanabe et al, 1980). In mild HIE, the background is normal or may be lacking in variability. In moderate to severe HIE, the background is always abnormal and demonstrates suppression of background amplitude. The degree of suppression correlates well with the severity of HIE. The worst case is a flat EEG or one with a burst-suppression pattern (Fig. 1.3). If the EEG remains suppressed for one week, 64 percent of patients will have neurologic impairment; after two weeks, 100 percent will be impaired. Epileptiform activity may be present as well, but it is not as predictive of outcome as is background suppression.

Treatment. The management of newborns with HIE requires immediate attention to derangements in several organs and the correction of acidosis. No therapeutic regimen has proved effective in treating the encephalopathy. Nevertheless, clinical experience and some studies indicate that control of seizures and reduction in cerebral edema increase the chance of a favorable outcome (Levene and Evans, 1985; Svenningsen et al, 1982).

Intravenous phenobarbital and phenytoin are equally effective (or ineffective) in controlling seizures due to HIE. The use of these drugs in newborns is detailed in a separate section. Following the initial load, daily determinations of serum concentration are needed to plan maintenance doses (Table 1.5). In prematures, protein binding of anticonvulsant drugs may be impaired and the free fraction concentration may be toxic, whereas the measured protein-bound fraction appears therapeutic.

If these two drugs prove ineffective, it is probably unwise and usually nonproductive to administer a polypharmacy of drugs.

Seizures usually cease spontaneously during the second week, and anticonvulsants should be stopped after a further week of control. The incidence of epilepsy among infants who had neonatal convulsions secondary to HIE is 30 to

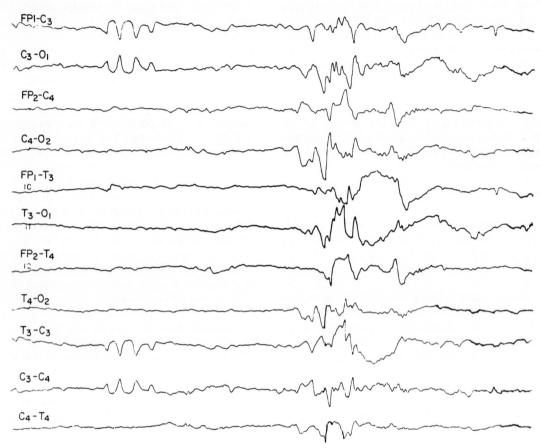

Figure 1.3 Burst suppression. Ten-second intervals of suppression are interrupted by bursts of slow and sharp waves in a term newborn with hypoxic-ischemic encephalopathy.

Table 1.5 ANTICONVULSANT DRUGS FOR CHILDREN

Drug	Initial Dose (mg/kg/day)	Maintenance (mg/kg/day)	Blood Concentration (μg/ml)	Half-Life (hrs)
Acetazolamide	10	10–50	*	24–72
Carbamazepine	5	15–20	4–12	14–27
Clonazepam	0.025	0.1–0.15	0.2–0.7*	20–40
Clorazepate	0.3	0.3–1	>1.2*	20–60
Ethosuximide	20	20–40	40–100	30–60
Methsuximide	20	20–40	*	*
Nitrazepam	0.2	0.5–1	*	18–30
Phenacemide	20	40–50	†	†
Phenytoin	5–7	5–7	10–20	5–14
Phenobarbital	3–5	3–5	10–40	37–73
Primidone	2–5	10–15	8–12	5–11
Trimethadione	20	30–60	*	16*
Valproic Acid	20	30–60	50–100	6–15

*Not clinically useful.
†Not established.

40 percent. There is no evidence that continued therapy prevents the subsequent development of epilepsy.

Intracranial pressure may be favorably influenced by the simple procedure of head elevation to 30 degrees and 10 percent fluid restriction. Mannitol has a potential benefit and no appreciable risk when given intravenously over 20 minutes at a dose of 0.25 g/kg and repeated every six hours during the first two days. Mannitol reduces intracranial pressure while at the same time increasing perfusion pressure. In contrast, the administration of corticosteroids reduces both intracranial pressure and perfusion pressure and should not be used (Levene and Evans, 1985).

Trauma and Intracranial Hemorrhage

Neonatal head trauma occurs most often in large term newborns of primiparous mothers. The usual clinical setting is a prolonged labor and difficult extraction due to fetal malposition or a precipitous delivery before the maternal cervix is sufficiently dilated. Intracranial hemorrhage may be subarachnoid, subdural, or intraventricular. Intraventricular hemorrhage is discussed in Chapter 4.

Primary Subarachnoid Hemorrhage

Clinical Features. This is the most common site of bleeding and probably originates from tearing of the superficial veins by shearing forces during a prolonged delivery with the head engaged. Mild HIE is often associated, but the newborn is usually well when an unexpected seizure occurs on the first or second day (Fenichel et al, 1984). Lumbar puncture is performed because of suspected sepsis and blood is found in the cerebrospinal fluid. Most such newborns will be neurologically normal later.

Diagnosis. A CT scan is useful to document the extent of hemorrhage. Blood is present in the interhemispheric fissure and the supratentorial and infratentorial recesses. Routine ultrasound does not reliably demonstrate subarachnoid hemorrhage. Epileptiform activity may be present on the EEG, but the background is not suppressed. This indicates that seizures are not due to HIE and the prognosis is more favorable.

Clotting studies should be performed to exclude the possibility of a coagulopathy.

Treatment. Seizures usually respond to phenobarbital or phenytoin. Specific therapy is not available for the hemorrhage, and post-hemorrhagic hydrocephalus is uncommon.

Subdural Hemorrhage

Clinical Features. Subdural hemorrhage is usually the consequence of a tentorial tear near its junction with the falx. This results from excessive vertical molding of the head in vertex presentation, anteroposterior elongation of the head in face and brow presentations, and prolonged delivery of the aftercoming head in breech presentation. Blood collects in the posterior fossa and may produce brainstem compression. The initial features are those of mild to moderate HIE. Clinical evidence of brainstem compression is delayed for twelve hours or longer and characterized by irregular respiration, abnormal cry, declining consciousness, hypotonia, seizures, and a tense fontanelle. Intracerebellar hemorrhage is sometimes associated (Serfontein et al, 1980). Mortality is high, and neurologic impairment among survivors is common.

Diagnosis. Subdural hemorrhage is readily visualized by CT and ultrasound.

Treatment. Small hemorrhages do not necessitate treatment, but surgical evacuation is required for large collections to relieve brainstem compression.

Hypoglycemia

A transitory, asymptomatic hypoglycemia can be detected in 11 percent of all newborns during the first hours post partum and before oral feeding is initiated. Hypoglycemia is not associated with neurologic impairment later in life. Symptomatic hypoglycemia may be secondary to cerebral stress or inborn errors of metabolism (Table 1.6).

Clinical Features. The time of onset of symptoms depends upon the underlying disorder. Early onset is generally associated with perinatal asphyxia or intracranial hemorrhage and late onset with inborn errors of metabolism. The syndrome includes any of the following symptoms: apnea, cyanosis, tachypnea, jitteriness, high-pitched cry, poor feeding, vomiting, apathy, hypotonia, seizures, and coma. Symptomatic hypoglycemia is often associated with later neurologic impairment.

Diagnosis. Neonatal hypoglycemia is defined as a whole blood glucose concentration of less than 20 mg/dl (1 mmol/L) in prematures and

Table 1.6 CAUSES OF NEONATAL HYPOGLYCEMIA

Primary Transitional Hypoglycemia
1. Complicated labor and delivery
2. Intrauterine malnutrition
3. Maternal diabetes
4. Prematurity

Secondary Transitional Hypoglycemia
1. Asphyxia
2. Central nervous system
3. Cold injuries
4. Sepsis

Persistent Hypoglycemia
1. Aminoacidurias
    a. Maple syrup urine disease
    b. Methylmalonic acidemia
    c. Propionic acidemia
    d. Tyrosinosis
2. Congenital hypopituitarism
3. Defects in carbohydrate metabolism
    a. Fructose-1,6-diphosphatase deficiency
    b. Fructose intolerance
    c. Galactosemia
    d. Glycogen storage disease, type I
    e. Glycogen synthase deficiency
4. Hyperinsulinism

low-birth-weight newborns, less than 30 mg/dl (1.5 mmol/L) in term newborns during the first seventy-two hours, and less than 40 mg/dl (2 mmol/L) in term newborns after seventy-two hours.

Treatment. Normal blood glucose concentrations can be restored by intravenous administration of glucose, but the underlying cause must be determined to provide definitive treatment.

Hypocalcemia

Hypocalcemia is defined as a blood concentration of less than 7 mg/dl (1.75 mmol/L). The onset of hypocalcemia in the first seventy-two hours post partum is associated with low birth weight, asphyxia, maternal diabetes, maternal hypoparathyroidism, and the DiGeorge syndrome: later onset hypocalcemia is seen in children fed evaporated cow's milk and other improper formulas, in maternal hypoparathyroidism, and in the DiGeorge syndrome.

Hypocalcemia occurs in less than 10 percent of stressed newborns and enhances the vulnerability to seizures, but it is rarely the primary cause (Robertson and Smith, 1975).

DiGeorge Syndrome

Clinical Features. This is a congenital hypoplasia of organs derived from the third and fourth pharyngeal pouches (thymus, parathyroid gland, and great vessels) of unknown cause (Conley et al, 1979). Multiple minor facial anomalies are associated. The presenting symptoms may be due to congenital heart disease, hypocalcemia, or both. Jitteriness and tetany usually begin in the first forty-eight hours. The peak onset of seizures is on the third day, but may be delayed for two weeks. Many affected newborns die of cardiac causes during the first month; survivors fail to thrive and are often affected by repeated infections because of the failure of cell-mediated immunity.

Diagnosis. Newborns who come to a physician's attention because of heart disease may be suspected of having hypocalcemia when a prolonged Q-T interval is detected on the electrocardiogram (EKG). Conversely, all newborns with symptoms of hypocalcemia should be examined for cardiac defects.

Treatment. Hypocalcemia generally responds to parathormone or to oral calcium and vitamin D.

Aminoacidopathies

Maple Syrup Urine Disease

The neonatal form of maple syrup urine disease (MSUD) is caused by complete absence of branched-chain ketoacid dehydrogenase. Leucine, isoleucine, and valine cannot be decarboxylated and they accumulate in blood, urine, and tissues (Fig. 1.4). Later-onset forms are described in Chapters 5 and 10. The defect is transmitted by autosomal recessive inheritance.

Clinical Features. Affected newborns appear healthy at birth, but symptoms of lethargy, feeding difficulty, and hypotonia develop after ingestion of protein. Seizures begin in the second week and are associated with signs of increased intracranial pressure (Lungarotti et al, 1982). Once seizures begin, they continue with increasing frequency and severity. Without therapy, opisthotonos, coma, and death follow within one month.

Diagnosis. Rapid screening of urine for MSUD can be accomplished by the addition of ferric chloride, which colors urine deep blue, or with 2,4-dinitrophenylhydrazine, which causes a cloudy, yellow precipitate. Specific diagnosis requires the demonstration of increased plasma concentrations of the three branch-chained amino acids or enzyme deficiency in peripheral leukocytes. Heterozygotes can be detected by diminished levels of enzyme activity.

Treatment. Exchange transfusions or perito-

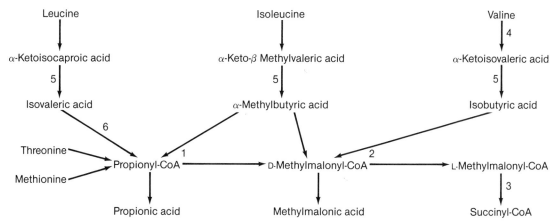

Figure 1.4 Branched-chain amino acid metabolism. *1*, Propionyl-CoA carboxylase (biotin cofactor). *2*, Methylmalonyl-CoA racemase. *3*, Methymalonyl-CoA mutase (adenosylcobalamin). *4*, Isovaleryl-CoA dehydrogenase. *5*, Branched-chain ketoacid dehydrogenase. (From Fenichel GM: Neonatal Neurology. Churchill Livingstone, New York, 1985.)

neal dialysis transiently lowers the plasma concentration of branch-chained amino acids and ketoacids. Administration of glucose and insulin provides a more prolonged reduction by promoting the uptake of amino acids into skeletal muscle.

A special diet, low in branched-chain amino acids, may be effective in preventing further encephalopathy and should be started immediately by nasogastric tube (Waisman et al, 1972).

Isovaleric Acidemia

Isovaleric acidemia is a fatty acid derived from leucine. Its conversion to propionyl-CoA is metabolized by the enzyme isovaleryl-CoA dehydrogenase (Fig. 1.4). It is transmitted by autosomal recessive inheritance, and the heterozygote state can be detected in cultured fibroblasts.

Clinical Features. The same enzyme defect may present as an acute, overwhelming disorder of the newborn or as a chronic, infantile form (de Sousa et al, 1986). Newborns are normal at birth, but within a few days become lethargic, refuse to feed, and vomit. The clinical syndrome is very similar to MSUD except that the urine is described as smelling like "sweaty feet" instead of maple syrup. Most affected newborns die within three weeks of ketoacidosis, pancytopenia, or intercurrent infection.

Diagnosis. Isovaleric acidosis is detected by the excretion of isovaleryl-lycine in the urine. Isovaleryl-CoA dehydrogenase activity can be assayed in cultured fibroblasts.

Treatment. A dietary regimen similar to that used for MSUD is beneficial. In addition, some children respond to supplementation with oral glycine, 800 mg/day, and others to oral L-carnitine, 200 mg/kg/day.

Glycine Encephalopathy

Glycine encephalopathy is due to a defect in the glycine cleaving system. It is inherited as an autosomal recessive trait.

Clinical Features. Affected newborns are normal at birth, but become irritable and refuse feeding during the first few days post partum. Progressive lethargy, hypotonia, respiratory disturbances, and myoclonic seizures follow. Some newborns survive the acute illness, but their subsequent course is characterized by mental retardation, epilepsy, and spasticity (Trauner et al, 1983).

Diagnosis. During the acute encephalopathy, the EEG demonstrates a burst-suppression pattern, which evolves into hypsarrhythmia during infancy. Diagnosis is established by the demonstration of hyperglycinemia in the absence of hyperammonemia or organic acidemia.

Treatment. Exchange transfusion provides only temporary relief of the encephalopathy, and dietary therapy has not proved successful in modifying the course. Diazepam, a competitor for glycine receptors, in combination with choline, folic acid, and sodium benzoate was useful in stopping seizures in two affected infants (Matalon et al, 1983).

Ketotic Hyperglycinemias

The ketotic hyperglycinemias constitute a heterogeneous group of disorders, all transmitted by autosomal recessive inheritance, in which there are defects in the further degradation of branch-chained amino acids (Fig. 1.4). *Propionic acidemia* (Wolf et al, 1981) and *methylmalonic acidemia* (Matsui et al, 1983) are the most frequently occurring disorders in this group.

Clinical Features. Considerable clinical variability may occur, depending upon the specific enzyme defect. In general, affected children are normal at birth and lethargy, irritability, and disturbed feeding develop during the first week. Severe metabolic acidosis follows, characterized by hypotonia, myoclonic and multifocal seizures, and progressive loss of consciousness. The mortality rate is high, and survivors are severely impaired mentally and physically.

Diagnosis. Ketotic hyperglycinemias should be considered in any newborn with metabolic acidosis, especially if associated with ketosis, hyperammonemia, and hyperglycinemia. Occasional newborns with propionic acidemia have hyperammonemia without ketoacidosis, suggesting an erroneous diagnosis of carbamyl phosphate synthetase deficiency.

Definitive diagnosis requires the demonstration of deficient enzyme activity in cultured fibroblasts or peripheral blood leukocytes.

Treatment. Newborns with overwhelming metabolic acidosis require peritoneal dialysis to remove toxic metabolites and cessation of all protein feeding. Once the initial crisis is over, a

diet restricted in protein to 1.0 to 1.5 g/kg/day can be initiated. Biotin supplementation is recommended for patients with propionic acidemia, and vitamin B_{12} supplementation for patients with methylmalonic acidemia.

Urea Cycle Disturbances

Carbamyl phosphate synthetase deficiency (CPS), *ornithine transcarbamylase deficiency* (OTC), *citrullinemia, argininosuccinic acidemia,* and *argininemia* (arginase deficiency) are the disorders secondary to defects in the enzyme systems responsible for urea synthesis (Fig. 1.5). Arginase deficiency does not produce symptoms in the newborn. OTC deficiency is an X-linked trait; all others are transmitted by autosomal recessive inheritance.

Clinical Features. The clinical features of urea cycle disorders are due to ammonia intoxication (Table 1.7). Progressive lethargy, vomiting, and hypotonia may develop on the first postpartum day, even before the initiation of protein feeding, and are followed by progressive loss of consciousness and seizures on subsequent days. Vomiting and lethargy correlate well with plasma ammonia concentrations above 200 μg/dl (120 μmol/L); coma above 300 μg/dl (180 μmol/L); and seizures above 500 μg/dl (300 μmol/L). Death follows quickly in untreated newborns.

Newborns with partial deficiency of CPS and

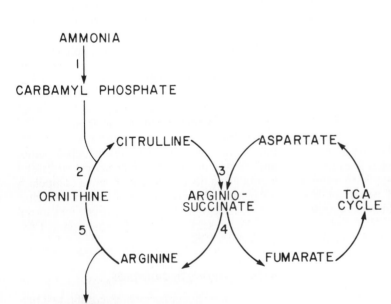

Figure 1.5 Ammonia metabolism. *1,* Carbamyl phosphate synthetase (CPS). *2,* Ornithine transcarbamylase (OTC). *3,* Argininosuccinate synthetase (AS). *4,* Argininosuccinate lyase (AL). *5,* Arginase. (From Fenichel GM: Neonatal Neurology. Churchill Livingstone, New York, 1985.)

Table 1.7 CAUSES OF NEONATAL HYPERAMMONEMIA

Liver Failure

Primary Enzyme Defects in Urea Synthesis
1. Argininosuccinic acidemia
2. Carbamyl phosphate synthetase deficiency
3. Citrullinemia
4. Ornithine transcarbamylase deficiency

Other Disorders of Amino Acid Metabolism
1. Glycine encephalopathy
2. Isovaleric acidemia
3. Methylmalonic acidemia
4. Multiple carboxylase deficiency
5. Propionic acidemia

Transitory Hyperammonemia of Prematurity

female carriers of OTC deficiency may become symptomatic when given a large protein load.

Diagnosis. The diagnosis of a urea cycle disturbance should be suspected in every newborn with a compatible clinical syndrome and hyperammonemia without organic acidemia. Definitive diagnosis requires identification of the specific enzyme defect in hepatic tissue or peripheral leukocytes.

Treatment. All newborns with inborn errors of urea synthesis require peritoneal dialysis to lower blood ammonia concentrations. In addition, waste nitrogen excretion can be promoted through pathways other than urea synthesis by administration of sodium benzoate and phenylacetic acid (Batshaw et al, 1981). Sodium benzoate promotes the synthesis of glycine from ammonia by converting glycine to hippuric acid, which is then excreted by the kidney. It should be used cautiously in newborns with hyperbilirubinemia. Phenylacetic acid enhances the excretion of glutamine, an alternate compound to urea for the removal of nitrogen. A favorable neurologic outcome depends upon early diagnosis and treatment (Msall et al, 1984). The longer the newborn remains in hyperammonemic coma, the lower the intelligence quotient (IQ).

Beyond the newborn period, normal plasma ammonia levels can be maintained on a low-protein diet with arginine supplementation. Episodic hyperammonemia may occur at the time of intercurrent illness and after a protein load. These episodes must be treated promptly with intravenous sodium benzoate, sodium phenylacetate and arginine, and nitrogen-free intravenous alimentation (Brusilow et al, 1984).

Herpes Simplex Encephalitis

Herpes genitalis (HSV-2) accounts for the majority of herpetic infections of the newborn. The most frequent cause of neonatal infection is contamination of the newborn during the second stage of labor by contact with maternal genital herpes. Among women with herpes genitalis, asymptomatic shedding of virus occurs with the same frequency at delivery (1.4 percent), whether or not episodes of symptomatic recurrence are noted during pregnancy (Arvin et al, 1986).

Transplacental infection is rare and produces malformations of the brain and eye resulting in microcephaly and micro-ophthalmia at birth.

Clinical Features. The clinical spectrum of perinatal infection is considerable (Nahmias et al, 1983). Among symptomatic newborns, two thirds have disseminated disease and one third have localized involvement of either the brain, eye, skin, or mouth. Whether disseminated or localized, approximately half of all infections involve the central nervous system. The overall mortality rate is 62 percent, and 50 percent of survivors have permanent neurologic impairment.

The onset of clinical manifestations may be as early as the fifth day, but is usually in the second week. A vesicular rash is present in 30 percent, usually on the scalp after vertex presentation and on the buttocks after breech presentation. Conjunctivitis, jaundice, and a bleeding diathesis may be present. The first symptoms of encephalitis are irritability and seizures. Seizures may be focal or generalized and are frequently refractory to therapy. Neurologic deterioration is progressive and characterized by coma and quadraparesis.

Diagnosis. The EEG is almost constantly abnormal and demonstrates a periodic pattern of slow waves or spike discharges (Mizrahi and Tharpe, 1982). Examination of the cerebrospinal fluid reveals lymphocytic leukocytosis, red blood cells, and an elevated protein concentration.

A rising antibody titer can be demonstrated by complement-fixation. Because of the passive transfer of antibodies, a diagnosis of neonatal herpes infection requires the demonstration of specific IgM-HSV antibodies. Viral antigens may be demonstrated in cytologic smears from vesicles by immunofluorescence using monoclonal or polyclonal antibodies.

Treatment. All women with genital herpes at term whose membranes are intact or ruptured for less than four hours should be delivered by cesarean section. Infected newborns are treated with acyclovir, but drug efficacy is still not established.

Mitochondrial Disorders

Pyruvate is at the center of intermediary metabolism. It is formed primarily from glucose by glycolysis and can be converted to lactate, alanine, acetyl-coenzyme A, or oxaloacetate. Pyruvate dehydrogenase (an enzyme complex) and pyruvate carboxylase are the enzymes that catalyze the entry of pyruvate into the tricarboxylic cycle. Disorders of pyruvate or the respiratory chain produce some elevation in the plasma concentration of lactic acid, if not symptomatic lactic acidosis. Several different syndromes are associated with defects in pyruvate metabolism and the respiratory chain (see Chapters 5, 7, and 10).

Clinical Features. The neonatal syndrome is characterized by overwhelming lactic acidosis. Lethargy, feeding difficulty, and apnea are initial signs. Rapid progression into coma is the rule. Seizures are rarely associated and, even then, are not a prominent feature.

Diagnosis. Lactic acidosis is profound and associated with hyperammonemia, hypoglycemia, pancytopenia, and aminoaciduria (Evans, 1986). Definitive diagnosis requires demonstration of the specific enzyme defect in cultured fibroblasts or other tissues.

Treatment. Initial therapy is directed at correcting acidosis by the administration of buffers. Specific therapy depends upon the enzyme defect.

Drug Withdrawal

Marijuana, alcohol, narcotic-analgesics, and hypnotic-sedatives are the drugs most commonly used during pregnancy. Marijuana and alcohol do not cause drug dependence in the fetus and are not associated with withdrawal symptoms. Hypnotic-sedatives, such as barbiturates, do not ordinarily produce withdrawal symptoms unless very large doses are ingested. Phenobarbital has a sufficiently long half-life in the newborn, so that sudden withdrawal does not occur.

The prototype of narcotic withdrawal in the newborn is that of heroin or methadone, but a similar syndrome occurs with codeine and propoxyphene. Withdrawal symptoms may occur in the newborn of even a nonaddicted mother using codeine as a cough suppressant (Mangurten and Benawra, 1980).

Clinical Features. Seventy percent of newborns exposed to heroin begin withdrawal during the first twenty-four hours and the remainder within forty-eight hours. The initial feature is a coarse tremor, present only during the waking state, which can shake an entire limb. This is followed by irritability; a shrill, high-pitched cry; and hyperactivity. The child seems hungry, but has difficulty feeding and vomits afterwards. Diarrhea and other symptoms of autonomic instability are common.

Myoclonic jerking is present in 10 to 25 percent of newborns undergoing withdrawal. It is not clear whether these movements are seizures or jitteriness. Definite seizures occur in less than 5 percent.

Diagnosis. The diagnosis should be suspected and anticipated in every newborn whose mother has a history of substance abuse. Even when such a history is not available, the combination of irritability, hyperactivity, and autonomic instability should provide a clue to diagnosis. Careful questioning of the mother concerning the use of prescription and nonprescription drugs is imperative. Specific drug identification is accomplished by blood and urine analyses.

Treatment. Symptoms remit spontaneously in three to five days, but there is appreciable mortality in untreated cases. Phenobarbital, 8 mg/kg/day, or chlorpromazine, 3 mg/kg/day, is equally effective in relieving symptoms and reducing mortality (Carin et al, 1983; Kahn et al, 1969). Morphine, meperidine, opium, and methadone are not sufficiently secreted in breast milk to cause or relieve addiction in the newborn.

Direct Drug Effects

Clinical Features. Local anesthetics used at delivery may reach the fetus either by accidental direct injection or the transplacental route. Fetal intoxication by local anesthetics generally produces internal and external ophthalmoplegia, bradycardia, and hypotonia. Seizures may occur during the first six hours.

Diagnosis. The combination of fixed, dilated pupils, ophthalmoplegia, and cardiac irregularities in a conscious child should always suggest the possibility of drug intoxication.

Treatment. Treatment is not needed, because drugs are eliminated spontaneously with good result.

Kernicterus

The terms kernicterus and bilirubin encephalopathy are used interchangeably to describe an acute encephalopathy with neurologic sequelae associated with elevated serum concentrations of bilirubin (Hansen and Bratlid, 1986). A significant concentration of bilirubin in an otherwise healthy term newborn is more than 20 mg/dl (340 μmol/L) of the serum indirect fraction. In sick prematures, 10 mg/dl (170 μmol/L) may be dangerous. The probability of brain damage correlates not only with the peak concentration of bilirubin but also with the duration of hyperbilirubinemia.

Clinical Features. The development of methods to prevent hemolytic disease and treat hyperbilirubinemia has markedly reduced the incidence of kernicterus. The group presently at greatest risk consists of the critically ill premature with respiratory distress syndrome, acidosis, and sepsis.

A consistent clinical syndrome has been described in newborns with kernicterus due to hemolytic disease (Van Praagh, 1961). Hypotonia, lethargy, and a poor sucking reflex are noted on the first day post partum. Fever, rigidity, and opisthotonic posturing develop in the next two days. Seizures may occur at this time, but are probably due to a concomitant hypoxic-ischemic encephalopathy rather than kernicterus. Tone gradually improves during the next month, but neurologic dysfunction becomes obvious in subsequent weeks and worsens progressively during infancy.

The typical clinical syndrome after the first year includes (1) extrapyramidal dysfunction, usually athetosis, which occurs in virtually every case (see Chapter 14); (2) disturbances of vertical gaze, upward more often than downward, in 90 percent; (3) high-frequency hearing loss in 60 percent; and (4) mental retardation in 25 percent.

Diagnosis. In newborns with hemolytic disease, a clinical diagnosis can be presumed on the basis of significant hyperbilirubinemia and a compatible evolution of symptoms. However, the diagnosis is difficult to establish in critically ill prematures in whom brain damage is more likely due to asphyxia and its consequences than from kernicterus.

Treatment. Kernicterus can be prevented by maintaining serum bilirubin concentrations below the toxic range. Once it has occurred, further damage can be limited, but not reversed, by lowering serum bilirubin concentrations.

Pyridoxine Dependency

This rare disorder, transmitted as an autosomal recessive trait, is caused by impaired glutamic decarboxylase activity (Lott et al, 1978).

Clinical Features. Multifocal clonic convulsions begin almost immediately after birth and progress rapidly to status epilepticus. However, a later onset, even after the first year, does not exclude the diagnosis (Goutieres and Aicardi, 1985). The seizures are refractory to standard anticonvulsants and respond only to pyridoxine. If pyridoxine supplementation is discontinued, seizures return within three weeks.

Diagnosis. In most cases, the diagnosis was suspected because a sibling had been affected by the same syndrome and died. In the absence of a positive family history, the diagnosis need only be considered in newborns with continuous seizures. The infantile-onset variety may be characterized by intermittent myoclonic seizures, focal clonic seizures, or generalized tonic-clonic seizures. The EEG is continuously abnormal because of generalized slowing and multifocal spike discharges. An intravenous injection of pyridoxine, 25 mg, stops the clinical seizure activity and often converts the EEG to normal in less than ten minutes.

Pyridoxine-responsive seizures also occur in newborns of mothers treated with isoniazid. The onset of seizures is in the third week post partum.

Treatment. A lifelong dietary supplement of pyridoxine, which varies from 2 to 30 mg/kg/day, is effective in preventing further seizures. The higher dose is used during infancy and the smaller dose in childhood. Subsequent psychomotor development is normal.

Incontinentia Pigmenti (Bloch-Sulzberger Syndrome)

Incontinentia pigmenti is a rare neurocutaneous syndrome involving the skin, teeth, eyes, and central nervous system. It is probably transmitted as an X-linked trait lethal in the hemizygous male, but autosomal dominant transmission has not been excluded (Curth and Warburton, 1965).

Clinical Features. The female-to-male ratio is 20:1. An erythematous and vesicular rash resembling epidermolysis bullosa is present on the flexor surfaces of the limbs and lateral aspect of the trunk at birth or soon thereafter. Neurologic disturbances occur in less than half of cases. In the newborn, the prominent feature is the onset of seizures on the second or third day, often confined to one side of the body. The rash persists for the first few months and is replaced by a verrucous eruption that lasts from weeks to months. Between six and twelve months, pigment is deposited in the previous area of rash in bizarre polymorphic arrangements. The pigment later regresses and may disappear completely.

Residual neurologic handicaps may include mental retardation, epilepsy, hemiparesis, and hydrocephalus. A rare associated neurologic disturbance is degeneration of anterior horn cells, producing clinical features similar to those of infantile spinal muscular atrophy (Larsen et al, 1987) (see Chapter 6).

Diagnosis. The character and evolution of the rash are essential for diagnosis.

Treatment. Neonatal seizures caused by incontinentia pigmenti ordinarily respond to standard anticonvulsant drugs.

Benign Familial Neonatal Convulsions

There are families in which several members have experienced neonatal convulsions that generally remit with age. The trait is transmitted by autosomal dominant inheritance, but a specific inborn error of metabolism has not been identified (Pettit and Fenichel, 1980).

Clinical Features. Multifocal clonic seizures begin shortly after birth in a child who otherwise appears normal. With or without treatment, the seizures usually stop spontaneously within three weeks. In 14 percent of newborns with benign familial convulsions, epilepsy develops later in life (Takebe et al, 1983).

Diagnosis. The syndrome should be suspected in any healthy newborn in whom seizures develop without apparent cause. Laboratory tests, including the EEG, are normal. A positive family history is critical to diagnosis, but may appear negative until grandparents are interviewed; parents are frequently unaware that they have experienced neonatal seizures.

Treatment. Standard anticonvulsant therapy should be administered. After four weeks of complete seizure control, the drug can be tapered and discontinued. If seizures return, a longer trial should be initiated.

TREATMENT OF NEONATAL SEIZURES

There is considerable evidence from animal studies that continuous seizure activity, even in the normoxemic brain, may cause brain damage by inhibition of protein synthesis and breakdown of polyribosomes. In human prematures, there is the additional concern that even subtle seizures markedly increase cerebral blood flow and cause intraventricular hemorrhage (Perlman and Volpe, 1983).

Although seizure control is clearly in the child's best interest, it is also clear that anticonvulsant drugs are potentially harmful to the immature brain. It is reasonable to assume that newborns with seizures that are difficult to control are in this state because they have already experienced brain damage. The use of toxic doses of multiple anticonvulsants is probably more harmful than the occasional seizure in a well-ventilated newborn and should be discouraged.

Phenobarbital

For most newborns, a therapeutic blood concentration of phenobarbital is 20 to 30 μg/ml (86 to 129 μmol/L). This can be achieved by a single intravenous loading dose of 20 mg/kg injected at a rate of 5 mg/min. Approximately 33 percent of all newborns with seizures respond to phenobarbital monotherapy at this blood concentration (Van Ormon and Darwish, 1985). Many asphyxiated newborns require and tolerate blood concentrations in excess of 30 μg/ml, and a loading dose of 30 mg/kg is reasonable (Donn et al, 1985). Phenobarbital monotherapy is effective in 85 percent of newborns with seizures when 40 mg/kg is administered in refractory cases (Gal et al, 1982).

The half-life of phenobarbital in newborns varies from 50 to 200 hours, and additional doses should be administered only on the basis of current blood concentration information. After the tenth day, the half-life shortens as the result of enzyme induction and steady state is easier to achieve.

Phenytoin

Phenytoin can be administered only intravenously. Oral doses are poorly absorbed in the newborn, and intramuscular doses are not absorbed at any age. A therapeutic blood concentration of 15 to 20 μg/ml (40 to 80 μmol/L) can be safely achieved by a single intravenous injection of 20 mg/kg at a rate of 0.5 mg/kg/minute (Painter et al, 1981). The half-life is long during the first week, and further administration should be based on current knowledge of blood concentration. Most newborns require a maintenance dose of 5 to 10 mg/kg/day.

Phenytoin may be more effective than phenobarbital in the management of tonic seizures, but otherwise provides little additional benefit for newborns with phenobarbital blood concentrations in excess of 40 μg/ml.

Paraldehyde

Paraldehyde is a safe and effective drug for transitory control of status epilepticus in newborns (Giacoia et al, 1984). Its half-life is approximately ten hours. Because a portion is excreted unchanged by the lungs, paraldehyde should be used only in well-ventilated term newborns.

Unfortunately, an intravenous preparation is no longer available, but it can be administered rectally mixed with equal parts of mineral oil.

Duration of Therapy

The treatment of seizures caused by an acute, self-limited encephalopathy, such as perinatal asphyxia, does not ordinarily require prolonged maintenance therapy. In most newborns, seizures stop when the acute encephalopathy is over. The incidence of later epilepsy among infants who had neonatal seizures due to perinatal asphyxia or trauma is approximately 30 percent (Watanabe et al, 1982). There is no evidence to suggest that continuous anticonvulsant therapy prevents the development of later epilepsy in newborns at risk. It is therefore reasonable to discontinue therapy after one week of complete seizure control. If seizures recur, anticonvulsant therapy can be reinitiated.

In contrast to newborns with seizures caused by acute encephalopathy, seizures caused by cerebral dysgenesis should be treated continuously. Eighty percent will be epileptic in childhood.

■ Paroxysmal Disorders of Infancy

The pathophysiology of paroxysmal disorders in infants is more varied than in newborns (Table 1.8). Seizures, especially febrile seizures, remain the major numerical cause, but apnea and syncope are relatively common as well. Infants with paroxysmal disorders are frequently referred for neurologic consultation because of the suspicion of seizures. The distinction is often difficult and relies more on obtaining a complete description

Table 1.8 PAROXYSMAL DISORDERS OF INFANCY

Apnea and Breathholding
1. Cyanotic
2. Pallid

Seizures
1. Febrile seizures
   a. Simple febrile
   b. Epilepsy
   c. Infectious
2. Afebrile seizures
   a. Generalized tonic-clonic seizures
   b. Partial seizures
3. Myoclonic seizures
   a. Infantile spasms
   b. Benign myoclonic epilepsy
   c. Severe myoclonic epilepsy
   d. Myoclonic status
   e. Lennox-Gastaut syndrome

Migraine
1. Benign paroxysmal vertigo (see Chapter 10)
2. Paroxysmal torticollis (see Chapter 14)
3. Cyclic vomiting

of the "spell" than on laboratory tests. There are times when it is impossible to determine the nature of an episode without personal observation. I have often asked parents to make tapes or motion pictures of hard-to-classify spells and have never been disappointed with the diagnostic clarity they provide. This is much more cost-effective than a hospitalization for "observation," during which time the spells are rarely observed by the doctor.

Ambulatory EEG is useful in selected infants to determine whether episodes of uncertain etiology are seizures. The technology of ambulatory EEG is described in the preceding section (p. 2). It allows continuous EEG recording for twenty-four to forty-eight hours at home and indicates whether the event-in-question is associated with epileptiform activity.

APNEA AND SYNCOPE

Infant apnea is defined as cessation of breathing for fifteen seconds or longer, or for less than fifteen seconds if accompanied by bradycardia (Spitzer and Fox, 1986). Premature newborns with respiratory distress syndrome may continue to have apneic spells as infants, especially if they are neurologically abnormal. Persistent apnea is often thought to be a seizure manifestation, but EEG monitoring in such children rarely demonstrates epileptiform activity in association with apneic spells or episodic tonic posturing. Some infants who have survived neonatal respiratory disease show a delayed progressive deterioration of brainstem function (Ellison and Farina, 1980). The mechanism is unknown, but the syndrome is characterized by frequent apnea with bradycardia and sudden infant death.

Breathholding spells occur in almost 5 percent of children (Lombroso and Lerman, 1967). They are a familial trait, probably transmitted by autosomal dominant inheritance with incomplete penetrance. A positive history is obtained in 23 percent of parents. Cyanotic and pallid varieties, which occur with equal frequency, are distinguished. Most children experience only one or the other, and some have both (Laxdal et al, 1969). Breathholding spells are involuntary responses to adverse stimuli. Children under four years of age cannot voluntarily hold their breath on request (Kuhns et al, 1979). Approximately 80 percent of spells begin before age eighteen months, and all spells start before age three years. The last episode is usually by age four and no later than age eight.

Cyanotic Syncope

Clinical Features. Cyanotic spells are usually provoked by anger, frustration, or fear. The infant's sibling takes away a toy; the child cries and then stops breathing in *expiration*. Cyanosis develops rapidly, followed quickly by limpness and loss of consciousness. Occasionally, cyanotic episodes are provoked by pain and these may not be preceded by crying.

If the attack lasts only a few seconds, the infant may resume crying upon awakening. Most spells, especially the ones referred for neurologic evaluation, are longer and are associated with tonic posturing of the body and clonic movements of the hands or arms. The eyes may roll upward as well. These movements are generally regarded as seizures by most observers, but are probably a brainstem release phenomenon not associated with abnormal electrical discharges.

After a short spell, there is rapid recovery and the child seems normal immediately; after a prolonged spell, the child first arouses and then goes to sleep.

Once an infant begins having breathholding spells, the frequency first increases for several months, then declines, and finally ceases.

Diagnosis. The typical sequence of crying, cyanosis, and loss of consciousness is critical for diagnosis. Many children with cyanotic syncope are misdiagnosed as having epilepsy because of lack of attention to the precipitating event. It is not sufficent to ask, "Did the child hold his breath?" The question conjures up the image of breathholding during inspiration. Instead, questioning should be focused on family history, precipitating events, absence of breathing, and facial color.

Between attacks, the EEG is always normal. During an episode, the EEG first shows diffuse slowing and then rhythmic slowing during the tonic-clonic activity.

Treatment. Treatment is not available to prevent future breathholding spells or to stop a spell in progress. The major function of the physician is to correctly identify the nature of the spell and explain that it is harmless. Children do not die during breathholding spells, and the episodes always cease spontaneously. (Does anyone know an adult who has breathholding spells?)

Pallid Syncope

Clinical Features. These are dramatic and frightening episodes usually provoked by a sudden, unexpected, painful event such as a bump on the head. The child rarely cries but, instead, becomes white and limp and loses consciousness. Parents invariably believe the child is dead and begin mouth-to-mouth resuscitation. After the initial limpness, the body may stiffen and be accompanied by clonic movements of the arms. As in cyanotic syncope, these movements represent a brainstem release phenomenon and not seizure activity. The duration of the spell is difficult to determine. It is very frightening to the observer, and seconds seem like hours. Afterwards, the child oftens falls asleep and is normal upon awakening.

Diagnosis. The pathophysiology of pallid syncope is reflex asystole (Stephenson, 1980). An attack can be provoked by initiating a vagal reflex by pressure on the eyeballs. However, I do not recommend provoking an attack as an office procedure; the diagnosis can be made by history alone.

Treatment. As with cyanotic spells, the major goal is to reassure the family that the child will not die during an attack. One needs to be very convincing. Atropine, 0.01 mg/kg/day, in two divided doses, has been recommended to prevent attacks, but is without experimental evidence of efficacy.

SEIZURES

Febrile Seizures

It is commonplace for an infant's first seizure to occur at the time of fever. Three explanations are possible: (1) an infection of the nervous system; (2) an underlying seizure disorder (epilepsy) in which the initial seizure is triggered by the stress of fever, but subsequent seizures may be afebrile; and (3) a simple febrile convulsion. Infections of the nervous system are dealt with in Chapters 2 and 4. The distinction between epilepsy and simple febrile convulsions is often difficult.

Clinical Features. Febrile seizures, not caused by infection or other definable cause, occur in approximately 4 percent of children. In only 2 percent of children whose first seizure is associated with fever will epilepsy develop by age seven (Nelson and Ellenberg, 1976), and in 7 percent by age twenty-five (Annegers et al, 1987). Factors associated with an increased risk for epilepsy are a prior abnormal neurologic or developmental state and complex seizures (defined as prolonged, focal, or multiple).

The infant who has a single, brief, generalized seizure during the rise of fever is likely to have experienced a simple febrile convulsion. "Brief" and "fever" are difficult to define. Parents do not use a stop clock, and when a child is having a seizure, seconds seem like minutes. Any child whose seizure is still in progress on arrival at the emergency room has had a prolonged seizure. Postictal sleep should not be counted as seizure time. Similarly, body temperature is never measured during a seizure and may be considerably different thirty minutes later.

Simple febrile convulsions are familial and probably transmitted by autosomal dominant inheritance with incomplete penetrance. One third of infants who experience a first simple febrile convulsion will have a second at the time of a subsequent febrile illness, and half of these will have a third febrile seizure. More than three episodes of simple febrile convulsions are unusual and suggestive of epilepsy. Infants with simple febrile convulsions do not have an underlying cerebral abnormality and are not at risk for later epilepsy or mental retardation (Ellenberg and Nelson, 1978). Following a first simple febrile convulsion, it is unusual for the second one to be prolonged; even when it is prolonged, the risk of subsequent epilepsy is not increased.

The small group of infants with epilepsy who present with a febrile seizure are important to identify as early as possible. Their diagnostic tests, drug therapy, and immunization schedules will be different from those of infants with simple febrile convulsions. Most such infants will be suspected of having epilepsy at the time of the first febrile seizure because the infant was neurologically abnormal or the seizure was complex.

In half this group, the diagnosis is established when the second seizure is nonfebrile.

Diagnosis. Any child who is thought to have an infection of the nervous system should undergo a lumbar puncture and examination of the cerebrospinal fluid. Approximately 15 percent of children with meningitis present with a febrile seizure, and infants may have no other signs of meningismus. However, a brief, generalized seizure from which the child recovers rapidly and completely is not caused by meningitis, especially if the fever subsides spontaneously or is otherwise explained.

Determinations of blood cell counts, glucose, calcium, electrolytes, urinalysis, and EEG on a routine basis are not cost-effective and should not be done (Gerber and Berliner, 1981). The decision for laboratory testing can be individualized to the circumstances of the specific case. An EEG should be performed in every infant who is neurologically abnormal or who has a family history of epilepsy. A CT scan is indicated in infants with focal seizures or focal deficits, even transitory, following the seizure.

Treatment. Since only one third of children with an initial febrile seizure will have a second seizure, it is unreasonable to treat every child. The low-risk group with a single, brief, generalized seizure should not be treated. There is no evidence that a second seizure, even if prolonged, will cause epilepsy or brain damage.

I recommend the following guidelines in other situations:

1. Infants with an abnormal neurologic state or a focal seizure are at high risk for epilepsy and should be started on prophylactic anticonvulsant therapy immediately.

2. When the initial febrile seizure is multiple or prolonged but the child recovers rapidly and completely, treatment is not indicated unless there is a positive family history of epilepsy.

3. Infants who have experienced two prolonged or more than three brief febrile seizures should be started on anticonvulsant therapy.

4. A family history of simple febrile convulsions is a relative contraindication to therapy.

Phenobarbital is the drug of choice. Valproic acid is equally effective in preventing recurrence of febrile seizures, but is not a preferred drug in this age group because of its potential for inducing fatal hepatotoxicity in one per six hundred treated infants (Dreifuss et al, 1987).

Nonfebrile Seizures

Disorders that produce nonfebrile tonic-clonic or partial seizures in infancy are not substantially different from those that cause nonfebrile seizures in childhood; see the section that follows. Major risk factors for the development of epilepsy in infancy and childhood are congenital malformations, neonatal seizures, and a family history of epilepsy (Nelson and Ellenberg, 1986).

A first partial motor seizure under the age of two is associated with a recurrence rate of 87 percent, whereas afterward the rate is 51 percent (Hirtz et al, 1984). The recurrence rate after a first nonfebrile, nonsymptomatic, generalized seizure is 60 to 70 percent at all ages (Elwes et al, 1985). As a rule, the earlier the age at onset of a nonfebrile seizure of any type, the more likely that the seizure is symptomatic rather than idiopathic.

Approximately 25 percent of children who have recurrent seizures during the first year, excluding neonatal seizures and infantile spasms, are developmentally or neurologically abnormal at the time of the first seizure (Matsumoto et al, 1983). The initial EEG has prognostic significance; a normal EEG is associated with a favorable neurologic outcome.

Infantile Spasms

Infantile spasm is an age-dependent myoclonic seizure that occurs with an incidence of 25 per 100,000 live births in the United States and Western Europe. An underlying etiology can be determined in approximately 75 percent of patients; congenital malformations and perinatal asphyxia are common causes, and tuberous sclerosis accounts for 20 percent of cases in some series (Table 1.9) (Riikonen, 1984). Despite considerable concern in the past, it is now established that pertussis immunization is not a cause of infantile spasms (Bellman et al, 1983). The combination of infantile spasms, hypsarrhythmia, and mental retardation is sometimes referred to as *West syndrome*.

Clinical Features. The peak age at onset is between four and seven months, and always before one year. The spasm is a flexor movement in 34 percent, an extensor movement in 23 percent, and mixed in the remainder (Kellaway et al, 1979).

Spasms generally occur in clusters, shortly after the infant awakens from sleep, and are not activated by stimulation. A rapid flexor spasm involving the neck, trunk, and limbs is followed by a tonic contraction sustained for two to ten seconds. Less severe flexor spasms are characterized only by dropping of the head and ab-

Table 1.9 NEUROCUTANEOUS DISORDERS CAUSING SEIZURES IN INFANCY

Tuberous Sclerosis
1. Seizure type
   a. Generalized
      (1) Infantile spasms
      (2) Lennox-Gastaut syndrome
      (3) Neonatal seizures
      (4) Tonic-clonic
   b. Partial
      (1) Simple motor
      (2) Complex
2. Cutaneous manifestations
   a. Abnormal hair pigmentation
   b. Adenoma sebaceum
   c. Depigmented areas
   d. Shagreen patch
   e. Café au lait spots

Neurofibromatosis
1. Seizure type
   a. Generalized tonic-clonic
   b. Partial complex
   c. Partial simple motor
2. Cutaneous manifestations
   a. Café au lait spots
   b. Axillary freckles
   c. Neural tumors

Sturge-Weber Syndrome
1. Seizure type
   a. Status epilepticus
   b. Epilepsia partialis continuans
   c. Partial simple motor
2. Cutaneous manifestation
   a. Hemifacial hemangioma

Incontinentia Pigmenti
1. Seizure type
   a. Neonatal seizures
   b. Generalized tonic-clonic
2. Cutaneous manifestations
   a. Erythematous bulla (newborn)
   b. Pigmentary whorls (infancy)
   c. Depigmented areas (childhood)

Linear Nevus Sebaceous Syndrome
1. Seizure type
   a. Infantile spasms
   b. Lennox-Gastaut syndrome
   c. Generalized tonic-clonic
2. Cutaneous manifestation
   a. Linear facial sebaceous nevus

duction of the arms or by flexion at the waist resembling colic. Extensor spasms resemble the second component of the Moro reflex: the head moves backward and there is sudden spreading of the arms. Whether flexor or extensor, the movement is almost always symmetric and brief.

Infants in whom the etiology is identifiable for spasms (symptomatic) are usually abnormal neurologically or developmentally when the spasms begin. Microcephaly is common in this group. Prognosis depends upon etiology, but as a rule the symptomatic group does poorly and experiences a high incidence of subsequent mental retardation and epilepsy.

Idiopathic cases are characteristically children who had been developing normally at the onset of spasms and have no history of prenatal or perinatal disorders. Neurologic examination, including head circumference, is normal. Approximately 40 percent of children with idiopathic spasms will be normal subsequently.

Diagnosis. There is often considerable delay from time of spasm onset to time of diagnosis. Infantile spasms are so unlike the usual perception of seizures that even experienced pediatricians may be slow to realize the significance of the movements. Colic is often considered and treated for several weeks before seizures are suspected.

Infantile spasms must be differentiated from benign myoclonus of early infancy, benign myoclonic epilepsy of infants, severe myoclonic epilepsy of infancy, and the Lennox-Gastaut syndrome (Table 1.10). The EEG is the single most important test for diagnosis. However, EEG findings vary with duration of recording, sleep state, and underlying disorder (Hrachovy et al, 1984). Hypsarrhythmia is the usual pattern recorded during the early stages of infantile spasms. It is characterized by a chaotic and continuously abnormal background of very high voltage and random slow waves and spikes. The spikes vary in location from moment to moment and at times become generalized, but are never repetitive. Typical hypsarrhythmia is most often recorded during wakefulness or active sleep. During quiet sleep, greater interhemispheric synchrony occurs and the background may have the appearance of burst-suppression.

The EEG may transiently normalize immediately upon arousal, but when spasms occur, either an abrupt attenuation of the background or high voltage slow waves appear concurrently.

Within a few weeks, the original chaotic pattern of hypsarrhythmia is replaced by greater interhemispheric synchrony. Epileptiform discharges change in their distribution from multifocal to generalized, and the generalized discharges are followed by attenuation of the record.

Treatment. There is general agreement that adrenocorticotropic hormone (ACTH) is an effective measure to stop infantile spasms, but it need not be used in every case. ACTH does not affect outcome in infants with spasms that are due to prenatal or perinatal brain abnormalities. In such infants, clonazepam or nitrazepam should be tried first and usually proves effective, at least temporarily (Dreifuss et al, 1986). Valproic acid may be effective as well, but is not a preferred drug in this age group because of an unacceptable rate of fatal hepatotoxicity (Dreifuss et al, 1987).

If clonazepam fails, ACTH therapy should be initiated. However, clonazepam should be continued in neurologically abnormal infants; ACTH usually provides only temporary respite from seizures and long-term anticonvulsant therapy will be needed. An ideal dose and duration of ACTH therapy have not been established. The protocol established by Snead and collaborators (1983) is frequently followed in the United States, although a Finnish study indicates that considerably smaller doses can be used with equal efficacy (Riikonen, 1984). ACTH gel, 150 units/M^2, is injected intramuscularly daily in two divided doses the first week, 75 units/M^2 daily the second week, 75 units/M^2 every other day the third and fourth weeks, and then tapered and discontinued over four weeks.

All infants with idiopathic infantile spasms who are neurologically and developmentally normal at the onset of spasms should be treated with ACTH using the same protocol. There is a sense, but no solid experimental data, that ACTH has a positive influence on prognosis in this group.

Among all infants treated with ACTH, approximately one third relapse during or after the course of treatment. In symptomatic more often than idiopathic cases, the infant either fails to respond to the initial course of ACTH therapy or relapses afterwards. The overall relapse rate is approximately 33 percent. A second course proves effective in 75 percent of cases in which the first course was successful, albeit at the price of increased adverse reactions.

High-dose pyridoxine should be considered

Table 1.10 EEG APPEARANCE IN MYOCLONIC SEIZURES OF INFANCY

Seizure Type	EEG Appearance
Infantile spasms	Hypsarrhythmia
	Slow spike and waves
	Burst-suppression
Benign myoclonus	Normal
Benign myoclonic epilepsy	Spike and wave (3 Hz)
	Polyspike and wave (3 Hz)
Severe myoclonic epilepsy	Polyspike and wave (>3 Hz)
Lennox-Gastaut syndrome	Spike and wave (2–2.5 Hz)
	Polyspike and wave (2–2.5 Hz)

in the treatment of infantile spasms when ACTH fails initially or relapses occur (Blennow and Stark, 1986). Some cases of infantile spasms or other seizures of infancy may be atypical presentations of pyridoxine-dependent seizures (Goutieres and Aicardi, 1985). However, in most cases the anticonvulsant properties of pyridoxine and ACTH are unrelated to their physiologic functions. The recommended dose of pyridoxine is 30 to 40 mg/kg/day.

Benign Myoclonus of Infancy

Clinical Features. Many reports of patients with infantile spasms include a small number with normal EEGs. Such infants cannot be distinguished from others with infantile spasms by clinical features: age at onset and appearance of movements are the same. The spasms occur in clusters, frequently at mealtime. Clusters increase in intensity and severity over a period of weeks or months and then abate spontaneously. After three months the spasms usually stop altogether, and while occasional episodes may recur, there are no spasms after age two (Lombroso and Fejerman, 1977). Affected infants are normal neurologically and developmentally and remain so afterwards. Benign myoclonus is used as a descriptive term because the spasms are thought to be a nonconvulsive involuntary movement.

Diagnosis. A normal EEG distinguishes this group from other causes of myoclonus in infancy. The CT scan is normal as well.

Treatment. Some infants have been treated with ACTH, benzodiazepines, or barbiturates; others have received no treatment. All did equally well. Treatment is not needed, and ACTH is probably contraindicated because of adverse side effects.

Benign Myoclonic Epilepsy

Clinical Features. This form of epilepsy is a rare disorder of uncertain etiology. A genetic basis is presumed because one third of patients have family members with epilepsy. Onset is between four months and two years. Affected infants are neurologically normal at onset of seizures and remain so afterwards. The seizures are characterized by brief myoclonic attacks, which may be restricted to head nodding, or they may be so severe as to throw the infant to the floor. The head drops to the chest, eyes roll upward, arms are thrown upward and outward, and legs flex (Dravet et al, 1985a). Myoclonic seizures may be single or repetitive, but consciousness is not lost. No other seizure types are observed in infancy, but generalized tonic-clonic seizures may occur in adolescence.

Diagnosis. During a seizure, the EEG demonstrates generalized 3 Hz spike-wave or polyspike-wave discharges. Sensory stimuli do not activate seizures. The pattern is consistent with a primary, generalized epilepsy.

Treatment. Valproic acid is effective in providing complete seizure control. If left untreated, seizures may persist for years. The use of valproic acid is potentially dangerous in this age group because of hepatotoxicity, but barbiturates and benzodiazepines are not effective.

Severe Myoclonic Epilepsy

Clinical Features. Affected infants are normal up to the time of seizure onset between two and ten months. A family history of epilepsy is present in 25 percent of cases. The first seizures are frequently febrile, usually prolonged, and can be generalized or focal clonic in type. Febrile and nonfebrile seizures recur, sometimes as status epilepticus (Dravet et al, 1985b). Generalized myoclonic seizures make their appearance after age one. At first mild and difficult to recognize as a seizure manifestation, they later become frequent and repetitive and disturb function. Partial complex seizures with secondary generalization may occur as well.

Coincident with the onset of myoclonic seizures are the slowing of development and the gradual appearance of ataxia and hyperreflexia.

Diagnosis. The initial differential diagnosis is febrile seizures. Because of the coincident age at onset, many will experience their first febrile seizure after pertussis immunization and subsequent neurologic deterioration will be incorrectly blamed on the immunization.

Because the febrile seizures are usually prolonged and sometimes focal, the suspicion of epilepsy should be high. A specific diagnosis is not possible until the appearance of myoclonic seizures in the second year.

Interictal EEG is at first normal. Paroxysmal abnormalities appear in the second year and are characterized by generalized spike-wave and polyspike-wave complexes with a frequency greater than 3 Hz. Discharges are activated by photic stimulation, drowsiness, and quiet sleep.

Treatment. The seizures are resistant to therapy with anticonvulsant drugs. Valproic acid and benzodiazepines should be tried first and carbamazepine added if necessary.

Lennox-Gastaut Syndrome

Lennox-Gastaut syndrome is characterized by the triad of seizures (atypical absence, atonic, and myoclonic), slow spike-wave complexes on EEG, and mental retardation. Most are secondary to underlying brain damage, but some are primary epilepsies. Some authorities reserve the term *myoclonic-astatic epilepsy* for cases of Lennox-Gastaut syndrome that are due to primary epilepsy.

Clinical Features. The peak age at onset is three to five years with less than half of cases beginning before age two. An underlying cause can be identified in approximately 60 percent: neurocutaneous disorders, perinatal disturbances, and postnatal brain injuries are most common. Twenty percent of children with the Lennox-Gastaut syndrome have a history of infantile spasms, sometimes with a seizure-free interval before development of the syndrome (Kurokawa et al, 1980).

Although the syndrome can begin in a normal child, most children are identified as neurologically abnormal prior to onset. The first seizures may be generalized tonic-clonic or focal clonic, but are usually tonic. Tonic seizures are characterized by stiffening of the body, upward deviation of the eyes, dilation of the pupils, and an alteration in respiratory pattern. The seizures frequently occur during sleep, and enuresis may be associated.

Atypical absence seizures occur in almost every case. In addition to the stare, there is trembling of the eyelids and mouth, followed by loss of facial tone so that the head leans forward and the mouth hangs open. Atonic seizures are characterized by sudden dropping of the head or body, at times throwing the child to the ground. More than 90 percent of patients are mentally retarded by age five.

Diagnosis. An EEG is essential for diagnosis. The characteristic feature during atypical absence or atonic seizures is a generalized burst of 2 to 2.5 Hz spike-wave complexes. Tonic seizures are associated with 1 Hz slow waves followed by generalized rapid discharges without postictal depression.

In addition to EEG, a thorough evaluation is needed to look for an underlying cause. Special attention should be given to skin manifestations suggesting a neurocutaneous syndrome (see Table 1.9). CT is useful for the diagnosis of congenital malformations, postnatal disorders, and neurocutaneous syndromes.

Treatment. Seizures are difficult to control. Valproic acid and clonazepam are the drugs most often effective (Gomez and Klass, 1983). ACTH may provide transitory relief of seizures.

MIGRAINE

Clinical Features. Migraine attacks are uncommon in infancy, but when they occur, the clinical features are often "paroxysmal" and suggest the possibility of seizures. Cyclic vomiting is probably the most common manifestation. Attacks of vertigo (see Chapter 10) or torticollis (see Chapter 14) may be especially perplexing, and some infants have attacks in which they rock back and forth and appear to be in discomfort.

Diagnosis. Migrainous vertigo (benign paroxysmal vertigo) is sufficiently stereotyped in presentation to be recognizable as a migraine variant. Other syndromes often remain undiagnosed until the episodes evolve into a typical migraine pattern. A positive family history of migraine in one parent, usually the mother, is essential for diagnosis.

Treatment. Antimigraine drugs are generally not used in infants.

■ Paroxysmal Disorders of Childhood

Children, like infants, with paroxysmal disorders are generally thought to have seizures until proven otherwise. Indeed, seizures are the most common paroxysmal disorder requiring medical consultation. Syncope, especially presyncope, is considerably more common, but is generally diagnosed and managed at home unless associated symptoms suggest a seizure.

The prevalence of migraine in childhood is ten times greater than that of epilepsy. Migraine syndromes that may suggest epilepsy are described in Chapters 2, 3, 10, 11, 14, and 15.

Sleep disorders often have a paroxysmal quality and may be confused with complex partial seizures. Such seizures are often activated by sleep, adding to the similarity.

SYNDROMES SIMULATING SEIZURES

Syncope

Syncope is loss of consciousness due to a transitory decline in cerebral blood flow. This may be caused by an irregular cardiac rate or rhythm or by alterations of blood volume or distribution.

Clinical Features. Syncope is a common event in otherwise healthy children, and the incidence is even greater in the second decade. The mechanism is a vasovagal reflex by which an emotional experience produces peripheral pooling of blood. The reflex may also be stimulated by overextension or sudden decompression of viscera and by the Valsalva maneuver. Fainting in a hot, crowded church is especially common, when the worshiper rises to stand after prolonged kneeling.

Healthy children do not faint while lying down and rarely while seated. Fainting from anything but standing or arising suggests the possibility of a cardiac arrhythmia and requires further investigation.

The child may first feel faint (described as faint, dizzy, or light-headed) or may lose consciousness without warning. Color drains from the face, and the skin becomes cold and clammy. With loss of consciousness, the child falls to the floor. Consciousness may be regained rapidly, or there may be stiffening of the body and clonic movements of the arms. The latter is not a seizure. Afterwards, there may be a short period of confusion, but not a prolonged postictal period. Recovery is complete within minutes.

Diagnosis. The critical factors in distinguishing syncope from seizures are the precipitating factors and the child's appearance. Seizures do not produce pallor and cold, clammy skin. Laboratory investigations are not cost-effective when syncope occurs in expected circumstances and examination is normal. Recurrent orthostatic syncope requires investigation of autonomic function, and any suspicion of cardiac abnormality deserves EKG monitoring.

Treatment. Infrequent syncopal episodes of obvious cause do not require treatment.

Hyperventilation Syndrome

Hyperventilation induces alkalosis by altering the proportion of blood gases. This is more readily accomplished in children than adults.

Clinical Features. During times of emotional upset, respiratory rate and depth may increase insidiously, first appearing like sighing and then as obvious hyperventilation. This is associated with tingling of the fingers that disturbs the patient further and may induce greater hyperventilation. Headache is associated. If hyperventilation is allowed to continue, the patient may lose consciousness.

Diagnosis. The observation of hyperventilation as a precipitating factor of syncope is essential to diagnosis. Often, patients are unaware that they were hyperventilating and probing questions are needed to elicit history in the absence of a witness.

Treatment. An attack in progress can be aborted by having the patient breathe into a paper bag.

Narcolepsy-Cataplexy

Narcolepsy-cataplexy is a sleep disorder characterized by an abnormally short latency from sleep onset to rapid eye movement (REM) sleep. REM sleep is attained in less than twenty minutes instead of the usual ninety minutes. Normal REM is characterized by dreaming and severe hypotonia. In narcolepsy-cataplexy, these phenomena occur during wakefulness.

Clinical Features. Age at onset may be from early childhood to middle adult life, but 60 percent of cases begin before age twenty (Kales et al, 1982). There are four components to the syndrome:

1. *Narcolepsy* refers to short sleep attacks. Three or four attacks occur each day, most often during monotonous activity, and are difficult to resist. Half of patients are easy to arouse from a sleep attack, and 60 percent feel refreshed afterwards. Narcolepsy is usually a life-long condition.

2. *Cataplexy* is a sudden loss of muscle tone induced by laughter, excitement, or startle. Almost all patients who have narcolepsy have cataplexy as well. The patient may collapse to the floor and then arise immediately. Partial paralysis, affecting just the face or hands, is more frequent than total paralysis. Two to four attacks occur daily, usually in the afternoon. They are embarrassing, but do not cause physical harm.

3. *Sleep paralysis* occurs in the transition between sleep and wakefulness. There is generalized hypotonia and, although mentally awake, the patient is unable to move any body part. Partial paralysis is less frequent. The attack may end spontaneously or upon being touched. Two thirds of patients with narcolepsy-cataplexy also experience sleep paralysis once or twice each week. Occasional episodes of sleep paralysis may occur in people who do not have narcolepsy-cataplexy.

4. *Hypnagogic hallucinations* are vivid, usually frightening, visual and auditory perceptions occurring at the transition between sleep and wakefulness—as if dreaming while awake. They

are reported as an associated event in half of patients with narcolepsy-cataplexy. Less than one episode occurs each week.

Diagnosis. The syndrome should be recognizable by history. However, the symptoms are embarrassing or sound "crazy" to the patient and considerable prompting is often needed to elicit a full history.

Difficulty may be encountered in distinguishing narcolepsy from other causes of excessive daytime sleepiness. The multiple sleep latency test is the standard for diagnosis. Patients with narcolepsy enter REM sleep within a few minutes of falling asleep.

Treatment. Symptoms of narcolepsy-cataplexy are very distressing, and in many cases emotional problems develop. Realization that narcolepsy is not a mental disorder is very comforting. The best treatment, when possible, is a program of "sleep hygiene" (Freemon, 1985):

1. Go to bed and arise at the same time each day, including weekends.

2. Avoid long daytime naps; instead, schedule brief naps.

3. Avoid shift or night work.

Amphetamine or methylphenidate is often prescribed for narcolepsy but should be given with caution because of potential abuse. Cataplexy can be treated with trihexyphenidyl, 2 mg three times a day, or imipramine, 50 mg three times a day.

Night Terrors

Night terrors are a partial arousal from non-REM sleep.

Clinical Features. The onset usually occurs before age four and almost always by age six. Two hours after falling asleep, the child awakens in a terrified state, does not recognize people, and is inconsolable. An episode usually lasts for five to fifteen minutes, but can last an hour. During this time, the child screams incoherently, may run if not restrained, and then goes back to sleep. Afterwards, there is no memory of the event.

Most children experience an average of one or more episodes each week. Night terrors stop by age eight in half of children but continue into adolescence in a third (DiMario and Emery, 1986).

Diagnosis. Half of children with night terrors are also sleepwalkers, and many have a family history of either sleepwalking or night terrors. The diagnosis should be made by history alone. A sleep laboratory evaluation may be helpful in unusual circumstances when the possibility of seizures cannot be excluded.

Treatment. Treatment is usually not needed, and regular bedtime sedation should be avoided except when spells are very frequent and intolerable to the family.

Familial Paroxysmal Choreoathetosis

This disorder is transmitted by autosomal dominant inheritance. It is often regarded as a form of "reflex" epilepsy because the paroxysms are stimulus-provoked and often responsive to prophylactic treatment with anticonvulsant drugs. However, the EEG does not demonstrate epileptiform activity, even during an attack (Lance, 1977).

Clinical Features. The age of onset varies from infancy to the third decade. The paroxysms, which are precipitated by sudden movement or startle, usually last less than two minutes, but can continue for several hours. Each attack may include dystonia, choreoathetosis, or ballismus (see Chapter 14). One or both sides of the body can be affected. Some patients have an "aura" described as tightness or tingling of the face or limbs. Attack frequency varies from once or twice each week to more than one hundred per day. Consciousness is always preserved during attacks. The disorder does not affect normal life span.

In some families, attacks are prolonged, not necessarily provoked by startle, and poorly responsive to anticonvulsants. The mechanism of choreoathetosis in such families is probably not epileptic.

Diagnosis. Approximately one quarter of cases are sporadic, some may be new mutations, and others are not genetic and due to identifiable cerebral disorders (see Table 14.1).

Ictal and interictal EEG are normal or demonstrate diffuse background slowing. An EEG does not predict which patients will respond to anticonvulsant therapy.

Treatment. Phenytoin or phenobarbital in ordinary anticonvulsant doses are effective in most cases.

MIGRAINE AND EPILEPSY

A link between migraine and epilepsy is suggested because (1) they are both familial, paroxysmal, and associated with transitory neurologic disturbances, (2) there is an increased incidence of epilepsy in migraineurs and migraine in epileptics, (3) headache can be a seizure manifestation, and (4) abnormal electroencephalograms are common in both disorders.

Clinical Features. In children who have epilepsy and migraine, both disorders may share a common aura and one may provoke the other. Basilar migraine (see Chapter 10) and benign occipital epilepsy best exemplify the fine line between epilepsy and migraine. Both are characterized by seizures, headache, and epileptiform activity.

Diagnosis. Asymptomatic central spikes are observed in 9 percent of children with migraine as compared with 1.9 percent of healthy children. Fourteen-and-six positive spikes, a normal adolescent pattern, occurs twice as commonly in children with migraine as compared with age-matched controls.

Treatment. Children who have both epilepsy and migraine must be treated for each condition separately.

STARING SPELLS

Daydreaming is a pleasant escape for people of all ages. Children feel the need for escape most acutely when in school and may stare vacantly out the window to the place they would rather be. Daydreams can be hard to break, and a child may not respond to verbal commands. Many dreamers are seen by neurologists, and EEG may be recommended. Sometimes the EEG shows sleep-activated central spikes or another abnormality not related to staring and inappropriate anticonvulsant drug therapy is started.

Absence (petit mal) and complex partial seizures are characterized by staring. They have characteristic clinical and EEG features that establish the diagnosis. Precise diagnosis should be made in every case before treatment is initiated.

Absence Epilepsy

The term petit mal has been used generically for all small seizures in which consciousness is not lost. Such use is not helpful and may lead to the wrong choice of anticonvulsant drug. Absence is now the preferred term for generalized seizures characterized by staring. Absence epilepsy is a genetic disorder, transmitted as an autosomal dominant trait with age-dependent penetrance (Berkovic et al, 1987). The EEG is

characteristic, and specific drug therapy is available.

Clinical Features. The peak age of onset is usually between four and eight, with a range between three and twelve. Absence never begins after age twenty, but may persist from childhood into the seventh and eighth decades (Gastaut et al, 1986). Girls are affected more often than boys. Affected children are otherwise healthy.

The reported incidence of epilepsy in families of children with absence varies from 15 to 40 percent. Concurrence in monozygotic twins is 75 percent for seizures and 85 percent for a 3 Hz spike-wave. Absence attacks are almost never secondary to an underlying disease.

Typical attacks last five to ten seconds and occur up to one hundred times each day. The child stops ongoing activity, stares vacantly, sometimes with rhythmic movements of the eyelids, and then resumes activity. There is never an aura or a period of postictal confusion. Longer seizures may last up to a minute and are indistinguishable by observation alone from complex partial seizures. Associated features may include myoclonus, increased or decreased postural tone, picking at clothes, turning of the head, and conjugate movements of the eyes. Occasional children and adults present to emergency rooms in a confusional state caused by absence status (see Chapter 2).

Approximately 50 percent of children with absence have had at least one generalized tonic-clonic convulsion. Some actually present for medical care because of a tonic-clonic seizure, even though absence attacks have occurred undiagnosed for months or years. Children with both absence and tonic-clonic seizures may be divided into two groups: (1) those with only 3 Hz spike-wave on EEG, and (2) those with 3 Hz spike-wave and a cortical focus. The first group has only absence epilepsy, which, if uncontrolled, spreads to lower brainstem structures, causing a generalized tonic-clonic convulsion. Most children in this group, like those who have only absence, will stop having seizures of both kinds after age twenty. The second group has a more complex epilepsy than simple absence and is likely to continue having tonic-clonic seizures in adult life.

Diagnosis. The EEG is pathognomonic. Bilaterally synchronous and symmetric paroxysms of 3 Hz spike-wave complexes appear concurrent with the clinical seizure (Fig. 1.6). The amplitude of discharge is greatest in the fronto-central regions. Although the discharge begins

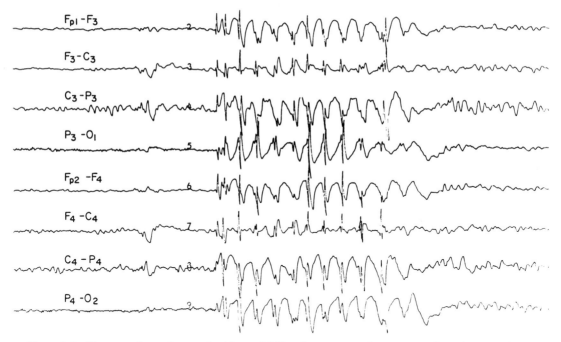

Figure 1.6 Absence epilepsy. A generalized burst of 3 Hz spike-wave complexes appears during hyperventilation.

with a frequency of 3 Hz, it may slow to 2 Hz at it ends. Hyperventilation almost always activates the discharge. The interictal EEG is normal.

Although the EEG pattern of discharge is stereotyped, variations on the theme in the form of multiple spike and wave discharges are also acceptable. During sleep, the discharges often lose their stereotypy and become polymorphic in form and frequency, but remain generalized.

Once a clinical-EEG correlation is made, it is unnecessary to look for an underlying disease. Subacute sclerosing panencephalitis and thalamic tumor may present with typical absence, but this is so uncommon as to be negligible.

Absence epilepsy is distinguished from two other primary generalized epilepsies in which absence occurs, *myoclonic absence* and *juvenile myoclonic epilepsy* (see Myoclonic Seizures), by the absence of myoclonic seizures (Berkovic et al, 1987).

Treatment. Ethosuximide and valproic acid are both equally effective in the treatment of absence, and each provides complete relief of seizures in 80 percent of cases. Ethosuximide is the treatment of choice because of its lower incidence of serious side effects. The EEG becomes normal if treatment is successful, and it is useful to repeat the EEG to confirm the seizure-free state.

Patients with only 3 Hz spike-wave on EEG should first be treated with ethosuximide alone, even if a tonic-clonic seizure occurred prior to initiation of therapy. If tonic-clonic seizures recur after therapy is initiated, then either phenobarbital can be added or valproic acid can be substituted for ethosuximide. Other drugs that may be useful in the treatment of refractory absence include clonazepam, trimethadione, and methsuximide (see Table 1.5).

Complex Partial Seizures

Complex partial seizures are unusual during the first decade and are generally less common in children than adults. They arise in the cortex, most often the temporal lobe, but can originate from the frontal or parietal lobes as well.

Clinical Features. Complex partial seizures may occur spontaneously or may be activated by sleep. Most last one to two minutes and rarely less than thirty seconds (Holmes, 1986). An aura is reported in less than 30 percent of children. It is usually a nondescript, unpleasant feeling, but might also be a stereotyped auditory hallucination or abdominal discomfort. The first manifestation of the seizure can be staring, automatic behavior, tonic extension of one or both arms, or loss of body tone. Staring is always associated with a change in facial expression and followed by automatic behavior. Automatisms vary from facial grimacing and fumbling movements of the fingers to walking, running, and resisting restraint. Automatic behavior in a given patient tends to be similar from seizure to seizure.

The seizure usually terminates with a period of postictal confusion, disorientation, or lethargy. Transitory aphasia is sometimes present. Secondary generalization is likely to occur at some time in untreated patients, especially if medication is abruptly withdrawn.

Partial complex status epilepticus is a rare event manifested by impaired consciousness, staring alternating with wandering eye movements, and automatisms of the face and hands. Such patients may present to the emergency room in a confused or delirious state (see Chapter 2).

Diagnosis. The etiology of complex partial seizures is heterogeneous, and a cause is often not determined. Brain tumor was thought to be an unusual cause in children, but magnetic resonance imaging (MRI) is likely to demonstrate a low-grade glioma in many otherwise normal children with hard-to-control seizures. MRI should be performed in all such cases.

An EEG should be recorded in both the waking and sleeping states. Hyperventilation and photic stimulation are not useful as provocative measures. A single EEG may be normal in the interictal period, but repeated EEGs usually reveal either a spike or slow-wave focus in the frontal or temporal lobe or multifocal abnormalities. During the seizure there are repetitive focal spike discharges in the involved area of cortex, which change to spike-slow wave complexes and then slow waves with amplitude attenuation as the seizure ends.

Treatment. Carbamazepine, phenytoin, primidone, and phenobarbital are effective for seizure control, but carbamazepine has become the treatment of choice because of fewer cognitive and behavioral disturbances (see Table 1.5). Phenacemide, which had previously been discarded as an anticonvulsant because of adverse side effects, has recently been reappraised and found to be safe and useful in children with intractable complex partial seizures (Coker, 1986). My own experience with phenacemide in similar cases has been positive as well.

Temporal lobectomy should be considered when seizures are refractory to anticonvulsant drugs (Meyer et al, 1986). In highly selected cases, as many as 80 percent may become seizure-free.

MYOCLONIC SEIZURES

Myoclonus is a brief, involuntary, muscle contraction (jerk) that may represent (1) a seizure manifestation, as in infantile spasms; (2) a physiologic response to startle or to falling asleep; or (3) an involuntary movement either alone or in combination with tonic-clonic convulsions (see Table 14.8). It is often difficult to distinguish myoclonic seizures from myoclonus (the movement disorder) on clinical grounds alone. Essential myoclonus and other disorders in which myoclonus is clearly not a seizure manifestation are discussed in Chapter 14.

Myoclonic Absence

Myoclonic absence is a rare epilepsy, probably distinct from absence epilepsy, in which 85 percent of patients are boys. It is probably not a homogeneous entity, but may be genetic in some cases and symptomatic of underlying brain disorders in others.

Clinical Features. Age at onset is between two and twelve years with the peak at seven. A family history of epilepsy is present in 25 percent of cases. Unlike absence epilepsy, 40 percent of affected children are mentally subnormal before the onset of seizures.

Seizures last ten to sixty seconds and occur several times each day. They are characterized by a combination of absence and intense rhythmic, bilateral myoclonus affecting the muscles of the shoulders, arms, and legs. Consciousness is not lost, and the child may be aware and disturbed by the jerking. Other seizures types do not usually occur.

Myoclonic absence sometimes persists into adult life and other times ceases spontaneously. Some children, though intellectually normal before the onset of seizures, are retarded later.

Diagnosis. Myoclonic absence is thought to be intermediary between primary and secondary epilepsy, but an underlying cause has not been determined. The EEG demonstrates the same 3 Hz spike-wave pattern associated with simple absence.

Treatment. The seizures are refractory to treatment. Occasional success may be achieved with a combination of valproic acid and ethosuximide.

Juvenile Myoclonic Epilepsy
(Janz Syndrome)

Juvenile myoclonic epilepsy (Janz syndrome) is a hereditary disorder, probably polygenic, in which up to 40 percent of patients have a positive family history of epilepsy. Seizures in affected relatives may be tonic-clonic, myoclonic absence, or simple absence (Delgado-Escueta and Enrile-Bacsal, 1984).

Clinical Features. The age at onset is between twelve and eighteen years in 75 percent of cases. The characteristic feature is a brief, bilateral, but not always symmetric, flexor jerk of the arms which may be repetitive. The jerk sometimes affects the legs, causing the patient to fall. Consciousness is usually retained so that the patient is aware of the jerking movement. Seizures are precipitated by sleep deprivation, alcohol ingestion, and awakening from nocturnal or daytime sleep.

Most patients also have generalized tonic-clonic seizures, and 10 percent have absence but are otherwise normal neurologically. As a rule, the potential to have seizures of one type or another continues throughout adult life.

Diagnosis. Seizures are accompanied by generalized polyspike discharges followed by a slow wave. The polyspike discharge is concurrent with the clinical seizure, and the slow wave occurs afterwards. Seizures are sometimes precipitated by photic stimulation or eye closure. The interictal record may be normal or may show 3.5 to 6 Hz multispike-wave complexes.

Treatment. Valproic acid is the treatment of choice and provides complete relief of all seizures in 75 percent of cases. Some patients require a second drug for control of tonic-clonic seizures.

Progressive Myoclonic Epilepsy

The term progressive myoclonic epilepsy is used to cover several progressive disorders of the nervous system characterized by (1) myoclonus; (2) seizures that may be tonic-clonic, tonic, or myoclonic; (3) progressive mental deterioration; and (4) cerebellar ataxia, involuntary movements, or both. Some of these disorders are due to specific lysosomal enzyme deficiencies, whereas others are probably mitochondrial disorders (Table 1.11).

Table 1.11 PROGRESSIVE MYOCLONIC EPILEPSIES

Ceroid lipofuscinosis, juvenile form (see Chapter 5)
Cherry-red spot–myoclonus
Glucosylceramide lipidosis (Gaucher III) (see Chapter 5)
Lafora disease
Mitochondrial encephalomyopathies (see Chapter 5)
Ramsay Hunt syndrome (see Chapter 10)
Unverricht-Lundborg syndrome

Lafora Disease

This is a rare hereditary disease probably transmitted by autosomal recessive inheritance.

Clinical Features. Onset is between six and nineteen years of age with the mean at age eleven. Tonic-clonic or myoclonic seizures are the presenting symptoms in 80 percent of cases. Myoclonus becomes progressively worse, may be segmental or massive, and is made worse by movement. Mental retardation begins early and is relentlessly progressive. Ataxia, spasticity, and involuntary movements occur late in the course. Death occurs five to six years from onset.

Diagnosis. The EEG is normal at first and then shows the development of nonspecific generalized polyspike discharges that are not activated by sleep. The background becomes progressively disorganized and epileptiform activity more constant. Photosensitive discharges are a regular feature late in the course.

Antemortem diagnosis is accomplished by demonstrating periodic acid–Schiff (PAS)-positive inclusion bodies consisting of polyglucasan material in liver or sweat gland biopsies (Carpenter and Karpati, 1981).

Treatment. The seizures become refractory to most anticonvulsant drugs, but the combination of valproic acid, clonazepam, and phenobarbital should be tried. Treatment of the underlying disease is not available.

Unverricht-Lundborg Syndrome

This term is used for a heterogeneous group of disorders that are clinically similar to Lafora disease, except that the rate of deterioration is slower, death occurs during adolescence, and Lafora inclusion bodies are not present. The syndrome is most often reported in Finland.

A combination of valproic acid, clonazepam, and phenobarbital is effective for seizure control (Iivanainen and Himberg, 1982).

Cherry-Red Spot–Myoclonus Syndrome

Cherry-red spot–myoclonus syndrome is a sialidosis with an isolated deficit in neuraminidase (Rapin et al, 1978).

Clinical Features. The disorder is similar to the Ramsay-Hunt syndrome (see Chapter 10) except for the presence of the cherry-red spot and blindness. Age at onset is usually adolescence. The initial complaint may be loss of vision, cerebellar ataxia, myoclonus, or tonic-clonic seizures. All four symptoms are present eventually. Mental deterioration does not occur. The disorder is disabling because of frequent seizures and ataxia but is not fatal.

Diagnosis. Liver biopsy reveals mucopolysac-charide-like inclusions in Kupffer cells and hepatocytes.

Treatment. Seizures often respond to standard anticonvulsants drugs. 5-Hydroxytryptophan, 300 mg daily, may stop the myoclonus and allow better function (Gascon et al, 1986).

PARTIAL SEIZURES

This section covers several different seizure types of focal cortical origin other than complex partial seizures. Such seizures may be purely motor or purely sensory or may affect higher cortical function. The most common partial seizure disorder is benign (Rolandic) epilepsy of childhood. Partial seizures are also secondary to underlying diseases, which can be focal, multifocal, or generalized.

All seizures that originate in the cortex may sometimes discharge into the brainstem, causing a tonic-clonic convulsion (secondary generalization). If the discharge remains focal for a few seconds, the patient experiences a focal seizure or an *aura* before losing consciousness. Often, the secondary generalization occurs so rapidly that a tonic-clonic seizure is the presenting symptom. The cortical origin of the seizure is only detectable on EEG.

Benign (Rolandic) Epilepsy of Childhood

This is a genetic disorder thought to be transmitted as an autosomal dominant trait. Forty percent of close relatives have a history of febrile seizures or epilepsy. Benign occipital epilepsy of childhood may be caused by the same genetic trait.

Clinical Features. The age at onset is three to thirteen years with the majority between five and ten. Seizures almost always stop spontaneously by age fourteen. Even without drug therapy, 10 percent have only one seizure, 70 percent have infrequent seizures, and only 20 percent have frequent seizures. Seventy percent of children experience only nocturnal seizures; 15 percent, only when awake; and 15 percent, both awake and asleep.

The typical seizure wakes the child from sleep. Paresthesias occur on one side of the mouth, followed by ipsilateral twitching of the face, mouth, and pharynx, resulting in speech arrest and drooling. Consciousness is preserved. The seizure lasts for one or two minutes. Daytime seizures do not generalize, but nocturnal seizures in children younger than five years old often spread to the arm or evolve into a generalized tonic-clonic convulsion.

Diagnosis. Neurologic examination is normal, as is CT or MRI. Interictal EEG demonstrates unilateral or bilateral spike discharges in the central or centrotemporal region. The spikes are typically of high-voltage and are activated by drowsiness and sleep (Fig. 1.7). The frequency of spike discharge does not correlate with subsequent course.

Treatment. Treatment is not needed if seizures are infrequent and only nocturnal. A single bedtime dose of phenobarbital or phenytoin is usually satisfactory for seizure control. After two years of treatment, medication can be withdrawn and 80 percent will remain seizure-free. Those who resume having seizures should be treated until age fourteen. All children will eventually stop having seizures whether they are treated or not (De Romanis et al, 1986).

Benign Occipital Epilepsy of Childhood

Clinical Features. Age at onset is between two and nine years, generally below five (Beaumanoir, 1983). One third of patients have a positive family history of epilepsy, frequently Rolandic epilepsy.

The initial seizure manifestation can consist of (1) visual hallucinations, usually flashing lights or spots; (2) blindness, hemianopia, or complete amaurosis; or (3) visual illusions, such as micropsia, macropsia, or metamorphopsia. More than one manifestation may occur simultaneously. The visual aura may be followed by unilateral clonic seizures, complex partial seizures, or generalized tonic-clonic seizures. Afterwards, the patient may have migraine-like headaches and nausea. Attacks occur when one is awake or asleep, but the greatest frequency is at the transition from wake to sleep.

Diagnosis. Neurologic examination is normal, as is CT or MRI. The interictal EEG demonstrates unilateral or bilateral high-amplitude occipital spike discharges that are inhibited by eye opening and enhanced by light sleep. During a seizure, there is rapid firing of spike discharges in one or both occipital lobes.

These cases may be difficult to distinguish from basilar migraine (see Chapter 10). Reports

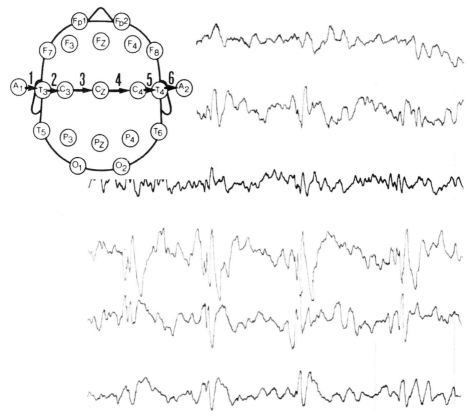

Figure 1.7 Rolandic epilepsy. Spike and spike-wave complexes originate from the right central electrode during drowsiness and sleep. (From Epstein CM, Andriola MR: Introduction to EEG and Evoked Potentials. JB Lippincott, Philadelphia, 1983.)

of basilar migraine with occipital spikes are probably benign occipital epilepsy and not migraine. Such cases respond to anticonvulsant drugs and not antimigraine agents.

Treatment. Complete seizure control is accomplished in the majority of patients with standard anticonvulsant drugs. Typical seizures never persist beyond adolescence, and only 5 percent have other types of seizures in adult life.

Aphasia

Speech arrest and aphasia occur during some complex partial seizures and with absence status. In addition, there is a disorder peculiar to children in which acquired aphasia is associated with epileptiform activity on EEG: the *Landau-Kleffner syndrome*. The cases are probably not homogeneous, but a typical clinical profile has emerged.

Clinical Features. Age at onset ranges from two to eleven years with 75 percent beginning between three and eight. The first symptom may be aphasia or epilepsy (Beaumanoir, 1985).

Aphasia is initially characterized by auditory verbal agnosia. The child has difficulty understanding what is said, spontaneous speech is reduced, and there is the appearance of deafness or autism. Seizures, which may be partial or generalized, occur in 70 percent of children. Status epilepticus is sometimes the presenting feature. Hyperactivity and personality change are noted in half of cases and may be caused by aphasia. Intelligence is not affected, and neurologic examination is otherwise normal.

Recovery of language is more likely to occur if the syndrome begins before age seven. Seizures generally cease by age ten and always by age fifteen.

Diagnosis. The Landau-Kleffner syndrome may be confused with autism, hearing loss, and psychotic behavior. The occurrence of seizures separates this syndrome from other considerations. The EEG demonstrates multifocal cortical spike discharges with a predilection for the temporal and parietal lobes. An injection of intravenous diazepam may normalize the EEG and improve speech transiently. However, this should not suggest that aphasia is caused by epileptiform activity. Rather, they both reflect an underlying cerebral disorder.

Treatment. Standard anticonvulsant drugs such as carbamazepine and phenytoin are usually effective in controlling the seizures, but may not improve speech.

Epilepsia Partialis Continuans

Focal motor seizures that do not stop spontaneously are termed epilepsia partialis continuans. It is an ominous symptom and almost always indicates an underlying cerebral disorder. The seizure may last for hours, days, or months.

Clinical Features. Focal jerking frequently begins in one body part, usually one side of the face or one hand, and then spreads to contiguous parts. Trunk muscles are rarely affected. The rate and intensity of the seizure vary at first, but then become more regular and persist in sleep. The affected limbs become paretic and almost always remain so afterwards (see Chapter 11).

Diagnosis. Possible causes include infarction, hemorrhage, tumor, and inflammation. A poorly defined entity of childhood that presents with epilepsia partialis continuans is *Rasmussen syndrome.* Affected children have focal motor seizures that defy treatment and progress to first affect both limbs on one side of the body before affecting the limbs on the other side. Progressive hemiplegia and other neurologic deficits develop, and there is often no recovery even after seizures have stopped. The syndrome is thought to be secondary to a low-grade smoldering encephalitis, but evidence to support such a notion is lacking.

The EEG demonstrates continuous spike discharges originating in one portion of the cortex with spread to contiguous areas and a mirror focus on the other side. Secondary generalization may occur.

A CT scan or MRI should be performed in every case, and arteriography is indicated if there is evidence of vascular disease.

Treatment. Every effort should be made to stop the seizures using intravenous anticonvulsant drugs (see "Treatment of Status Epilepticus" later on). Pentobarbital coma is often required. Even then, seizures return when coma is lifted.

GENERALIZED TONIC-CLONIC SEIZURES

Generalized tonic-clonic seizures are the most common seizure of childhood. They are dramatic and frightening events that invariably demand medical attention. Seizures that are prolonged or repeated without recovery are termed *status epilepticus.* The diagnostic considerations in a child who presents with a generalized tonic-clonic seizure are summarized in Table 1.12.

Clinical Features. The age of onset is anytime after the neonatal period. Symptomatic cases may occur at any age, but the onset of primary generalized epilepsy without absence is usually the second decade. With absence, age at onset shifts to the first decade.

The initial feature is sudden loss of consciousness. The child falls to the floor and the body stiffens. This is followed by repetitive jerking (clonic) movements of the limbs; at first these movements are rapid and rhythmic and then become slower and less rhythmic as the seizure abates. The eyes roll backward in the orbit; breathing is rapid and deep, causing saliva to froth at the lips; and there may be urinary and bowel incontinence. Such seizures are followed by a postictal sleep from which arousal is difficult. Afterwards, the child appears normal, but may have sore limb muscles and a painful tongue, bitten during the seizure.

Diagnosis. A first, generalized tonic-clonic seizure requires laboratory evaluation. The extent of evaluation must be individualized. Important determining factors include (1) body temperature, (2) neurologic examination, (3) family history, and (4) known precipitating factors. An eyewitness report of focal features at the onset of the seizure, or the recollection of an aura, indicates a partial seizure with secondary generalization.

During the seizure, the EEG demonstrates generalized repetitive spikes during the tonic phase and then periodic bursts of spikes during the clonic phase. The clonic portion is usually obscured by movement artefact. As the seizure ends, there is slowing of the background and amplitude attenuation.

Between seizures, brief generalized spike or spike-wave discharges may occur that are polymorphic in appearance. Discharge frequency is

Table 1.12 DIAGNOSTIC CONSIDERATIONS FOR A FIRST NONFEBRILE TONIC-CLONIC CONVULSION AFTER AGE TWO

Primary generalized epilepsy
Partial seizure with secondary generalization
Acute encephalopathy encephalitis (see Chapter 2)
Progressive disorders of the nervous system (see Chapter 5)
Isolated unexplained seizure

sometimes increased by drowsiness and light sleep. The presence of focal discharges indicates that the tonic-clonic seizure was secondarily generalized.

Cerebrospinal fluid is normal following a brief, tonic-clonic seizure due to primary epilepsy. However, prolonged or repeated seizures may cause a leukocytosis of up to 80 cells/cubic mm with a polymorphonuclear predominance (Schmidley and Simon, 1981). Protein concentration can be mildly elevated, but glucose is normal.

Treatment. Phenobarbital, phenytoin, and carbamazepine are each equally effective as prophylactic agents to prevent further seizures. Status epilepticus must be treated with intravenous drugs (see "Treatment of Status Epilepticus").

Pseudoseizures

"Hysterical" seizures are an effective method of seeking attention and secondary gain. They more often occur in adolescence than childhood and in people with epilepsy. Pseudoseizures often begin when true seizures come under control and the secondary gain of epilepsy is lost.

Clinical Features. Pseudoseizures rarely simulate true seizures and are easily distinguished by an experienced observer (Gulick et al, 1982). They may be manifest by a rich variety of motor and behavioral phenomenon, but three broad patterns are often observed:

1. Unilateral or bilateral motor activity characterized by tonic posturing and tremulousness in which the patient's movements are thrashing or jerking rather than tonic-clonic, different movements may occur simultaneously.

2. Behavioral or emotional changes in which distress or discomfort is expressed, followed by semipurposeless, but not stereotyped, behaviors such as fumbling with objects or walking.

3. Periods of unresponsiveness.

Attacks may be precipitated and ended by suggestion. Patients do not hurt themselves and do not have incontinence.

Diagnosis. Pseudoseizures usually occur at home and are believed to be real. If the child has epilepsy, the seizures are reported by telephone to the physician and drug schedules are needlessly revised, often to the patient's detriment. The possibility of pseudoseizures must be considered in children with epilepsy in whom frequent seizures develop after an initial period of control.

Children who do not have epilepsy and in whom pseudoseizures develop are frequently brought to an emergency room and may be started on anticonvulsant drugs before any investigations are initiated. It is then difficult to stop the medications and obtain a baseline EEG. Most pseudoseizures are diagnosed by observation alone. When question remains, ambulatory EEG, and especially EEG-video monitoring, provides accurate diagnosis (King et al, 1982).

Treatment. Pseudoseizures are managed best by determining the secondary gain provided by seizures and offering alternate methods of satisfaction. They usually stop when the nature of the attacks is understood by care-providers.

■ Anticonvulsant Drug Therapy

The goal of anticonvulsant therapy is to maximize normal function by balancing seizure control against drug toxicity.

INDICATIONS TO START THERAPY

Prophylactic therapy should be initiated whenever there is a reasonable expectation that seizures will recur. The risk of recurrence after a first unexplained and untreated tonic-clonic seizure in individuals of all ages is 62 percent within one year and 72 percent within two years (Elwes et al, 1985). Among children younger than seven years of age after a single unexplained nonfebrile seizure, 61 percent have a second seizure: 90 percent within one year and almost all within two years (Hirtz et al, 1984). After a second seizure, 90 percent of children have a third seizure. When children of all ages and with partial or generalized nonfebrile seizures are considered together, the untreated recurrence rate is considerably lower (Shinnar et al, 1986). This can be explained by the relatively high prevalence of benign (Rolandic) epilepsy of childhood.

The majority of individuals who have a first nonfebrile seizure can be expected to have more seizures, but a significant minority have a single unexplained seizure that does not require therapy. Epileptiform activity on EEG, a family history of epilepsy, and an abnormal neurologic or developmental examination are factors that support initiating therapy after a single seizure.

In contrast to nonfebrile seizures, the risk of recurrence after a first febrile convulsion is relatively small (see "Febrile Seizures").

DISCONTINUING THERAPY

Children who have an acute encephalopathy (e.g., anoxia, head trauma, encephalitis) and associated seizures need to be treated with anticonvulsant drugs. When the acute encephalopathy is over and seizures have stopped, anticonvulsant therapy should be discontinued. Only a minority of children will later have epilepsy, and they can be treated when seizures recur. There is no evidence that continuous anticonvulsant therapy will prevent the development of epilepsy in such cases.

As a rule, children being treated for epilepsy should be maintained seizure-free four years before attempts are made to discontinue therapy (Emerson et al, 1981; Thurston et al, 1982). Two years may be sufficient in selected cases such as benign epilepsy of childhood (Shinnar et al, 1985). The risk factors that predict a recurrence of seizures after therapy is discontinued include (1) seizures that were hard to control at onset, (2) an EEG demonstrating epileptiform activity when drugs are discontinued, and (3) a child who is neurologically or developmentally abnormal.

PRINCIPLES OF THERAPY

Always start with a single drug. Approximately 75 percent of children with epilepsy can be fully controlled with monotherapy (Reynolds and Shorvon, 1981). Even those patients who are never controlled are likely to do better on monotherapy than polytherapy (Schmidt, 1983). There are several problems with polytherapy: (1) drugs compete with each other for protein binding sites, (2) one drug can increase the rate and pathway of catabolism of a second drug, (3) drugs have cumulative toxicity, and (4) compliance is more difficult.

When there is a need to use more than one drug, choose drugs that have different spectrums of activity or mechanism of action. Change only one drug at a time. If several changes are made simultaneously, it is not possible to determine which drug is responsible for a beneficial or an adverse effect.

Do not administer anticonvulsant drugs more often than three times each day. An acceptable steady state can be attained with many drugs using a twice-a-day regimen and some once a day. Compliance usually falls when drugs are taken more than twice each day. It is especially difficult for children to take medicine at school.

BLOOD CONCENTRATIONS

The development of techniques to measure blood concentrations of anticonvulsant drugs has been an important advance in the treatment of epilepsy. It is customary to measure protein-bound fractions even though the free-fraction is responsible for efficacy and toxicity. While the ratio of free-to-bound fractions is relatively constant, some drugs, such as valproic acid, have a greater affinity for binding protein than others and will displace them when used together. This raises the free concentration of the displaced drug and may cause toxicity even though the measured protein-bound fraction is "therapeutic."

Reference values of drug concentrations are guidelines. Some patients are seizure-free with concentrations that are below the reference value, and others are unaffected by apparent toxic concentrations.

Most anticonvulsants follow first-order kinetics; blood levels increase proportionately with increases in oral dose. The major exception is phenytoin, which follows zero-order kinetics. The drug is maximally metabolized until the responsible enzyme system is saturated, and then a small increment in oral dose produces large increments in blood concentration.

The half-lives of anticonvulsants listed in Table 1.5 are at steady state. Half-lives are generally longer when a patient is first exposed to a drug. Steady state is usually achieved after five half-lives. Similarly, five half-lives are required to eliminate a drug after it has been discontinued. Drug half-lives vary from individual to individual and frequently are shortened by the concurrent use of other drugs.

Some anticonvulsants are metabolized to active metabolites that have anticonvulsant and toxic properties. With the exception of phenobarbital derived from primidone, these metabolites are not usually measured. Active metabolites may provide seizure control or cause toxicity when the blood concentration of the parent compound is low.

ADVERSE REACTIONS

Many anticonvulsant drugs are irritating to the gastric mucosa and produce nausea and vomiting. When this occurs, symptoms may be relieved by smaller doses at more frequent intervals, using enteric coated preparations and administering the drug after meals.

Toxic adverse reactions are dose-related. All anticonvulsant drugs cause sedation when blood concentrations are excessive. Subtle cognitive and behavioral disturbances, which are appreciated only by the patient or family, often occur at low blood concentrations. The patient's observation of toxicity should not be discounted because the blood concentration is within the therapeutic range. As doses are increased, serious impairments of attention span, memory, and interpersonal relations are observed. This is especially common with barbiturates, but can occur with any drug.

Idiosyncratic reactions are not dose-related. They may occur on the basis of hypersensitivity (usually manifested as rash, fever, and lymphadenopathy), but may also be caused by the production of toxic metabolites. Idiosyncratic reactions are not always predictable, and the patient's observation should be respected, even when the reaction was not previously reported.

SELECTION OF AN ANTICONVULSANT DRUG

The drugs most often selected for the treatment of tonic-clonic and partial seizures are carbamazepine, phenobarbital, and phenytoin. Clonazepam, phenacemide, primidone, and valproic acid are used in refractory cases.

The initial drugs selected for the treatment of absence and myoclonic seizures are ethosuximide and valproic acid. Secondary drugs are benzodiazepines (clonazepam, clorazepate, and nitrazepam), methsuximide, and trimethadione. The ketogenic diet is an alternative to drug therapy.

Acetazolamide is used as an adjunct to therapy in children with refractory absence or myoclonic epilepsy and is sometimes administered the week before menses in women with catamenial epilepsy.

ACTH and pyridoxine are each used to provide transitory relief of intractable seizures in infants (see "Infantile Spasms"), but are not ordinarily used in older children.

Acetazolamide (Diamox, Lederle)

Indications. Adjunct therapy for absence, myoclonic, and catamenial epilepsy.

Administration. The initial dose for children with absence or myoclonic seizures is 10 mg/kg/day. Increments of 10 mg/kg to a total of 50 mg/kg/day in two divided doses may be used.

In women with catamenial epilepsy, 250 mg/day is administered for the week preceding the expected time of menses.

Adverse Reactions. Toxic reactions include tingling of the fingers and polyuria. Idiosyncratic reactions are rare.

Carbamazepine (Tegretol, Geigy)

Indications. Tonic-clonic and partial seizures. Atypical absence may be exacerbated (Snead and Hosey, 1985).

Administration. Absorption from the gastrointestinal tract is slow and variable. Generic preparations tend to be absorbed more rapidly and cleared quickly. Approximately 85 percent is protein-bound. Carbamazepine induces its own metabolism and the initial dose should be 25 percent of maintenance dose to avoid toxicity. The usual maintenance dose is 15 to 20 mg/kg/day to provide a blood concentration of 4 to 12 μg/ml (17 to 51 μmol/L). Half-life at steady state is 5 to 27 hours, and dosing three times a day is usually required in children.

Concurrent use of erythromycin, propoxyphene, verapamil, and cimetidine interferes with carbamazepine metabolism and causes toxicity.

Adverse Effects. A depression of peripheral leukocytes is expected, but rarely sufficient (absolute neutrophil count <1,000) to warrant discontinuation of therapy. An initial white blood cell count should be performed six weeks after therapy is started, at least once a year thereafter, and at times of febrile illness.

Cognitive disturbances within the therapeutic range are minimal as compared with the use of phenytoin or phenobarbital. Sedation, ataxia, and nystagmus occur at toxic blood concentrations.

Clonazepam (Klonopin, Roche)

Indications. Infantile spasms, myoclonic seizures, absence, and partial seizures (Ishikawa et al, 1985).

Administration. The initial dose is 0.025 mg/kg/day in two divided doses. Increments of 0.025 mg/kg are recommended every three to five days as needed and tolerated. The usual maintenance dose is 0.1 mg/kg/day in three divided doses. Most children cannot tolerate doses greater than 0.15 mg/kg/day. Therapeutic blood concentrations are 0.02 to 0.07 μg/ml; 47 percent is protein-bound and half-life is 20 to 40 hours.

Adverse Effects. Toxic effects within the therapeutic range include sedation, cognitive impairment, hyperactivity, and excessive salivation. Idiosyncratic reactions are unusual.

Clorazepate (Tranxene, Abbott)

Indications. Adjunct therapy for refractory myoclonic and partial seizures. Clorazepate should not be used as a primary anticonvulsant.

Administration. The smallest capsule, 3.75 mg, is given once each day and increased by one capsule every three days as needed and tolerated. Maintenance doses of 1 to 3 mg/kg/day in three divided doses are recommended (Berchou et al, 1983). Total dose is limited by toxicity and blood concentration measurements are not useful.

Toxicity. Sedation occurs within the therapeutic range and limits usefulness. Higher doses cause ataxia, diplopia, and impairment of cognitive function.

Ethosuximide (Zarontin, Parke-Davis)

Indications. Treatment of choice for absence, also useful for myoclonic absence.

Administration. The drug is absorbed rapidly, and peak blood concentrations appear within four hours. It is not bound to plasma proteins. Half-life is 30 hours in children and up to 60 hours in adults. The initial dose is 20 mg/kg/day in three divided doses after meals to avoid gastric irritation. Increments of 10 mg/kg/day are administered as needed and tolerated to provide a blood concentration above 40 μg/ml (280 μmol/L).

Adverse Effects. Ethosuximide does not interact with other anticonvulsants because it is not protein-bound. Idiosyncratic reactions include dystonia and a lupus-like syndrome. Aplastic anemia is a rare complication. Common toxic reactions include nausea, abdominal pain, headache, and sedation. Gastrointestinal symptoms occur within the therapeutic range and limit usefulness.

Methsuximide (Celontin, Parke-Davis)

Indications. A secondary drug for absence and myoclonic seizures if ethosuximide and valproic cannot be used.

Administration. Methsuximide is rapidly absorbed and reaches peak blood concentrations within two hours. However, active metabolites rather than the parent compound are probably responsible for efficacy and toxicity. Some of

these accumulate for thirty to forty hours. The initial dose is 20 mg/kg/day in three divided doses. Increments of 10 mg/kg/day are administered as needed and tolerated. Blood concentration measurements of the parent compound are not helpful.

Adverse Reactions. Drowsiness is the most common side effect, but gastric irritation and personality change may occur as well.

Nitrazepam (Mogadon, Roche)

Indications. Infantile spasms and myoclonic seizures.

Administration. This drug is not approved for use in the United States. Half-life is eighteen to thirty hours. Initial dose is 0.2 mg/kg/day in two divided doses. Biweekly increments of 0.3 mg/kg are administered as needed until a maintenance dose of 0.5 to 1.0 mg/kg/day is achieved (Dreifuss et al, 1986).

Adverse Effects. Drowsiness, hypotonia, and increased secretions are the usual side effects.

Phenacemide (Phenurone, Abbott)

Indications. Intractable complex partial seizures.

Administration. This drug has not been tested as initial monotherapy, but can be effective when other drugs have failed. Therapy should be initiated at a dose of 20 mg/kg/day in three divided doses and increased biweekly by 10 mg/kg/day. The usual maintenance dose is 40 to 50 mg/kg/day.

Adverse Reactions. The drug has an undeserved reputation for serious toxicity (Coker, 1986). Dose-related hepatotoxicity is the major concern. The actual incidence is lower than for valproic acid, and regular monitoring of hepatic enzymes should prevent irreversible liver damage. Aplastic anemia has been attributed to phenacemide as well, but the evidence is not compelling.

Phenytoin (Dilantin, Parke-Davis)

Indications. Tonic-clonic seizures, partial seizures, status epilepticus.

Administration. Oral absorption is slow and unpredictable in newborns, erratic in infants, and probably not reliable until three to five years. Even in adults there is considerable individual variability. The bioavailability of many generic preparations is poor. Once absorbed, phenytoin is 70 to 95 percent protein-bound. A typical maintenance dose is 7 mg/kg/day in newborns and 5 mg/kg/day in children. Half-life is up to sixty hours in term newborns, up to 140 hours in prematures, five to fourteen hours in children, and ten to thirty-four hours in adults. Capsules are usually taken in two divided doses, but tablets are more rapidly absorbed and may require dosing three times a day.

Phenytoin can be rapidly loaded by giving three times the maintenance dose by either the oral or intravenous route (see "Treatment of Status Epilepticus"). Intramuscular injections are not absorbed and should not be used.

Blood concentration below 10 µg/ml (40 µmol/L) are metabolized by first-order kinetic, but higher concentrations are by zero-order kinetics. The usual therapeutic range is 10 to 20 µg/ml (40 to 80 µmol/L) and once within that range, dosage increments must be small.

Adverse Reactions. The major adverse reactions are hypersensitivity, gum hypertrophy, and hirsutism. Hypersensitivity reactions usually occur with six weeks of initiating therapy and are characterized by rash, fever, and lymphadenopathy. Once such a reaction has occurred, the drug should be discontinued. Concurrent use of antihistamines is not appropriate management. Continued use of the drug may produce a Stevens-Johnson syndrome or a lupus-like disorder.

Gum hypertrophy is caused by a combination of phenytoin metabolites and plaque on the teeth. In individuals with good oral hygiene, there is less risk for gum hypertrophy to develop. The importance of good oral hygiene should be discussed at the onset of therapy.

Hirsutism is more a problem for girls than boys and is a valid reason for discontinuing therapy in favor of another drug.

Memory impairment, decreased attention span, and personality change may occur at therapeutic concentrations, but less often and less severely than with phenobarbital.

Phenobarbital

Indications. Tonic-clonic and simple partial seizures.

Administration. Oral absorption is slow, and daily doses are better given with the evening meal than at bedtime if seizures are hypnagogic. Intramuscular absorption requires one to two hours and should not be used for rapid loading (see "Treatment of Status Epilepticus"); 50 percent is protein-bound, and 50 percent is free.

Initial and maintenance doses are 3 to 5 mg/ kg/day. Half-life is forty-six to 136 hours in adults, thirty-seven to seventy-three hours in children, and sixty-one to 173 hours in term newborns. Because of the very long half-life at all ages, once-a-day dosing is usually satisfactory, and steady-state blood concentrations should be measured after two weeks of therapy. Therapeutic blood concentrations are 10 to 40 µg/ml (40 to 160 µmol/L).

Adverse Effects. The most common and limiting side effect in children is hyperactivity. Adverse behavioral changes occur in half of children ages two to ten. Parents should be warned of this possibility at the onset of therapy. Behavioral changes are dose-related, and other barbiturates that are converted to phenobarbital produce the same adverse effects at equivalent phenobarbital blood concentrations.

Drowsiness and cognitive dysfunction, rather than hyperactivity, are the usual adverse effects after age ten. However, in one randomized trial of phenobarbital against carbamazepine, psychological testing was not adequate to demonstrate any behavioral or cognitive difference between the two drugs (Mitchell and Chavez, 1987). Infants tolerate the drug well, and it remains a drug of choice for oral use in newborns and infants. Idiosyncratic reactions are unusual.

Primidone (Mysoline, Ayerst)

Indications. Tonic-clonic and partial seizures.

Administration. This drug is metabolized to at least two active metabolites, phenobarbital and phenyl-ethyl-malonamide (PEMA). Primidone half-life is six to twelve hours, and PEMA half-life is twenty hours. The usual maintenance dose is 10 to 15 mg/kg/day, but the initial dose should be 25 percent of maintenance or there is intolerable sedation. A therapeutic blood concentration of primidone is 8 to 12 µg/ml (36 to 52 µmol/L). The blood concentration of phenobarbital derived from primidone is generally four times greater, but this ratio is altered when other anticonvulsant drugs are administered concurrently.

Adverse Reactions. These are the same as for phenobarbital, except that the risk of intolerable sedation from the first tablet is great.

Trimethadione (Tridione, Abbott)

Indications. Simple absence, myoclonic absence, myoclonic seizures. This older drug has effectively been displaced by ethosuximide and valproic acid, but should not be discarded. It may be effective in children who are refractory to other anticonvulsants.

Administration. Trimethadione is metabolized to the active metabolite 5,5-dimethyl-2,4-oxazolidindione (DMO). The half-life of trimethadione is sixteen hours and the half-life of DMO is ten days. The initial dose is 20 mg/kg in three divided doses, the dose is increased incrementally as tolerated and needed to 60 mg/kg/day. The maintenance dose is usually limited by toxicity. Measuring blood concentrations of the parent compound is not as helpful as measuring blood concentrations of DMO, which must be kept above 700 μg/ml.

Adverse Reactions. The most common toxic effects are sedation and blurring of vision on exposure to bright light. The serious idiosyncratic complication is bone marrow suppression during the first six months of therapy and monthly erythrocyte and leukocyte counts are mandatory during that time.

Valproic Acid (Depakene, Abbott)

Indications. Myoclonic seizures, simple absence, myoclonic absence, myoclonus, and tonic-clonic seizures. It is especially useful for mixed seizure disorders.

Administration. Oral absorption is rapid, and half-life is six to fifteen hours. Three-times-a-day dosing is needed to achieve constant blood concentrations. An enteric-coated capsule (Depakote) slows absorption and allows twice-a-day dosing in many individuals.

The initial dose is 20 mg/kg/day. Increments of 10 mg/kg/day are administered to provide a blood concentration of 50 to 100 μg/ml (350 to 700 μmol/L). Protein binding is 95 percent at blood concentrations of 50 μg/ml, and 80 percent at 100 μg/ml. Therefore, doubling the blood concentration increases the free-fraction eightfold. Blood concentrations close to 100 μg/ml are usually required. Depakene has a strong affinity for plasma proteins and displaces other anticonvulsant drugs.

Adverse Reactions. Valproic acid has dose-related and idiosyncratic hepatotoxicity. Dose-related hepatotoxicity is harmless and characterized by increased concentrations of serum transaminases. Other dose-related effects are pancreatitis and hyperammonemia. Both may be associated with nausea and vomiting, but are reversible when the drug is discontinued.

The major idiosyncratic reaction is fatal liver necrosis caused by the production of an aberrant and toxic metabolite. In children younger than two years of age on monotherapy with valproic acid, the incidence of fatal hepatic necrosis is 1:600. In children over two years of age, the incidence is 1:30,000 (Dreifuss et al, 1987). There are no reported cases of fatal hepatotoxicity in children over ten years of age treated with valproic acid alone.

The clinical manifestations of idiosyncratic hepatotoxicity are similar to Reye syndrome (see Chapter 2). It may begin after one day of therapy or be delayed for as long as six months. There is no reliable way to monitor for idiosyncratic hepatotoxicity or to predict its occurrence.

TREATMENT OF STATUS EPILEPTICUS

Immediate Management

Status epilepticus is a medical emergency and necessitates prompt attention. Initial assessment should be rapid and includes cardiorespiratory function, history leading up to status, and neurologic examination. A controlled airway must be established immediately and mechanical ventilation made available. Venous access is established next. Blood is withdrawn for glucose, electrolytes, and anticonvulsant concentrations when applicable. Other tests (i.e., toxic screen) are performed as indicated. After blood is withdrawn, an intravenous infusion of saline is started for the administration of anticonvulsant drugs. An intravenous bolus of 1 ml/kg of a 50 percent glucose solution is then administered.

Drug Treatment

The ideal drug for treating status epilepticus is one that acts rapidly, has a long duration of action, and does not produce sedation. Diazepam is used widely for this purpose, but is inadequate because the duration of action is brief. In addition, children who are given intravenous diazepam after a prior load of barbiturate may experience respiratory depression. If diazepam is chosen as a first drug, the dose is 0.2 mg/kg, not to exceed 10 mg at a rate of 1 mg/minute. If benzodiazepines are preferred, lorazepam is probably preferable to diazepam because of its longer action (Crawford et al, 1987). The usual dose in children twelve years or younger is 0.1 mg/kg; 0.07 mg/kg is used in adolescents.

My own preference is intravenous phenytoin because of its very long duration of action.

Fifteen mg/kg are injected at a rate not to exceed 0.5 mg/kg/minute. Newborns and infants generally require 20 mg/kg. The slow rate of administration is used to avoid cardiac arrhythmias.

Phenytoin is usually effective unless status is caused by severe, acute encephalopathy. When phenytoin fails, several alternatives are available; my preference is first paraldehyde and then pentobarbital coma.

Paraldehyde is a general anesthetic; 70 to 80 percent is metabolized in the liver, and the remainder is excreted unchanged by the lungs. It can only be used in well-ventilated patients with adequate liver function. A 5 percent solution in 5 percent dextrose is infused drop by drop, titrating the seizures until they stop. If seizures recur, pentobarbital coma is indicated.

The patient should have been transferred by now from the emergency room to an intensive care unit, intubated, and mechanically ventilated. An arterial line is placed and the patient monitored for blood pressure, cardiac rhythm, body temperature, and blood oxygen saturation.

With an EEG monitor recording continuously, 10 mg/kg boluses of pentobarbital are infused until a burst-suppression pattern appears on the EEG. Coma may be maintained safely for up to three days with a continuous infusion of 3 mg/kg/hour. The EEG should be checked several times each day for burst-suppression. Longer periods of pentobarbital coma are associated with pulmonary edema.

References

1. Albani M, Bentele KHP, Budde C, et al: Infant sleep apnea profile: preterm vs. term infants. Eur J Pediatr 143:261, 1985.
2. Annegers JF, Hauser WA, Shirts SB, et al: Factors prognostic of unprovoked seizures after febrile convulsions. N Engl J Med 316:493, 1987.
3. Arvin AM, Hensleigh PA, Prober CG, et al: Failure of antepartum cultures to predict the infant's risk of exposure to herpes simplex virus at delivery. N Engl J Med 315:796, 1986.
4. Batshaw ML, Thomas GH, Brusilow SW: New approaches to the diagnosis and treatment of inborn errors of urea synthesis. Pediatrics 68:290, 1981.
5. Beaumanoir A: Infantile epilepsy with occipital focus and good prognosis. Eur Neurol 22:43, 1983.
6. Beaumanoir A: The Landau-Kleffner syndrome. In Roger J, Dravet C, Bureau M, et al, eds. Epileptic Syndromes in Infancy, Childhood and Adolescence. John Libbey Eurotext Ltd, London, 1985, p 181.
7. Bellman MH, Ross EM, Miller DL: Infantile spasms and pertussis immunization. Lancet 1:1031, 1983.
8. Berchou RC, Rodin EA, Russell ME: Clorazepate therapy for refractory seizures. Neurology 31:1483, 1983.
9. Bergman I, Painter MJ, Hirsch RP, et al: Outcome in neonates with convulsions treated in an intensive care unit. Ann Neurol 14:642, 1983.
10. Berkovic SF, Andermann FA, Andermann E, et al: Concepts of absence epilepsies: Discrete syndromes or biological continuum? Neurology 37:993, 1987.
11. Blennow G, Starck L: High dose B$_6$ treatment in infantile spasms. Neuropediatria 17:7, 1986.
12. Bridgers SL, Ebersole JS, Ment LR, et al: Cassette electroencephalography in the evaluation of neonatal seizures. Arch Neurol 43:49, 1986.
13. Brusilow SW, Danney M, Waber LJ, et al: Treatment of episodic hyperammonemia in children with inborn errors of urea synthesis. N Engl J Med 310:1630, 1984.
14. Carin I, Glass L, Parekh A, et al: Neonatal methadone withdrawal. Effect of two treatment regimens. Am J Dis Child 137:1166, 1983.
15. Carpenter S, Karpati G: Sweat gland duct cell in Lafora disease: Diagnosis by skin biopsy. Neurology 31:1564, 1981.
16. Clancy R, Malin S, Laraque D, et al: Focal motor seizures heralding stroke in full-term neonates. Am J Dis Child 139:601, 1985.
17. Coker SB: The use of phenacemide for intractable partial complex epilepsy in children. Pediatr Neurol 2:230, 1986.
18. Conley ME, Beckwith JB, Mancer JFK, et al: The spectrum of the DiGeorge syndrome. J Pediatr 94:883, 1979.
19. Coulter DL, Allen RJ: Benign neonatal sleep myoclonus. Arch Neurol 39:191, 1982.
20. Crawford TO, Mitchell WG, Snodgrass SR: Lorazepam in childhood status epilepticus and serial seizures. Effectiveness and tachyphylaxis. Neurology 37:190, 1987.
21. Curth HO, Warburton D: The genetics of incontinentia pigmenti. Arch Dermatol 92:229, 1965.
22. Danner R, Shewmon A, Sherman MP: Seizures in an atelencephalic infant. Is the cortex essential for neonatal seizures? Arch Neurol 42:1014, 1985.
23. De Romanis F, Feliciani M, Ruggieri S: Rolandic paroxysmal epilepsy: a long term study in 150 children. Ital J Neurol Sci 7:77, 1986.
24. de Sousa C, Chalmers RA, Stacey TE, et al: The response to L-carnitine and glycine therapy in isovaleric acidemia. Eur J Pediatr 144:451, 1986.
25. Delgado-Escueta AV, Enrile-Bacsal F: Juvenile myoclonic epilepsy of Janz. Neurology 34:285, 1984.
26. DiMario FJ Jr, Emery ES: The natural history of night terrors. Ann Neurol 20:440, 1986.
27. Donn SM, Grasela TH, Goldstein G: Safety of a higher loading dose of phenobarbital in the term newborn. Pediatrics 75:1061, 1985.
28. Dravet C, Bureau M, Roger J: Benign myoclonic epilepsy in infants. In Roger J, Dravet C, Bureau M, et al, eds. Epileptic Syndromes in Infancy, Childhood and Adolescence. John Libbey Eurotext Ltd, London, 1985a, p 51.
29. Dravet C, Bureau M, Roger J: Severe myoclonic epilepsy in infants. In Roger J, Dravet C, Bureau M, et al, eds. Epileptic Syndromes in Infancy, Childhood and Adolescence. John Libbey Eurotext Ltd, London, 1985b, p 58.
30. Dreifuss FE, Farwell J, Holmes G, et al: Infantile spasms: Comparative trial of nitrazepam and corticotropin. Arch Neurol 43:1107, 1986.
31. Dreifuss FE, Santilli N, Langer DH, et al: Valproic acid hepatic fatalities: A retrospective review. Neurology 37:379, 1987.

32. Ellenberg JH, Nelson KB: Febrile seizures and later intellectual performance. Arch Neurol 35:17, 1978.

33. Ellison PH, Farina MA: Progressive central nervous system deterioration: A complication of advanced chronic lung disease of prematurity. Ann Neurol 8:43, 1980.

34. Elwes RDC, Chesterman P, Reynolds EH: Prognosis after a first untreated tonic-clonic seizure. Lancet 2:752, 1985.

35. Emerson R, D'Souza BJ, Vining EP, et al: Stopping medication in children with epilepsy. N Engl J Med 304:1125, 1981.

36. Evans OB: Lactic acidosis in childhood: Part II. Pediatr Neurol 2:5, 1986.

37. Fenichel GM: Hypoxic-ischemic encephalopathy in the newborn. Arch Neurol 40:261, 1983.

38. Fenichel GM: Difficulty in clinical identification of neonatal seizures: An EEG monitor study. Yale J Biol Med 60:139, 1987.

39. Fenichel GM, Olson BJ, Fitzpatrick JE: Heart rate changes in convulsive and nonconvulsive apnea. Ann Neurol 7:577, 1980.

40. Fenichel GM, Webster DL, Wong WKT: Intracranial hemorrhage in the term newborn. Arch Neurol 41:30, 1984.

41. Finer NN, Robertson CM, Richards RT, et al: Hypoxic-ischemic encephalopathy in term-neonates: Perinatal factors and outcome. J Pediatr 98:112, 1981.

42. Freemon FR: The treatment of narcolepsy and cataplexy. Comp Ther 11:44, 1985.

43. Gal P, Toback J, Boer HR, et al: Efficacy of phenobarbital monotherapy in treatment of neonatal seizures—relationship to blood levels. Neurology 32:1401, 1982.

44. Gascon G, Wallenberg B, Daif AK, et al: Successful treatment of action myoclonus with 5-hydroxytryptophan in cherry red spot–myoclonus syndrome. Ann Neurol 20:440, 1986.

45. Gastaut H, Zifkin BG, Mariani E, et al: The long-term course of primary generalized epilepsy with persisting absences. Neurology 36:1021, 1986.

46. Gerber MA, Berliner BC: The child with a "simple" febrile seizure. Appropriate diagnostic evaluation. Am J Dis Child 135:431, 1981.

47. Giacoia, GP, Gessner PK, Zaleska MM, et al: Pharmacokinetic of paraldehyde disposition in the neonate. J Pediatr 104:291, 1984.

48. Goldberg RN, Goldman SL, Ramsay RE, et al: Detection of seizure activity in the paralyzed neonate using continuous monitoring. Pediatrics 69:583, 1982.

49. Gomez MR, Klass DW: Epilepsies of infancy and childhood. Ann Neurol 13:113, 1983.

50. Goutieres F, Aicardi J: Atypical presentations of pyridoxine-dependent seizures: A treatable cause of intractable epilepsy in infants. Ann Neurol 17:117, 1985.

51. Gulick TA, Spinks IP, King DW: Pseudoseizures: Ictal phenomena. Neurology 32:24, 1982.

52. Hansen TWR, Bratlid D: Bilirubin and bilirubin toxicity. Acta Paediatr Scand 75:513, 1986.

53. Henderson-Smart DJ, Pettigrew AG, Campbell DJ: Clinical apnea and brainstem function in preterm infants. N Engl J Med 308:353, 1983.

54. Hirtz DG, Ellenberg JH, Nelson KB: The risk of recurrence of nonfebile seizures in children. Neurology 34:637, 1984.

55. Holden KR, Mellits ED, Freeman JM: Neonatal seizures: I. Correlation of prenatal events with outcomes. Pediatrics 70:165, 1982.

56. Holmes G: Partial seizures in children. Pediatrics 77:725, 1986.

57. Holmes G, Rowe J, Hafford J, et al: Prognostic value of the electroencephalogram in neonatal asphyxia. EEG Clin Neurophysiol 53:60, 1982.

58. Hrachovy RA, Frost JD Jr, Kellaway P: Hypsarryhthmia: Variations on a theme. Epilepsia 25:317, 1984.

59. Iivanainen M, Himberg J-J: Valproate and clonazepam in the treatment of severe progressive myoclonus epilepsy. Arch Neurol 39:236, 1982.

60. Ishikawa A, Sakuma N, Nagashima T, et al: Clonazepam monotherapy for epilepsy in childhood. Brain Dev 7:610, 1985.

61. Kahn EJ, Neumann LL, Polk GA: The course of the heroin withdrawal syndrome in newborns treated with phenobarbital or chlorpromazine. J Pediatr 75:495, 1969.

62. Kales A, Cadieux RJ, Soldatos CR, et al: Narcolepsy-cataplexy: I. Clinical and electrophysiologic characteristics. Arch Neurol 39:164, 1982.

63. Kellaway P, Hrachovy RA: Status epilepticus in newborns: A perspective on neonatal seizures. In Delgado-Escueta AV, Wasterlain C, Treiman DM, et al, eds. Advances in Neurology. Volume 34: Status Epilepticus. Raven Press, New York, 1983, p 93.

64. Kellaway P, Hrachovy RA, Frost JD, et al: Precise characterization and quantification of infantile spasms. Ann Neurol 6:214, 1979.

65. King DW, Gallagher BB, Murvin AJ, et al: Pseudoseizures: Diagnostic evaluation. Neurology 32:18, 1982.

66. Kuhns LR, Berger PE, Zieroff E, et al: Duration of voluntary apnea in children. Radiology 132:355, 1979.

67. Kurokawa T, Goya N, Fukuyama Y, et al: West syndrome and Lennox-Gastaut syndrome: A survey of natural history. Pediatrics 65:81, 1980.

68. Lance JW: Familial paroxysmal dystonic choreoathetosis and its differentiation from related syndromes. Ann Neurol 2:285, 1977.

69. Larsen R, Ashwal S, Peckham N: Incontinentia pigmenti: Association with anterior horn cell degeneration. Neurology 37:446, 1987.

70. Laxdal T, Gomez MR, Reiher J: Cyanotic and pallid syncopal attacks in children (breath-holding spells). Dev Med Child Neurol 11:755, 1969.

71. Levene MI, Evans DH: Medical management of raised intracranial pressure after severe birth asphyxia. Arch Dis Child 60:12, 1985.

72. Lombroso CT, Fejerman N: Benign myoclonus of early infancy. Ann Neurol 1:138, 1977.

73. Lombroso CT, Lerman P: Breathholding spells (cyanotic and pallid infantile syncope). Pediatrics 39:563, 1967.

74. Lott IT, Coulombre T, DiPaolo RV, et al: Vitamin B_6 dependent seizures: Pathology and chemical findings in brain. Neurology 28:47, 1978.

75. Lungarotti MS, Calabro A, Signorini E, et al: Cerebral edema in maple syrup urine disease. Am J Dis Child 136:648, 1982.

76. Mangurten HH, Benawra R: Neonatal codeine withdrawal in infants of nonaddicted mothers. Pediatrics 65:159, 1980.

77. Matalon R, Naidu S, Hughes JR, et al: Nonketotic hyperglycinemia: Treatment with diazepam—a competitor for glycine receptors. Pediatrics 71:581, 1983.

78. Matsui SM, Mahoney MJ, Rosenberg LE: The natural history of the inherited methylmalonic acidemias. N Engl J Med 308:857, 1983.

79. Matsumoto A, Watanabe K, Sugiura M, et al: Prognostic factors of convulsive disorders in the first year of life. Brain Dev 5:469, 1983.

80. Meyer FB, Marsh WR, Laws ER Jr, et al: Temporal lobectomy in children with epilepsy. J Neurosurg 64:371, 1986.
81. Mitchell WG, Chavez JM: Carbamazepine versus phenobarbital for partial onset seizures in children. Epilepsia 28:56, 1987.
82. Mizrahi EM, Tharpe BR: A characteristic EEG pattern in neonatal herpes simplex encephalitis. Neurology 32:1215, 1982.
83. Msall M, Batshaw ML, Suss R, et al: Neurologic outcome in children with inborn errors of urea synthesis. Outcome of urea-cycle enzymopathies. N Engl J Med 310:1500, 1984.
84. Nahmias AJ, Keyserling HL, Kerrick GM: Herpes simplex. In Remington JS, Klein JO, eds. Infectious Diseases of the Fetus and Newborn Infant. 2nd edition. WB Saunders Co, Philadelphia, 1983, p 636.
85. Nelson KB, Broman SH: Perinatal risk factors in children with serious motor and mental handicaps. Ann Neurol 2:371, 1977.
86. Nelson KB, Ellenberg JH: Predictors of epilepsy in children who have experienced febrile seizures. N Engl J Med 295:1029, 1976.
87. Nelson KB, Ellenberg JH: Apgar scores as predictors of chronic neurologic disability. Pediatrics 68:36, 1981.
88. Nelson KB, Ellenberg JH: Antecedents of seizure disorders in early childhood. Am J Dis Child 140:1053, 1986.
89. Painter MJ, Pippenger C, Wasterlain C, et al: Phenobarbital and phenytoin in neonatal seizures: Metabolism and tissue distribution. Neurology 31:1107, 1981.
90. Perlman JM, Volpe JJ: Seizures in the preterm infant: effects on cerebral blood flow velocity, intracranial pressure, and arterial blood pressure. J Pediatr 102:288, 1983.
91. Pettit RE, Fenichel GM: Benign familial neonatal seizures. Arch Neurol 37:47, 1980.
92. Rapin I, Goldfischer S, Katzman R, et al: The cherry-red spot–myoclonus syndrome. Ann Neurol 3:234, 1978.
93. Reynolds EH, Shorvon D: Monotherapy or polytherapy for epilepsy. Epilepsia 22:1, 1981.
94. Riikonen R: Infantile spasms: Modern practical aspects. Acta Paediatr Scand 73:1, 1984.
95. Robertson NRC, Smith MA: Early neonatal hypocalcemia. Arch Dis Child 50:604, 1975.
96. Sarnat HB, Sarnat MS: Neonatal encephalopathy following fetal distress: A clinical and electroencephalographic study. Arch Neurol 33:696, 1976.
97. Schmidley JW, Simon RP: Postictal pleocytosis. Ann Neurol 9:81, 1981.
98. Schmidt D: Reduction of two drug therapies in intractable epilepsy. Epilepsia 24:368, 1983.
99. Serfontein GL, Rom S, Stein S: Posterior fossa subdural hemorrhage in the newborn. Pediatrics 65:40, 1980.
100. Sher PK, Brown SB: Gelastic epilepsy. Onset in the neonatal period. Am J Dis Child 130:1126, 1976.
101. Shinnar S, Vining EPG, Mellits ED, et al: Discontinuing antiepileptic medication in children with epilepsy after two years without seizures. N Engl J Med 313:976, 1985.
102. Shinnar S, Zeitlin-Gross L, Moshe SL, et al: The low risk of seizure recurrences following a first unprovoked seizure in children and adolescence: a prospective study. Ann Neurol 20:388, 1986.
103. Snead OC, Benton JW, Myers GJ: ACTH and prednisone in childhood seizure disorders. Neurology 33:966, 1983.
104. Snead OC, Hosey LC: Exacerbation of seizures in children by carbamazepine. N Engl J Med 313:916, 1985.
105. Spitzer AR, Fox WW: Infant apnea. Pediatr Clin North Am 33:561, 1986.
106. Stephenson JBP: Reflex anoxemic seizures and ocular compression. Dev Med Child Neurol 22:380, 1980.
107. Svenningsen NW, Blennow G, Lindroth M, et al: Brain-oriented intensive care treatment in severe neonatal asphyxia. Arch Dis Child 57:176, 1982.
108. Takebe Y, Chiba C, Kimura S: Benign familial neonatal convulsions. Brain Dev 5:319, 1983.
109. Thurston JH, Thurston DL, Hixon BB, et al: Prognosis in childhood epilepsy. Additional follow-up of 148 children 15 to 23 years after withdrawal of anticonvulsant therapy. N Engl J Med 306:831, 1982.
110. Trauner DA, Page T, Greco C, et al: Progressive neurodegenerative disorder in a patient with nonketotic hyperglycinemia. J Pediatr 98:272, 1983.
111. Van Orman CB, Darwish HZ: Efficacy of phenobarbital in neonatal seizures. Can J Neurol Sci 12:95, 1985.
112. Van Praagh R: Diagnosis of kernicterus in the neonatal period. Pediatrics 28:870, 1961.
113. Waisman HA, Smith BA, Brown ES, et al: Treatment of branched-chain ketoacidurias (BCKA) during acute illness. Clin Pediatr 11:360, 1972.
114. Watanabe K, Kuroyanagi M, Hara K, et al: Neonatal seizures and subsequent epilepsy. Brain Dev 4:341, 1982.
115. Watanabe K, Miyazaki S, Hara K, et al: Behavioral state cycles, background EEGs and prognosis of newborns with perinatal asphyxia. EEG Clin Neurophysiol 49:618, 1980.
116. Wolfe B, Hsia YE, Sweetman L, et al: Propionic acidemia: A clinical update. J Pediatr 99:835, 1981.

2 Altered States of Consciousness

The terms used in this text to describe states of decreased consciousness are provided in Table 2.1. With the exception of "coma," these definitions are not standard. However, they are more precise and therefore more useful than terms such as "semicomatose" and "semistuporous." The term *encephalopathy* is used to describe a diffuse disorder of the brain in which at least two of the following three symptoms are present: (1) altered states of consciousness, (2) altered cognition or personality, and (3) seizures. *Encephalitis* is an encephalopathy accompanied by cerebrospinal fluid pleocytosis.

It is an important caveat that lack of responsiveness does not always equal lack of consciousness. For example, infants with botulism (see Chapter 6) may have such severe hypotonia and ptosis that they cannot move their limbs or eyelids in response to stimulation. They appear in coma or stupor, but are actually alert. The locked-in syndrome (a brainstem disorder in which the individual can process information, but not respond) and catatonia are other examples of diminished responsiveness in the alert state.

Freemon (1976) has described "two roads" to coma. The "high-road" is characterized by increased neuronal excitability. The patient becomes restless, then confused; next, tremor, hallucinations, and delirium (an agitated-confusional state) develop. Myoclonic jerks may be noted. Seizures herald the end of delirium and are followed by stupor or coma. Table 2.2 summarizes the differential diagnosis of "the high-road." Tumors and other mass lesions are not expected causes. Instead, the diagnosis is more heavily weighted in favor of metabolic, toxic, and inflammatory disorders.

The "low-road" is characterized by decreased neuronal excitability and lacks an agitated stage. Instead, there is progressive deterioration from lethargy to obtundation, stupor, and coma. The differential diagnosis is considerably larger and includes mass lesions and other causes of increased intracranial pressure (Table 2.3).

It is clear from comparing Tables 2.2 and 2.3 that considerable overlap exists between conditions that present with agitation-confusion and with lethargy-coma. Therefore, the disorders responsible for each are described together in the text to prevent repetition.

■ Diagnostic Approach to Delirium

Any child with the acute behavioral changes of delirium (agitation, confusion, delusions, or hallucinations) should be assumed to have an organic encephalopathy until proven otherwise. Delirium is usually caused by a toxic or metabolic disorder diffusely affecting both cerebral hemispheres. Schizophrenia should not be a consideration in a prepubertal child with acute delirium. Delusions are fixed beliefs that cannot be altered by reason. Paranoid delusions of

Table 2.1 STATES OF DECREASED CONSCIOUSNESS

Lethargy	Difficulty in maintaining the aroused state
Obtundation	Responsive to stimulation other than pain*
Stupor	Responsive only to pain*
Coma	Unresponsive to pain

*Responsive indicates cerebral alerting and not just reflex withdrawal.

42

Table 2.2 CAUSES OF AGITATION
AND CONFUSION

Epileptic
1. Absence status (see Chapter 1)
2. Complex partial seizure (see Chapter 1)

Infectious Disorders
1. Viral infections
   a. Aseptic meningitis
   b. Encephalitis
   c. Reye syndrome
   d. Postinfectious encephalomyelitis
2. Systemic infections
   a. Fever
   b. Sepsis

Metabolic Disorders
1. Hyponatremia
2. Hypoglycemia
3. Systemic carnitine deficiency
4. Thyroid disorders
5. Uremia

Migraine
1. Acute confusional
2. Aphasic
3. Transient global amnesia

Psychologic
1. Panic disorder
2. Schizophrenia

Toxic
1. Prescription drugs
2. Substance abuse
3. Toxins

Vascular
1. Congestive heart failure
2. Embolism
3. Hypertensive encephalopathy
4. Lupus erythematosus
5. Subarachnoid hemorrhage
6. Vasculitis

schizophrenia are logical to the patient and frequently part of an elaborate system of irrational thinking in which the patient feels menaced. Delusions associated with organic encephalopathy are less logical, not systematized, and tend to be stereotyped.

A hallucination is the perception of sensory stimuli that are not present. Visual hallucinations are almost always caused by organic encephalopathy, and auditory hallucinations, especially if accusatory, usually indicate a psychiatric illness. Stereotyped auditory hallucinations that represent a recurring memory are an exception and suggest temporal lobe seizures.

HISTORY AND PHYSICAL EXAMINATION

Children who present with delirium, even with stable vital function, must be assessed rapidly, because the potential for deterioration to states of diminished consciousness is always present. Careful history must be obtained of (1) the events leading to the behavioral change, (2) drug or toxic exposure (prescription drugs are more often at fault than substances of abuse, and a medicine cabinet inspection should be ordered in every home the child has visited), (3) personal or family history of migraine or epilepsy, (4) recent or concurrent fever, infectious disease, or systemic illness, and (5) previous history of encephalopathy.

Examination of the eyes, in addition to determining the presence or absence of papilledema, provides other clues to etiology. Drug or toxic exposure is suggested by small or large pupils that respond poorly to light, nystagmus, or impaired eye movements. Fixed deviation of the eyes in one lateral direction may indicate that (1) the encephalopathy has focal features, (2) seizures are a cause of the confusional state, or (3) seizures are part of the encephalopathy.

The general and neurologic examinations should specifically include a search for evidence of trauma, needle marks on the limbs, meningismus, and cardiac disease.

LABORATORY INVESTIGATIONS

Laboratory evaluation should be individualized, and every test is not essential for each clinical situation. The first step is to obtain blood and urine. Studies of potential interest include culture, complete blood count, sedimentation rate, toxic screen, glucose, electrolytes, calcium and phosphorus, urea nitrogen, ammonia, liver function tests, and T_4 and thyroid-stimulating hormone. If possible, an uncontrasted head computerized tomogram (CT) should be obtained while these results are pending. If sedation is required to perform the study, a short-acting benzodiazepine is preferred. Nondiagnostic blood studies and a normal CT scan are an indication for lumbar puncture looking for infection, hemorrhage, and increased intracranial pressure. A manometer should always be available to measure cerebrospinal fluid pressure.

An electroencephalogram (EEG) can be very useful in the evaluation of delirious patients and should be performed at an opportune time. It is almost always abnormal in acute organic encephalopathies and normal in psychiatric illness (Obrecht et al, 1979). The minimal finding is slowing of the posterior rhythm; more severe encephalopathies are characterized by diffuse

Table 2.3   CAUSES OF LETHARGY AND COMA

Epilepsy
1. Postictal state (see Chapter 1)
2. Status epilepticus (see Chapter 1)

Hypoxia-Ischemia
1. Cardiac arrest
2. Cardiac arrhythmia
3. Congestive heart failure
4. Near drowning
5. Neonatal (see Chapter 1)
6. Hypotension
   a. Autonomic dysfunction
   b. Dehydration
   c. Hemorrhage
   d. Pulmonary embolism

Increased Intracranial Pressure
1. Cerebral abscess (see Chapter 4)
2. Cerebral edema (see Chapter 4)
3. Cerebral tumor (see Chapters 4 and 10)
4. Herniation syndromes (see Chapter 4)
5. Hydrocephalus (see Chapters 4 and 18)
6. Intracranial hemorrhage
   a. Spontaneous (see Chapter 4)
   b. Traumatic

Infectious Disorders
1. Infections of the brain
   a. Bacterial meningitis (see Chapter 4)
   b. Fungal meningitis (see Chapter 4)
   c. Viral encephalitis
   d. Reye syndrome
2. Postinfectious encephalomyelitis
3. Postimmunization encephalopathy
4. Systemic infections
   a. Fever
   b. Sepsis-toxic shock
   c. Shock-encephalopathy syndrome

Metabolic and Systemic Disorders
1. Inborn errors of metabolism
   a. Neonatal presentation (see Chapter 1)
   b. Disorders of pyruvate metabolism (see Chapter 5)

   c. Urea cycle disorder, heterozygote (see Chapter 1)
   d. Glycogen storage disorders (see Chapter 1)
   e. Systemic carnitine deficiency
2. Renal disease
   a. Uremic encephalopathy
   b. Hypertensive encephalopathy
   c. Dialysis encephalopathy
   d. Complications of immunosuppression
3. Hepatic disease
4. Disorders of osmolality
   a. Hypernatremia
   b. Hyperglycemia
   c. Hyponatremia
   d. Hypoglycemia
5. Endocrine disorders
   a. Adrenal insufficiency
   b. Hypoparathyroidism
   c. Thyroid disorders
6. Other metabolic disorders
   a. Burn encephalopathy
   b. Parenteral hyperalimentation
   c. Hypomagnesemia
   d. Vitamin B complex deficiency

Toxic
1. Prescription drugs
2. Substance abuse
3. Toxins

Trauma
1. Concussion
2. Contusion
3. Intracranial hemorrhage
   a. Epidural hematoma
   b. Subdural hematoma
   c. Intracerebral hemorrhage
4. Neonatal (see Chapter 1)

Vascular
1. Hypertensive encephalopathy
2. Intracranial hemorrhage-nontraumatic (see Chapter 4)
3. Lupus erythematosus (see Chapter 11)
4. Vasculitis (see Chapter 11)

theta and *delta* slowing, absence of faster frequencies, and intermittent rhythmic *delta* (Fig. 2.1). Specific abnormalities may include (1) epileptiform activity consistent with absence or complex partial status, (2) triphasic waves indicating hepatic or uremic encephalopathy (Fig. 2.2), and (3) periodic lateralizing epileptiform discharges in one temporal lobe suggesting herpes encephalitis.

■ Diagnostic Approach to Lethargy and Coma

The approach to children with states of diminished consciousness is very similar to the approach suggested for delirium, except for a greater sense of urgency. Progressive decline in state of consciousness can be caused by diffuse or multifocal disturbances of the cerebral hemispheres or by focal injury to the brainstem. The anatomic site of abnormality can often be determined by physical examination.

HISTORY AND PHYSICAL EXAMINATION

The historical data to be obtained are the same as for delirium, except that mass lesions are now an important consideration. Further inquiry must be made concerning trauma or preceding symptoms of increasing intracranial pressure.

Physical examination is directed at determining both the anatomic site of disturbed cerebral

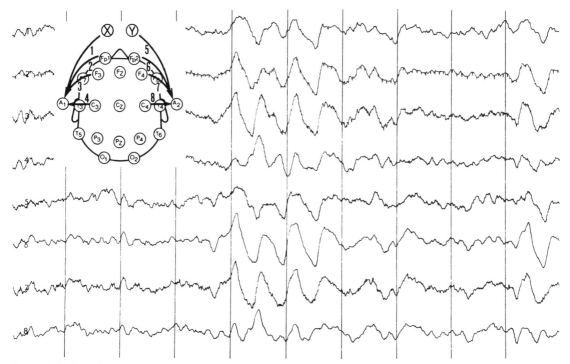

Figure 2.1 Frontal intermittent rhythmic activity. Bursts of slow waves with frontal predominance are a nonspecific abnormality in early encephalopathy. (From Epstein CM, Andriola MR: Introduction to EEG and Evoked Potentials. JB Lippincott, Philadelphia, 1983.)

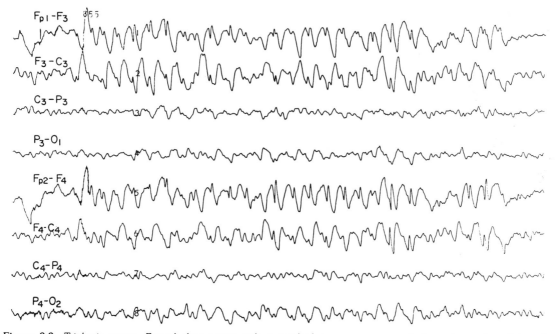

Figure 2.2 Triphasic waves. Frontal slow waves with a notched appearance are a feature of uremic and hepatic encephalopathy.

function and its etiology. The important variables in locating the site of abnormality are (1) state of consciousness, (2) pattern of breathing, (3) pupillary size and reactivity, (4) eye movements, and (5) motor responses (Plum and Posner, 1980). Lethargy and obtundation are generally caused by mild depression of hemispheric function. Stupor and coma are characteristic of much more extensive disturbance of hemispheric function or involvement of the diencephalon and upper brainstem. Derangements of the dominant hemisphere may have a greater effect on consciousness than derangements of the non-dominant hemisphere.

Cheyne-Stokes respiration, in which periods of hyperpnea alternate with periods of apnea, results from an extensive, usually bilateral diencephalic disturbance with the brainstem intact. Hypothalamic and midbrain damage causes a sustained, rapid, and deep hyperventilation (central neurogenic hyperventilation). Abnormalities within the medulla and pons affect the respiratory centers and cause several different patterns of respiratory control:

1. *Apneustic breathing*, a pause at full inspiration.

2. *Ataxic breathing*, haphazard breaths and pauses without a predictable pattern.

3. *Ondine's curse*, failure of automatic breathing when asleep.

The pupillary light reflex is usually retained in metabolic disturbances, and its absence in a comatose patient indicates a structural abnormality. The major exception is drugs (see "Delirium" later on in this chapter). A fixed dilated pupil in an alert patient is always caused by topical administration of mydriatics. In comatose patients, hypothalamic damage causes unilateral pupillary constriction and a Horner syndrome; midbrain lesions cause midposition fixed pupils; pontine lesions cause small but reactive pupils; and lateral medullary lesions cause a Horner syndrome.

Tonic lateral deviation of both eyes indicates a seizure originating in the hemisphere opposite to the direction of gaze or a destructive lesion in the hemisphere in the direction of gaze. Ocular motility in comatose patients can be assessed by instilling ice water sequentially fifteen minutes apart in each ear to chill the tympanic membrane. Ice water in the right ear causes both eyes to rapidly deviate to the right and then slowly return to the midline. The first phase is a brainstem reflex, and its presence demonstrates the bilateral integrity of the brainstem. Abduction of the right eye with failure of left eye adduction demonstrates a lesion in the

medial longitudinal fasciculus (*see* Chapter 15). The second phase requires a corticopontine pathway originating in the left hemisphere and terminating in the right pontine lateral gaze center. Its presence demonstrates unilateral hemispheric function.

Careful observation must be made of trunk and limb position at rest, spontaneous movements, and response to noxious stimuli. Spontaneous movement of all limbs generally indicates a mild depression of hemispheric function without structural disturbance. Monoplegia or hemiplegia, except in the postictal state, suggests a structural disturbance of the contralateral hemisphere. An extensor response of the trunk and limbs to a noxious stimuli is termed *decerebrate rigidity*. The most severe form is called *opisthotonos*: the neck is hyperextended and the teeth clenched; the arms adducted, hyperextended, and hyperpronated; and the legs extended with the feet plantar flexed. Decerebrate rigidity indicates brainstem compression and should be considered an ominous sign whether present at rest or in response to noxious stimuli. Flexion of the arms and extension of the legs is termed *decorticate rigidity*. It is uncommon in children except following head injury and indicates hemispheric dysfunction with brainstem integrity.

LABORATORY INVESTIGATIONS

Laboratory investigations are similar to those described for the evaluation of delirium. Head CT with contrast enhancement should be performed promptly in order to exclude the possibility of mass lesion and herniation. It is a great error to send a child whose condition is uncertain for a CT scan without a physician in attendance who knows how to monitor deterioration and intervene appropriately.

■ Hypoxia and Ischemia

Hypoxia and ischemia usually occur together. Prolonged hypoxia causes personality change first and then loss of consciousness; acute anoxia results in immediate loss of consciousness.

PROLONGED HYPOXIA

Clinical Features. Prolonged hypoxia can result from severe anemia (oxygen-carrying capacity reduced by at least half), congestive heart failure, chronic lung disease, and neuromuscular disorders.

The best studied model of prolonged, mild hypoxia is ascent to high altitudes. Mild hypoxia causes impaired memory and judgment, confusion, and decreased motor performance. With greater degrees of hypoxia, there is obtundation, multifocal myoclonus, and sometimes focal neurologic signs such as monoplegia and hemiplegia. Children with chronic cardiopulmonary disease may experience an insidious alteration in behavioral state as arterial oxygen concentration slowly declines.

Neuromuscular disorders that weaken respiratory muscles, such as muscular dystrophy, often produce nocturnal hypoventilation as a first symptom of respiratory insufficiency. This is characterized by frequent awakenings and fear of sleeping (see Chapter 7).

Diagnosis. Children with chronic cardiopulmonary disorders are often given sedation for diagnostic studies and may become depressed during long hospitalizations. Personality change is sometimes attributed to these factors rather than hypoxia. Arterial P_{O_2} values below 40 mm Hg are regularly associated with obvious neurologic disturbances, but minor mental disturbances may occur at concentrations of 60 mm Hg, especially when hypoxia is chronic.

Treatment. Encephalopathy usually reverses when PA_{O_2} is increased, but persistent cerebral dysfunction can occur in mountain climbers after returning to sea level (West, 1986), and permanent cerebral dysfunction may develop in children with chronic hypoxia (O'Dougherty et al, 1985). As a group, children with chronic hypoxia from congenital heart disease have a lower intelligence quotient (IQ) than nonhypoxic children. The severity of mental decline is related to duration of hypoxia.

Children with neuromuscular disorders who become symptomatic during sleep can be treated overnight with mouth-intermittent positive pressure ventilation (see Chapter 7).

ACUTE ANOXIA-ISCHEMIA

The usual circumstance of acute anoxia-ischemia is cardiac arrest or sudden hypotension. Anoxia without ischemia occurs with suffocation (near-drowning, choking). Prolonged anoxia always leads to bradycardia and cardiac arrest. Consciousness is lost within six to eight seconds of cerebral circulatory failure, but may take somewhat longer when anoxia occurs without ischemia. In adults, hippocampal and Purkinje cells begin to die after four minutes of total anoxia-ischemia and ten minutes is believed to

be the outside limit of brain viability. Exact timing may be difficult in clinical situations when ill-defined intervals of anoxia and hypoxia occur. Remarkable survivals are sometimes associated with near-drowning in water cold enough to lower cerebral temperature and metabolism.

The pattern of hypoxic-ischemic brain injury in newborns is different and depends to a large degree upon brain maturity (see Chapter 1).

Clinical Features. Consciousness is lost within eight seconds of circulatory failure, but may take longer when anoxia occurs without ischemia. Presyncopal symptoms of lightheadedness and visual disturbances sometimes precede loss of consciousness. Convulsions and extensor rigidity follows.

There has been considerable effort to identify predictors of outcome after hypoxic-ischemic events. In adults following cardiac arrest, only 13 percent regain independent function in the first year post arrest (Levy et al, 1985). Outcome in children is somewhat better because of a lower incidence of pre-existing cardiopulmonary disease. Absence of pupillary responses on initial examination is an ominous sign; none such patients recover independent function. Twenty-four hours post arrest, patients with poor prognosis are identified by lack of motor responses in the limbs and eyes. In contrast, a favorable outcome can be predicted for patients who rapidly develop eye movements that are roving or conjugate and limb withdrawal to pain.

Two delayed syndromes of neurologic deterioration are reported following anoxia. The first is *delayed postanoxic encephalopathy*, the appearance of apathy or confusion one to two weeks after apparent recovery. This is followed by motor symptoms, usually rigidity or spasticity, and may progress to coma or death. Demyelination is the suggested mechanism. The other syndrome is *postanoxic action myoclonus*. This usually follows a severe episode of anoxia-ischemia due to cardiac arrest. All voluntary activity initiates disabling myoclonus (see Chapter 14). Symptoms of cerebellar dysfunction are present as well.

Diagnosis. In the first seventy-two hours following severe hypoxia, CT demonstrates changes secondary to cerebral edema but has no prognostic value (Fitch et al, 1985). The EEG varies from mild slowing of the posterior rhythm, to generalized theta-delta slowing, to burst-suppression or absence of activity. The latter are always associated with poor neurologic outcome or death, but lesser abnormalities are not useful in predicting prognosis (Kuroiwa and Celesia, 1980).

Treatment. The principles of managing patients who have sustained hypoxic-ischemic encephalopathy do not differ substantially from the principles of caring for other comatose patients. Oxygenation, circulation, and blood glucose concentration must be maintained. Intracranial pressure must be lowered sufficiently to allow satisfactory cerebral perfusion (see Chapter 4). Seizures are managed with anticonvulsant drugs (see Chapter 1). Anoxia is invariably associated with lactic acidosis, and acid-base balance must be restored.

Barbiturate coma is frequently utilized to slow cerebral metabolism, but neither clinical nor experimental evidence indicates a beneficial effect following cardiac arrest (Dearden, 1985). Hypothermia is clearly useful to prevent brain damage during the time of hypoxia-ischemia, but has questionable value after the event.

Postanoxic action myoclonus can be treated effectively with valproic acid.

PERSISTENT VEGETATIVE STATE

This term is used interchangeably with *neocortical death* to describe patients, who after recovery from coma, return to a state of wakefulness without cognition. Brainstem functions such as respiration and circulation are intact, and with good nursing care survival is indefinite. A persistent vegetative state occurs in 12 percent of adults who survive nontraumatic coma, but is probably less common in children (Campbell, 1984). The usual causes in order of declining frequency are anoxia-ischemia, metabolic or encephalitic coma, and head trauma. Recovery is rare when the vegetative state has persisted for one month in adults. The prognosis may be better in children, but there is little reason for hope after three months.

The term *irreversible coma* has recently been introduced for legal rather than medical purposes to allow the termination of life support in patients who do not meet the definition of brain death. There is no neurologic basis to distinguish persistent vegetative state (in which life support cannot be terminated) from irreversible coma.

BRAIN DEATH

Standards for the diagnosis of brain death have evolved, but recent guidelines established by a presidential commission have been endorsed by major specialty societies and are now generally accepted (President's Commission,

1981). The important features of the report are summarized in Table 2.4. Caution was urged in applying the criteria to children younger than five years, but subsequent experience supports their validity from term birth through childhood (Moshe and Alvarez, 1986; Vernon and Holzman, 1986). Absence of cerebral blood flow is the earliest and most definitive validation of brain death. EEG activity may still be present twenty-four hours after cerebral blood flow ceases, but always becomes isoelectric subsequently (Drake et al, 1986).

■ Infectious Disorders

VIRAL ENCEPHALITIS

Encephalitis usually affects the meninges as well as the brain, and the term meningoencephalitis may be more accurate. However, it is useful for viral diagnosis to distinguish encephalitis from aseptic meningitis, because most viruses produce one or the other, but not both. An annual incidence of 7.4/100,000 for encephalitis and 10.9/100,000 for aseptic meningitis remained relatively constant in one Minnesota county over a thirty-year period (Beghi et al, 1984). Both conditions were more common in the summer, in childhood, and in males. The diagnosis of viral encephalitis remains primarily a clinical decision, and specific viral identification is established in only 15 to 20 percent of cases (Beghi et al, 1984; Kennard and Swash, 1981).

Table 2.4 THE DIAGNOSIS OF BRAIN DEATH

An experienced physician must determine that:
1. Cessation of all brain function has occurred
   a. Cerebral functions are absent—coma
   b. Brain stem reflexes are absent
      (1) Pupillary light reflex
      (2) Corneal reflex
      (3) Oculocephalic reflex
      (4) Oculovestibular reflex
      (5) Oropharyngeal reflex
      (6) Respiratory reflexes
2. Cessation of brain function is irreversible
   a. Sufficient cause is established
   b. Possibility of recovery is excluded
3. A period of observation is appropriate
   a. With confirmatory test,* minimum period is six hours
   b. Without confirmatory test
      (1) If cause is not anoxia, minimum period is twelve hours.
      (2) If cause is anoxia, minimum period is twenty-four hours.

*Confirmatory tests include cerebral angiography, radioisotope cerebral blood flow study, and EEG.

The classification of viruses undergoes frequent change, but a constant first step is the separation of viruses with a DNA nucleic acid core from those with an RNA core. The only DNA virus that produces acute, postnatal encephalitis in immunocompetent hosts is herpes simplex. RNA viruses causing encephalitis are myxoviruses (influenza and measles encephalitis), arboviruses (St. Louis encephalitis, eastern equine encephalitis, western equine encephalitis, and LaCrosse-California encephalitis), retroviruses (acquired immune deficiency syndrome [AIDS] encephalitis), and rhabdoviruses (rabies). RNA viruses (coxsackie, ECHO, mumps, and lymphocytic choriomeningitis virus) are also responsible for aseptic meningitis.

In addition to acute viral infections of the brain and meninges, encephalopathies also occur following systemic viral infections. These are thought to be an "allergic" response of the brain to infection that results in demyelination.

Aseptic Meningitis

The term aseptic meningitis is used to define a syndrome of meningismus and cerebrospinal fluid leukocytosis without bacterial or fungal infection. It is a benign, self-limited disease with complete recovery anticipated in 95 percent of cases.

Clinical Features. Twenty percent of patients have a history of antecedent respiratory infection or gastrointestinal illness. The onset of symptoms is abrupt and characterized by fever, headache, and stiff neck. Irritability, lethargy, and vomiting are frequently associated. "Encephalitic" symptoms are not part of the syndrome, but febrile convulsions may occur in predisposed infants. Systemic illness is uncommon, but when present may suggest specific viral disorders (parotitis-mumps, myalgia-coxsackie, rash-ECHO and Lyme disease, diarrhea-enteroviruses).

The acute illness usually lasts for less than one week, but malaise and headache may continue for several weeks afterwards. Communicating hydrocephalus is an unusual long-term sequela.

Diagnosis. In most cases of aseptic meningitis, the cerebrospinal fluid contains 10 to 200 leukocytes, but cell counts of 1,000 or greater may occur with lymphocytic choriomeningitis. The response is primarily lymphocytic, but polymorphonuclear leukocytes may predominate early in the course. Protein concentration is generally between 50 and 100 mg/dl (0.5 to 1 g/L) and glucose concentration normal, but may

be slightly reduced in mumps and lymphocytic choriomeningitis.

Most cases of aseptic meningitis occur in the spring or summer and enteroviruses (Coxsackie and ECHO) are responsible for most cases in children. Mumps and poliomyelitis remain important causative agents in countries where immunization is not mandatory. Nonviral causes of aseptic meningitis are rare, but must be considered; these include Lyme disease, systemic lupus erythematosus, migraine, and irritation of the meninges from blood, drugs, and contrast materials.

Lyme disease, caused by a spirochete (*Borrelia bergdorferi*), is endemic in the eastern half of the United States (Reik et al, 1986). A preceding skin lesion (erythema chronicum migrans) is characteristic, but not always present. Most patients have only aseptic meningitis, which clears completely in six weeks, but some develop encephalitis and may have persistent neurologic impairment. An antibody titer to the causative organism is diagnostic.

Patients with a personal or family history of migraine may experience attacks of severe headache associated with stiff neck and focal neurologic disturbances such as hemiparesis and aphasia (Bartleson et al, 1981; Brattstrom et al, 1984). Cerebrospinal fluid examination reveals a pleocytosis of five to 300 cells that are mainly lymphocytes and a protein concentration of 50 to 100 mg/dl (0.5 to 1 g/L). It is not clear whether such attacks are migraine provoked by intercurrent aseptic meningitis or whether they represent a "meningitic" form of migraine. Recurrent attacks in some patients suggest that the mechanism is wholly migrainous.

Bacterial meningitis is the major concern in children presenting with meningismus. While cerebrospinal fluid examination provides several clues that differentiate bacterial from viral meningitis, it is still reasonable to initiate antibiotic therapy for every child with a clinical syndrome of aseptic meningitis until a negative cerebrospinal fluid culture is obtained (see Chapter 4). This is especially true in children who have received antibiotic therapy prior to examination of the cerebrospinal fluid.

Treatment. Treatment of viral aseptic meningitis is symptomatic. Bed rest in a quiet environment and mild analgesics provide satisfactory relief of symptoms in the majority of cases.

Herpes Simplex Encephalitis

Two similar strains of herpes simplex virus (HSV) are pathogenic to humans. HSV-1 is associated with oral-facial infections and HSV-2 with genital infections. Both are worldwide in distribution (Corey and Spear, 1986). Forty percent of children have antibodies to HSV-1, but antibodies to HSV-2 are not routinely detected until puberty. HSV-1 is the important causative agent of acute postneonatal herpes simplex encephalitis, and HSV-2 of encephalitis in the newborn (see Chapter 1).

Initial oral-facial infection with HSV-1 may be asymptomatic. The virus replicates in the skin, infecting nerve fiber endings and then the trigeminal ganglia. Further replication occurs within the ganglia before the virus enters a latent stage during which time it cannot be recovered from the ganglia. Reactivation occurs during time of stress, especially intercurrent febrile illness, and virus ordinarily retraces its neural migration to the skin of the face, but may occasionally spread proximally to the brain causing encephalitis. The immunocompetence of the host maintains the virus in a latent state. An immunocompromised state results in frequent reactivation and severe, widespread infection.

Herpes simplex is the single most common cause of nonepidemic encephalitis and accounts for 10 to 20 percent of all cases. The annual incidence is estimated at 2.3 cases per million population. Thirty-one percent of cases occur in children (Whitley et al, 1982).

Clinical Features. Primary infection is often the cause of encephalitis in children. Only 22 percent of patients give a history of recurrent labial herpes infection. The typical initial features are an acute onset of fever, headache, lethargy, nausea, and vomiting. Eighty percent of patients show focal neurologic disturbances (hemiparesis, cranial nerve deficits, visual field loss, aphasia, and focal seizures), and the remainder show behavioral changes or generalized convulsions without clinical evidence of focal neurologic deficits. However, both groups have focal abnormalities on neuroradiographic studies or EEG. The acute stage of encephalitis lasts for approximately one week. Recovery takes several weeks and is often incomplete.

Herpes meningitis (Corey and Spear, 1986) is usually associated with genital lesions and caused by HSV-2. The clinical features are similar to aseptic meningitis due to other viruses.

Diagnosis. Prompt diagnosis of herpes simplex encephalitis is important because treatment is available. Cerebrospinal fluid pleocytosis is present in 97 percent of cases. The median count is 130 white blood cells (WBC)/cu mm (range 0 to 1,000). Up to 500 RBC/cu mm may be present as well. Median protein concentration is 80 mg/dl (0.8 g/L), but 20 percent may have normal protein concentrations and 40 percent are in excess of 100 mg/dl (1 g/L). Glucose concentration is usually normal, but measures less than half of blood glucose in 7 percent of cases (Whitley et al, 1982).

A presumptive diagnosis of herpes encephalitis requires evidence of focal abnormality on neuroradiographic studies or EEG. The EEG demonstrates focal abnormalities in 81 percent of biopsy-proven cases compared with 59 percent for CT and 50 percent for radioisotope scan. The EEG is always abnormal but may demonstrate nonspecific generalized slowing of the background. Focal polymorphic delta in one temporal lobe superimposed upon the slow background raises the suspicion of herpes encephalitis, but the presence of periodic lateralizing epileptiform discharges (PLEDs) is virtually diagnostic (Fig. 2.3) (Ch'ien et al, 1977).

Magnetic resonance imaging (MRI) may prove to be the most sensitive early indicator of herpes encephalitis (Schroth et al, 1987). T_2-weighted studies reveal increased signal intensity in one or both temporal lobes.

Brain biopsy with virus isolation by tissue culture is the only method for definitive diagnosis, but is not a standard of practice. Herpes infection may be patchy, and it is possible to remove an unaffected portion of temporal lobe (Landry et al, 1982). Most physicians begin treatment on the basis of a compatible clinical history and an EEG, CT scan, or MRI that supports the clinical impression.

Treatment. Acyclovir has replaced vidarabine as the treatment of choice (Whitley et al, 1986). The dosage is 10 mg/kg every eight hours, infused in 100 ml of standard intravenous fluid over a one-hour period. Mortality is 28 percent and is highest in patients who are already in coma when treatment is initiated. In 38 percent of patients, function returns to normal. Prognosis is best for noncomatose children younger than ten years of age.

Measles (Rubeola) Encephalitis

Compulsory immunization has almost eliminated natural measles infection in the United States. The risk of encephalitis from natural disease is one per 1,000. During the first twenty years of the measles vaccine program, it is estimated that 52 million cases of measles, 5,200 deaths, and 17,400 cases of mental retardation were prevented (Bloch et al, 1985). The mech-

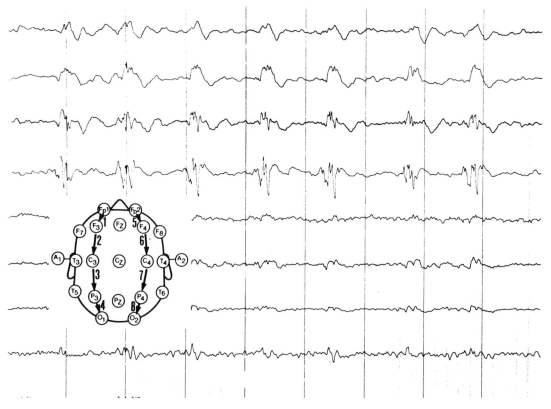

Figure 2.3 Periodic lateralizing epileptiform discharges (PLEDs). This pattern is often seen in conditions with acute focal cerebral necrosis, such as herpes encephalitis. (From Epstein CM, Andriola MR: Introduction to EEG and Evoked Potentials. JB Lippincott, Philadelphia, 1983.)

anism of measles encephalitis has been contested, but there is reason to believe that both direct viral infection and allergic demyelination are at fault (Johnson et al, 1984). A chronic form of measles encephalitis (subacute sclerosing panencephalitis) is described in Chapter 5.

Clinical Features. Measles is a neurotropic virus and EEG abnormalities are present in half of cases, even without clinical symptoms of encephalopathy (Gibbs et al, 1959). Symptoms of encephalitis begin one to eight days after the appearance of rash, but can be delayed for three weeks. The onset is usually abrupt and is characterized by lethargy or obtundation, which may rapidly progress to coma. Generalized seizures occur in half of patients. The spectrum of neurologic disturbances includes hemiplegia, ataxia, and involuntary movement disorders. Acute transverse myelitis may be present as well (see Chapter 12). Neurologic morbidity (mental retardation, epilepsy, and paralysis) is high, but does not correlate with the severity of acute encephalitis.

Measles encephalitis may occur as a consequence of measles immunization. The incidence is estimated to be one per million doses. Fever and rash occur seven to twelve days after immunization and are quickly followed by lethargy and irritability (Peltola and Heinon, 1986). Generalized seizures may occur. The systemic features and the encephalopathy always have their onset during the second week following immunization; symptoms that occur earlier are not related to immunization. Recovery is complete. While there is clearly an increased risk of febrile convulsions following measles immunization, there is no evidence of permanent neurologic disturbances (Centers for Disease Control, 1984; Pollock and Morris, 1983).

Diagnosis. Examination of cerebrospinal fluid reveals a lymphocytic pleocytosis. The number of lymphocytes is usually highest in the first few days, but rarely exceeds 100/cu mm. Protein concentrations are generally between 50 and 100 mg/dl (0.5 to 1 g/L), and glucose concentration is normal.

Treatment. Treatment is supportive. Anticonvulsant drugs usually provide satisfactory seizure control.

Arboviral (Arthropod-Borne) Encephalitis

This group of viruses is classified on the basis of ecology rather than structure. Tics and mosquitos are the usual vectors, and epidemics occur in the spring and summer. Each encephalitis has a defined geographic area (Leads from MMWR, 1985). Japanese encephalitis is the most widespread internationally. Arboviruses account for 10 percent of all encephalitis reported annually in the United States.

St. Louis Encephalitis

Clinical Features. St. Louis encephalitis is endemic in the western United States and epidemic in the Mississippi valley and Atlantic states. The vector in both regions is a mosquito, and birds are the major reservoir.

The spectrum of neurologic illness varies from aseptic meningitis to severe encephalitis, leading to death within days. The mortality rate for recent epidemics has been declining. Headache, vomiting, and states of decreased consciousness are typical features. Stiff neck and seizures are less common, and focal neurologic disturbances are rare. The usual duration of illness is one to two weeks. As a rule, children recover completely but adults may be left with mental or motor impairment.

Diagnosis. Cerebrospinal fluid examination reveals a lymphocytic pleocytosis of 50 to 500 cell/cu mm and a protein concentration between 50 and 100 mg/dl (0.5 to 1 g/L). Glucose concentration is normal.

The virus is difficult to culture, and diagnosis requires a fourfold or greater increase in complement fixation and hemagglutination inhibition antibody titers between acute and convalescent sera.

Treatment. Treatment is supportive. An effective antiviral agent is not available.

Eastern Equine Encephalitis

Clinical Features. Eastern equine encephalitis is a perennial infection of horses in southern New Jersey. The mortality rate is high. Human cases are sporadic and follow epidemics in horses. Most occur in the mid-Atlantic states, but occasional patients are reported from Massachusetts to Florida. Wild birds serve as a reservoir and mosquitos as a vector.

Onset is usually abrupt and characterized by high fever, headache, and vomiting, followed by drowsiness, coma, and seizures (Scully et al, 1984). The full syndrome evolves in two days. Signs of meningismus are usually present. Mortality rates in some past epidemics have been as high as 65 percent, but are now considerably lower. Mortality is highest in young children, and mental impairment, seizures, and disturbed motor function are expected in survivors.

Diagnosis. The cerebrospinal fluid pressure is usually elevated and examination reveals 200 to 2,000 WBC/cu mm, of which half are polymorphonuclear leukocytes. Diagnosis relies upon the demonstration of a fourfold or greater rise in complement fixation and neutralizing antibody titers between acute and convalescent sera.

Treatment. Treatment is supportive. An effective antiviral agent is not available.

Western Equine Encephalitis

Clinical Features. This is a very rare disorder. Wild birds serve as a reservoir and mosquitos as a vector. All recent cases have been reported from North Dakota, South Dakota, and Canada. Twenty to 30 percent of cases occur in infants.

In infants, the infection is characterized by irritability, fever, meningismus, bulging of the fontanelle, seizures, and coma. Older children may have a "flu-like" syndrome before demonstrating symptoms of meningoencephalitis. The inital symptom is usually behavioral change, including delirium, which is followed by drowsiness and coma. Focal abnormalities lateralizing to one temporal lobe may be present on the EEG and radioisotope scan suggesting herpes encephalitis (Bia et al, 1980).

Symptoms last for one to two weeks, and although overall mortality is 10 percent, most fatal cases involve infants. Fifty percent of surviving infants have permanent mental impairment and seizures.

Diagnosis. Cerebrospinal fluid pleocytosis is first a mixture of polymorphonuclear leukocytes and lymphocytes and then lymphocytes alone. Protein concentration is between 50 and 100 mg/dl (0.5 to 1 g/L). Diagnosis relies on the demonstration of a fourfold or greater rise in complement-fixing or neutralizing antibodies between acute and convalescent sera.

At presentation, western equine encephalitis may be difficult to distinguish from herpes encephalitis without brain biopsy.

Treatment. Treatment is supportive. An effective antiviral agent is not available.

California-LaCrosse Encephalitis

LaCrosse virus is the most common cause of encephalitis by California serogroup viruses in the United States.

Clinical Features. Prior to 1984, most cases were reported from Wisconsin and Minnesota. Recent epidemics have occurred in Indiana and sporadic cases are reported throughout the Midwest and western New York. Small woodland mammals serve as a reservoir and the mosquito as the vector.

Most cases of encephalitis occur in children, and asymptomatic infection is common in adults. The initial feature is a "flu-like" syndrome that lasts for two or three days. Encephalitis is heralded by headache followed by seizures and rapid progression to coma (Chun et al, 1968). Focal neurologic disturbances are present in 20 percent of cases. Symptoms begin to resolve three to five days after onset, and most children recover without neurologic sequelae. Fatalities are uncommon and are usually restricted to infants.

Diagnosis. Examination of cerebrospinal fluid reveals a mixed pleocytosis with lymphocytes predominating. The usual count is 50 to 200 cells/cu mm, but range may be from 0 to 600. The virus is difficult to culture, and diagnosis depends upon the demonstration of a fourfold or greater increase in hemagglutination inhibition and neutralizing antibody titers between acute and convalescent sera.

Treatment. Treatment is supportive. An effective antiviral agent is not available.

Japanese B Encephalitis

Japanese B encephalitis is a major cause of encephalitis in Asia and is an important health hazard to nonimmunized travelers during summer months.

Clinical Features. The initial features are two to three days of malaise, fever, and headache or irritability. This is followed by meningismus, confusion, and delirium. During the second or third week, photophobia and generalized hypotonia develop. Seizures may occur at any time. Finally, rigidity, a mask-like facies, and brainstem dysfunction ensue. Mortality rates are very high among indigenous populations and lower among Western travelers. This may be accounted for by difference in the age of the exposed populations.

Diagnosis. Cerebrospinal fluid pleocytosis varies from 20 to 500 cells/cu mm. It is initially mixed, but later lymphocytes predominate. Protein concentration is usually between 50 and 100 mg/dl (0.5 to 1 mg/L), and glucose concentration is normal. Diagnosis depends upon the demonstration of a fourfold or greater elevation of complement-fixing antibodies between acute and convalescent sera.

Treatment. Treatment is supportive. An effective antiviral agent is not available, but immunization provides effective protection.

Acquired Immune Deficiency Syndrome Encephalitis

AIDS is a new human viral disease caused by retroviruses identified initially as human T-lymphotropic virus III (HTLV-III) and lymphadenopathy-associated virus (LAV), and now called human immunodeficiency virus (HIV). It is spread in adults by sexual contact, intravenous drug abuse, and blood transfusion. Childhood cases usually occur in offspring born to women with AIDS and in those receiving blood products, such as prematures and hemophiliacs.

Clinical Features. Children with AIDS demonstrate failure to thrive and acquire opportunistic infections of the lungs, mucous membranes, and brain (Epstein et al, 1985). An immunocompromised state should be suspected in every child with an opportunistic infection.

In addition to causing opportunistic infections, HIV attacks the brain, producing a subacute encephalitis, and the spinal cord, producing transverse myelitis (see Chapter 12). The encephalitis is characterized by loss of developmental milestones, dementia, weakness, and spasticity. Some children have involuntary movement disorders, and seizures may occur anytime during the course (Belman et al, 1986). Death usually occurs a few months after onset.

Diagnosis. Criteria for the diagnosis of AIDS includes (1) opportunistic infections, (2) appropriate risk factors, (3) defective cell-mediated immunity, (4) polyclonal hypergammaglobulinemia, and (5) positive antibody titer. Treatable infections (*Toxoplasma* abscess, cryptococcal meningitis, *Candida* meningitis) must be excluded before HIV encephalitis is diagnosed.

The cerebrospinal fluid abnormalities are minimal and not constant. Protein concentration is 50 to 100 mg/dl (0.5 to 1 g/L), glucose concentration is normal or slightly decreased, but monocytic pleocytosis is uncommon. In some children, progressive calcification of the basal ganglia is demonstrable on CT scan.

Treatment. Azidothymidine (AZT) is recommended for palliation of advanced adult cases but has not been used in children (Fischl et al, 1987). Mortality in symptomatic children has been 100 percent. Not all newborns with positive antibody titers have become symptomatic.

Cat-Scratch Disease

The responsible etiologic agent has not been identified, but is presumed to be a virus.

Clinical Features. This is a benign, self-limited disease transmitted to children by a cat bite or scratch. A small, sometimes unidentifiable, papule appears at the inoculation site that may persist for one or two weeks. Lymphadenopathy develops proximal to the site of injury and persists for several weeks. Most children are either asymptomatic or have tender nodes, low-grade fever, and rash. Encephalitis is an unusual complication.

Neurologic manifestations follow systemic symptoms by one to five weeks (Lyon, 1971). The onset is characterized by generalized seizures and coma without antecedent symptoms. Focal neurologic deficits are uncommon. Recovery is rapid, usually within one week, and generally complete.

In addition to encephalopathy, cat-scratch disease has also been implicated as a possible cause of focal arteritis and stroke (Selby and Walker, 1979). In such cases, cerebral infarction with hemiplegia and aphasia may occur in the absence of encephalopathy.

Diagnosis. The diagnosis is primarily based upon the history of a cat scratch or bite, followed by lymphadenopathy and then encephalopathy. Examination of the cerebrospinal fluid demonstrates a mild lymphocytic pleocytosis, generally 0 to 50 cu mm, and normal or slightly elevated protein concentration. During the encephalopathy, the EEG is always abnormal as a result of mild slowing of the background rhythms. A skin test for cat-scratch disease is available but is of limited diagnostic value.

Treatment. Treatment is supportive. An effective antiviral agent is not available.

Reye Syndrome

Reye syndrome is a systemic disorder of mitochondrial function that occurs during or following viral infection. There is convincing evidence that the disorder occurs more often when salicylates are administered during viral illness for relief of symptoms (Hurwitz et al, 1985). The realization that mitochondrial dysfunction results from the combination of viral infection and salicylates has led to decreased use of salicylates in children and a marked decline in the incidence of Reye syndrome.

Clinical Features. In the United States, sporadic cases are generally associated with varicella (chickenpox) or nonspecific respiratory infections; small epidemics are associated with influenza B infection. When varicella is the precipitating infection, the initial stage of Reye syndrome occurs three to six days after the appearance of rash.

The clinical course is relatively predictable and has been divided into four stages:

Stage I. Vomiting, confusion, and lethargy.

Stage II. Agitation, delirium, decorticate posturing, and hyperventilation.

Stage III. Coma and decerebrate posturing.

Stage IV. Flaccidity, apnea, and dilated fixed pupils.

The progression from stage I to IV may be explosive and may evolve in less than twenty-four hours. More commonly, the period of recurrent vomiting and lethargy lasts for a day or longer. Most children with vomiting and chemical evidence of hepatic dysfunction following varicella or respiratory infection have liver biopsy features of Reye syndrome (Lichtenstein et al, 1983), despite normal cerebral function. This has been designated as Reye stage 0. Stages I and II represent increasing degrees of encephalopathy with metabolic dysfunction and edema. Stages III and IV indicate generalized increased intracranial pressure and herniation.

Focal neurologic disturbances and meningismus are not part of the syndrome. Fever is not a prominent feature, and hepatomegaly occurs in half of patients late in the course.

Outcome is variable; as a rule, however, infants do worse than older children, and progression to grades III and IV at all ages is associated with a high death rate and impaired neurologic function in survivors.

Diagnosis. Typical blood abnormalities are hypoglycemia, hyperammonemia, and increased concentration of hepatic enzymes. Serum bilirubin remains normal and jaundice does not occur. Acute pancreatitis is sometimes associated and can be identified by increased concentrations of serum amylase.

The cerebrospinal fluid is normal except for increased pressure. The EEG is always abnormal and consistent with a diffuse encephalopathy.

Liver biopsy is definitive. Light microscopy reveals panlobular accumulation of small intracellular lipid droplets and depletion of succinic acid dehydrogenase in the absence of other abnormalities. Electron microscopic changes include characteristic mitochondrial abnormalities, peroxisomal proliferation and swelling, proliferation of smooth endoplasmic reticulum, and glycogen depletion.

Conditions that mimic Reye syndrome are systemic carnitine deficiency, ornithine transcarbamylase deficiency, and valproic acid hepatotoxicity. These inborn errors of metabolism should be assumed and sought for in any child with recurrent Reye syndrome or a family history of similar illness. Metabolic products of valproic acid are mitochondrial poisons that have been used to produce an experimental model of Reye syndrome.

Treatment. Stage I and II disease should be watched closely in a pediatric intensive care unit and treated with intravenous hypertonic (10 to 15 percent) glucose solutions at normal maintenance volumes. Stages III and IV require treatment of increased intracranial pressure (see Chapter 4), and all would agree with the following measures: elevation of the head, controlled mechanical ventilation, and mannitol (Shaywitz et al, 1986; Trauner, 1986). Corticosteroids are of limited benefit and should not be used routinely. Intracranial pressure monitors and pentobarbital coma continue to be advocated by some authorities, although they have never been demonstrated to affect outcome. Fortunately, this once common and deadly disease has almost disappeared with discontinuation of salicylate therapy for children.

BACTERIAL SEPSIS

Endotoxic shock is frequently associated with bacterial sepsis. It may complicate meningitis or systemic infections. Encephalopathy is caused by fever, metabolic alterations, and hypotension.

Gram-Negative Sepsis

Clinical Features. The onset of symptoms may be explosive and characterized by fever or hypothermia, chills, hyperventilation, hemodynamic instability, and mental changes (irritability, delirium, or coma). Multiple organ failure follows (1) renal shutdown due to hypotension, (2) hypoprothrombinemia due to vitamin K deficiency, (3) thrombocytopenia due to nonspecific binding of immunoglobulin, (4) disseminated intravascular coagulation with infarction or hemorrhage in several organs, and (5) progressive respiratory failure (Karakusis, 1986).

Diagnosis. Sepsis must always be considered in the differential diagnosis of shock and blood cultures must be obtained. When shock is the initial manifestation, gram-negative sepsis is likely. Shock secondary to *Staphylococcus aureus* is more likely to occur during the course of infection and not as a presenting symptom.

Treatment. Septic shock is a medical emergency. Antibiotic therapy should be initiated promptly at maximal doses. Hypotension must be treated by restoration of intravascular volume and each factor contributing to coagulopathy addressed. Mortality is high even with optimal treatment.

Toxic Shock Syndrome

Toxic shock syndrome is a potentially lethal illness caused by infection or colonization with some strains of *Staphylococcus aureus* (Chesney et al, 1982).

Clinical Features. The onset is abrupt and characterized by high fever, hypotension, vomiting, diarrhea, myalgia, headache, and a desquamating rash. Multiple organ failure may occur during the time of desquamation. Serious complications include cardiac arrhythmia, pulmonary edema, and oliguric renal failure. Initial encephalopathic features are agitation and confusion. This may be followed by lethargy, obtundation, and generalized tonic-clonic seizures.

The majority of cases have occurred in menstruating girls who use tampons, but this syndrome is also a complication of influenza and influenza-like illness in children with staphylococcal colonization of the respiratory tract (MacDonald et al, 1987).

Diagnosis. There is no diagnostic laboratory test, and the diagnosis is based upon the typical clinical and laboratory findings. Over half of patients have sterile pyuria, immature granulocytic leukocytes, coagulation abnormalities, hypocalcemia, low serum albumin and total protein concentrations, and elevated concentration of blood urea nitrogen, transaminase, bilirubin, and creatine kinase (Tofte and Williams, 1982). *S. aureus* is cultured from infected sites.

Treatment. Hypotension usually responds to volume restoration with physiologic saline. Some patients require vasopressors or fresh frozen plasma. Antibiotic therapy should be initiated promptly with an effective agent against *S. aureus*.

Hemorrhagic Shock and Encephalopathy Syndrome

This recently described syndrome of infants is presumed to be caused by sepsis, but the etiology is unknown (Whittington et al, 1985).

Clinical Features. Most affected children are younger than one year of age, but cases are described up to twenty-six months. One third of children have mild prodromal symptoms of vomiting. For most, the onset is explosive; a previously well child is found unresponsive and in convulsions. Fever of 38° to 39° C is a constant feature. Marked hypotension with poor peripheral perfusion is followed by profuse watery or bloody diarrhea with metabolic acidosis and compensatory respiratory alkalosis. Disseminated intravascular coagulopathy develops and bleeding is noted from every venipuncture site.

Mortality is very high; mental and motor impairment in survivors has been constant.

Diagnosis. The syndrome resembles toxic shock, gram-negative sepsis, heatstroke, and Reye syndrome. Abnormal renal function occurs in every case, but serum ammonia remains normal, hypoglycemia is unusual, and blood cultures yield no growth.

Cerebrospinal fluid is normal except for increased pressure. CT demonstrates small ventricles and loss of sulcal marking due to cerebral edema. The EEG background is diffusely slow.

Treatment. Affected children require intensive care with ventilatory support, volume replacement, correction of acid-base and coagulation disturbances, anticonvulsant therapy, and control of cerebral edema.

POSTINFECTIOUS ENCEPHALOMYELITIS

Demyelinating disorders that occur during or after systemic viral illnesses are called "postinfectious" and presumed to be caused by an allergic reaction. The nervous system is not thought to be infected. Either central or peripheral myelin may be affected, but there is considerable controversy as to whether both can be affected simultaneously. Examples of postinfectious disorders appear in several chapters of the text and include the Guillain-Barré syndrome (see Chapter 7), acute cerebellar ataxia (see Chapter 10), transverse myelitis (see Chapter 12), brachial neuritis (see Chapter 13), optic neuritis (see Chapter 16), and Bell's palsy (see Chapter 17). An increased incidence of some postinfectious disorders is encountered in immunocompromised populations and provides further support for the allergic hypothesis.

The cause-and-effect relationship between viral infection and many of these syndromes is virtually impossible to establish if a latency period of thirty days is allowed between viral infection and onset of neurologic dysfunction. The average school-aged child experiences four to six "viral illnesses" each year, so that 33 to 50 percent of children will report a viral illness thirty days before any life event. A greater than 50 percent incidence of viral illness, thirty days prior to onset, is not reported for any syndrome listed above.

Some systemic viral infections, such as measles, cause encephalitis by direct cerebral infection and simultaneously produce demyelination on an allergic basis. Such encephalopathies are not truly "postinfectious." Reye syndrome should be considered separately as well, since the encephalopathy is caused by mitochondrial dysfunction and not demyelination.

Clinical Features. Magnetic resonance imaging has expanded the spectrum of clinical features associated with postinfectious encephalopathy by allowing the demonstration of very small demyelinating lesions. Lethargy and weakness are at one end of the spectrum and coma at the other.

The encephalopathy is often preceded by lethargy, headache, and vomiting. It is not clear whether these "systemic features" are symptoms of a viral illness or early encephalopathy. The onset of neurologic symptoms is abrupt and characterized by declining states of consciousness and seizures. In some cases, the generalized encephalopathy is preceded by optic neuritis, transverse myelitis, or both (see "Devic Syndrome," Chapter 12). Some children never have focal neurologic signs, while others have hemiplegia, quadriplegia, ataxia, and cranial nerve dysfunction (Sriram and Steinman, 1984).

Mortality is highest in the first week, and although recovery among survivors is variable, the degree of recovery may be astonishing.

Diagnosis. Magnetic resonance imaging is diagnostic. T2-weighted images reveal a marked increase in signal intensity throughout the white matter (Fig. 2.4). Adrenoleukodystrophy must be excluded in boys.

The cerebrospinal fluid is frequently normal. Occasional abnormalities are a mild lymphocyte pleocytosis and elevation of protein concentration.

Treatment. Most children with severe encephalopathies are treated with corticosteroids,

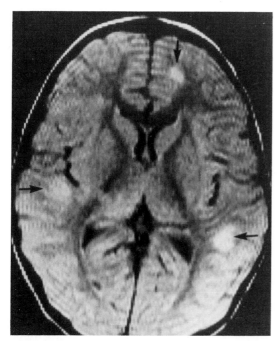

Figure 2.4 Postinfectious demyelination of the cerebral hemispheres. Areas of increased signal intensity are seen in both hemispheres (arrows).

despite the absence of conclusive evidence that such treatment is beneficial.

■ Postimmunization Encephalopathy

Three types of vaccines are in general use in the United States: (1) live-attenuated viruses, (2) whole or fractionated killed organisms, and (3) toxoids.

Live-attenuated virus vaccines (measles, mumps, rubella, varicella, and oral poliomyelitis) are intended to produce a mild and harmless infection with subsequent immunity. However, even under ideal circumstances of vaccine preparation and host resistance, the child may develop symptoms of the natural disease and experience its known neurologic complications. Measles is the only live-attenuated virus vaccine that causes encephalopathy (see "Measles Encephalitis").

Whole killed organisms (pertussis, influenza, rabies, and parenteral poliomyelitis) and fractionated killed organisms (hepatitis B and *Haemophilus influenzae*) do not reproduce their natural disease, but may produce encephalopathy by other mechanisms. Pertussis is the only whole killed vaccine presently implicated as a cause of encephalopathy. Rabies vaccine had

been an important cause of encephalomyelitis in the past, but the present vaccine, prepared from virus grown on human diploid cells, has been implicated only as a rare cause of polyneuropathy (Bernard et al, 1982). Several case reports have suggested that influenza immunization may cause encephalopathy, but considering the millions of doses administered, the number of cases reported is less than might be expected by chance alone. Toxoids are produced by inactivation of toxins produced by bacteria. Diphtheria and tetanus toxoids are the only ones presently in use, and neither is associated with encephalopathy. New pertussis vaccines presently being used in Japan are toxoids of one or more toxins elaborated by the pertussis organism. It is not clear whether or not these new vaccines have a lower incidence of encephalopathy than the whole cell vaccine.

Pertussis Vaccine Encephalopathy

Clinical Features. Febrile seizures are the single most common adverse reaction to pertussis immunization. More than half of children with postimmunization febrile seizures have a personal or family history of simple febrile convulsions (Hirtz et al, 1983; Stetler et al, 1985). The third immunization is associated with the greatest risk of provoking simple febrile convulsions, since the child is then at an age when the risk of such convulsions is greatest (Pollack and Morris, 1983).

A National Childhood Encephalopathy Study (NCES) in the United Kingdom identified all children aged two months to three years admitted to hospital with encephalopathy or encephalitis and using a case-control technique estimated that the vaccine-attributed risk is approximately 1/110,000 doses-administered (95 percent confidence limit 1/360,000 to 1/44,000), and the risk of permanent brain damage in a previously healthy child is 1/310,000 doses-administered (95 percent confidence limit 1/5,000,000 to 1/54,000). The relative-risk for permanent brain damage was based on only eleven children, of whom only five had unexplained encephalopathies. If those cases with other identified causes of encephalopathy are eliminated from the calculation, the 95 percent confidence limits become so broad as to make the 1/310,000 estimate meaningless.

An accepted sequence of events for the diagnosis of pertussis vaccine encephalopathy is the onset of prolonged, generalized tonic-clonic seizures and states of decreased consciousness within seventy-two hours of immunization. All other causes must be excluded. The encephalopathy is severe at onset and followed by recovery. There is no evidence that (1) killed vaccine can cause prolonged, deleterious effects or that (2) chronic neurologic disturbances can become manifest later in the absence of an acute encephalopathy.

Diagnosis. Pertussis vaccine encephalopathy has no specific features and cannot be distinguished on clinical grounds from encephalopathies of other cause. The mechanism is unknown, but cannot be demyelination; there are no naturally occurring bacterial diseases that produce demyelination of the central nervous system.

The cerebrospinal fluid may be normal or may demonstrate a mild lymphocytic pleocytosis and elevation of protein content. The EEG should be abnormal during the acute encephalopathy.

Treatment. Treatment is supportive.

■ Metabolic Encephalopathies

INBORN ERRORS OF METABOLISM

Inborn errors of metabolism that produce states of decreased consciousness are associated with hyperammonemia, hypoglycemia, or organic aciduria. Neonatal seizures are a presenting feature in most of these conditions (see Chapter 1), but some may not be symptomatic until infancy or childhood. Inborn errors with later onset encephalopathy include (1) pyruvate dysmetabolism and respiratory chain disorders (see Chapters 5, 6, and 10); (2) hemizygotes for ornithine carbamylase deficiency and heterozygotes for carbamyl phosphate synthetase deficiency (see Chapter 1); (3) glycogen storage diseases (see Chapter 1); and (4) systemic carnitine deficiency.

Systemic Carnitine Deficiency

L-Carnitine is an essential cofactor for the transfer of long-chain fatty acids across the inner mitochondrial membrane. The transfer requires the conversion of acyl-CoA to acylcarnitine. If carnitine is deficient, toxic levels of acyl-CoA accumulate and impair the citric acid cycle, gluconeogenesis, the urea cycle, and fatty-acid oxidation (Rebouche and Engel, 1983; Stumpf et al, 1985). Insufficient serum or tissue carnitine concentrations may occur as a result of (1) primary genetic disorders of carnitine metabolism, (2) secondary to other inborn errors of metabolism, and (3) secondary to acquired systemic disorders (Table 2.5).

Primary Carnitine Deficiency

Primary carnitine deficiency is transmitted by autosomal recessive inheritance. A systemic and a myopathic form are recognized. It is not clear whether the two forms are genetically distinct.

Clinical Features. Primary systemic carnitine deficiency is a disease of infancy and early childhood. It is characterized by attacks of vomiting, confusion, lethargy and coma provoked by intercurrent illness or fasting. Recurrent attacks are the rule, and mortality is considerable in the absence of prompt treatment. Between attacks, the child may appear normal. Some families have constant cardiomyopathy.

Primary muscle carnitine deficiency is manifested by mild to moderate proximal weakness (see Chapters 6 and 7).

Diagnosis. The acute attacks resemble Reye syndrome clinically and chemically: hypoglycemia, hypoprothrombinemia, hyperammonemia, elevated concentrations of liver enzymes, and fatty deposition in hepatocytes are present.

The deficiency is diagnosed by demonstration of low carnitine concentrations in blood or tissues. Blood carnitine concentrations in patients with primary carnitine deficiency are less than 20 μmol/mg noncollagen protein and those with secondary deficiency have higher, but less than normal, concentrations.

Table 2.5 DIFFERENTIAL DIAGNOSIS OF CARNITINE DEFICIENCY

Primary Genetic Carnitine Deficiency
1. Systemic
2. Muscle

Secondary to Other Metabolic Errors
1. Aminoacidurias
   a. Propionic acidemia
   b. Methylmalonic acidemia
   c. Isovaleric acidemia
   d. Glutaric aciduria
2. Disorders of pyruvate metabolism
   a. Pyruvate dehydrogenase deficiency
   b. Pyruvate carboxylase deficiency
   c. Multiple carboxylase deficiency
3. Disorders of the respiratory chain

Secondary to Acquired Disorders
1. Hemodialysis
2. Total parenteral nutrition
3. Malnutrition
4. Pregnancy
5. Reye syndrome
6. Valproic acid hepatotoxicity

Treatment. Dietary supplementation with L-carnitine is recommended for children with primary carnitine deficiency. The initial dose is 50 mg/kg/day, which is increased as tolerated until the desired blood concentration is attained. Adverse effects include nausea, vomiting, diarrhea, and abdominal cramps.

During an acute attack, a diet rich in medium-chain triglycerides and low in long-chain triglycerides should be provided in addition to carnitine. General supportive care is required for hypoglycemia and hypoprothrombinemia.

RENAL DISORDERS

In children with chronic renal failure, an acute or chronic uremic encephalopathy, hypertensive encephalopathy, dialysis encephalopathy, and neurologic complications of the immunocompromised state may develop.

Acute Uremic Encephalopathy

Clinical Features. In children with acute renal failure, symptoms of cerebral dysfunction develop over several days. *Asterixis*, a flapping tremor at the wrist when the arms are extended and the wrists flexed, is often the initial feature. This is followed by periods of confusion and headache, sometimes progressing to delirium, and then lethargy. The patient becomes weak and tremulous and experiences muscle cramps. Myoclonic jerks and tetany may be present. If uremia continues, decreasing consciousness and seizures follow.

Diagnosis. The mechanism is multifactorial and does not correlate with concentrations of blood urea nitrogen alone. Hyperammonemia and disturbed equilibrium of ions between the intracellular and extracellular spaces are probably important factors.

Late stages may be confused with hypertensive encephalopathy, but initial features occur in the absence of increased intracranial pressure. The EEG is abnormal early in the course and demonstrates slowing of the background rhythms and periodic triphasic waves.

Treatment. Hemodialysis reverses the encephalopathy and should be performed as quickly as possible after diagnosis.

Chronic Uremic Encephalopathy

Clinical Features. Chronic renal failure may cause a stereotyped encephalopathy, even in the absence of hemodialysis (Foley et al, 1981; Rotundo et al, 1982). All affected children have renal failure during the first year, usually from congenital renal hypoplasia. Age at onset is between one and nine years. Growth failure is a constant feature prior to onset of encephalopathy. Three stages are described:

Stage 1 consists of delayed motor development, dysmetria and tremor, or ataxia. Examination during this stage reveals hyperreflexia, mild hypotonia, and extensor plantar responses. Within six to twelve months, all patients progress to stage 2.

Stage 2 is characterized by myoclonus of the face and limbs, partial motor seizures, dementia, and then generalized seizures. Facial myoclonus and lingual apraxia make speech and feeding difficult, and limb myoclonus interferes with ambulation. The duration of stage 2 is variable and may last from months to years.

In *stage 3*, there is progressive bulbar failure, a vegetative state, and death.

Diagnosis. This is a clinical diagnosis. Initially, the EEG reveals progressive slowing and then the development of superimposed epileptiform activity. CT demonstrates progressive cerebral atrophy. The disorder may be difficult to distinguish from dialysis encephalopathy.

Hyperparathyroidism with hypercalcemia has been noted in some children with this syndrome, but parathyroidectomy does not reverse the process (Geary et al, 1980). It has been suggested that the syndrome may be caused by aluminum toxicity from antacids administered as phosphate binders (Sedman et al, 1984). Aluminum plasma concentrations should be determined during stage 1 and, if elevated, aluminum ingestion discontinued.

Treatment. Hemodialysis and renal transplantation have not altered the course in most patients.

Hypertensive Encephalopathy

The mechanism of hypertensive encephalopathy remains controversial, but the result is damage to small arterioles which leads to patchy areas of ischemia and edema. Therefore, focal neurologic deficits are relatively common.

Clinical Features. The initial features are transient attacks of cerebral ischemia and headache. Such symptoms may be dismissed as part of uremic encephalopathy, despite the warning signs of focal neurologic deficits. Headache persists and is accompanied by visual disturbances and vomiting. Seizures and states of diminished consciousness follow. The seizures are frequently focal at onset and then secondarily generalized. Examination reveals papilledema and retinal hemorrhages.

Diagnosis. Clinical judgment is critical to diagnosis. Hypertensive encephalopathy can be distinguished from other encephalopathies associated with renal disease by the greater elevation of blood pressure and the presence of focal neurologic disturbances.

Treatment. Treatment consists of aggressive efforts to reduce hypertension and anticonvulsant therapy. Measures to reduce cerebral edema are required in some patients.

Dialysis Encephalopathy

Chronic dialysis may be associated with acute, transitory neurologic disturbances attributed to the rapid shift of fluids and electrolytes between intracellular and extracellular spaces. Most common are vascular headaches and seizures. Seizures usually occur toward the end of dialysis or up to twenty-four hours later and may be preceded by lethargy and delirium.

In contrast, progressive encephalopathies associated with dialysis are often fatal. There are two important causes: (1) encephalitis secondary to immunosuppression and (2) the dialysis dementia syndrome. Opportunistic infections in the immunodeficient host are usually due to cytomegalovirus, toxoplasmosis, and mycoses.

Dialysis Dementia Syndrome

Clinical Features. The mean interval of onset of symptoms is four years after commencing dialysis (range one to seven years), and subsequent progression of symptoms varies from weeks to years (O'Hare et al, 1983). All patients demonstrate a characteristic speech disturbance either as an initial feature or later in the course. It begins as intermittent hesitancy of speech (stuttering and slurring) and may progress to aphasia. Agraphia and apraxia may be present as well. Subtle changes in personality occur early in the course and give the appearance of depression. Progressive dementia follows, which may be preceded by a phase of hallucinations and agitation.

Myoclonic jerking of the limbs is often present before the onset of dementia. First noted during dialysis, it soon becomes continuous and interferes with normal activity. Generalized tonic-clonic seizures develop in most patients and become more frequent and severe as the encephalopathy progresses. Complex partial seizures may be observed, but focal motor seizures are not expected.

Neurologic examination reveals the triad of speech arrest, myoclonus, and dementia. In addition, many patients show symmetric proximal weakness (myopathy) or distal weakness and sensory loss (neuropathy) with loss of tendon reflexes.

Diagnosis. EEG changes correlate well with disease progress. A characteristic early feature is the appearance of paroxysmal high-amplitude delta activity in the frontal areas, despite a normal posterior rhythm. Eventually, the background becomes generally slow and frontal triphasic waves are noted. Epileptiform activity develops in all patients with dialysis dementia and is the critical EEG feature that differentiates dialysis dementia from uremic encephalopathy. The activity consists of sharp, spike, or polyspike discharges that may have a periodic quality.

Treatment. There is considerable evidence that aluminum toxicity may be an important contributory cause, but no single factor has been established as etiologic. Excess aluminum may be derived from orally administered aluminum gels or from the dialysate. Removal of aluminum from dialysate prevents the appearance of new cases and progression in some established cases, even if oral gels are still administered.

Early renal transplantation is the obvious choice to prevent development of the syndrome, but does not always provide relief in established cases.

Benzodiazepines are useful in treating myoclonus and seizures, and may improve the speech disturbance as well.

HEPATIC ENCEPHALOPATHY

Fulminant hepatic failure in children is caused by viral hepatitis, drugs and toxins, and Reye syndrome (Rogers and Rogers, 1980). The encephalopathy that accompanies hepatic failure cannot be explained by abnormalities of any single factor, such as ammonia, but is due to multifactorial metabolic derangements. Severe viral hepatitis with marked elevation of unconjugated bilirubin may even lead to kernicterus in older children (Ho et al, 1980).

In children with chronic choleastatic liver disease, demyelination of the posterior columns and peripheral nerves may develop as a result of vitamin E deficiency. The major features are ataxia, areflexia, and gaze paresis, without evidence of encephalopathy (see Chapter 10).

Clinical Features. Malaise and fatigue are early symptoms that accompany features of hepatic failure: jaundice, dark urine, abnormal liver function tests. Nausea and vomiting occur when hepatic failure is fulminant. The onset of coma may be spontaneous or induced by gastrointestinal bleeding, infection, high-protein intake, and excessive use of tranquilizers or diuretics. The first features are a change in affect and disturbed sleep. These are followed by drowsiness, hyperventilation, and the appearance of asterixis. Hallucinations sometimes occur during early stages, but more often there is continuous progression to coma. Seizures and decerebrate rigidity develop as the patient becomes comatose.

Diagnosis. In hepatic coma, the EEG is not specific but is always abnormal and suggests a metabolic encephalopathy: loss of posterior rhythm, generalized slowing of background, and frontal triphasic waves (see Fig. 2.2).

Biochemical markers of liver failure include a sharp rise in transaminase activity (SGOT and SGPT), elevated prothrombin time, mixed hyperbilirubinemia, and a decline in serum albumin concentration.

Treatment. The goal of treatment is to maintain cerebral, renal, and cardiopulmonary function until liver regeneration can occur. Cerebral function is impaired, not only by abnormal concentrations of metabolites but also by cerebral edema.

DISORDERS OF OSMOLALITY

The osmolality of a solution is determined by the number of particles in solution. Sodium salts, glucose, and urea are the primary osmoles of the extracellular space, potassium salts of the intracellular space, and plasma proteins of the intravascular space. Because cell membranes are permeable to water and osmotic equilibrium must be maintained, the volume of intracellular fluid is determined by the osmolality of the extracellular space.

Hypernatremia and hyperglycemia are the major causes of serum hyperosmolality, and hyponatremia of serum hypo-osmolality.

Hypernatremia

Hypernatremia is usually caused by dehydration in which water loss exceeds sodium loss and by overhydration with hypertonic saline. It

is a medical emergency and, if not corrected promptly, may lead to permanent brain damage and death.

Clinical Features. Hypernatremic dehydration may be a consequence of vomiting or diarrhea, especially if water intake is restricted. Iatrogenic hypernatremia is usually caused by overzealous correction of hyponatremia. Acute alterations in sodium concentration are much more likely to cause encephalopathy than are equivalent concentrations attained slowly. Symptoms of hypernatremia are all referable to the nervous system and include irritability, lethargy progressing to coma, and seizures. The presence of focal neurologic deficits suggests the possibility of cerebral venous sinus thrombosis.

Diagnosis. Symptomatic hypernatremia develops at sodium concentrations above 160 mEq/L (160 mmol/L). The EEG demonstrates the nonspecific slowing associated with metabolic encephalopathies. Focal slowing of EEG or focal abnormalities on examination warrant CT to look for venous sinus thrombosis.

Chronic or recurrent episodes of hypernatremia may result from hypodipsia, a rare condition encountered in children with underlying congenital or acquired brain disorders (Hammond et al, 1986). Hypodipsia is caused by lack of thirst. The syndrome is usually associated with a defect in secretion of the antidiuretic hormone arginine vasopressin.

Treatment. Rapid water replacement can lead to cerebral edema. The recommended approach is to correct abnormalities of intravascular volume before correcting the water deficit (Finberg, 1973).

Hyperglycemia

The major cause of symptomatic hyperglycemia in children is diabetic ketoacidosis. Nonketotic, hyperglycemic coma, associated with mild or non–insulin-requiring diabetes, is unusual in children.

Clinical Features. The syndrome develops acutely in children who have neglected to take prescribed doses of insulin or who have a superimposed infection. Initial features are polydypsia, polyuria, and fatigue. Hyperventilation is present to compensate for the metabolic acidosis. Lethargy rapidly progresses to coma. Ketoacidosis is the leading cause of death in children with diabetes and mortality rates are still as high as 10 percent.

Cerebral edema is an early and constant feature of diabetic ketoacidosis (Krane et al,

1985). Its severity correlates with changes in level of consciousness and may contribute to death in some cases. Other, less common, neurologic complications are venous sinus thrombosis and intracerebral hemorrhage (Atluru, 1986). Both are associated with focal or generalized seizures.

Diagnosis. Diabetic ketoacidosis is diagnosed by the combination of a blood glucose level above 400 mg/dl (22 mmol/L), the presence of serum and urinary ketones, an arterial pH less than 7.25, and serum bicarbonate less than 15 mmol/L.

Treatment. Intravenous normal saline or Ringer's solution is given first to correct hypovolemia. This is followed by 0.45 percent saline solution with potassium salts added. Regular intravenous boluses of crystalline insulin are given to reduce blood glucose concentrations.

Hyponatremia

Hyponatremia may result from water retention, sodium loss, or both. Water retention is often caused by the syndrome of inappropriate antidiuretic hormone secretion (SIADH) and sodium loss by renal disease, vomiting, and diarrhea. Permanent brain damage from hyponatremia is uncommon, but may occur if the serum sodium concentration is allowed to remain below 115 mEq/L for several hours (Arieff, 1986).

SIADH

This syndrome occurs in association with a variety of neurologic disorders that include head trauma, infections, and intracranial hemorrhage.

Clinical Features. Most patients with SIADH have a pre-existing loss of consciousness from their underlying neurologic disorder. In such patients, hyponatremia is the only feature of SIADH. In those who are alert, lethargy develops from the hyponatremia but rarely progresses to coma or seizures.

Diagnosis. In caring for children with acute intracranial disorders, one must be vigilant to the possibility of SIADH; repeated determinations of serum sodium concentration are required. Once hyponatremia is documented, urinary sodium concentration must be measured. Urinary sodium is usually greater than 20 mEq/L (20 mmol/L) and parallels intake. Definitive diagnosis requires the demonstration of inappropriately high plasma concentrations of arginine vasopressin in the presence of hyponatremia.

Treatment. All signs of SIADH respond to fluid restriction. An intake of 50 to 75 percent of maintenance is generally satisfactory.

Sodium Loss

Clinical Features. Hyponatremic encephalopathy is caused by the movement of water into the brain. Symptoms of nausea, vomiting, muscular twitching, and lethargy appear when the serum sodium concentration falls below 125 mEq/L (125 mmol/L). A further decline below 115 mEq/L (115 mmol/L) is associated with seizures and coma.

Diagnosis. Hyponatremia should be recognized as a potential problem in children with vomiting or diarrhea and with renal disease. Serum and urinary sodium concentrations are both decreased.

Treatment. The treatment of acute symptomatic hyponatremia remains controversial. Rapid correction is important, but only to mildly hypotonic concentrations (Ayus et al, 1985). Sudden corrections of greater than 20 mEq/L (20 mmol/L) are associated with seizures, hypernatremic encephalopathy, and the possibility of central pontine myelinolysis (Norenberg, 1983). Half-normal saline should be administered at a rate that requires at least twenty-four hours for complete correction.

Hypoglycemia

Symptomatic hypoglycemia after the neonatal period is usually associated with insulin use in the treatment of diabetes mellitus. Sepsis and inborn errors of metabolism account for only a minority of cases.

Clinical Features. Clinical features are not precisely predictable from blood glucose concentration (Malouf and Brust, 1985). Hypoglycemia does not usually become symptomatic until blood concentrations below 50 mg/dl (2.8 mmol/L) are attained. The rate of fall may be important in determining the clinical picture. Dizziness and tremor may occur at blood concentrations below 60 mg/dl (3.1 mmol/L) and serve as a warning of insulin overdose. Greater declines in blood glucose concentration result in confusion, delirium, and loss of consciousness. Sudden hemiplegia, usually transitory and sometimes shifting between the two sides, is a rare feature of hypoglycemia. The mechanism is unknown, and CT shows no evidence of infarction.

Diagnosis. Hypoglycemia should always be suspected in diabetic children with an altered mental status or level of decreased consciousness. Blood glucose concentration should be measured promptly.

Treatment. Diabetic children should be encouraged to carry a source of sugar for use at the first symptom of hypoglycemia. Children who are comatose from hypoglycemia should be corrected promptly with intravenous glucose solutions. Complete recovery is the rule.

ENDOCRINE DISORDERS

Adrenal Disorders

Adrenal hypersecretion is associated with agitation or depression, but does not produce coma. Adrenal failure is seen during sepsis, after the abrupt withdrawal of corticosteroid therapy, and is secondary to adrenal hemorrhage. Initial symptoms are nausea, vomiting, abdominal pain, and fever. Lethargy progresses to coma and is associated with hypovolemic shock. Prompt intravenous infusions of fluids, glucose, and corticosteroids are life-saving.

Parathyroid Disorders

The neurologic features of hyperparathyroidism are all related to hypercalcemia. Weakness and myopathy are relatively common. Alterations in mental status occur in 50 percent of patients and include apathy, delirium, paranoia, and dementia. Apathy and delirium occur at serum calcium concentrations greater than 11 mg/dl (2.75 mmol/L), psychosis and dementia at concentrations of 16 mg/dl (4.0 mmol/L) and greater.

Seizures are the major manifestation of hypoparathyroidism and hypocalcemia. They may be generalized or focal and are often preceded by tetany (see Chapter 1). Hypocalcemic seizures do not respond to anticonvulsant drugs and must be treated with calcium replacement.

Thyroid Disorders

Hyperthyroidism produces exhilaration bordering on mania and may be associated with seizures and chorea. Thyroid storm (crisis) is a life-threatening event characterized by restlessness, cardiac arrhythmia, vomiting, and diarrhea. Delirium is an early feature, but may progress to coma.

Acquired hypothyroidism affects both the central and peripheral nervous systems. Peripheral effects include neuropathy and myopathy. Central effects are cranial nerve abnormalities, ataxia, psychoses, dementia, seizures, and

coma. Delusions and hallucinations occur in more than half of long-standing cases. Myxedema coma, a rare manifestation of long-standing hypothyroidism in adults, is even more uncommon in children. It is characterized by profound hypothermia without shivering.

OTHER METABOLIC ENCEPHALOPATHIES

Several, less frequent, causes of metabolic encephalopathy are listed in Table 2.3. Some are attributable to derangements of a single substance, most are multifactorial.

In 5 percent of children with burns covering 30 percent of body surface, an encephalopathy develops that may be intermittent. Onset may be days to weeks after the burn. Altered mental states (delirium or coma) and seizures (generalized or focal) are the major features. Multiple metabolic alterations are present, and the encephalopathy cannot usually be attributed to a single factor (Mohnot et al, 1982).

Encephalopathies that occur during total parenteral hyperalimentation are generally due to hyperammonemia caused by excessive loads of amino acids (Grazer et al, 1984).

Hypomagnesemia in infancy may be caused by prematurity, maternal deficiency, maternal or infant hypoparathyroidism, high-phosphorus diets, exchange transfusion, intestinal disorders, and specific defects in magnesium absorption. These conditions are often associated with hypocalcemia. Excessive use of diuretics causes hypomagnesemia in older children. Symptoms develop below plasma concentrations of 1.2 mg/dl (0.5 mmol/L) and include jitteriness, hyperirritability, and seizures. Further decline in serum magnesium concentrations leads to obtundation and coma.

Deficiency of one or more B vitamins may be associated with lethargy or delirium, but only thiamine deficiency causes coma. Thiamine deficiency is relatively common in alcoholic adults and produces Wernicke's encephalopathy, but is uncommon in children. Subacute necrotizing encephalopathy is a thiamine deficiency-like state in children (see Chapters 5 and 10).

■ Migraine

Migraine is remarkable for producing a large variety of neurologic syndromes and is discussed in several chapters. Among its less common manifestations are a confusional state, an amnestic state, and coma.

ACUTE CONFUSIONAL MIGRAINE

Clinical Features. A confused and agitated state resembling toxic-metabolic psychosis occurs as a migraine variant in children between the ages of five and sixteen. Most are ten years or older. Attacks are characterized by a relatively rapid evolution of symptoms. The child becomes delirious and appears to be in pain, but does not complain of headache. Impaired awareness of environment, retarded responses to painful stimuli, hyperactivity, restlessness, and combative behavior are evident. The duration of an attack is usually three to five hours and may last as long as twenty. Eventually, the child falls into a deep sleep, appears normal upon awakening, and has no memory of the episode. Confusional attacks tend to recur over a relatively brief period of days or months and then evolve into typical migraine episodes (Ehyai and Fenichel, 1978).

Diagnosis. Migraine is always a clinical diagnosis and should be arrived at only after other possibilities are excluded. It relies heavily upon a positive family history of migraine, but not necessarily of confusional migraine. During or shortly after a confusional attack, the EEG demonstrates unilateral temporal or occipital slowing (Emery, 1977).

Treatment. The acute attack should be treated with intramuscular chlorpromazine, 1 mg/kg. Effective prophylaxis may be accomplished with propranolol (see Chapter 3).

MIGRAINE COMA

Migraine coma is a rare but extreme form of migraine that can be fatal (Fitzsimons and Wolfenden, 1985).

Clinical Features. The major features of this syndrome are (1) recurrent episodes of coma precipitated by trivial head injury and (2) apparent meningitis associated with life-threatening cerebral edema. Migraine coma has been reported in a kindred with *familial hemiplegic migraine* (see Chapter 11), but a similar syndrome may occur in sporadic cases as well. Coma develops following trivial head injury and is associated with fever. Intracranial pressure is increased due to cerebral edema, which can be localized to one hemisphere and cause sufficient midline shift to produce herniation. States of decreased consciousness may last for several days. Recovery is then complete.

Diagnosis. Coma following even trivial head injury causes concern for intracranial hemorrhage. A CT scan must be performed unless there is a history of prior attacks and the diagnosis of migraine coma already established. The initial scan may be negative, especially if done immediately. Later scans demonstrate generalized or focal edema.

Examination of the cerebrospinal fluid reveals increased pressure and a pleocytosis of up to 100 cells/cu mm. The combination of fever, coma, and cerebrospinal fluid pleocytosis suggests viral encephalitis, and herpes may be queried if edema is localized to one temporal lobe.

Treatment. Patients who have experienced migraine coma should be treated with a prophylactic agent to prevent further attacks (see Chapter 3). The major treatment goal during the acute attack is to decrease intracranial pressure by reducing cerebral edema (see Chapter 4).

TRANSIENT GLOBAL AMNESIA

Transient global amnesia is a syndrome in adults characterized by sudden inability to form new memories with repetitive questioning of events and no other neurologic symptoms or signs. Migraine is the probable cause when such attacks occur in children or in more than one family member (Dupuis et al, 1987).

Clinical Features. Attacks last from twenty minutes to several hours, and retrograde amnesia is present upon recovery. Many adults with this syndrome have a prior history of migraine (Crowell et al, 1984), and a similar syndrome may be seen in children with migraine following trivial head injury (Haas and Ross, 1986). The attacks are similar to acute confusional migraine except that there is less delirium and more isolated memory deficiency.

Diagnosis. A personal or family history of migraine is essential for diagnosis. The CT scan is normal, but the EEG may demonstrate slowing of the background rhythm in one temporal lobe.

Treatment. Management is the same as for classic migraine (see Chapter 3).

■ Psychologic Disorders

Panic disorders and schizophrenia may present with the acute onset of symptoms suggesting delirium or confusion and need to be distinguished from acute organic encephalopathies.

PANIC DISORDER

Clinical Features. Panic attacks were thought to be confined to adult life, but now are recognized to occur in adolescence and school-aged children (Herskowitz, 1986). This is an agitated state caused by anxiety. Principal features are paroxysmal dizziness, headache, and dyspnea. Hyperventilation is often associated and results in further dizziness, paresthesias, and lightheadedness. Attacks may be provoked by phobias, such as going to school. They can last for minutes to hours and recur daily.

Diagnosis. Panic attacks simulate cardiac or neurologic disease, and many children will undergo extensive, but unnecessary, medical evaluation before the correct diagnosis is reached. Panic disorder should be suspected in children with recurrent attacks of hyperventilation, dizziness, or dyspnea.

Treatment. Antidepressant drugs have varying degrees of efficacy. Imipramine has the best success rate. Initial dosages are less than used for depression (0.25 mg/kg/day), but higher dosages may be needed if concurrent depression must be treated as well.

SCHIZOPHRENIA

Clinical Features. Schizophrenia is a disorder of adolescence or early adult life and should not be suspected in prepubertal children. Affected individuals are without antecedent history of affective disorder. An initial feature is often declining work performance simulating dementia. Intermittent depersonalization may occur early in the course (not knowing where or who one is) and suggest complex partial seizures.

Thoughts move with loose association from one idea to another, until they become incoherent. Delusions and hallucinations are common and usually have paranoid features. Motor activity can be either lacking, with the patient remaining stationary, or excessive and purposeless. This combination of symptoms in an adolescent may be difficult to distinguish clinically from drug encephalopathy.

Diagnosis. Diagnosis is established by careful evaluation of mental status. Family history may be positive for schizophrenia. Neurologic examination is normal as are laboratory investigations. A normal EEG in an awake child with the clinical picture of an acute encephalopathy should always point to psychologic disturbances, including schizophrenia.

Treatment. Schizophrenia is generally considered to be a chemical disorder of the brain. It is incurable, but many of the symptoms are alleviated by antipsychotic drugs. The classes of drugs most often used in children are phenothiazines and haloperidol.

■ Toxic Encephalopathies

Accidental poisoning with drugs and chemicals left carelessly within reach are relatively common in children from ages one to four. Between ages four and ten, there is a trough in the frequency of poisoning, and then an increasing frequency of intentional poisoning with substances of abuse and prescription drugs.

PRESCRIPTION DRUGS

Most intentional overdoses are with prescription drugs, as they are readily available. Delirium or coma may be due to toxic effects of psychoactive drugs (anticonvulsants, antidepressants, antipsychotics, and tranquilizers), hypoglycemia (insulin and oral hypoglycemic agents), and acid-base disturbances (salicylates).

The encephalopathies that occur when drugs cause disorders of osmolality or organ failure are described in the section on Metabolic Encephalopathies.

Clinical Features. Psychoactive drugs are readily available in many households and are a frequent cause of poisoning. As a rule, toxic doses produce lethargy, nystagmus or ophthalmoplegia, and loss of coordination. Higher concentrations result in coma and seizures. Involuntary movements may occur as an idiosyncratic or dose-related effect.

Diazepam is remarkably safe when taken alone, and there are no instances of coma or death from overdose. Other benzodiazepines are reasonably safe as well.

Tricyclic antidepressants are the most widely prescribed drug in the United States and account for 25 percent of serious overdoses (Braden et al, 1986). The major features are coma, hypotension, and anticholinergic effects (flushing, dry skin, dilated pupils, tachycardia, decreased gastrointestinal motility, and urinary retention). Seizures and myocardial depression may be present as well.

The onset of symptoms following phenothiazine or haloperidol administration may be delayed for six to twenty-four hours and symptoms may be intermittent (Knight and Roberts, 1986). Extrapyramidal disturbances are a prominent feature (see Chapter 14), as are symptoms of anticholinergic poisoning. Fatalities are uncommon and probably caused by cardiac arrhythmia.

Diagnosis. Laboratory identification of most drugs can be accomplished within two hours. A drug screen of the urine should be performed in all cases of unidentified coma or delirium. If an unidentified product is found in the urine, further identification may be possible in the plasma. Blood concentration should be determined when a known drug is ingested.

Treatment. The degree of supportive care needed is individualized to the severity of the poisoning. Every child needs an intravenous line and careful monitoring of cardiorespiratory status. A continuous electrocardiogram (EKG) is often required because of concern for arrhythmia. Unabsorbed drug must be removed from the stomach by lavage and repeated doses of activated charcoal (30 mg every six hours) administered to prevent absorption and increase drug clearance. Extrapyramidal symptoms are treated with intravenous diphenhydramine, 2 mg/kg, and cardiac arrhythmias caused by phenothiazines with intravenous phenytoin, 15 mg/kg.

SUBSTANCE ABUSE

Alcohol remains the most commonly abused substance in the United States. More than 90 percent of high school seniors have used alcohol one or more times and 6 percent are daily drinkers (Kulberg, 1986). Approximately 6 percent of high school seniors use marijuana daily, but less than 0.1 percent are regular users of hallucinogens or opiates. The use of cocaine, stimulants, and sedatives has been increasing in recent years. Daily use of stimulants is reported by up to 1 percent of high school seniors.

Clinical Features. The American Psychiatric Association defines the diagnostic criteria for substance abuse to include (1) a pattern of pathologic use with inability to stop or reduce use, (2) impairment of social or occupational functioning, which includes school performance in children, and (3) persistence of the problem for one month or longer.

The clinical features of acute intoxication vary with the substance used. Almost all disturb judgment, intellectual function, and coordination. Alcohol and sedatives then lead to drowsiness, sleep, and obtundation. In contrast, hallucinogens result in bizarre behavior, which includes hallucinations, delusions, and muscle rigidity. Drugs such as phencyclidine (angel dust) and lysergic acid diethylamide (LSD) produce a clinical picture that simulates schizophrenia.

The usual picture of marijuana intoxication is euphoria and a sense of relaxation at low doses and a "dream-like" state with slow response-time at higher doses. Very high blood concentrations produce depersonalization, disorientation, and sensory disturbances. Hallucinations and delusions are unusual with marijuana and should suggest mixed-drug use.

Amphetamine abuse should be considered when an agitated state is coupled with peripheral evidence of adrenergic toxicity: mydriasis, flushing, diaphoresis, and reflex bradycardia secondary to peripheral vasoconstriction.

Cocaine affects the brain and heart. Early symptoms include euphoria, mydriasis, headache, and tachycardia. Higher doses produce emotional lability, nausea and vomiting, flushing, and a syndrome that simulates paranoid schizophrenia. Life-threatening complications are hyperthermia, seizures, and cardiac arrhythmia.

Diagnosis. The major challenge is to differentiate acute substance intoxication from schizophrenia. Important clues are a history of substance abuse obtained from family or friends, associated autonomic and cardiac disturbances, and alterations in vital signs. Urine and plasma screens are generally successful in detecting the substance or its metabolites.

Treatment. Management of acute substance abuse depends upon the substance used and the amount ingested. Treating physicians must always be alert to the possibility of multiple drug or substance exposure. An attempt should be made to empty the gastrointestinal tract of substances taken orally. Supportive care is generally required to support cardiorespiratory function and correct metabolic disturbances. Intravenous diazepam is useful for hallucinations and seizures produced by stimulants and hallucinogens. Standard cardiac drugs are used to combat arrhythmias.

The most vexing problem with substance abuse is generally not the acute management of intoxication, but rather breaking the habit. This requires patient motivation and long-term inpatient and outpatient treatment.

POISONS

Most accidental poisonings occur in small children who ingest common household products. The ingestion is usually discovered quickly because the child becomes sick and vomits. Insecticides, herbicides, and products containing hydrocarbons or alcohol are frequently implicated. Clinical features vary with the specific agent ingested. Optimal management requires proper identification of constituent poisons, estimation of amount ingested, interval since exposure, cleansing of the gastrointestinal tract, specific antidotes when available, and supportive measures.

■ Trauma

Trivial head injuries, without loss of consciousness, are commonplace in children and almost constant in toddlers. Migraine should be suspected whenever transitory neurologic disturbances (e.g., confusion, amnesia, blindness, ataxia, hemiplegia) follow trivial head injuries. Important causes of significant head injuries are child abuse in infants, sports and play injuries in children, and motor vehicle accidents in adolescence.

Neonatal head injuries generally present with seizures and are considered in Chapter 1. Loss of consciousness is the major feature of postnatal head injuries. Mild head injuries are characterized by temporary loss of consciousness without evidence of focal neurologic disturbances. Such events are usually termed *concussion*. Severe head injuries are characterized by prolonged intervals of coma associated with brain swelling and intracranial hemorrhage.

MILD HEAD INJURIES

Clinical Features. Mild closed head injuries are associated with temporary loss of consciousness and the absence of localizing neurologic signs. The child may just be "stunned" without definite loss of consciousness or obtunded for several hours, but never in coma. Once the conscious state is attained, the child is invariably tired and sleeps long and soundly if left undisturbed. As a rule, recovery is complete but may be followed by amnesia for the event and an interval before and after. The length of the amnestic interval correlates with the severity of injury.

Many children will complain of headache and dizziness for several days or weeks following concussion. Memory disturbances and irritability may be present as well. The severity and duration of these symptoms approximate the severity of injury, but sometimes seem disproportional.

Focal or generalized seizures, sometimes status epilepticus, may occur one or two hours following mild head injury (Snoek et al, 1984). This may even occur in children who did not experience loss of consciousness. Such seizures rarely indicate later epilepsy.

Diagnosis. A CT scan is not needed for every child with mild head injury, but has almost become standard practice. It may be cost-effective in reducing the number of hospital admissions. If CT is not performed, then skull radiographs may be useful to at least eliminate the possibility of depressed skull fracture. An EEG should be performed if there is any question that the head injury occurred as part of a seizure or if neurologic disturbances are disproportionate to the severity of injury.

Treatment. Mild head injuries do not require treatment and the only purpose of hospitalization is to observe the child for delayed hemorrhage or cerebral edema. There is no standard of practice to determine the need for hospitalization, but suspicion of child abuse, skull fracture, and abnormal vital signs are the most compelling reasons (Dershewitz et al, 1983).

If the child does not need hospitalization, it is unreasonable to ask the parents to awaken the child at regular intervals and perform neurologic examinations. Normal children are difficult to arouse from sleep, and a child who has had a head injury and spent several hours in an emergency room will sleep all the sounder. A child who does not need hospital observation does not need home observation.

SEVERE HEAD INJURIES

Shaking Injuries

Clinical Features. Shaking is a common method of child abuse in infants. An unconscious infant is brought to the emergency room with a bulging fontanelle. Seizures may have precipitated the hospital visit. History is fragmentary and inconsistent among informants. Typically, the child has been left in the care of a babysitter or the mother's "boy-friend."

There is no external evidence of injury, but ophthalmoscopic examination reveals retinal and optic nerve sheath hemorrhages (Lambert et al, 1986). Many of the hemorrhages may be old, suggesting repeated shaking injuries. Death may result from uncontrollable increased intracranial hemorrhage. In such cases, postmortem examination demonstrates evidence of blunt injury, which was not demonstrable antemortem (Duhaime et al, 1987). It is likely that all "shaking injuries" have some component of direct blunt injury as well.

Diagnosis. The CT scan reveals a swollen brain, but may not demonstrate subdural collections of blood if bleeding is recent. Subdural tap should be performed whether or not subdural blood is observed on CT. It is both diagnostic and therapeutic.

Treatment. Bilateral subdural taps should be performed immediately with the intention of removing as much blood as possible. The amount available for drainage through a subdural tap is only a small percentage of the total volume in the subdural space. The goal of subdural tap is not to remove all subdural blood, but rather to remove a sufficient quantity to relieve increased intracranial pressure and to aid reabsorptive mechanisms. Taps are repeated daily until the removable volume begins to decline; then an every-other-day schedule of subdural taps allows continued reduction of the accumulated fluid. Subdural-peritoneal shunt may be required, if permanent effusion develops.

Transfusion may be needed, if peripheral hematocrit is low and falling.

Protective service must be sought to prevent repeated injuries. Overall, the neurologic and visual outcome is poor. Most children will be left with considerable handicap.

Closed Head Injuries

Clinical Features. Loss of consciousness is not always immediate; a lucid period of several minutes may intervene between injury and onset of neurologic deterioration (Snoek et al, 1984). The Glasgow Coma Scale is used widely to quantify the degree of responsiveness following head injuries (Table 2.6). Scores of 8 or less correlate well with severe injury.

Acute brain swelling and intracranial hemorrhage account for the clinical manifestations. Increased intracranial pressure is always present and may lead to herniation if uncontrolled. Focal neurologic deficits suggest intracerebral hemorrhage.

Table 2.6   GLASGOW COMA SCALE*

Eye Opening (E)	
spontaneous	4
to speech	3
to pain	2
none	1
Best Motor Response (M)	
obeys	6
localizes	5
withdraws	4
abnormal flexion	3
abnormal extension	2
none	1
Verbal Response (V)	
oriented	5
confused conversation	4
inappropriate words	3
incomprehensible sounds	2
none	1

*Coma score = E + M + V.

Epidural and subdural hematomas are almost impossible to distinguish on clinical grounds alone. Progressive loss of consciousness is a consistent feature, and both may be associated with a lucid interval between time of injury and neurologic deterioration. Supratentorial epidural hematomas are usually temporal or temporoparietal in location. The blood may be arterial in origin (tearing of the middle meningeal artery), venous, or both. Skull fracture is present in 75 percent of cases. Infratentorial epidural hematoma is venous in origin and produces signs of brainstem compression.

Supratentorial subdural hematomas are venous in origin, frequently bilateral and usually occur without associated skull fracture. Posterior fossa subdural hemorrhage is most often seen in newborns (see Chapter 1) and older children with posterior skull fractures. Both cause symptoms by compression of adjacent structures and increasing intracranial pressure.

Mortality rates in children with severe head injury vary from 10 to 35 percent, depending upon the series (Bruce et al, 1979). Low mortality rates are sometimes associated with higher percentages of survivors with chronic vegetative states. Duration of coma is the best guide to long-term morbidity (Filley et al, 1987). Permanent neurologic impairment is constant when coma persists for one month or longer.

Diagnosis. A CT scan should be performed as rapidly as possible after closed head injuries. Brain swelling and subarachnoid hemorrhage with blood collecting along the falx are typical findings. Epidural, subdural, and intracerebral hemorrhage may be detected as well. Immediately after injury, epidural and subdural hematomas appear as regions of increased density between the brain and scalp. Epidural hematoma has a characteristic lens-shaped appearance (Fig. 2.5), while subdural hematoma is convex towards the skull and concave towards the brain. Some acute surface hematomas are briefly isodense and may be unobserved. With time, density decreases in all.

Intracerebral hemorrhage is usually superficial, but may also extend deep into the brain. Frontal or temporal lobe contusion is common. Discrete deep hemorrhages without a superficial extension are probably not traumatic in origin.

Children with head injuries must be kept with the neck immobilized until radiographic examination for fracture-dislocation of the cervical spine is done, since the force of a blow to the skull is frequently propagated to the neck. Attention must also be paid to possible limb and organ injury when head injury occurs in a motor vehicle accident.

Treatment. Children with severe head injuries must be managed in an intensive care unit. Essential support includes controlled ventilation, prevention of hypotension, and sufficient reduction in brain swelling to maintain cerebral perfusion. Methods to reduce cerebral edema are reviewed in Chapter 3. Pentobarbital coma does not affect outcome (Ward et al, 1985).

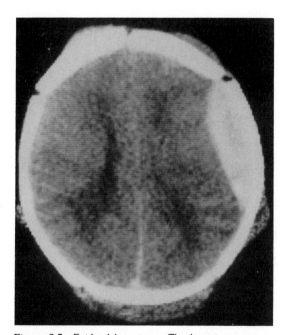

Figure 2.5 Epidural hematoma. The hematoma appears as a lens-shaped density just below the skull.

Epidural hematoma and acute expanding subdural hematoma warrant immediate surgery. Small subdural collections that do not produce a mass effect can be left in place until the patient's condition is stabilized and the options then considered.

Phenytoin is routinely administered intravenously to prevent seizures, despite evidence that it is probably ineffective in this regard (Young et al, 1983a,b).

Open Head Injuries

Skull fractures, other than linear fractures, are associated with an increased risk of infection. A fracture is *depressed* if the inner table fragment is displaced by at least the thickness of the skull. Depressed fractures are *compound* if the scalp is lacerated and *penetrating* if the dura is torn (Jennett and Teasdale, 1981). Depressed fractures of the skull vault may injure the underlying brain and tear venous sinuses. The result is hemorrhage into the brain and subdural space. Treatment includes elevation of depressed fragments, debridement and closure of the scalp laceration, and systemic penicillin.

Basal skull fractures with dural tear may result in leakage of cerebrospinal fluid from nose or ear and meningitis. Such leaks usually develop within three days of injury. The timing and need for dural repair are somewhat controversial, but all agree with the need for intravenous antibiotic coverage.

Posttraumatic Epilepsy

In 53 percent of patients with penetrating head injuries, posttraumatic epilepsy will develop (Salazar et al, 1985). Half will continue to have seizures as long as fifteen years after injury. Two thirds will have seizure onset during the first year post injury, and 90 percent by five years, but onset is delayed by ten to fifteen years in 7 percent. Patients with focal neurologic deficits and large cerebral lesions at the time of injury have the greatest risk for posttraumatic epilepsy. Initial seizures are generalized in 70 to 80 percent of cases.

Posttraumatic epilepsy is much less common with closed head injuries (Annegers et al, 1980). The five-year incidence after severe head trauma (brain contusion, intracranial hemorrhage, or 24 hours of unconsciousness or amnesia) is 11.5 percent, and after moderate head trauma (skull fracture or 30 minutes to 24 hours of unconsciousness or amnesia) is 1.6 percent. Mild head injuries (less than 30 minutes of unconsciousness or amnesia) is not associated with an increased incidence of posttraumatic epilepsy.

■ Hypertensive Encephalopathy

Hypertensive encephalopathy occurs when increases in systemic blood pressure exceed the limits of cerebral autoregulation. The consequences are cerebral edema and increased intracranial pressure.

Clinical Features. Children with hypertensive encephalopathy almost always have chronic renal disease and are undergoing chronic dialysis. The initial symptoms are usually severe generalized headache followed by progressive decline in consciousness or bizarre behavior. Other symptoms include vomiting, seizures, and myoclonic jerking of the limbs. Focal neurologic deficits may occur and should not detract from confidence in the diagnosis (Del Giudice and Aicardi, 1979).

Diagnosis. Because the syndrome occurs in children on chronic renal dialysis awaiting transplantation, the differential diagnosis includes disorders of osmolality, uremic encephalopathy, and dialysis encephalopathy. The EEG is always abnormal, but not specific. Generalized slowing of the background is a constant feature; paroxysmal discharges are sometimes associated. Periodic complexes may be present.

Treatment. Hypertensive encephalopathy is a medical emergency and should be treated by prompt reduction of blood pressure.

References

1. Annegers JF, Grabow JD, Groover RV, et al: Seizures after head trauma: A population study. Neurology 30:683, 1980.
2. Arieff AI: Hyponatremia, convulsions, respiratory arrest, and permanent brain damage after elective surgery in healthy women. N Engl J Med 314:1529, 1986.
3. Atluru VL: Spontaneous intracerebral hematomas in juvenile diabetic ketoacidosis. Pediatr Neurol 2:167, 1986.
4. Ayus JC, Krothapalli RK, Arieff AI, et al: Changing concepts in treatment of severe symptomatic hyponatremia. Rapid correction and possible relation to central pontine myelinolysis. Am J Med 78:897, 1985.
5. Bartleson JD, Swanson JW, Whisnant JP: A migrainous syndrome with cerebrospinal fluid pleocytosis. Neurology 31:1257, 1981.
6. Beghi E, Nicolosi A, Kurland LT, et al: Encephalitis and aseptic meningitis, Olmsted county, Minnesota, 1950–1981: I. Epidemiology. Ann Neurol 16:283, 1984.
7. Belman AL, Lantos G, Horoupian D, et al: AIDS: Calcification of the basal ganglia in infants and children. Neurology 36:1192, 1986.
8. Bernard KW, Smith PW, Kader EJ, et al: Neuroparalytic illness and human diploid cell rabies vaccine. JAMA 248:3136, 1982.
9. Bia FJ, Thornton GF, Main AJ, et al: Western equine encephalitis mimicking herpes simplex encephalitis. JAMA 244:367, 1980.
10. Bloch AB, Orenstein WA, Stetler HC, et al: Health impact of measles vaccination in the United States. Pediatrics 76:524, 1985.
11. Braden NJ, Jackson JE, Walson PD: Tricyclic antidepressant overdose. Pediatr Clin North Am 33:287, 1986.
12. Brattstrom L, Hindfelt B, Nilsson O: Transient neurological symptoms associated with mononuclear pleocytosis of the cerebrospinal fluid. Acta Neurol Scand 70:104, 1984.
13. Bruce DA, Raphaely RC, Goldberg AI, et al: Pathophysiology, treatment, and outcome following severe head injury in children. Child Brain 5:174, 1979.
14. Campbell AGM: Children in a persistent vegetative state (editorial). Br Med J 289:1022, 1984.
15. Centers for Disease Control: Adverse Events Following Immunization. Surveillance Report No. 2, 1982–1984. Issued December 1986.
16. Chesney PJ, Crass BA, Polyak MB, et al: Toxic shock syndrome: Management and long-term sequelae. Ann Intern Med 96:847, 1982.
17. Ch'ien LT, Boehm RM, Robinson H, et al: Characteristic early electroencephalographic changes in herpes simplex encephalitis. Arch Neurol 34:361, 1977.
18. Chun RWM, Thompson WH, Grabow JD, et al: California arbovirus encephalitis in children. Neurology 18:369, 1968.
19. Corey L, Spear PG: Infections with herpes simplex viruses (parts 1 and 2). N Engl J Med 314:686, 749, 1986.
20. Crowell GF, Stump DA, Biller J, et al: The transient global amnesia-migraine connection. Arch Neurol 41:75, 1984.
21. Dearden NM: Ischaemic brain. Lancet 2:255, 1985.
22. Del Guidice E, Aicardi J: Atypical aspects of hypertensive encephalopathy in childhood. Neuropediatria 10:150, 1979.
23. Dershewitz RA, Kaye BA, Swisher CN: Treatment of children with posttraumatic transient loss of consciousness. Pediatrics 72:602, 1983.
24. Drake B, Ashwal S, Schneider S: Determination of cerebral death in the pediatric intensive care unit. Pediatrics 78:107, 1986.
25. Duhaime A-C, Gennarelli TA, Thibault LE, et al: The shaken baby syndrome. A clinical, pathological, and biomedical study. J Neurosurg 66:409, 1987.
26. Dupuis MJM, Pierre Ph, Gonsette RE: Transient global amnesia and migraine in twin sisters (letter). J Neurol Neurosurg Psychiatry 50:816,1987.
27. Ehyai A, Fenichel GM: The natural history of acute confusional migraine. Arch Neurol 35:368, 1978.
28. Emery ES: Acute confusional states in children with migraine. Pediatrics 60:110, 1977.
29. Epstein LG, Sharer LR, Joshi VV, et al: Progressive encephalopathy in children with acquired immune deficiency syndrome. Ann Neurol 17:488, 1985.
30. Filley CM, Cranberg LD, Alexander MP, et al: Neurobehavioral outcome after closed head injury in childhood and adolescence. Arch Neurol 44:194, 1987.

31. Finberg L: Hypernatremic (hypertonic) dehydration in infants. N Engl J Med 289:196, 1973.
32. Fischl MA, Richman DD, Grieco MH, et al: The efficacy of azidothymidine (AZT) in the treatment of patients with AIDS and AIDS-related complex. A double-blind, placebo-controlled trial. N Engl J Med 317:185, 1987.
33. Fitch SJ, Gerald B, Magill HL, et al: Central nervous system hypoxia in children due to near drowning. Radiology 156:647, 1985.
34. Fitzsimon RB, Wolfenden WH: Migraine coma. Meningitic migraine with cerebral oedema associated with a new form of autosomal dominant cerebellar ataxia. Brain 108:555, 1985.
35. Foley CM, Polinsky MS, Gruskin AB, et al: Encephalopathy in infants and children with chronic renal disease. Arch Neurol 38:656, 1981.
36. Freemon FR: Two roads to coma: The Scottish hypothesis. Med Hypotheses 2:82, 1976.
37. Geary DF, Fennell RS, Andriola M, et al: Encephalopathy in children with chronic renal failure. J Pediatr 96:41, 1980.
38. Gibbs FA, Gibbs EL, Carpenter PR, et al: Electroencephalographic abnormality in "uncomplicated" childhood diseases. JAMA 171:1050, 1959.
39. Grazer RE, Sutton JM, Friedstrom S, et al: Hyperammonemic encephalopathy due to essential amino acid hyperalimentation. Arch Intern Med 144:2278, 1984.
40. Haas DC, Ross GS: Transient global amnesia triggered by mild head trauma. Brain 109:251, 1986.
41. Hammond DN, Moll GW, Robertson GL, et al: Hypodipsic hypernatremia with normal osmoregulation of vasopressin. N Engl J Med 315:433, 1986.
42. Herskowitz J: Neurologic presentations of panic disorder in childhood and adolescence. Dev Med Child Neurol 28:617, 1986.
43. Hirtz DG, Nelson KB, Ellenberg JH: Seizures following childhood immunizations. J Pediatr 102:14, 1983.
44. Ho K-C, Hodach R, Varma R, et al: Kernicterus and central pontine myelinolysis in a 14-year-old boy with viral hepatitis. Ann Neurol 8:633, 1980.
45. Hurwitz ES, Barrett MJ, Bregman D, et al: Public Health Service study of Reye's syndrome and medications. JAMA 257:1905, 1987.
46. Jennett B, Teasdale G: Management of Head Injuries. FA Davis, Philadelphia, 1981, p 193.
47. Johnson RT, Griffin DE, Hirsch RL, et al: Measles encephalomyelitis—clinical and immunologic studies. N Engl J Med 310:137, 1984.
48. Karakusis PH: Considerations in the treatment of septic shock. Med Clin North Am 70:933, 1986.
49. Kennard C, Swash M: Acute viral encephalitis. Its diagnosis and outcome. Brain 104:129, 1981.
50. Knight ME, Roberts RJ: Phenothiazine and butyrophone intoxication in children. Pediat Clin North Am 33:299, 1986.
51. Krane EJ, Rockoff MA, Wallman JK, et al: Subclinical brain swelling in children during treatment of diabetic ketoacidosis. N Engl J Med 312:1147, 1985.
52. Kulberg A: Substance abuse: Clinical identification and management. Pediatr Clin North Am 33:325, 1986.
53. Kuroiwa Y, Celesia GC: Clinical significance of periodic EEG patterns. Arch Neurol 37:15, 1980.
54. Lambert SR, Johnson TE, Hoyt CS: Optic nerve and retinal hemorrhages associated with the shaken baby syndrome. Arch Ophthalmol 104:1509, 1986.
55. Landry ML, Booss J, Hsiung GD: Duration of vidarabine therapy in biopsy-negative herpes simplex encephalitis. JAMA 247:332, 1982.
56. Leads from the MMWR: Arboviral infections of the central nervous system. JAMA 253:3231, 1985.
57. Levy DE, Caronna JJ, Singer BH, et al: Predicting outcome from hypoxic-ischemic coma. JAMA 253:1420, 1985.
58. Lichtenstein PK, Heubi JE, Daugherty CC, et al: Grade I Reye's syndrome. A frequent cause of vomiting and liver dysfunction after varicella and upper-respiratory-infection. N Engl J Med 309:133, 1983.
59. Lyon LW: Neurologic manifestations of cat-scratch disease. Arch Neurol 25:23, 1971.
60. MacDonald KL, Osterholm MT, Hedberg CW, et al: Toxic shock syndrome. A newly recognized complication of influenza and influenzalike illness. JAMA 257:1053, 1987.
61. Malouf R, Brust JCM: Hypoglycemia: Causes, neurological manifestations, and outcome. Ann Neurol 17:421, 1985.
62. Mohnot D, Snead OC, Benton JW Jr: Burn encephalopathy in children. Ann Neurol 12:42, 1982.
63. Moshe SL, Alvarez LA: Diagnosis of brain death in children. J Clin Neurophysiol 3:239, 1986.
64. Norenberg MD: A hypothesis of osmotic endothelial injury. A pathogenetic mechanism in central pontine myelinolysis. Arch Neurol 40:66, 1983.
65. Obrecht R, Okhomina FOA, Scott DF: Value of EEG in acute confusional states. J Neurol Neurosurg Psychiatry 42:75, 1979.
66. O'Dougherty M, Wright FS, Loewenson RB, et al: Cerebral dysfunction after chronic hypoxia in children. Neurology 35:42, 1985.
67. O'Hare JA, Callaghan NM, Murnaghan DJ: Dialysis encephalopathy. Clinical, electroencephalographic and interventional aspects. Medicine 62:129, 1983.
68. Peltola H, Heinonen OP: Frequency of the true adverse reactions to measles-mumps-rubella vaccine. A double-blind-controlled trial in twins. Lancet 1:939, 1986.
69. Plum F, Posner JB: The Diagnosis of Stupor and Coma. 3rd edition. FA Davis Co, Philadelphia, 1980, p 19.
70. Pollock TM, Morris J: A 7-year survey of disorders attributed to vaccination in North West Thames region. Lancet 1:753, 1983.
71. President's Commission: Guidelines for the determination of death. JAMA 246:2184, 1981.
72. Rebouche CJ, Engel AG: Carnitine metabolism and deficiency syndromes. Mayo Clin Proc 58:533, 1983.
73. Reik L, Burgdorfer W, Donaldson IO: Neurologic abnormalities in Lyme disease without erythema chronicum migrans. Am J Med 81:73, 1986.
74. Rogers EL, Rogers MC: Fulminant hepatic failure and hepatic encephalopathy. Pediatr Clin North Am 27:701, 1980.
75. Rotundo A, Nevins TE, Lipton M, et al: Progressive encephalopathy in children with chronic renal disease. Kidney Int 21:486, 1982.
76. Salazar AM, Jabbari B, Vance SC, et al: Epilepsy after penetrating head injury. I. Clinical correlates. A report of the Vietnam Head Injury Study. Neurology 35:1406, 1985.
77. Selby G, Walker GL: Cerebral arteritis in cat-scratch disease. Neurology 29:1413, 1979.
78. Schroth G, Gawehn J, Thron A, et al: Early diagnosis of herpes simplex encephalitis by MRI. Neurology 37:179, 1987.
79. Scully RE, Mark EJ, McNeely BU: Case records of the Massachusetts General Hospital: Weekly clinicopathological conference, case 50-1984. N Engl J Med 311:1559, 1984.

80. Sedman AB, Wilkening GN, Warady BA, et al: Encephalopathy in childhood secondary to aluminum toxicity. J Pediatr 105:836, 1984.

81. Shaywitz BA, Lister G, Duncan CC: What is the best treatment for Reye's syndrome? Arch Neurol 43:730, 1986.

82. Snoek JW, Minderhould JM, Wilmink JT: Delayed deterioration following mild head injury in children. Brain 107:15, 1984.

83. Sriram S, Steinman L: Postinfectious and postvaccinial encephalomyelitis. Neurol Clin North Am 2:341, 1984.

84. Stetler HC, Orenstein WA, Bart KJ, et al: History of convulsions and use of pertussis vaccine. J Pediatr 107:175, 1985.

85. Stumpf DA, Parker Jr WD, Angelini C: Carnitine deficiency, organic acidemias, and Reye's syndrome. Neurology 35:1041, 1985.

86. Tofte RW, Williams DN: Clinical and laboratory manifestations of toxic shock syndrome. Ann Intern Med 96:843, 1982.

87. Trauner DA: What is the best treatment for Reye's syndrome? Arch Neurol 43:729, 1986.

88. Vernon DD, Holzman BH: Brain death: Considerations for pediatrics. J Clin Neurophysiol 3:251, 1986.

89. Ward JD, Becker DP, Miller JD, et al: Failure of prophylactic barbiturate coma in the treatment of severe head injury. J Neurosurg 62:383, 1985.

90. West JB: Do climbs to extreme altitude cause brain damage? Lancet 2:387, 1986.

91. Whitley RJ, Alford CA, Hirsch MS, et al: Vidarabine versus acyclovir therapy in herpes simplex encephalitis. N Engl J Med 314:144, 1986.

92. Whitley RJ, Soong S-J, Linneman C Jr, et al: Herpes simplex encephalitis. Clinical assessment. JAMA 247:317, 1982.

93. Whittington LK, Roscelli JD, Parry WH: Hemorrhagic shock and encephalopathy: Further description of a syndrome. J Pediatr 106:599, 1985.

94. Young B, Rapp RP, Norton JA, et al: Failure of prophylactically administered phenytoin to prevent early posttraumatic seizures. J Neurosurg 58:231, 1983.

95. Young B, Rapp RP, Norton JA, et al: Failure of prophylactically administered phenytoin to prevent late posttraumatic seizures. J Neurosurg 58:236, 1983.

3 Headache

■ Approach to Headache

Parents seek medical attention for a child with headache, not so much looking for relief of pain as to be assured that the headache is not a malevolent sign of intracranial disease such as brain tumor. If this is the understood purpose for consultation, then it may not be necessary in all cases to identify the cause of headache. The paramount goal is to provide assurance that headache is not a sign of serious illness. There are circumstances in which this is the only possible achievement. It is not possible to explain the basis of every headache, unless one finds comfort in using the term psychogenic as a synonym for idiopathic. It is possible, usually by history and physical examination alone, but sometimes with the aid of diagnostic studies, to distinguish headaches that are only painful from those that are harmful. This distinction can usually be made by identifying the structure or structures that are generating pain.

SOURCES OF PAIN

Pain-sensitive structures of the head and neck are summarized in Table 3.1. The major pain-sensitive structures inside the skull are blood vessels. Mechanisms that stimulate pain from blood vessels are vasodilation, inflammation, and traction-displacement. Traction-displacement of intracranial arteries is the major source of headache with increased intracranial pressure (see Chapter 4). The brain parenchyma, its ependymal lining, and meninges are insensitive to pain. Cranial nerves V, IX, and X carry pain fibers, and distortion of the intracranial portion of these nerves can produce pain. However, this is an uncommon event in children.

The innervation of pain from supertentorial intracranial vessels is transmitted by the trigeminal nerve, whereas pain from infratentorial intracranial vessels is transmitted by the first three cervical nerves. Arteries in the superficial portion of the dura are innervated by the ophthalmic division of the trigeminal nerve and refer pain to the eye and forehead. The middle meningeal artery is innervated by the second and third division of the trigeminal nerve and refers pain to the temple. Cerebral arteries are innervated by all three divisions of the trigeminal nerve and refer pain to the eye, forehead, and temple. In contrast, pain from all structures in the posterior fossa is referred to the occiput and neck.

Several different extracranial structures are pain-sensitive. Major scalp arteries are present around the eye, forehead, and temple and produce pain when dilated or stretched. Cranial bones are insensitive, but periosteum, especially in the sinuses and near the teeth, is painful when inflamed. The inflamed periosteum is usually tender to palpation or to other forms of physical stimulation. Muscles attached to the skull become a source of pain when there is prolonged contraction. The largest group of such muscles are the neck extensors, which attach to the occipital ridge, the masseter muscles, and the frontalis muscle. The mechanism of muscle pain

Table 3.1 SOURCES OF HEADACHE PAIN

Intracranial
    Cerebral and dural arteries
    Large veins and venous sinuses
Extracranial
    Extracranial arteries
    Periosteum/sinuses
    Muscles attached to skull
    Cervical roots
    Cranial nerves

is not fully understood, but is generally regarded to be caused by prolonged overcontraction. The extraocular muscles are a source of muscle contraction pain in patients with heterophoria. When an imbalance exists, especially in convergence, long periods of close work cause difficulty in maintaining conjugate gaze and pain is felt in the orbit.

Pain from the cervical roots and cranial nerves is generally due to mechanical traction from injury or malformation. Pain follows this nerve distribution: the neck and back of the head up to the vertex for the cervical roots, and the face for the cranial nerves.

DESCRIPTIONS OF PAIN

In most cases, history is everything in the attempt to diagnose the cause of headache. Yet in children, especially very young ones, the person experiencing pain is incapable of describing it. A young child asked to describe the quality of pain usually responds with sullen silence and looks imploringly at his mother to answer the foolish question. Encouraging remarks from the mother, such as "Don't look at me," or "Talk to the doctor, he needs to know," do not stimulate a response. To the young child, the only quality of pain is that it hurts and this should be self-evident. The doctor then tries to help the child with a litany of words that can be used to describe pain, e.g., throbbing, pulsating, tight, or sharp. Realizing that he has been identified as uncooperative with the authorities, the child seeks approval by confessing to all.

It is rarely productive to ask a child younger than ten years of age how often headaches occur or how long they last. Children of this age who wear wrist watches use them as a status symbol or as jewelry and do not consult them as a measure of time. For small children, as for Einstein, time is relative and cannot be expressed in absolute numbers.

One then turns to the parents to determine how long and how often headache has been occurring. Parents are usually quite helpful in this regard. The exception is the parent who replies, either through conviction or to impress you with the severity of the situation, that the child who is sitting comfortably before you has had a headache every day for the past six months or one year. At this point the temptation is great, but should be avoided, to ask the child if he or she is in pain at that very moment. The child must answer yes or make the mother appear a liar. The better question is, "How many different kinds of headache do you have?" The usual response is that there are two kinds of headache: the bad headache, of which the child complains spontaneously, and the mild headache, of which the child complains when asked, "Are you having a headache?" When such history is obtained, the physician should direct further inquiry to the bad headache and give short shrift to the other. An alternate explanation for the complaint of daily headaches of one year's duration is that the child has a flurry of headaches over a period of a week or two, then after a prolonged headache-free interval experiences another flurry of daily headaches.

Helpful responses to traditional questions concerning the history of headache can be obtained from children aged ten to twelve years or older (Table 3.2). There are several typical patterns of headache that, when present, allow recognition of either the source or mechanism of pain. Throbbing temporal pain is usually vascular in origin; steady, tight pain, especially in the occipital region or in a band around the head, is likely to be muscular in origin. Periosteal pain, especially inflammation of the sinuses, is localized and tender to palpation. Cervical root and cranial nerve pain have a radiating or shooting quality. Confusion arises when there are several mechanisms of pain experienced concurrently. It is common for individuals with migraine to also have a tension headache and for individuals with sinusitis to experience vascular headache as well.

A continuous, low-intensity, chronic headache, in the absence of associated symptoms or signs, is likely to be psychogenic. Intermittent headaches, especially those associated with nausea, from which the child recovers completely and is normal between attacks, is likely to be migraine. The recent onset of a severe headache, unlike anything previously experienced, from which the child never returns to a normal baseline, is probably due to significant intracranial disease.

Table 3.2 DIAGNOSTIC FEATURES OF HEADACHE

Length of illness
Frequency and duration
Location
Quality
Time of day
Associated features
Factors that precipitate
Factors that relieve

Most headaches are bilateral. Unilateral headache suggests migraine, intracranial mass lesions that are displacing local vessels without producing generalized increased intracranial pressure, and unilateral sinusitis. Time of onset may indicate a stressful period for a child, such as school or visitation by a separated parent.

EVALUATION

It is now commonplace for children referred to a pediatric neurologist for headache to present with a head computerized tomogram (CT) or at least a report of a normal CT. The only question asked by the primary physician was, "Does this child have a brain tumor?" Unfortunately, the normal CT neither explained nor cured the headache. Obtaining a routine CT or electroencephalogram (EEG) on every child who presents with headache is not cost-effective, and these tests are not a substitute for adequate history and physical examination.

If the history is typical for migraine and examination is normal, there is no reason to perform laboratory tests. As a rule, CT is unlikely to be helpful in a child with intermittent headaches who is normal in the interval. The first step in evaluation is to determine the source of pain. If the source is clearly extracranial, there is no reason to image the brain but there may be reason to image extracranial sources of pain, such as the sinuses or cervical spine. If the source of pain cannot be identified, laboratory investigations are warranted.

■ Migraine

Migraine is the most common cause of headache in children referred for neurologic consultation. It is a hereditary disorder transmitted by autosomal dominant inheritance. A positive migraine history in at least one parent is reported 90 percent of the time if both parents are personally interviewed and 80 percent of the time when only one parent is interviewed (Bille, 1962). The prevalence of migraine is 2.5 percent under the age of seven (both sexes equally affected), 5 percent from age seven to puberty (female to male ratio of 3:2), 5 percent in postpubertal males, and 10 percent in postpubertal females (Deubner, 1982; Sillanpaa, 1983). The prevalence in preschool children is probably higher than the recorded figure, because migraine symptoms in preschool children

tend to be atypical and are rarely identified as migraine at the time. The higher incidence of migraine in pubertal females as compared with that in males is probably related to the triggering effect of the menstrual cycle on migraine attacks.

TRIGGERING FACTORS

Among individuals with a predisposition to migraine, individual attacks are usually provoked by an idiosyncratic triggering factor. Common triggering factors are stress, exercise, head trauma, allergy, diet, and the premenstrual decline in circulating estrogen.

Stress and Exercise

When life-stress or exercise is the triggering factor, the onset of migraine symptoms may occur during stress or exercise or during the period of relaxation that follows. Therefore, stress is rarely a factor in provoking attacks upon awakening, but is likely to be contributory when attacks occur during school or shortly after returning home. Although there is no established "personality type" of migrainous school-aged children, those who are intense and fastidious about their performance place themselves under greater stress and more often implicate stress as a triggering factor.

Head Trauma

Head trauma probably provokes migraine attacks by causing sudden stretching (or other distortion) of cranial arteries. Trivial blows to the head during competitive sports are significant triggering factors because they occur on a background of vigorous exercise and stress (Matthews, 1972). A severe migraine attack—headache, vomiting, transitory neurologic deficits—following a head injury frequently suggests the possibility of intracranial hemorrhage. Unnecessary diagnostic tests can be avoided if the cause-and-effect relationship between head trauma and migraine is appreciated and the diagnosis of migraine established.

Transient cerebral blindness, as well as other transitory neurologic deficits, sometimes occur after head trauma in children with migraine (see Chapter 16). In some of these children, electroconvulsive discharges from the occipital lobes are recorded during the first twenty-four hours after the injury.

Allergy and Diet

An allergic basis for migraine has been considered because some migraineurs have attacks only during certain seasons of the year and others report the precipitation of attacks by the ingestion of specific foods. Although an allergic basis for migraine has not been substantiated and there is no evidence that children with migraine are more prone to allergies than other children (Bille, 1962), it is reasonable to assume that an allergic reaction, like any other stress, may serve as a triggering factor in a genetically predisposed individual.

Menstrual Cycle

The higher rate of prevalence of migraine among postpubertal girls as compared either with prepubertal children of both sexes or postpubertal boys supports the observation that hormonal changes in the normal female cycle serve to trigger attacks of migraine. The widespread use of oral contraceptives has provided some insight into the relationship between the female hormonal cycle and migraine. Oral contraceptives increase the frequency and intensity of migraine attacks in women with a previous history of migraine and may serve to precipitate the initial attack in genetically predisposed women who have previously been migraine-free (Kudrow, 1975; Whitty et al, 1966). Among women taking oral contraceptives, the greatest increase in frequency of migraine occurs at midcycle. Recent evidence suggests that the decline in concentration of circulating estrogens is the critical factor in precipitating an attack (Dalton, 1976; Somerville, 1971).

CLINICAL SYNDROMES

There are three major headache syndromes associated with migraine: classic migraine, common migraine, and cluster headache. It is not clear whether or not classic and common migraine are a variable expression of the same genetic defect: different members of the same kindred may manifest symptoms of classic or common migraine. Cluster headache is probably a distinct genetic entity with a relatively uniform presentation of symptoms within the same family (Ekbom, 1970). However, a common link between cluster headache and other forms of migraine is suggested by the occasional occurrence of classic migraine symptoms during an attack of cluster headache (Medina and Diamond, 1977).

In addition to the headache syndromes of migraine, there are also migraine equivalents in which the cardinal features are transitory disturbances in neurologic function. Headache is a minor feature or not present at all. Migraine equivalent syndromes are discussed in several other chapters (Table 3.3). They are variants of classic and common migraine, never of cluster.

Classic Migraine

Classic migraine is a biphasic event. In the initial phase, a wave of excitation followed by depression of cortical function spreads over both hemispheres from back to front. This is associated with decreased regional cerebral blood flow and transitory neurologic disturbances. Whether these disturbances are primarily due to ischemia or neuronal depression is uncertain. The second phase is ordinarily, but not necessarily, associated with increased blood flow in both the internal and external carotid circulation. It is associated with headache, nausea, and sometimes vomiting. The mechanism of headache and the nausea remains uncertain, but is probably not explained by increased blood flow alone.

During any individual attack, the major clinical symptoms may be related only to the first phase (migraine equivalents), only to the second phase (headache and vomiting), or both. The most common symptoms of the initial phase are visual aberrations: the perception of sparkling lights or colored lines, blind spots, blurred vision, hemianopia, transitory blindness, micropsia, and visual hallucinations. With proper interviewing techniques, visual symptoms can be identified in 41 percent of children with migraine (Hachinski et al, 1973). The visual symptoms tend to be stereotyped for each child and may be perceived in one eye, in one field, or without localization.

Visual hallucinations and other visual distortions may be associated with impairment of time

Table 3.3 MIGRAINE EQUIVALENTS

Acute confusional migraine (see Chapter 2)
Transient global amnesia (see Chapter 2)
Basilar migraine (see Chapter 10)
Benign paroxysmal vertigo (see Chapter 10)
Hemiplegic migraine (see Chapter 11)
Paroxysmal torticollis (see Chapter 14)
Ophthalmoplegic migraine (see Chapter 15)
Cyclic vomiting

sense and body image. This symptom complex in migraine has been referred to as "the Alice-in-Wonderland syndrome" (Golden, 1979). More extreme disturbances in mental states—amnesia, confusion, and psychosis—are discussed in the sections on confusional migraine and transient global amnesia (see Chapter 2).

After visual aberrations, dysesthesias of the limbs and perioral region are the next most common sensory symptoms in classic migraine. The occurrence of focal motor deficit, usually hemiplegia or ophthalmoplegia, is referred to as complicated migraine. Such deficits, although alarming, are transitory; normal function usually returns within twenty-four hours and always within seventy-two hours.

A migraine attack may terminate at the end of the initial phase and headache is not experienced. Alternatively, the initial phase may be brief or asymptomatic and then headache is the presenting symptom. The pain is frequently dull at first, and then becomes throbbing, pulsating, or pounding. Severe headache that is maximal at onset is not migraine. Pain is unilateral in approximately two thirds of patients and bilateral in the remainder. It is most intense in the region of the eye, forehead, and temple. Eventually, the pain becomes constant and diffuse as tension headache is superimposed upon migraine. The headache lasts two to six hours and is associated at least with nausea and sometimes vomiting. Anorexia and photophobia are concomitant symptoms. The child appears ill and needs to lie down. The onset of vomiting frequently heralds the end of the attack. As discomfort diminishes, the fatigued child falls into a deep sleep. Normal function is resumed upon awakening.

Most patients experience one to four attacks each month. However, there may be long intervals in which the child is symptom-free and other intervals in which attacks occur more than once each week. Those with frequent headaches are probably experiencing a life-stress.

Common Migraine

Common migraine differs from classic migraine because the symptoms are more variable and do not regularly evolve in a biphasic mode of neurologic aura and headache. Consequently, the attacks are less readily identified as migrainous in nature. A pre-headache phase is not prominent. Visual disturbances, such as described for classic migraine, may occur, but the more typical symptoms are personality change, malaise, dizziness, and nausea. Recurrent vomiting may be the only manifestation of common migraine in preschool children.

The headache may be unilateral in location and pounding in quality, but more often the child has difficulty in localizing the pain and describing its quality. When the headache is prolonged, the pain is not of uniform intensity; instead, intermittent severe headaches are superimposed on a background of chronic discomfort in the neck and other pericranial muscles (Olesen, 1978). There is difficulty separating common migraine from tension headache. The child appears sick, wants to lie down, and is sensitive to light and sound. Nausea and vomiting may occur repeatedly, but do not herald the termination of the attack, and can be more prominent than the headache.

Cluster Headache

Cluster headache is considerably less common than migraine and is generally regarded to be genetically distinct. The prevalence of cluster headache in the United States is 0.4 percent for men and 0.08 percent for women (Kudrow, 1980). Approximately 85 percent of patients are males. The onset occurs almost exclusively after age ten, but may occur in those as young as age three (Kudrow, 1980). Eighty percent of patients have clusters of headaches over a period of weeks or months separated by intervals of one to two years. The other 20 percent have chronic headache; such headaches are considered to be the cluster type despite the lack of "clustering" because of associated features (Pearce, 1980).

Headache is the initial symptom; pain is always unilateral and the same side of the head is affected in each attack. It begins behind and around one eye, then spreads to the entire hemicranium. During an attack, the patient cannot lie still, but typically walks the floor in anguish. Pain is always intense and may be described as throbbing or constant. The scalp may seem edematous and tender. One third of patients experience sudden intense jabs of pain suggesting tic douloureux. Nausea and vomiting are not associated, but symptoms of hemicranial autonomic dysfunction—injection of the conjunctiva, tearing of the eye, Horner syndrome, sweating, flushing of the face, and stuffiness of the nose—develop ipsilateral to the headache. The duration of an attack may be as brief as ten minutes or as long as four hours, but thirty minutes to two hours is typical. As a rule, only one attack occurs each day but several attacks within twenty-four hours is not unusual. A cluster of daily attacks lasting four to eight weeks may occur once or twice a year, often in the autumn or spring. Patients are headache-free in the interim.

Alcohol ingestion is a common trigger of cluster headaches, but only during the period of susceptibility.

DIAGNOSIS

The diagnosis of migraine is based on clinical observation and cannot be confirmed or refuted by laboratory tests. Salient features are a family history of migraine and some combination of recurrent headache, nausea, or neurologic disturbances. There should be reluctance to make the diagnosis if both parents are questioned and family history is negative. Motion sickness is present in 45 percent and somnambulism in 30 percent of children with migraine (Barabas et al, 1983a, 1983b).

Electroencephalography

The most frequent EEG abnormality during a classic migraine attack is a slow wave focus in the temporal lobe of one hemisphere. During a basilar attack, the most common abnormality is occipital slowing, especially intermittent rhythmic delta. Between attacks, the EEG is usually normal. Asymptomatic central spikes are observed in 9 percent of the children with migraine as compared with 1.9 percent of healthy children, suggesting a common link between Rolandic epilepsy (see Chapter 1) and migraine (Kinast et al, 1982). Fourteen-and-six positive spikes, a normal adolescent pattern, occur twice as commonly in children with migraine as age-matched controls (Jay, 1982). Its increased prevalence in children with migraine is of uncertain significance.

TREATMENT

The essential caveat for the treatment of migraine in children is that irrespective of treatment, about one half of all patients have more than a 50 percent reduction in headache frequency in the six months following the initial visit to a neurologist (Prensky and Sommer, 1979). Once the child's parents are convinced that headache is due to migraine and not brain tumor, they are less anxious, the child is more relaxed, and headaches either decrease in frequency or are discussed less often. The therapeutic efficacy of neurologic consultation has the dual effect of making drug evaluation difficult while at the same time reinforcing the neurologist's notion that the drug regimen selected is useful.

There are two approaches to migraine therapy: treatment of the acute attack and prophylaxis. Whichever approach is selected, it is important to develop in the patient and family a sense of "learning how to live with migraine":

1. Avoid, when possible, those activities that are known to trigger attacks.
2. When attacks occur, give in and go to bed.
3. Use as little medication as possible, because repeated dosages only lead to further gastrointestinal upset.
4. Do not use narcotics or other addicting drugs. The treatment should be less harmful than the attack.

Treating the Acute Attack

Although aspirin and other common analgesics may provide relief of pain in children who suffer from only mild headaches, non-narcotic analgesics do not provide adequate relief of pain for most patients; antimigraine agents should be prescribed. Two oral antimigraine agents are available to treat the acute attack: ergotamine and isometheptene. Parenteral therapy with ergot or chlorpromazine may be required for severe intractable migraine.

Ergotamine

Ergotamine is the drug most often prescribed for the acute treatment of migraine. The response is variable and should never be used for the purpose of diagnosis. Ergotamine preparations are commercially available for administration by the parenteral, oral, rectal, sublingual, and inhalation routes. Sublingual administration is preferred, not because it is more effective, but because it is convenient to take and less likely to produce gastric upset. The sublingual dose is 2 mg. It should be taken as early as possible in the evolution of the attack, preferably before headache is established. A second tablet may be taken twenty minutes after the first, during a single attack. Repeated administration should be discouraged, as it intensifies nausea and vomiting.

Isometheptene

Isometheptene mucate is a sympathomimetic agent commercially available as *Midrin*, a compound containing 65 mg of isometheptene mucate, 325 mg of acetaminophen, and 100 mg of the antihistamine dichloralphenazone. Midrin is more effective than placebo or ergotamine in reducing the nausea and vomiting of migraine, but is not more effective in treating headache (Yuill et al, 1972). The usual dosage is two capsules at the onset of an attack.

Chlorpromazine

Adult migraineurs, and sometimes adolescents, may present to an emergency room in a prolonged, severe migraine attack seeking relief from pain. Narcotics are frequently administered, but are inappropriate as they may lead to addiction.

Intramuscular chlorpromazine, 1 mg/kg, is a safe and effective alternative. In one study, 96 percent of adult migraineurs presenting to an emergency room were relieved of pain and nausea within one hour of injection (Iserson, 1983). The only adverse reaction is orthostatic hypotension, but this is less likely to occur in children than in adults.

Migraine Prophylaxis

An extraordinary number of agents with diverse pharmacologic properties have been administered daily to migraineurs in an effort to prevent attacks. These agents include, but are not limited to, hormones, serotonin agonists and antagonists, tranquilizers, antidepressants, antihistamines, anticonvulsants, calcium channel blocking agents, vasoconstrictors, and vasodilators. For many of these agents, double-blind control trials in adults have demonstrated significant improvement in frequency of migraine as compared with placebo. Unfortunately, success in the treated group rarely exceeds 50 percent and statistical significance is achieved because patients on placebo have done worse than might be expected.

Propranolol is the only agent that consistently demonstrates greater efficacy than placebo and has been the drug of choice in migraine prophylaxis. Calcium channel blocking agents have undergone recent trials in children and adults and appear to be a promising group of agents.

Propranolol

Propranolol is a beta-adrenergic blocking agent that was serendipitously found useful in preventing migraine attacks in patients being treated for cardiovascular disease. This observation led to several control trials in which propranolol was found effective in 55 to 84 percent of patients (Rosen, 1983). The dose in children is 2 mg/kg in three divided doses (Ludvigsson, 1974). Adverse reactions—hypotension, pulse rate reduction, and provocation of underlying asthma—may occur at low dosages. For this reason, propranolol should be started at less than one-half the therapeutic dose and slowly increased as tolerated. Depression is a common complication, necessitating discontinuation of therapy, and parents should be warned of this reaction when the drug is started. Plasma levels of propranolol are not useful in determining the effective dose for migraine (Cortelli et al, 1985).

Patients who respond to propranolol do not develop tolerance. However, if the drug is abruptly stopped after six to twelve months of therapy, some patients will have rebound headaches of increased frequency (Diamond, 1976). Others will continue to demonstrate the benefits achieved during therapy.

Calcium Channel Blocking Agents

Calcium channel blocking agents are vasodilators that prevent the influx of calcium into vascular smooth muscle. They have been used extensively for coronary artery disease and are effective dilators of the cerebral vasculature as well. Specific agents that have been tested in migraine are listed in Table 3.4. Cyproheptadine and nifedipine have been studied in children, and a mg/kg dose is available. Nimodipine (not yet available in the United States), flunarizine, and verapamil have not been tested in children with migraine and the dosages provided in Table 3.4 are for adults. Calcium channel blocking agents as a group have little or no toxicity in children with a normal cardiovascular system.

Table 3.4 CALCIUM CHANNEL BLOCKING AGENTS

Cyproheptadine	0.2–0.4 mg/kg
Nifedipine	1 mg/kg
Flunarizine	5 mg b.i.d.
Nimodipine	40 mg t.i.d.
Verapamil	80 mg t.i.d.

Cyproheptadine should be an especially potent prophylactic agent for migraine. It is not only a calcium channel blocking agent but also an antihistamine with mild to moderate antiserotonin activity. However, in large clinical trials, fewer than 50 percent of patients reported improvement (Lance et al, 1970). In contrast, 80 percent improvement rates are reported for flunarizine (Louis, 1981), verapamil (Markley et al, 1984; Solomon et al, 1983) and nifedipine (Meyer and Hardenberg, 1983). However, all of these reports are based on very small numbers of patients. A two-week to three-week delay is expected between the onset of treatment and the anticipated result.

Treating Cluster Headache

The treatment of cluster headache is usually directed at suppressing recurrent headaches rather than treating a headache in progress. The inhalation of 100 percent oxygen at a rate of 7 liters/minute is effective in relieving an acute attack in 82 percent of patients (Kudrow, 1981).

Methysergide Maleate

Methysergide maleate, a serotonin agonist, was popularized as a prophylactic agent for migraine and for cluster in 1964 (Graham, 1964). Methysergide is effective in preventing attacks in more than 50 percent of migraineurs. The dose in adults is 2 mg three times a day after meals to avoid gastric upset. A mg/kg dose has not been established for children. Unfortunately, retroperitoneal fibrosis, as well as other fibrotic syndromes, occur in patients taking the medication regularly for periods greater than one year. The fibrosis is ordinarily reversible when medication is stopped. Methysergide maleate can be used safely for periods of less than six months and is particularly useful for short-term therapy in patients with cluster headache. It is effective in 70 percent of patients (Curran et al, 1967).

Prednisone

Prednisone is effective in suppressing bouts of cluster headache in three quarters of patients who are unresponsive to methysergide (Kudrow, 1980). An initial dose of 1 mg/kg is administered for the first five days and then tapered over the following two weeks. If headaches reappear during the tapering process, the dose is increased and maintained at a level sufficient to keep the patient headache-free. If the bout of cluster is prolonged, prednisone should be tapered before the appearance of adverse side effects.

Lithium Carbonate

Lithium is used in patients with the chronic form of cluster in whom headache never ceases. Increasing doses are used to achieve a blood concentration of 1.2 mEq/L (1.2 mmol/L). Most patients have at least a partial response to lithium, but only 50 percent are relieved completely.

■ Nonmigrainous Vascular Headaches

Other than migraine, vascular headache may be caused by traction or displacement of intracranial vessels, vasodilation of intracranial or extracranial vessels, and vasculitis. Traction and displacement of intracranial vessels is the primary mechanism of headache in patients with increased intracranial pressure and is discussed in Chapter 4.

VASODILATIVE HEADACHES

Table 3.5 lists several conditions that cause vasodilation in either the internal carotid circulation, the external carotid circulation, or both, and result in headache. The list is not intended to be exhaustive, but focuses instead on headaches that are likely to be encountered in childhood and adolescence. Vasodilative headaches are generally bitemporal or diffuse and described as pounding, throbbing, or pulsating. The pain is made worse by sudden jarring or movement of the head. There may be difficulty in differentiating migrainous from nonmigrainous vas-

Table 3.5 NONMIGRAINOUS
VASODILATIVE HEADACHE

Fever
Drugs and toxins
Alcohol
Marijuana
Caffeine withdrawal
Food additives
Effort headache
Orgasmic headache
Hypertension
Post-traumatic headache

cular headaches by the description of pain. Further, many factors that trigger vascular headache in nonmigrainous individuals also trigger migraine in migraineurs. Severe vascular headache of any cause is often compounded by tension headache.

Fever

Clinical Features. Fever is the most common cause of vascular headache. The degree of vasodilation parallels the rise of body temperature. Vasodilation is both intracranial and extracranial. Headache is bitemporal or diffuse in location and throbbing in quality.

Diagnosis. The association between fever and headache is ordinarily self-evident and does not lead to diagnostic studies unless infection of the nervous system or subarachnoid hemorrhage is suspected. Suspicion is raised when headache or personality change is disproportionate to the degree of fever and when meningismus is present.

Treatment. Aspirin or acetaminophen is effective for combating both fever and headache, but aspirin is contraindicated in children because of the possibility of Reye syndrome (see Chapter 2).

Drugs and Toxins

Many psychotropic drugs, analgesics, and cardiovascular agents have vasodilating properties. Drug-induced headache should be suspected in a child who has vascular headache in relation to the administration of any drug.

Alcohol Headache

Ethyl alcohol produces vasodilation and may precipitate migraine or cluster headache in a predisposed individual. Hangover headache is probably due to vasodilation as well, but the mechanism is not fully understood. Acetaldehyde, an oxidation product of alcohol, is an established cause of vascular headache and may be responsible for the suffering of hangover.

Most hangover headaches are treated with time. Concurrent gastritis prevents the use of oral medication.

Marijuana

Marijuana is a peripheral vasodilator and produces a sensation of warmth, injection of the conjunctivae, and sometimes frontal headache. The headache is mild and ordinarily experienced only during use. However, marijuana metabolites are present in the blood for several days after use and prolonged vasodilative headaches may be present chronically in children who are regular users.

Caffeine Withdrawal

Clinical Features. Many children, especially adolescents, drink large volumes of carbonated beverages containing caffeine each day. Caffeine has vasoconstricting properties and does not in itself cause headache. However, rebound vasodilation occurs when blood caffeine concentrations fall. It is commonplace for individuals who regularly drink large amounts of caffeine to notice a dull frontotemporal headache an hour or more after last use. More caffeine is taken to relieve the headache, and caffeine addiction is initiated (Greden et al, 1980). Withdrawal symptoms eventually become quite severe and include throbbing headache, anxiety, and malaise.

Diagnosis. Most people associate caffeine with coffee and are not cognizant of the caffeine content of soft drinks. Adolescent girls frequently use diet colas as a substitute for food and become caffeine-dependent.

Treatment. Caffeine addiction, like other addictions, is often hard to break. Some patients can be weaned off caffeine, but most require abrupt cessation and experience withdrawal symptoms. Hospitalization and sedation are sometimes necessary to help patients through withdrawal.

Food Additives

Clinical Features. Chemicals are added to food as preservatives and to enhance appearance. Ordinarily, the concentration is low and adverse effects occur only in individuals who are genetically sensitive. Nitrites are powerful vasodilators used widely to enhance the appearance of cured meats such as hot dogs, salami, bacon, and ham. Diffuse, throbbing headaches may occur just after ingestion.

Monosodium glutamate (MSG) is used primarily in Chinese cooking and may produce generalized vasodilation. A syndrome described in sensitive individuals includes both a throbbing bitemporal headache and a band headache, sometimes associated with pressure and tightness of the face and a burning sensation over the body (Schaumberg et al, 1969). Symptoms occur twenty to twenty-five minutes after MSG ingestion.

Diagnosis. The regular association between ingestion of a specific food and vascular headache quickly becomes self-evident to the patient.

Treatment. Headache can be prevented only by avoidance of the offending chemical. This may not be easy, since it is often difficult to determine which additives are present in prepared foods.

Benign Exertional Headache

Exertion, especially during competitive sports, is a known trigger for migraine in predisposed individuals (see "Migraine" earlier in this chapter). Physical exertion is more likely to produce headache when effort is prolonged and sufficient to sustain the pulse at twice its resting rate for ten minutes or longer (Diamond and Dalessio, 1982). Pain begins during or just following exercise and may last as long as four hours. It is throbbing in quality and bitemporal in location.

Diagnosis. The association between exertion and headache is easily recognized. Medical consultation is usually not requested unless the patient is a serious athlete whose performance is impaired.

Treatment. Exertional headache can sometimes be prevented by taking ergotamine or methysergide prior to activities that are known to induce benign exertional headache. Indomethacin, 25 mg three times daily, is also reported to reduce the incidence of attacks (Diamond and Dalessio, 1982).

Orgasmic Headache

Clinical Features. A dull muscle contraction headache, primarily occipital, but also in a band distribution, may be experienced as sexual excitement increases (Lance, 1982). It is not incapacitating and does not disrupt sexual activity. Benign exertional headache may also occur during prolonged sexual arousal. A more severe and dangerous headache is one which occurs just before and during the moment of orgasm. This headache, caused by sudden increase in blood pressure, is similar to the headache associated with pheochromocytoma. Blood pressure elevation during orgasm is considerable and can be associated with subarachnoid hemorrhage and stroke in patients with underlying risk factors.

The pain is explosive, but of short duration. It is usually located behind the eyes or in the temples and is throbbing in quality. Severe headache lasts only for minutes, but may be followed by a milder headache that can linger for hours. Orgasmic headache does not occur with every orgasm and is more often experienced during periods of frequent sexual activity, especially when orgasm is achieved twice within a brief period. Males are affected more commonly than females.

Diagnosis. Orgasmic headaches are sufficiently severe and alarming that some authorities suggest a contrasted CT scan in all patients (Diamond and Dalessio, 1982). A CT scan is clearly indicated if there is any suggestion of subarachnoid hemorrhage or focal neurologic disturbances. However, when orgasmic headache occurs infrequently, and episodes are separated by long intervals of time, the cost of CT is probably not warranted when neurologic examination is normal.

Treatment. There is no established method for preventing orgasmic headache other than decreasing the frequency of intercourse where frequency is clearly a factor. Ergot may be useful in some individuals and propranolol prophylaxis in others (Johns, 1986).

Hypertension

An acute rise in systemic blood pressure clearly causes the explosive throbbing headache associated with orgasm and pheochromocytoma. Several authorities have suggested that individuals with chronic hypertension may have low-grade occipital headache on awakening that diminishes as the patient gets up and begins activity. However, there is no convincing evidence that chronic hypertension is a cause of headache and in most individuals hypertension is a silent disease. The development of chronic headache in children with renal disease should not be ascribed to hypertension (see Chapter 2). Instead, alternative causes must be pursued. Headaches are common in patients on dialysis and may be due to tension, the precipitation of migraine attacks, and dialysis itself (Bana et al, 1972). Dialysis headache begins a few hours after the procedure is terminated and is characterized by mild bifrontal throbbing headache, which may be associated with nausea and vomiting.

Posttraumatic Headache

Several different kinds of headache may be associated with head trauma, including vascular headache, tension headache, and psychogenic headache. Vascular headache is experienced in 40 percent of patients in the first day or two after head injury. It is a diffuse pounding headache made worse by movement of the head or by coughing and straining. Dizziness may be associated. Posttraumatic vascular headaches subside spontaneously. Prolonged posttraumatic headaches are generally psychogenic, and are not vascular in origin (see Chapter 2).

VASCULITIS

Headaches due to vasculitis, especially temporal arteritis, are important in the differential diagnosis of vascular headaches in adults. Cerebral vasculitis is uncommon in childhood and usually occurs as part of a collagen vascular disease, secondary to a hypersensitivity reaction, or as part of an infection of the nervous system.

Connective Tissue Disorders

Headache is a relatively common feature of systemic lupus erythematosus and mixed connective tissue disease (Bronshvag et al, 1978; Meislin et al, 1968). In patients with connective tissue disease, it is not clear that neurologic symptoms, including headache, are caused by vasculitis of the cerebral arteries.

Clinical Features. Headache is not a presenting symptom of lupus in children. The common presenting symptoms are fever, arthritis, and skin rash. Symptoms referrable to the nervous system—seizures and mental changes—are the initial manifestation in less than 5 percent of affected children. Hepatosplenomegaly and lymphadenopathy are present in approximately 70 percent of children, twice as common as in adults.

Mixed connective disease is a syndrome with symptoms of lupus erythematosus, scleroderma, and polymyositis. It usually has a more benign course than lupus. Thirty-five percent of patients with mixed connective disease report vascular headaches. The headaches are only moderate in severity and generally do not interfere with activities of daily living. Headaches may be unilateral or bilateral, but are generally throbbing in quality. More than half of patients report visual aura, and some will have nausea and vomiting. Those with visual aura and vascular headaches may be classified as migraine, but it is statistically unlikely that such a high percentage of patients with mixed connective disease also have migraine.

Diagnosis. The diagnosis of connective tissue disease depends upon the combination of a compatible clinical syndrome and the demonstration of antinuclear antibodies in the blood. The presence of antinuclear antibodies in a child with headache who has no systemic symptoms of connective tissue disease should suggest the possibility of a hypersensitivity reaction.

Treatment. Children with connective tissue disease are ordinarily treated with corticosteroids. In many cases, headaches develop while the child is already taking corticosteroids and this should not be an indication to increase the dose. Headache is not a disabling symptom, it does not indicate a generalized encephalopathy, and it should be treated with analgesics.

Hypersensitivity Vasculitis

The important causes of hypersensitivity vasculitis in children are serum sickness, Henoch-Schönlein purpura (see Chapter 11), and amphetamine abuse (Matick et al, 1983). Patients with serum sickness and Henoch-Schönlein purpura have systemic symptoms that precede the headache. In contrast, amphetamine abusers may have only cerebral vasculitis and present with headache, encephalopathy, focal neurologic deficits, and subarachnoid hemorrhage.

Encephalitis

The vascular headache associated with viral encephalitis is caused in part by vasculitis and in part by vascular displacement and traction due to increased intracranial pressure (see Chapter 2). Encephalitis should be considered in children with acute onset of headache associated with personality change or seizures.

■ Muscle Contraction Headache

ACUTE TENSION HEADACHE

Clinical Features. Acute tension headache is an exceedingly common headache in people of all ages and both sexes. It is generally brought on by fatigue, exertion, and temporary life stress. The mechanism is prolonged contraction of muscles attached to the skull. The pain is described as constant, aching, and tight. It is localized mainly to the back of the head and neck, sometimes becomes diffuse, and may be described as a constricting band around the head. Vascular headache and acute tension headache may be concurrent. Nausea, vomiting, and other symptoms are not present.

Diagnosis. Acute tension headache should be separated from chronic tension headache, which has similar clinical features but persists for weeks, months, and years (see the discussion on psychogenic headache later on). Chronic tension headache is probably not a muscle contraction headache. Acute tension headache is self-diagnosed, and the individual never seeks medical attention.

Treatment. Pain is relieved by rest or relaxation and also responds to aspirin or acetaminophen.

WHIPLASH AND OTHER NECK INJURIES

Whiplash and other neck injuries produce pain by rupture of cervical disks, damage to soft tissue, injury to occipital nerves, and excessive muscle contraction. The muscle contraction component is an effort to splint the area of injury and thereby reduce further tissue damage. Constant contraction of the neck extensors produces a dull aching pain not only in the neck but also in the shoulders and upper arms. The head is generally kept in a fixed position. Nausea and vomiting are not associated.

Diagnosis. Following any neck or head injury, radiographs of the cervical spine are needed to determine the presence of fracture or dislocation. Shooting pains that radiate either to the occiput or down the arm and into the fingers suggest the possibility of disk herniation and require further study with myelography or CT.

Treatment. Muscle contraction headache following cervical spine injuries is relieved by lying or sitting with the head supported, the superficial application of heat to the painful muscles, muscle relaxants, and simple analgesics.

EYESTRAIN

Clinical Features. Prolonged ocular near-fixation in a child with a latent disturbance in convergence may cause dull aching pain behind the eyes that is quickly relieved when the eyes are closed. The pain is of muscular origin and caused by the continuous effort to maintain conjugate gaze. If work is continued despite ocular pain, acute tension headache may be superimposed.

Diagnosis. Children who complain of eyestrain are often thought to have refractive errors and eyeglasses are fitted. In fact, refractive errors do not cause eyestrain in children as presbyopia does in adults.

Treatment. Eyestrain is relieved by resting the eyes.

■ Other Extracranial Pain Syndromes

SINUSITIS

It is commonplace, when seeking a family history of migraine, for parents to identify their own episodic headache, preceded by scintillating scotoma and followed by nausea and vomiting, as sinusitis. It is a favored diagnosis by physicians and patients to describe most chronic or episodic headaches and is usually wrong.

Clinical Features. Children with sinusitis are usually sick. They are febrile, feel stuffy, and have difficulty maintaining a clear airway. Localized tenderness is present over the infected frontal or maxillary sinuses, and inflammation of the ethmoid or sphenoidal sinuses causes deep midline pain behind the nose. Pain is exaggerated by blowing the nose or by quick movements of the head, especially bending forward. Vascular headache due to fever may be concurrent.

Diagnosis. Radiographs reveal clouding of the sinuses and sometimes a fluid level. CT of the skull is exceptionally accurate in identifying sinusitis, but is usually an unnecessary expense.

Treatment. The primary objective of treatment is to allow the sinus to drain. This is usually accomplished with decongestants, but sometimes surgery is required. Antibiotics have limited usefulness if drainage is not established.

TEMPOROMANDIBULAR JOINT (TMJ) SYNDROME

Any discussion of TMJ syndrome must begin with the caveat that there remains considerable uncertainty concerning the association of temporomandibular joint disease and headache.

The temporomandibular joint syndrome has been described in children age eight years and older (Katzberg et al, 1985). The duration of symptoms before diagnosis is as long as five years and averages twenty-one months. It is not generally recognized as a disease of childhood. The primary disturbance is an arthritis of the joint that produces localized pain in the lower face and joint crepitus. Because of pain on one side, chewing is performed on the opposite side. Unfortunately, this has the unwanted effect of overuse of the affected side. The overused masseter muscle becomes tender and a muscle contraction headache ensues and is felt on the side of the face and at the vertex. The cause of arthritis is generally attributed to dental malocclusion, but a history of prior injury of the jaw is reported in one third of children with temporomandibular joint syndrome.

Diagnosis. Radiographs of the temporomandibular joint demonstrate some internal derangement in 94 percent of affected children and degenerative arthritis in 39 percent (Katzberg et al, 1985). Magnetic resonance imaging (MRI) of the joint using surface coils is said to provide the most effective technique of demonstrating disturbed joint architecture (Katzberg et al, 1986).

Treatment. Treatment for TMJ syndrome has not been established based upon controlled experiments. Placebos provide considerable benefit and extensive oral surgery is not indicated. Nonsteroidal inflammatory agents, heat to the tense muscles, and dental splints may all prove useful.

CHRONIC TENSION (PSYCHOGENIC) HEADACHE

It has been a recurring theme of this chapter that life-stress is a factor in triggering several different kinds of headache. Migraine is the most common chronic headache syndrome in children for which life-stress is a critical triggering factor. After migraine, tension headache is the next most common cause of chronic headache in children. When adults with chronic tension headache are asked about the onset of their symptoms, almost 50 percent date the onset before age twenty and 15 percent before age ten (Lance et al, 1965). Females are affected three times more frequently than males.

Unlike that of acute tension headache, which is muscular in origin, the mechanism of chronic tension headache is not well understood and probably arises from several different pain-sensitive structures. Almost all individuals with chronic tension headache suffer from depression and anxiety. The potential for suicide must be explored whenever there is evidence of serious depression. Chronic headache in children is often a response to a real life-stress situation such as physical and sexual abuse, pressure to succeed in activities for which the child is noncompetitive, and nonacceptance by peers. Secondary gain, in the form of avoidance of a difficult situation, is common.

Clinical Features. Pain is almost always bilateral and diffuse. The back of the head is more often painful than the front, and the site of most intense pain may shift during the course of the day. Much of the time, headache is dull and aching; sometimes it has a pounding vascular quality and then is more intense. Headache is generally present upon awakening and may continue all day. Most children describe an undulating course characterized by long periods in almost every day in which headache is present and shorter intervals when they are headache-free.

Chronic tension headache is not associated with nausea, vomiting, or transitory neurologic disturbances. When these associated features are present, they usually occur only a few times a month and suggest that the patient has both intermittent migraine and chronic tension headache. Neurologic examination should be normal.

Diagnosis. The diagnosis of chronic tension headache is to some extent a diagnosis of exclusion. It is important to be certain that chronic headache is not caused by migraine or increased intracranial pressure, conditions requiring specific treatment. Most children with chronic tension headache will have had a head CT scan before referral to a neurologist, and if not, it is reasonable that one be done. No matter how convinced the physician is that the child does not have increased intracranial pressure by history and physical examination, parents are rarely convinced by anything less than CT. It is difficult to investigate the cause of chronic tension headache until the specter of brain tumor has been laid to rest. An EEG is indicated in selected individuals in whom the intermittent nature of the headache or associated features suggest the possibility of epilepsy.

All children with chronic tension headache must be asked the question, "Do you have more than one kind of headache?" This is important to separate concurrent headache syndromes such as migraine and chronic tension headache. Once the diagnosis of chronic tension headache is established, the severity of depression must be analyzed. This is probably the most important factor in determining whether psychiatric consultation is indicated.

Treatment. Chronic tension headache is by definition difficult to treat or it wouldn't be a chronic headache. Most children who are moderately or severely depressed and all who are suicidal should be referred for psychotherapy. Many children have easily recognizable sources of anxiety that can be expressed or identified. Unfortunately, identification of the source of anxiety does not make it go away, although it is an important first step in resolving the conflict. In many children, headache is not caused by a single issue, rather headache is used in response to several different life-stresses and becomes a lifestyle. Many such children will benefit either from psychotherapy or physiologic techniques such as relaxation exercises or biofeedback.

Most patients will have tried and received no benefit from several over-the-counter analgesics before coming to a doctor. The use of more powerful analgesics or analgesic-muscle relaxant combinations will also prove to be of limited or no value. Antidepressants are the only class of drugs that are found to be beneficial for chronic tension headache. Increasing doses of amitriptyline at bedtime, as tolerated, have proved beneficial in clinical trials (Lance, 1982).

Benzodiazepines may be useful when anxiety is a more significant symptom than depression. Diazepam has been the one most often administered, but longer acting benzodiazepines such as alprazolam are becoming more popular. A small dose is first given at bedtime and then during daytime as well with sedation as a limiting factor.

SEIZURE HEADACHES

Diffuse headache caused by vasodilation of cerebral arteries is a frequent postictal symptom following a generalized tonic-clonic convulsion. In patients who have both epilepsy and migraine, one can trigger the other, so that concurrent headache and seizure activity are experienced frequently. Approximately 1 percent of epileptics report headache as a seizure manifestation (Young and Blume, 1983). This phenomenon has been termed "seizure headaches" (Swaiman and Frank, 1978). Most patients with seizure headaches are known epileptics, but some children present with headache as the only manifestation of their seizure disorder.

The association of migraine and epilepsy are discussed in Chapters 1 and 10.

Clinical Features. Several different syndromes are described in which headache is an epileptic manifestation. Headache may be the only symptom of seizure activity (Swaiman and Frank, 1978). In such children, headaches are paroxysmal, generally bifrontal, frequently accompanied by nausea and vomiting, and followed by lethargy and sleep. The sequence suggests migraine. However, there is no family history of migraine, nor can a triggering factor be identified for attacks. Attacks may occur during sleep or anytime during the day and last for several hours. The EEG demonstrates spike and wave discharges, and the regular administration of anticonvulsant drugs prevents further attacks.

Headache may also occur as a seizure manifestation in patients who are known to be epileptic. Such individuals usually have a long history of partial or generalized seizures prior to the development of headache. Associated ictal events depend upon the site of the cortical focus and may include auditory hallucinations, visual disturbances, vertigo, déja vu, and focal motor seizures. Headache is usually the initial manifestation of the seizure, but can also follow other partial seizure manifestations such as déja vu and vertigo. The headache may be described as throbbing, sharp, or without an identified quality. Complex partial seizures, simple partial seizures, or generalized tonic-clonic seizures follow the headache phase. Spike foci in patients with seizure headaches may arise in any region of the brain, but have a temporal lobe predominance.

Two children with seizure headaches were studied with depth electrodes prior to surgery (Laplante et al, 1983). Both were found to have seizure activity confined to the right hippocampus and amygdala during seizure headaches. In one, pain was localized to the vertex and associated with shortness of breath and lightheadedness. At times, the seizure progressed to aphasia but consciousness was preserved. The other child had frequent attacks of dizziness and tinnitus associated with the sudden onset of pain in the temporal region lasting for thirty to sixty seconds. Temporal lobe surgery provided complete relief of seizure activity in both patients.

Diagnosis. Most children with seizure headaches are diagnosed by the demonstration of interictal spike discharges on the EEG. The presence of interictal spike discharges, especially Rolandic spikes, in a child with headache does not necessarily mean that the headaches are a seizure manifestation. For example, children with migraine have a 9 percent incidence of Rolandic spikes. Children who have clinical syndromes of migraine, a positive family history of migraine, and have never had a clinical seizure should be considered to have migraine and not epilepsy despite the presence of interictal spike discharges.

An EEG is indicated in children with chronic paroxysmal headache who do not have a positive family history of migraine. If interictal spike discharges are demonstrated, an effort should be made to record a seizure headache using an ambulatory EEG monitor. The demonstration of continuous epileptiform activity during a headache provides reassurance that headache is a seizure manifestation and that anticonvulsant drugs are indicated. However, the side of the seizure focus does not necessarily match the location of the headache.

Treatment. The response to anticonvulsant therapy is usually considered diagnostic as well as therapeutic. Since the seizure focus is usually cortical in origin and most often originates from the temporal lobe, carbamazepine or phenytoin is recommended.

References

1. Bana DS, Yap AU, Graham JR: Headache during hemodialysis. Headache 12:1, 1972.
2. Barabas G, Ferrari M, Matthews WS: Childhood migraine and somnambulism. Neurology 33:948, 1983a.
3. Barabas G, Matthews WS, Ferrari M: Childhood migraine and motion sickness. Pediatrics 72:188, 1983b.
4. Bille B: Migraine in school children. Acta Paediatr 51:13, 1962.
5. Bronshvag MM, Prystowsky SD, Traviesa DC: Vascular headaches in mixed connective tissue disease. Headache 18:154, 1978.
6. Cortelli P, Sacquengna T, Albani F, et al: Propranolol plasma levels and relief of migraine. Relationship between plasma propranolol and 4-hydroxypropranolol concentrations and clinical effects. Arch Neurol 42:46, 1985.
7. Curran DA, Hinterberger H, Lance JW: Methysergide. Res Clin Stud Headache 1:74, 1967.
8. Dalton K: Migraine and oral contraceptives. Headache 15:247, 1976.
9. Deubner DC: An epidemiologic study of migraine and headache in 10-20 year olds. Headache 22:268, 1982.
10. Diamond S: Treatment of migraine with isometheptene, acetaminophen, and dichloralphenazone combination: A double-blind crossover trial. Headache 15:282, 1976.
11. Diamond S, Dalessio DJ: The Practicing Physician's Approach to Headache. 3rd edition. Williams & Wilkins, Baltimore, 1982, pp 72–74.
12. Ekbom K: A clinical syndrome of cluster headache and migraine. Acta Neurol Scand 46:1, 1970.
13. Golden GS: The Alice in Wonderland syndrome in juvenile migraine. Pediatrics 63:517, 1979.
14. Graham JR: Methysergide for prevention of headache: Experience in 500 patients over three years. N Engl J Med 270:67, 1964.
15. Greden JF, Victor BS, Fontaine P, et al: Caffeine-withdrawal headache: a clinical profile. Psychosomatics 21:411, 1980.
16. Hachinski VC, Prochawka J, Steele JC: Visual symptoms in the migraine syndrome. Neurology 23:570, 1973.
17. Iserson KV: Parenteral chlorpromazine treatment of migraine. Ann Emerg Med 12:756, 1983.
18. Jay GW: Epilepsy, migraine, and EEG abnormalities in children: A review and hypothesis. Headache 22:110, 1982.
19. Johns DR: Benign sexual headache within a family. Arch Neurol 43:1158, 1986.
20. Katzberg RW, Bessette RW, Tallents RH, et al: Normal and abnormal temporomandibular joint: MR imaging with surface coil. Radiology 158:183, 1986.
21. Katzberg RW, Tallents RH, Hayakawa K, et al: Internal derangement in the temporomandibular joint: findings in the pediatric age group. Radiology 154:125, 1985.
22. Kinast M, Leuders H, Rother AD, et al: Benign focal epileptiform discharges in childhood migraine (BFEDC). Neurology 32:1309, 1982.
23. Kudrow L: The relationship of headache frequency to hormone use in migraine. Headache 15:36, 1975.
24. Kudrow L: Cluster Headache: Mechanisms and Management. Oxford University Press, Oxford, 1980.
25. Kudrow L: Response of cluster headache attacks to oxygen inhalation. Headache 21:1, 1981.
26. Lance JW: Mechanism and Management of Headache. 4th edition. Butterworths, London, 1982, p 78.
27. Lance JW, Anthony M, Somerville B: Comparative trial of serotonin antagonists in the management of migraine. Br Med J 2:327, 1970.
28. Lance JW, Curran DA, Anthony M: Investigators into the mechanisms and treatment of chronic headache. Med J Aust 2:909, 1965.
29. Laplante P, Saint-Hilaire JM, Bouvier G: Headache as an epileptic manifestation. Neurology 33:1493, 1983.
30. Louis P: A double-blind placebo-controlled prophylactic study of flunarizine (sibelium) in migraine. Headache 21:235, 1981.
31. Ludvigsson J: Propranolol used in prophylaxis of migraine in children. Acta Neurol Scand 50:109, 1974.
32. Markley HG, Cheronis JCD, Piepho RW: Verapamil in prophylactic therapy of migraine. Neurology 34:973, 1984.
33. Matick H, Anderson D, Brumlik J: Cerebral vasculitis associated with oral amphetamine overdose. Arch Neurol 40:253, 1983.
34. Matthews WB: Footballer's migraine. Br Med J 2:325, 1972.
35. Medina JL, Diamond S: The clinical link between migraine and cluster headache. Arch Neurol 34:470, 1977.
36. Meislin A, Rothfield N: Systemic lupus erythematosus in childhood. Analysis of 42 cases with comparative data on 200 adult cases followed concurrently. Pediatrics 42:37, 1968.
37. Meyer JS, Hardenberg J: Clinical effectiveness of calcium entry blockers in prophylactic treatment of migraine and cluster headaches. Headache 23:266, 1983.
38. Olesen J: Some clinical features of the acute migraine attack. An analysis of 750 patients. Headache 18:268, 1978.
39. Pearce JMS: Chronic migrainous neuralgia: a variant of cluster headache. Brain 103:149, 1980.
40. Prensky AL, Sommer D: Diagnosis and treatment of migraine in children. Neurology 29:506, 1979.
41. Rosen JA: Observations on the efficacy of propranolol for the prophylaxis of migraine. Ann Neurol 13:92, 1983.
42. Schaumberg HH, Byck R, Gerstl R, et al: Monosodium L-glutamate. Its pharmacology and role in the Chinese restaurant syndrome. Science 163:826, 1969.
43. Sillanpaa M: Changes in the prevalence of migraine and other headaches during the first seven school years. Headache 23:15, 1983.

44. Solomon GD, Steel JG, Spaccavento LJ: Verapamil prophylaxis of migraine. A double-blind, placebo-controlled study. JAMA 250:2500, 1983.
45. Somerville BW: Role of progesterone in menstrual migraine. Neurology 21:853, 1971.
46. Swaiman KF, Frank Y: Seizure headaches in children. Dev Med Child Neurol 20:580, 1978.
47. Waters WE: Controlled clinical trial of ergotamine tartrate. Br Med J 2:325, 1970.
48. Whitty CWM, Hockaday J, Whitty MM: The effect of oral contraceptives on migraine. Lancet 1:856, 1966.
49. Young GB, Blume WT: Painful epileptic seizures. Brain 106:537, 1983.
50. Yuill GM, Swinburn WR, Liversedge LA: A double-blind crossover of isometheptene mucate compound and ergotamine in migraine. Br J Clin Pract 26:76, 1972.

4 Increased Intracranial Pressure

Increased intracranial pressure is not ordinarily a "presenting symptom" (Table 4.1). Most often, it is brought to attention because of headache, vomiting, personality change, and alterations in states of consciousness. Less frequently, the presenting complaint may be diplopia or the observation that one or both eyes are turning in. Finally, some children are referred for neurologic consultation because a primary physician believes the child has papilledema. Conditions causing increased intracranial pressure are described elsewhere in the book, especially in chapters on altered states of consciousness, headache, ataxia, and disorders of ocular motility. To avoid duplication, this chapter is restricted to conditions in which symptoms of increased intracranial pressure are initial and prominent features.

■ Pathophysiology

Once the cranial bones fuse during childhood, the contents of the skull are enveloped by a rigid box. Intracranial pressure is then the sum of the individual pressures exerted by the brain, blood, and cerebrospinal fluid. An increase in size of any of these three compartments must be accommodated by an equivalent decrease in size of one or both of the other compartments, if intracranial pressure is to remain constant. Because cerebral blood flow must be kept relatively constant to provide oxygen and nutrients, the major adaptive mechanisms available to relieve pressure are the compressibility of the brain and the rapid reabsorption of cerebrospinal fluid by arachnoid villi. Infants and young children, in whom the cranial bones are still unfused, have the additional adaptive mechanism of spreading the cranial bones apart to increase cranial volume.

THE CEREBROSPINAL FLUID

The choroid plexus accounts for at least 70 percent of cerebrospinal fluid production and the transependymal movement of fluid from brain to ventricular system accounts for the remainder. The average volumes of cerebrospinal fluid are 90 ml in children from ages four to thirteen years and 150 ml in adults. Rate of formation is approximately 0.35 ml/minute, or 500 ml/day (Cutler and Spertell, 1982). Therefore, approximately 14 percent of total volume turns over every hour. The rate at which cerebrospinal fluid is formed remains relatively constant and declines only slightly as cerebrospinal fluid pressure increases. In contrast, the rate of absorption increases linearly as cerebrospinal fluid pressure exceeds 70 mm H_2O. At a pressure of 200 mm, the rate of absorption is three times the rate of formation.

Table 4.1 PRESENTING FEATURES OF INCREASED INTRACRANIAL PRESSURE

Large head (see Chapter 18)
Bulging fontanelle
Failure to thrive
Setting-sun sign
Shrill cry
Diplopia (see Chapter 15)
Headache
Diplopia
Mental changes
Nausea and vomiting
Papilledema

Therefore, impaired absorption, and not increased formation, is the usual mechanism of progressive hydrocephalus. Choroid plexus papilloma is the only pathologic process in which formation overwhelms absorption. When absorption is impaired, efforts directed at decreasing the formation of cerebrospinal fluid are not likely to have a significant effect upon volume.

CEREBRAL BLOOD FLOW

The primary determinant of cerebral blood flow is systemic arterial pressure. Normal cerebral blood flow remains remarkably constant from newborn to adult life and is generally 50 to 60 ml/minute/100 g brain weight. Blood vessels on the surface and at the base of the brain are more richly innervated by autonomic nerve fibers than are vessels of any other organ. These nerve fibers allow the autoregulation of cerebral blood flow. Autoregulation refers to a buffering effect by which cerebral blood flow remains constant despite changes in systemic arterial perfusion pressure. Alterations in the arterial blood concentration of carbon dioxide have an important effect upon total cerebral blood flow. Hypercarbia dilates cerebral blood vessels and increases blood flow while hypocarbia constricts cerebral blood vessels and decreases flow. Alterations in blood oxygen content have the reverse effect, but are not as potent a stimulus for vasoconstriction or vasodilation as are alterations in blood carbon dioxide concentration.

Cerebral perfusion pressure is the difference between mean systemic arterial pressure and intracranial pressure. It can be reduced to dangerous levels either by reducing systemic arterial pressure or by increasing intracranial pressure. The autoregulation of the cerebral vessels is lost when cerebral perfusion pressure falls below 50 torr or when there is severe acidosis. Increased intracranial blood volume can be caused by arterial vasodilation or by obstruction of cerebral veins and venous sinuses. Increased intracranial blood volume, like increased cerebrospinal fluid volume, results in increased intracranial pressure.

CEREBRAL EDEMA

Cerebral edema is an increase in brain volume due to an increase in its water and sodium content. Edema may be localized or generalized; when generalized, it causes increased intracranial pressure. Cerebral edema is generally categorized as (1) *vasogenic*, (2) *cytotoxic*, or (3) *interstitial*.

Vasogenic edema is caused by increased capillary permeability and is encountered with brain tumor, abscess, infarction, trauma, and hemorrhage. The fluid is located primarily in the white matter and responds to treatment with corticosteroids. Osmotic agents have no effect on vasogenic edema, but can decrease the volume of normal brain tissue and in that way reduce total intracranial pressure.

Cytotoxic edema is caused by swelling of neurons, glia, and endothelial cells. It is usually due to hypoxia, ischemia, or infection of the nervous system. Increased fluid is located in both gray and white matter. Corticosteroids are not effective in decreasing edema, but osmotic agents may relieve intracranial pressure by reducing brain volume.

Interstitial edema is due to transependymal movement of fluid from ventricular system to brain. This occurs when cerebrospinal fluid absorption is blocked and the ventricles are enlarged. The fluid collects chiefly in the periventricular white matter. Agents alleged to reduce cerebrospinal fluid production, such as acetazolamide and furosemide, may be useful. Corticosteroids and osmotic agents are not effective (Fishman, 1980).

MASS LESIONS

Mass lesions (e.g., tumor, abscess, hematoma, arteriovenous malformation) produce increased intracranial pressure by (1) physically occupying space at the expense of other intracranial compartments, (2) provoking cerebral edema, (3) blocking the circulation and absorption of cerebrospinal fluid, (4) increasing blood flow, and (5) obstructing venous return.

■ Symptoms and Signs

The clinical features of increased intracranial pressure depend upon the age of the child and the rate at which pressure increases. Newborns and infants present a special case because increased pressure can be vented in part by expanding the volume of the skull. The rate at which intracranial pressure increases is important at all ages. Intracranial structures accommodate remarkably well to slowly increasing pressure, but sudden changes are intolerable and always result in some combination of headache, personality change, and states of decreasing consciousness.

INCREASED INTRACRANIAL PRESSURE IN INFANCY

Measurement of head circumference and palpation of the anterior fontanelle are rapid and readily available methods to assess intracranial volume and pressure. Head circumference is measured by determining its greatest anteroposterior circumference. Normal standards are different for premature and term newborns. Normal head growth in the term newborn is 2 cm/month for the first three months, 1 cm/month for the second three months, and 0.5 cm/month for the next six months. Excessive head growth is a major feature of increased intracranial pressure throughout the first year and even up to three years. However, normal head growth does not preclude the presence of increased intracranial pressure. In posthemorrhagic hydrocephalus, considerable ventricular dilation precedes any measurable change in head circumference by compressing the brain parenchyma (Volpe et al, 1977).

The palpable tension of the anterior fontanelle is an excellent measure of intracranial pressure. In a quiet child, a fontanelle that bulges above the level of the bone edges and is sufficiently tense to cause difficulty in determining where bone ends and fontanelle begins is always abnormal and indicates increased intracranial pressure. A full fontanelle, which is clearly distinguishable from the surrounding bone edges, may indicate increased intracranial pressure, but can also be caused by crying, edema of the scalp, subgaleal hemorrhage, and extravasation of intravenous fluids. The normal fontanelle is clearly demarcated from bone edges, falls below the surface, and pulsates under the examining finger.

While the size of the anterior fontanelle and its rate of closure are variable, increased intracranial pressure should be suspected when the metopic and coronal sutures are sufficiently separated to admit a fingertip.

When the separation of cranial sutures is no longer sufficient to decompress increased intracranial pressure, the infant experiences lethargy and vomiting and fails to thrive. Palsies of the sixth cranial nerve, impaired upward gaze (setting-sun sign), and disturbances of blood pressure and pulse may ensue. Papilledema is uncommon.

INCREASED INTRACRANIAL PRESSURE IN CHILDREN

Headache

Headache is one of the more constant symptoms of increased intracranial pressure at all ages. It is usually expressed in infants as irritability and refusal to eat. Traction and displacement of intracranial arteries is the major cause of headache from increased intracranial pressure (see Chapter 3). As a rule, pain fibers from supratentorial intracranial vessels are transmitted by the trigeminal nerve and referred to the eye, forehead, and temple. In contrast, infratentorial intracranial vessels are innervated by cervical nerves and pain is referred to the occiput and neck.

When there is generalized increased intracranial pressure, such as may occur from cerebral edema or obstruction of the ventricular system, headache is generalized and more often prominent in the morning upon awakening and rising to a standing position. Pain is constant, but may vary in intensity. Coughing, sneezing, straining, and other maneuvers that transiently increase intracranial pressure exaggerate the headache. The quality of pain is often difficult to describe. Vomiting in the absence of nausea, especially upon arising in the morning, is often a concurrent feature.

In the absence of generalized increased intracranial pressure, localized, or at least unilateral, headache can occur if a mass causes traction on contiguous vessels.

In children younger than ten years of age, symptoms of increased intracranial pressure can be temporarily relieved by the separation of sutures. Such children may have a symptom-free interval of several weeks following weeks or months of chronic headache and vomiting. The relief of pressure is always temporary and symptoms return with their prior intensity. An intermittent course of symptoms should not direct attention away from the possibility of increased intracranial pressure.

Any individual who was previously well and then experiences an acute, intense headache described as "the worst headache I ever had in my life" has surely suffered a subarachnoid hemorrhage. A small hemorrhage need not cause loss of consciousness, but still produces sufficient meningeal irritation to cause intense headache and some stiffness of the neck. Fever may be present as well.

Diplopia/Strabismus

Paralysis of one or both abducens nerves is a relatively common feature of generalized increased intracranial pressure and may be a more prominent feature than headache in children with pseudotumor cerebri (see Chapter 15).

Papilledema

Papilledema is passive swelling of the optic disk secondary to increased intracranial pressure (Table 4.2). The mechanism of swelling is uncertain, but generally is believed to be caused by obstruction of venous return from the retina and nerve head. It is usually bilateral and, when unilateral, suggests a mass lesion behind the affected eye. Early papilledema is asymptomatic, and only when it is advanced does the patient experience transitory obscuration of vision. Preservation of visual acuity separates papilledema from primary optic nerve disturbances such as optic neuritis, in which visual acuity is always profoundly impaired early in the course (see Chapter 16).

The observation of papilledema in a child with headache or diplopia confirms the diagnosis of increased intracranial pressure. However, the diagnosis of papilledema is not always easy and congenital variations of disk appearance may confuse the issue. The earliest sign of papilledema is loss of spontaneous venous pulsations in the vessels around the disk margin. Spontaneous venous pulsations are said to occur in approximately 80 percent of normal eyes, but this is closer to 100 percent in children. Spontaneous venous pulsations cease when intracranial pressure exceeds 200 mm H$_2$O. Therefore, papilledema is not present, if spontaneous

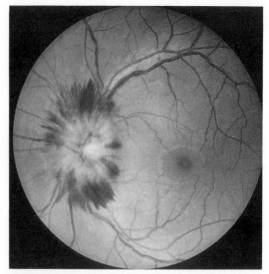

Figure 4.1 Acute papilledema. The optic disk is swollen with peripapillary nerve fiber layer hemorrhages.

venous pulsations are present, no matter how obscure the disk margin may appear. Conversely, when spontaneous venous pulsations are lacking in children, papilledema should be suspected even though the disk margin is flat and well visualized.

As edema progresses, the disk swells and is raised above the plane of the retina, causing obscuration of the margin and tortuosity of the veins (Fig. 4.1). Associated features include small flame-shaped hemorrhages and nerve fiber infarcts known as "cotton-wool" (Fig. 4.2).

Table 4.2 DIFFERENTIAL DIAGNOSIS OF SWOLLEN DISK

Congenital disk elevation
Increased intracranial pressure
Ischemic neuropathy
Juvenile diabetes
Optic glioma
Papillitis
Retinitis
Retrobulbar mass
Uveitis

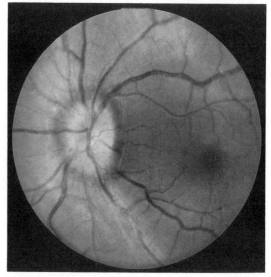

Figure 4.2 Established papilledema. The optic disk is elevated with opacification of the nerve fiber layer around the disk margin and retinal folds (Paton's lines) temporally.

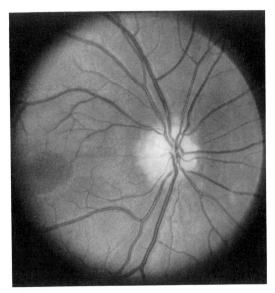

Figure 4.3 Drusen. The disk margin is indistinct, and the physiologic cup is absent. Yellowish, globular bodies are present on the surface.

If the process continues, the retina surrounding the disk becomes edematous so that the disk appears greatly enlarged and retinal exudates radiate from the fovea. Eventually, the hemorrhages and exudates clear, but optic atrophy ensues and blindness may be permanent. Even if increased intracranial pressure is relieved during the early stages of disk edema, four to six weeks are required before the retina appears normal again.

Congenitally elevated disks that give the false impression of papilledema are usually caused by hyaline bodies (drusen) within the nerve head. The actual drusen are not observable during the first decade, and therefore only the elevated nerve head is apparent. Drusen continue to grow and can be seen in older children and in their parents (Fig. 4.3). Drusen are inherited as an autosomal dominant trait and tend to occur more often in whites than other racial groups. Anomalous nerve head elevations should be easily distinguished from papilledema because spontaneous venous pulsations are present.

HERNIATION SYNDROMES

Increased intracranial pressure may cause portions of the brain to shift from their normal location into other compartments, causing compression of structures already occupying that space. Such shifts may occur under the falx cerebri, through the tentorial notch, and through the foramen magnum (Table 4.3).

Falx Herniation

Herniation of one cingulate gyrus under the falx cerebri is common when one hemisphere is enlarged. The major feature is compression of the internal cerebral vein and the anterior cerebral artery, resulting in still greater increased intracranial pressure because of reduced venous outflow and arterial infarction.

Unilateral (Uncal) Transtentorial Herniation

The tentorial notch allows structures to pass from the posterior to the middle fossa. Under normal circumstances, it is filled with the brainstem, the posterior cerebral artery, and the third nerve. Unilateral transtentorial herniation characteristically occurs when enlargement of one temporal lobe causes the uncus or hippocampus to bulge into the tentorial notch. Falx herniation is usually associated. Because intracranial pressure must be considerable to cause such a shift, states of decreased consciousness are present even prior to the actual herniation and continue to decline further as the brainstem is compressed. Direct pressure on the oculomotor nerve causes ipsilateral dilation of the pupil; sometimes the contralateral pupil is dilated because the displaced brainstem compresses the opposite oculomotor nerve against the incisura of the tentorium. Contralateral homonymous

Table 4.3 HERNIATION SYNDROMES

Unilateral (Uncal) Transtentorial Herniation
1. Decreasing states of consciousness
2. Respiratory irregularity
3. Dilated and fixed pupil
4. Homonymous hemianopia
5. Increased blood pressure, slow pulse
6. Decerebrate rigidity

Bilateral (Central) Transtentorial Herniation
1. States of decreasing consciousness
2. Pupillary constriction or dilation
3. Impaired upward gaze
4. Irregular respiration
5. Decerebrate or decorticate rigidity

Cerebellar (Downward) Herniation
1. Neck stiffness or head tilt
2. States of decreasing consciousness
3. Impaired upward gaze
4. Irregular respirations
5. Lower cranial nerve palsies

hemianopia is a constant feature but is impossible to test in an unconscious patient because of compression of the ipsilateral posterior cerebral artery. With further pressure on the midbrain, both pupils become dilated and fixed, respirations become irregular, decerebrate posturing is noted, and death results from cardiorespiratory collapse.

Bilateral (Central) Transtentorial Herniation

Central herniation is usually associated with generalized cerebral edema. Both hemispheres are displaced downward and the diencephalon and midbrain are pushed caudally through the tentorial notch. The diencephalon becomes edematous and the pituitary stalk may be avulsed. The clinical features are states of decreasing consciousness, pupillary constriction and then dilation, impaired upward gaze, irregular respiration, disturbed control of body temperature, decerebrate or decorticate posturing, and death.

Cerebellar Herniation

Increased pressure in the posterior fossa may cause upward herniation of the cerebellum through the tentorial notch or downward displacement of one or both cerebellar tonsils through the tentorial notch. Upward displacement causes compression of the midbrain, resulting in impairment of upward gaze, dilated or fixed pupils, and respiratory irregularity. Downward cerebellar herniation causes compression of the medulla, resulting in states of decreasing consciousness, impaired upward gaze, and lower cranial nerve palsies. One of the earliest features of cerebellar herniation into the foramen magnum is neck stiffness or head tilt as an effort is made to relieve the pressure by enlarging the surface area of the foramen magnum.

■ Monitoring Intracranial Pressure

The value of continuous intracranial pressure monitoring remains controversial (Miller, 1985; Ropper, 1985). Three types of intracranial pressure monitors are presently in use. The oldest technique is *ventriculostomy*. A catheter is placed in the frontal horn of the lateral ventricle and connected to a pressure transducer. It provides a direct measure of ventricular pressure. The normal range of intraventricular pressure is between 0 and 15 mm Hg, but is usually no higher than 5 mm Hg in infants (Welch, 1980). The disadvantages of the technique are that the brain must be punctured, the ventricle is difficult to locate when there is cerebral edema, and infection rates up to 22 percent are recorded (Aucoin et al, 1986), especially in patients with open head injuries or intracranial hemorrhage.

A second technique is the *subarachnoid screw*, of which the Richmond bolt is used most commonly. A hole is drilled in the skull, the dura and arachnoid opened, and the bolt twisted into the drilled hole so that it lies beneath the inner table of the skull and against the brain. The bolt must remain in perfect position or faulty measurements are obtained (Miller et al, 1986). Unfortunately, the bolt may be difficult to stabilize in young children whose skull is thin. The overall infection rate is 7.5 percent and these are mainly confined to patients with head injuries and intracranial hemorrhage.

The third and newest technique is the *subdural cup catheter*. A Silastic ribbon with a central lumen is placed in the subdural space through a burr hole. On one side of the ribbon is a cup that lies against the arachnoid and acts as a pressure transducer. This device is probably more accurate and less likely to become blocked than the Richmond bolt, but infection rates of up to 15 percent are recorded. Risk of infection with any technique of monitoring is lower if the device is used for three days or less.

The most important question to be asked in deciding whether or not to implant a monitoring device is "will the results of monitoring affect management?" In many situations, including Reye syndrome in which monitoring is used extensively, there is no evidence that intracranial pressure monitoring alters outcome. The symptomatology and prognosis of increased intracranial pressure depends as much or more on its cause as on the level of pressure attained.

■ Medical Treatment

Several measures to lower increased intracranial pressure are available, even in circumstances where surgical intervention is required (Table 4.4).

HEAD ELEVATION

Elevating the head 30 degrees above horizontal decreases intracranial pressure by improving

Table 4.4 MEDICAL MEASURES TO DECREASE
INTRACRANIAL PRESSURE

Elevation of head
Hyperventilation
Osmotic diuretics
Mannitol
Glycerol
Corticosteroids
Hypothermia
Pentobarbital coma

jugular venous drainage. Systemic blood pressure is not affected, so that the overall result is increased cerebral perfusion. The effect of head elevation on intracranial pressure has been measured in normal and asphyxiated newborns using a continuous wave Doppler technique (Emery and Peabody, 1983). Pressure is higher in the dependent position and lower in the elevated position in both groups, but the effect is greater in asphyxiated newborns.

HYPERVENTILATION

Intracranial pressure is reduced within seconds of initiating hyperventilation. The mechanism is vasoconstriction secondary to hypercarbia. The goal is to lower the arterial pressure of carbon dioxide from 40 to 25 torr. Further reduction may cause ischemia and is contraindicated. Vasoconstriction is not maintained as long as hyperventilation is continued. However, as the vessels redilate and blood flow returns to normal, "rebound," in which blood flow increases above baseline, does not occur.

OSMOTIC DIURETICS

Mannitol and glycerol are the two osmotic diuretics most widely used in the United States. Mannitol, 0.25 g/kg, is given intravenously as a 20 percent solution. Much larger doses were previously recommended, but the lower dose is equally effective and produces less rebound. Mannitol does not cross the blood-brain barrier. It remains in the plasma and creates an osmotic gradient that draws water from brain into capillaries. Onset of action is within thirty minutes, and the peak effect is generally one to two hours after administration. The effect is short-lasting, and infusions must be given three to six times each day in order to keep serum osmolality below 320 mOsm/L (320 nmol/L). Because repeated infusions of mannitol produce dehydration as well as fluid and electrolyte imbalance, it is generally used for only two or three days. Rebound may occur when mannitol is discontinued.

Glycerol, 1 g/kg, is given intravenously as a 10 percent solution three or four times a day. The onset of action is within thirty minutes, and the effect usually lasts twenty-four hours or longer. Like mannitol, dehydration and electrolyte disturbances may follow repeated administration. Rebound is less prominent than with mannitol.

CORTICOSTEROIDS

Corticosteroids such as dexamethasone are effective in the treatment of vasogenic edema. The intravenous dose is 0.1 to 0.2 mg/kg every six hours. Onset of action is twelve to twenty-four hours, and peak action may be delayed even longer. The mechanism is uncertain. Cerebral blood flow is not affected. Corticosteroids are most useful for reducing edema surrounding mass lesions.

HYPOTHERMIA

Hypothermia decreases cerebral blood flow and is frequently used concurrently with pentobarbital coma. Body temperature is generally kept between 27° and 31° C. It is not clear how much is gained by hypothermia in addition to other measures that decrease cerebral blood flow such as head elevation, hyperventilation, and pentobarbital coma.

PENTOBARBITAL COMA

Barbiturates reduce cerebral blood flow, decrease edema formation, and lower the metabolic rate of the brain (Steer, 1982). These effects do not occur at anticonvulsant plasma concentrations, but require brain concentrations sufficient to produce a burst-suppression pattern on the electroencephalogram (EEG) (Fig. 4.4). Barbiturate coma is particularly useful in patients with increased intracranial pressure secondary to hypoxia-ischemia and disorders of mitochondrial function such as Reye syndrome. Pentobarbital is preferable to phenobarbital because it produces less cardiotoxicity. However, both drugs may reduce cardiac output and produce hypotension. Plasma concentrations do not adequately reflect brain concentrations. Conse-

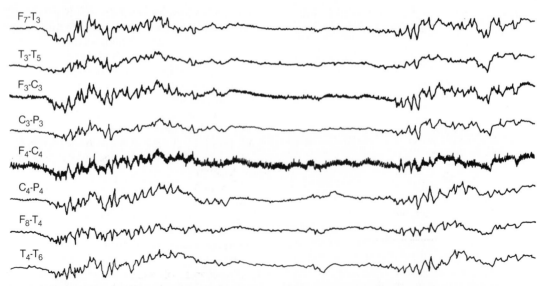

Figure 4.4 Burst-suppression in pentobarbital coma. Long intervals of amplitude suppression are interrupted by bursts of mixed frequencies.

quently, an EEG monitor is imperative to determine brain concentrations as reflected by a burst-suppression pattern.

Pentobarbital is given as 10 mg/kg boluses until the desired EEG pattern is obtained. Hypotension, when it occurs, is generally not observed until 40 to 60 mg/kg are administered. It is important to remember that barbiturates tend to accumulate and the dose needed to maintain barbiturate coma is 3 mg/kg/hour. Coma can be maintained safely for up to three days. During barbiturate coma, there is gastroparesis and medications given through a nasogastric tube are not adequately absorbed, but may remain in the stomach and then undergo rapid absorption when coma is lifted.

■ Hydrocephalus

Hydrocephalus is a condition marked by excessive volume of intracranial cerebrospinal fluid. It is termed *communicating* or *noncommunicating*, depending upon whether or not there is communication of cerebrospinal fluid between the ventricular system and subarachnoid space. Congenital hydrocephalus occurs in approximately one per thousand total births. It is generally associated with other congenital malformations and may be caused by genetic disturbances or intrauterine disorders such as infection and hemorrhage. Often, a cause cannot be determined. Because congenital hydro-

cephalus almost always presents as macrocephaly, it is discussed in Chapter 18.

Acquired hydrocephalus may be caused by brain tumor, intracranial hemorrhage, or infection. Solid brain tumors generally produce hydrocephalus by obstructing the ventricular system, while nonsolid tumors such as leukemia impair the reabsorptive mechanism in the subarachnoid space. Choroid plexus papilloma is unique among tumors because hydrocephalus may be produced by excessive formation of cerebrospinal fluid.

Intracranial hemorrhage and infection may produce communicating and noncommunicating hydrocephalus and also may increase intracranial pressure through the mechanisms of cerebral edema and impaired venous return. Because several factors contribute to increased intracranial pressure, acquired hydrocephalus is discussed by etiology in the sections that follow.

■ Brain Tumor

Primary tumors of the posterior fossa and middle fossa are discussed in Chapters 10, 15, and 16 (Table 4.5). This section deals with tumors of the cerebral hemispheres.

Tumors of glial origin comprise approximately 40 percent of supratentorial tumors in infancy and childhood (Gjerris et al, 1985). The common glial tumors of childhood in order of frequency are astrocytoma, ependymoma, and

Table 4.5 BRAIN TUMORS IN CHILDREN

Posterior Fossa Tumors
1. Medulloblastoma (see Chapter 10)
2. Astrocytoma (see Chapter 10)
3. Ependymoma (see Chapter 10)
4. Brainstem glioma (see Chapter 15)
5. Hemangioblastoma (see Chapter 10)

Middle Fossa Tumors
1. Sellar and parasellar tumors (see Chapter 16)
2. Optic glioma (see Chapter 16)

Hemispheric Tumors
1. Neuroepithelial
   a. Astrocytoma
   b. Oligodendroglioma
   c. Ependymoma
   d. Primitive neuroectodermal tumors
2. Pineal region tumors
   a. Pineal-parenchymal tumors
      (1) Pineoblastoma
      (2) Pineocytoma
   b. Germ cell tumors
      (1) Embryonal cell carcinoma
      (2) Teratoma
      (3) Germinoma
   c. Glial tumors
      (1) Astrocytoma
      (2) Ganglioglioma
3. Choroid plexus papilloma
4. Angiomas
5. Meningioma
6. Dysplasias
7. Metastatic tumors

oligodendroglioma. A mixture of two or more cell types is the rule. Oligodendroglioma occurs exclusively in the cerebral hemispheres, whereas astrocytoma and ependymoma may be found in either a supratentorial or infratentorial location.

Oligodendroglioma is rare in childhood and generally not encountered until adolescence. These tumors are slow-growing, tend to calcify, and generally present as seizures rather than increased intracranial pressure.

HEMISPHERIC ASTROCYTOMAS

Hemispheric astrocytomas are graded by histologic appearance into three classes: low-grade, anaplastic, and glioblastoma multiforme. Anaplastic tumors and glioblastoma multiforme are referred to as high-grade tumors. Glioblastoma multiforme accounts for fewer than 10 percent of childhood supratentorial astrocytomas and is more likely to occur in adolescence than in infancy.

Clinical Features. The initial manifestations of glial tumors in children depend upon location and may include seizures, hemiparesis, and movement disorders affecting one side of the body. Seizures are the most common initial manifestation. Tumors infiltrating the basal ganglia and internal capsule are less likely to cause seizures than those closer to cortical structures. A mass effect may not be present early in the course because slow-growing, infiltrating tumors can be accommodated by surrounding neural structures. Such tumors may cause only seizures for several years before causing weakness of the contralateral limbs.

Headache is a relatively common complaint and may be focal if the tumor is producing localized displacement of vessels without increasing intracranial pressure. A persistent focal headache usually correlates well with tumor location.

Symptoms of increased intracranial pressure—generalized headache, nausea, and vomiting—are an initial manifestation of hemispheric astrocytoma in only 37 percent of children, but are a feature at time of diagnosis in 79 percent. Increased intracranial pressure is likely to occur in rapidly growing tumors that provoke edema of the hemisphere. A mass effect is produced that causes collapse of one ventricle, shift of midline structures, and pressure on the aqueduct. When herniation occurs, or if there is dilation of the lateral ventricles due to pressure on the aqueduct, the early features of headache, nausea, vomiting, and diplopia are followed by generalized weakness or fatigability, lethargy, and states of decreased consciousness.

Papilledema is constant in children with generalized increased intracranial pressure except those under two years of age who may develop macrocephaly instead. When papilledema is present, abducens palsy is usually associated. Other neurologic findings depend upon the site of the tumor and could include hemiparesis, hemisensory loss, or homonymous hemianopia.

Diagnosis. Hemispheric astrocytomas are readily identified by computerized tomography (CT). Contrast enhancement is mandatory when brain tumor is suspected. Magnetic resonance imaging (MRI) is a more powerful tool and is essential for the demonstration of low-grade gliomas. It is no better than CT for the diagnosis of high-grade tumors.

Low-grade gliomas appear as low-density or cystic areas that are enhanced when contrast is injected (Fig. 4.5). Cerebral edema is identified as a low-density area surrounding the tumor which does not demonstrate contrast enhancement. High-grade gliomas have patchy areas of

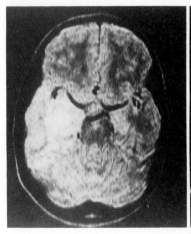 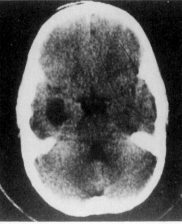

Figure 4.5 Low-grade glioma, magnetic resonance imaging (left) and computed tomography (right). An area of increased signal intensity in the right temporal lobe is revealed on MRI; this appears as a cystic lesion on CT.

low and high density, sometimes evidence of hemorrhage, and cystic degeneration. Marked contrast enhancement is noted, often in a ring pattern. When a mass effect is present, there is shift of midline structures, deformity of the ipsilateral ventricle, and swelling of the affected hemisphere with obliteration of sulcal markings (Fig. 4.6). A mass effect can be identified in 50 percent of low-grade astrocytomas, 90 percent of anaplastic tumors, and 100 percent of glioblastoma multiforme (Weisberg, 1980).

Treatment. All children with increased intracranial pressure due to hemispheric astrocytoma should be treated for vasogenic cerebral edema with dexamethasone. Headache and nausea are frequently relieved within twenty-four hours, and neurologic deficits are often improved as well. Surgical resection of the tumor is the next step in treatment. Complete removal is rarely possible—with the exception of cystic cerebral astrocytoma, which resembles cerebellar astrocytomas in having a mural nodule within the cyst. In these tumors, the five-year survival rate following surgery alone is 90 percent (Palma et al, 1983).

Postoperative radiation is recommended for all grades of astrocytomas. The five-year survival rate for children with low-grade astrocytoma is increased from 25 percent to over 50 percent by the addition of radiation therapy (Schulte, 1984). Patients with anaplastic astrocytomas have less than a 30 percent five-year survival rate even with radiation, and those with glioblastoma multiforme have less than a 3 percent five-year survival (Duffner et al, 1986).

Because the five-year survival is poor with high-grade astrocytomas, several chemotherapy protocols have been tried (Allen, 1985). The most promising regimen is one in which eight drugs (vincristine, hydroxyurea, procarbazine, CCNU, cisplatin, cytosinarabinoside, high-dose methylprednisolone, and cyclophosphamide) are all administered in one day repeatedly for two or three weeks. Although this approach does provide some short-term benefits, long-term survival is unaffected.

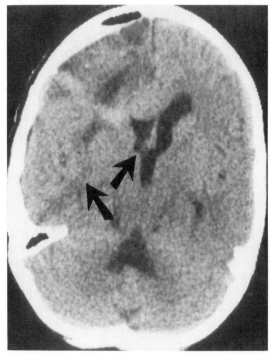

Figure 4.6 Mass effect. Invasive tumor of left hemisphere (arrow) compresses the lateral ventricle on that side (arrow) and causes herniation under the falx.

EPENDYMOMA

Ependymomas are tumors derived from cells that line the ventricular system and may be found either in a supratentorial or infratentorial location. Infratentorial ependymoma is discussed in Chapter 10 because it may present as ataxia. However, symptoms of increased intracranial pressure are the first manifestation in 90 percent of children with posterior fossa ependymoma and papilledema is present in 75 percent at the time of initial examination. Approximately 60 percent of children with ependymoma are younger than five years old at the time of diagnosis and only 4 percent are older than fifteen years (Dohrmann et al, 1976). As a rule, children with infratentorial ependymoma are younger than children with supratentorial ependymoma.

The expected location of supratentorial ependymoma is in relationship to the third and lateral ventricles. However, ependymal tumors may arise within the hemispheres at a site distant from the ventricular system. Such tumors are thought to be derived from ependymal cell rests.

Clinical Features. Symptoms of increased intracranial pressure are less prominent in supratentorial tumors than infratentorial tumors. Common presenting symptoms are focal weakness, seizures, and visual disturbances. Papilledema is a common physical finding in all patients with ependymoma. Hemiparesis, hyperreflexia, and hemianopia are typical features, but some children present only with ataxia. The average duration of symptoms before diagnosis is seven months, but can be as little as one month in malignant tumors and as long as several years in low-grade tumors.

Diagnosis. Tumor density on CT is usually greater than brain density, and contrast enhancement is present. Small cysts within the tumor are relatively common. Approximately one third of supratentorial ependymomas contain calcium.

Tumors within the third ventricle cause marked dilation of the lateral ventricles with edema of the hemispheres and obliteration of sulcal markings. High-grade tumors are likely to seed the subarachnoid space, producing metastases in the spinal cord and throughout the ventricular system. In such cases, tumor cells may line the lateral ventricles and produce a "cast" of contrast enhancement around the ventricles.

Treatment. Surgical resection is the first step in management, but is never curative. Low-grade supratentorial ependymomas are associated with a low risk of metastases and should be treated with local radiation. Children with high-grade supratentorial tumors should receive at least whole brain radiation and complete craniospinal radiation should be considered as well (Cohen and Duffner, 1984). Several studies of chemotherapy are in progress. A significant increase in long-term survival has not been demonstrated. Overall, the five-year survival rate in all children with ependymoma is only 28 percent (Duffner et al, 1986). Children with tumors that are supratentorial in location or of low grade for malignancy have a better prognosis than do children in whom the tumors are infratentorial in location or anaplastic.

PRIMITIVE NEUROECTODERMAL TUMORS (PNET)

PNETs are relatively rare tumors of childhood consisting of small, undifferentiated, darkly staining cells, that have neuronal, glial, and mesenchymal elements. These tumors resemble medulloblastoma, but are always located in the cerebral hemispheres (Ashwal et al, 1984).

Clinical Features. Age at onset may be anytime during childhood, but is usually the first decade. Males and females are affected equally. Because these tumors are highly malignant, the progression of symptoms is rapid and time to diagnosis is usually less than three months. Approximately one half of children present with features of increased intracranial pressure. Other manifestations are determined by tumor site. Two thirds of tumors are located in the frontal or parietal lobe. Seizures, monoparesis, hemiplegia, and ophthalmoplegia are initial manifestations in approximately 10 percent of patients. Hydrocephalus or head enlargement is unusual as a presenting feature.

Diagnosis. With and without contrast enhancement, CT is an effective method for determining tumor location and size. PNETs appear as poorly defined, infiltrating and lobular masses, sometimes containing multiple cysts and hemorrhage. The tumor mass is surrounded by cerebral edema, and midline structures are frequently shifted under the falx.

Treatment. Cerebral edema may be relieved by the use of dexamethasone. Complete tumor resection is rarely accomplished, but partial resections are helpful to relieve tumor burden. Perioperative mortality rates range from 22 to 50 percent. Radiation therapy is usually employed postoperatively, but its value is not firmly established. Several chemotherapeutic trials are ongoing, including the eight-drugs-in-one-day protocol developed for malignant astrocytomas.

Unfortunately, the mean survival of all patients is only twenty-six months. Long-term survivals have been attributed to complete surgical removal of the tumor. However, the tumor does metastasize throughout the subarachnoid space of brain and spinal cord; tumor recurrence is possible even when the primary is believed to be fully resected.

PINEAL REGION TUMORS

Tumors found in the pineal region may be derived from several different histologic types. Germ cell tumors are the most common, then tumors of the pineal parenchyma, and finally other histologic types. The incidence of pineal region tumors is ten times higher in Japan than in the United States or Western Europe. As a group, pineal region tumors are more common in boys than girls and generally become symptomatic during the second decade.

Clinical Features. Because these tumors are in a midline location, where they can invade or compress the third ventricle or aqueduct, symptoms of increased intracranial pressure are common. The onset of pressure symptoms may be acute and accompanied by midbrain dysfunction (Packer et al, 1984). Midbrain dysfunction due to pressure by pineal region tumors on the periaqueductal gray is usually referred to as *Parinaud's syndrome:* supranuclear palsy of upward gaze with preservation of downward gaze and retraction-convergence nystagmus when upward gaze is attempted. Eventually, there may be paralysis of both upward and downward gaze and loss of accommodation. Pupillary light reflexes may be lost as well and the pupils remain mid-dilated.

Tumors growing into or compressing the anterior hypothalamus produce loss of vision, diabetes insipidus, precocious puberty, and emaciation. Precocious puberty occurs almost exclusively in males. Extension of tumor into the posterior fossa produces multiple cranial neuropathies and ataxia, and lateral extension causes hemiparesis.

Diagnosis. With or without contrast, CT accurately images tumor location and the presence of secondary hydrocephalus but cannot distinguish histologic types. As a rule, germinomas are isodense and noncalcified and have irregular margins. Contrast enhancement is not homogeneous. Teratomas appear lobulated, and have both hyperdense and multicystic areas. Calcification may be present, and contrast enhancement is not uniform. Tumors that spread into the ventricular system and have intense contrast enhancement are likely to be malignant. Tumors that contain abundant amounts of calcium are likely to be benign.

Cerebrospinal fluid concentrations of alphafetoprotein and human chorionic gonadotropin may be useful markers of specific histologic types and may also be used to quantify response to treatment. Embryonal cell carcinomas secrete alpha-fetoprotein and human chorionic gonadotropin. Choriocarcinomas secrete human chorionic gonadotropin and not alpha-fetoprotein. Other tumors of the pineal region do not usually secrete either of these proteins. While it was hoped that histologic type could be determined by cerebrospinal fluid assay, the secretion of these proteins is not sufficiently reliable to obviate the need of surgical biopsy for histologic identification.

Treatment. Stereotactic biopsy is essential to establish histologic type and plan therapy. Ventricular drainage may be needed to relieve hydrocephalus. Germinomas are highly radiosensitive, and five-year survival rates of 50 to 80 percent are reported. Other tumors of the pineal region are less radiosensitive. Complete surgical removal of pineal region tumors has been discouraged in the past because mortality and morbidity rates have been prohibitive. Improved surgical techniques are now allowing successful removal in many cases (Schulte et al, 1987).

CHOROID PLEXUS PAPILLOMA

Choroid plexus papilloma is an unusual tumor, representing between 1 and 4 percent of childhood brain tumors. It generally occurs in young children and may be present at birth.

Clinical Features. Choroid plexus tumors are usually located in one lateral ventricle. They present with symptoms and signs of increased intracranial pressure due to hydrocephalus. Communicating hydrocephalus may be caused by excessive production of cerebrospinal fluid by the tumor, but noncommunicating hydrocephalus due to obstruction of the ventricular foramen is more common. If the tumor is pedunculated, its movement may cause intermittent ventricular obstruction by a ball-valve mechanism. The usual course is one of rapid progression with only a few weeks from onset of symptoms to diagnosis.

Infants usually have macrocephaly and are thought to have congenital hydrocephalus. Older children present with nausea, vomiting, diplopia, headaches, and weakness. Papilledema is the rule.

Diagnosis. Because affected children have clear evidence of increased intracranial pressure, CT is usually the first test performed. The tumor is visualized within one ventricle as a mass of increased density with marked contrast enhancement. Hydrocephalus of one or both lateral ventricles is visualized as well. Choroid plexus papillomas are highly vascular and angiography should be performed prior to surgery. Many tumors bleed spontaneously, and the spinal fluid may be xanthochromic or grossly bloody. The concentration of protein in the cerebrospinal fluid is usually elevated.

Treatment. Complete surgical extirpation is the treatment of choice. Operative mortality may be as high as 16 percent because the tumor has a tendency to hemorrhage (Guidetti and Spallone, 1981). If the tumor is removed completely, hydrocephalus is relieved without the need of a shunt and recurrences are unusual.

METASTATIC TUMORS

Cerebral metastatic disease is unusual in childhood. Tumors with the highest frequency of producing cerebral metastases are osteogenic sarcoma and rhabdomyosarcoma in patients younger than fifteen years of age and testicular germ cell tumors after age fifteen (Graus et al, 1983). The cerebral hemispheres are more often affected than are posterior fossa structures. Pulmonary involvement always precedes cerebral metastasis.

Brain metastasis is rarely present at the time of initial cancer diagnosis.

OTHER TUMORS

Other brain tumors of childhood are listed in Table 4.5. These are rare tumors. The symptoms and signs caused by different hemispheric tumors are similar and generally produce some combination of increased intracranial pressure, seizures, and hemiparesis. CT is useful in each case to identify the presence of tumor. Complete surgical excision is the treatment of choice when

possible; if not, partial resection or biopsy is performed to relieve tumor burden and to establish tissue diagnosis. Radiation is administered following partial resection and especially when there is evidence of malignancy.

■ Intracranial Arachnoid Cysts

Primary arachnoid cysts are cavities within the arachnoid filled with cerebrospinal fluid. The cause of cyst formation is uncertain, but is generally considered a minor disturbance in arachnoid formation and not a pathologic process (Naidich et al, 1986). Arachnoid cysts are identified in 0.5 percent of postmortem examinations: two thirds are supratentorial and one third infratentorial.

Clinical Features. Age at onset is almost always during infancy, but can be delayed until adolescence. Presenting manifestations are related to cyst size. Small cysts are asymptomatic and discovered only incidentally. Large cysts produce symptoms by compression of adjacent structures or by increasing intracranial pressure. Focal neurologic disturbances vary with location, but are most often hemiparesis or seizures when the cyst is supratentorial and ataxia when infratentorial. Compression of the parietal lobe from early infancy may result in undergrowth of contralateral limbs.

Increased intracranial pressure can be caused by mass effect or hydrocephalus and is associated with cysts in all locations. Presenting features include macrocephaly, headache, and behavioral change.

Diagnosis. It has become commonplace for children with headache, learning or behavioral disorders, and suspected seizures to undergo CT examination. Many will have incidental arachnoid cysts. A cause-and-effect relationship should be considered only if the cyst is large and if it clearly explains the symptoms.

Treatment. Simple drainage of the cyst often results in reaccumulation of fluid and recurrence of symptoms. The definitive procedure is to shunt the cyst into the peritoneal space (Harsh et al, 1986).

■ Intracranial Hemorrhage

HEAD TRAUMA

Head trauma is a major cause of intracranial hemorrhage from the newborn period through childhood and adolescence. It is associated with intracerebral hemorrhage, subarachnoid hemorrhage, subdural hematoma, and epidural hematoma. Increased intracranial pressure is a constant feature of intracranial hemorrhage and also occurs following concussion without hemorrhage from cerebral edema. Intracranial hemorrhage from head trauma is discussed in Chapter 2.

INTRAVENTRICULAR HEMORRHAGE OF THE NEWBORN

Intraventricular hemorrhage is primarily a disorder of liveborn prematures with respiratory distress syndrome. The autoregulation of cerebral blood flow, which maintains local tissue needs by alterations in cerebrovascular resistance, is impaired in prematures with respiratory distress syndrome. During episodes of systemic hypotension, cerebral blood flow is decreased and there is a potential for cerebral infarction. Such infarctions usually occur symmetrically in the white matter adjacent to the lateral ventricles

and are termed *periventricular leukomalacia.* Low-density lesions in the periventricular white matter can be identified on CT at 40 weeks conceptional age in 89 percent of newborns with a birthweight less than 1500 g (McCarton-Daum et al, 1983).

During episodes of systemic hypertension, there is increased cerebral blood flow, and hemorrhage occurs first in the subependymal germinal matrix and then bursts through the ependymal lining into the lateral ventricle. The predilection of the germinal matrix for hemorrhage during episodes of increased cerebral blood flow has not been fully explained. The likely explanation is the existence of prior ischemic injury which weakens the capillary walls and their supporting structures, making them vulnerable to rupture during episodes of increased cerebral blood flow (Fig. 4.7). Echo-dense lesions consistent with periventricular leukomalacia can be detected by ultrasound in 36 percent of prematures with intraventricular hemorrhage (McMenamin et al, 1984).

Intraventricular hemorrhage also occurs in term newborns, but the mechanism of hemorrhage at term is different than at preterm.

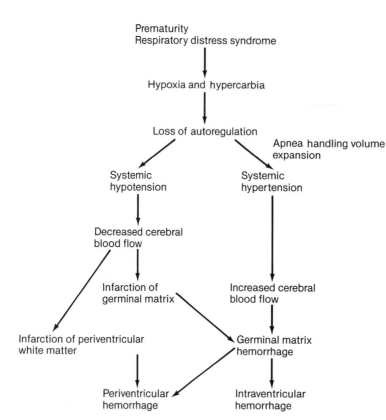

Figure 4.7 Pathophysiology of periventricular-intraventricular hemorrhage. (From Fenichel GM: Neonatal Neurology. Churchill Livingstone, New York, 1985.)

Intraventricular Hemorrhage of Prematures

The true incidence of intraventricular hemorrhage in the premature has been established by routine use of ultrasound. In newborns weighing less than 1500 g, the incidence is approximately 40 percent. A grading system has been developed to quantify the severity of hemorrhage (Table 4.6).

Clinical Features. The routine use of ultrasound in all newborns with birth weights of 1800 g or less has resulted in the diagnosis of intraventricular hemorrhage in asymptomatic newborns. Only 54 percent of newborns with intraventricular hemorrhage are predicted by clinical symptoms and signs, and these are generally the ones with grade III and IV hemorrhages (Lazzara et al, 1980).

In some prematures, there is rapid deterioration of neurologic state characterized by decreasing states of consciousness, severe hypotonia, and respiratory insufficiency. Within minutes to hours there is obvious evidence of increased intracranial pressure: a bulging fontanelle, decerebrate posturing, loss of pupillary reflexes, and respiratory arrest. Hypothermia, bradycardia, hypotension, and a 10 percent fall in hematocrit may be associated.

More commonly, the hemorrhage presents in a subacute fashion with stepwise progression of symptoms over a period of hours or even days. The initial symptoms are subtle and are characterized by a change in behavior, diminished spontaneous movement, and either an increase or decrease in appendicular tone. The fontanelle remains soft, and vital signs are stable. These first symptoms may correspond to grade I hemorrhage. Some newborns will then stabilize and have no further difficulty. Others undergo clinical deterioration characterized by hypotonia and states of declining consciousness. This deterioration probably corresponds to the presence of blood in the ventricles. The child becomes lethargic or obtunded and then may stabilize. If continued bleeding causes acute ventricular dilation, apnea and coma follow. Seizures occur

when blood dissects into the cerebral parenchyma.

All newborns with intraventricular hemorrhage are at risk for developing progressive hydrocephalus. The likelihood is much greater among children with grade III and IV hemorrhage and least likely among children with grade I and II hemorrhage. Initial ventricular dilation is probably due to plugging of the arachnoid villi and impaired reabsorption of cerebrospinal fluid (Hill et al, 1982). The ventricles are able to enlarge continuously by compression of the brain without causing a measurable change in head circumference. Therefore, weekly ultrasound studies are imperative to follow the progression of hydrocephalus. Approximately one half of prematures with intraventricular hemorrhage never demonstrate ventricular dilation. Among those with ventricular dilation, half develop progressive hydrocephalus and the other half have normal pressure hydrocephalus (Hill and Volpe, 1981). Among those infants with normal pressure hydrocephalus, progressive hydrocephalus develops in half even after two months of stable ventricular size. In the other half, or one quarter of the total group with posthemorrhagic ventricular dilation, progressive hydrocephalus never develops.

Diagnosis. Ultrasound is essential for the diagnosis of intraventricular hemorrhage in the newborn. CT is equally effective, but ultrasound is preferred because it can be performed in the intensive care nursery, study time is briefer, and there is no radiation.

Prevention. Prevention is the only treatment for intraventricular hemorrhage of prematurity. It could be accomplished by preventing prematurity and by the delivery of mothers prior to term at specialized perinatal centers. Most intraventricular hemorrhage occurs during the first three days post partum, but the initial subependymal hemorrhage may be present immediately after birth. Optimal care of the premature with respiratory distress syndrome during the early hours post partum is critical to outcome and can best be accomplished in a specialized neonatal unit. Optimal care includes the maintenance of normal tensions of carbon dioxide and oxygen, normal osmolality and viscosity, normal perfusion pressure without episodic hypertension, good ventilatory control, and avoiding the routine use of heparin to maintain the patency of vascular catheters.

In addition, several interventions for the prevention of intraventricular hemorrhage have been tested either in humans or in animal mod-

---

Table 4.6 GRADES OF INTRAVENTRICULAR HEMORRHAGE IN PREMATURES

1. Isolated subendymal hemorrhage
2. Intraventricular hemorrhage without ventricular dilation
3. Intraventricular hemorrhage with ventricular dilation
4. Intraventricular hemorrhage with ventricular dilation and hemorrhage into the parenchyma of the brain

els. The one most widely tested in humans is the administration of phenobarbital to all prematures. Initial studies using small groups of children provided inconsistent results. A large, multicentered, double-blind control study demonstrated that phenobarbital did not have a protective effect and might actually increase the risk of intraventricular hemorrhage (Kuban et al, 1980).

Intramuscular vitamin E, given as soon as possible after delivery and followed by oral supplementation on the second and fourth days post partum, has been found useful in one double-blind control study to prevent intraventricular hemorrhage, especially in newborns weighing less than 1000 g (Speer et al, 1984). It is suggested that vitamin E protects the cerebral microcirculation from the effects of asphyxia.

Treatment. Once intraventricular hemorrhage has occurred, treatment is directed at preventing or stabilizing progressive posthemorrhagic hydrocephalus. It is difficult to assess the efficacy of treatment for posthemorrhagic hydrocephalus because it is not clear that ventricular dilation is an important cause of chronic neurologic impairment. All newborns with progressive posthemorrhagic hydrocephalus have also experienced asphyxial encephalopathy, germinal matrix hemorrhage, and periventricular leukomalacia. Neurologic morbidity at one year correlates better with the degree of parenchymal damage than with ventricular size (Allan et al, 1984).

Children with progressive intraventricular dilation require a ventriculoperitoneal shunt. However, early shunt placement, while the ventricles still contain blood, has a high incidence of shunt failure and infection. Therefore, several methods have been tried to prevent posthemorrhagic hydrocephalus in order to either delay the time of shunt surgery or to obviate the need for it.

The procedure that has undergone the greatest scrutiny is *serial lumbar puncture*. A major problem is the technical difficulty of performing repeated lumbar punctures on a small premature. Contradictory results on the efficacy of serial lumbar punctures have been reported by different groups. While the value of the technique is not established, the method is recommended for at least temporary amelioration of posthemorrhagic hydrocephalus if, in response to the procedure, a decrease in ventricular size is documented by ultrasound (Kreusser et al, 1985).

An alternate approach to serial lumbar punc-

ture is *external ventricular drainage*. A catheter is placed in one lateral ventricle, and the fluid is drained into a closed collecting system. This method is technically easier than serial lumbar punctures but carries the risk of producing ventriculitis.

A final approach is the use of *chemical agents* such as acetazolamide and furosemide, which are presumed to reduce the production of spinal fluid (Shinnar et al, 1985). Acetazolamide is started at a dose of 25 mg/kg/day for one day and then increased by 25 mg/kg/day each day to a maximum of 100 mg/kg/day. A metabolic acidosis may occur at the maintenance dose of 100 mg/kg/day. Base replacement with a systemic alkalizer must be initiated simultaneously to maintain the serum bicarbonate level greater than 18 mEq/L (18 mmol/L). Furosemide is started at a dose of 1 mg/kg/day in three divided doses and may be increased to 3 mg/kg/day. The results with this protocol are encouraging, but the number of treated infants reported is not sufficiently large to support a definite conclusion.

The neurologic outcome for newborns following intraventricular hemorrhage is clearly linked to the grade of hemorrhage. Following grade II hemorrhage, up to 75 percent of children may have normal intellectual and motor development whereas virtually all children with grade IV hemorrhage have some neurologic morbidity. However, some children are normal following grade III hemorrhage and others are impaired following grade I hemorrhage (Williamson et al, 1983). Neurologic outcome is determined by multiple factors, of which asphyxia and periventricular infarction probably play an important role.

Intraventricular Hemorrhage at Term

Unlike intraventricular hemorrhage in the premature, which originates almost exclusively from the germinal matrix, intraventricular hemorrhage at term may originate from the veins of the choroid plexus, from the germinal matrix, or both.

Clinical Features. Term newborns with intraventricular hemorrhage may be divided into two groups. More than half are delivered with difficulty, frequently from breech position, and have suffered some degree of intrauterine asphyxia (Fenichel et al, 1984). These babies are usually bruised and require resuscitation. At first, they appear to be improving and then multifocal seizures occur on the second day post partum.

The fontanelle is tense, and the cerebrospinal fluid is bloody.

The other half have experienced neither trauma nor asphyxia and appear normal at birth. Then, during the first hours post partum, apnea, cyanosis, and a tense fontanelle develop. The mechanism of hemorrhage is not understood.

Posthemorrhagic hydrocephalus is common in both groups, and 35 percent will require shunt placement (Scher et al, 1982).

Diagnosis. Ultrasound is as useful for diagnosis of intraventricular hemorrhage in the term newborn as in the premature.

Treatment. Term newborns with intraventricular hemorrhage are treated in the same manner as prematures with intraventricular hemorrhage.

ARTERIAL ANEURYSMS

Arterial aneurysms are vestiges of the embryonic circulation and are present in a rudimentary form prior to birth. Only rarely do they rupture during infancy. More often, they become symptomatic after age ten and usually after age twenty. Symptomatic arterial aneurysms in childhood may be associated with coarctation of the aorta or polycystic kidney disease. Aneurysms tend to be located at the bifurcation of major arteries at the base of the brain.

Clinical Features. The first manifestation is usually subarachnoid hemorrhage. The presentation may be catastrophic—sudden loss of consciousness, tachycardia, hypotension, and evidence of increased intracranial pressure. However, in most patients the first bleeding from an aneurysm is not catastrophic but is a "warning leak" that may go unrecognized. The warning leak is characterized by severe headache, stiff neck, and low-grade fever. Occasionally, aneurysms produce neurologic signs by exerting pressure on adjacent cranial nerves. The oculomotor nerve is most frequently affected, resulting in disturbances of gaze and pupillary function.

Physical activity is not related to time of rupture. Aneurysmal size is the only predictor of rupture; those smaller than 1 cm in diameter have a low probability of rupture (Weibers et al, 1981).

The patient's state of consciousness is the most important predictor of survival (Kassell and Torner, 1984). Approximately 50 percent of patients die during the first hospitalization, some from the initial hemorrhage during the first fourteen days. Untreated, another 30 percent die from recurrent hemorrhage in the next ten years.

Diagnosis. On the day of aneurysmal rupture, CT demonstrates intracranial hemorrhage in 96 percent of patients. However, the blood is rapidly reabsorbed and can be demonstrated in only 64 percent of patients on the fifth day after rupture. In some patients, the aneurysm can be visualized using CT with contrast enhancement.

Lumbar puncture is often performed because the patient has a stiff neck, headache, and fever suggesting bacterial meningitis. The fluid is usually grossly bloody and therefore diagnostic of subarachnoid hemorrhage. Unfortunately, blood in the cerebrospinal fluid is often attributed to a traumatic tap when time is not taken to centrifuge the fluid and examine it for xanthochromia. Once a diagnosis of subarachnoid hemorrhage is established, either by CT or by lumbar puncture, four-vessel cerebral arteriography is essential. All vessels must be visualized in order to determine the aneurysmal site and the presence of multiple aneurysms.

Treatment. The initial goals of therapy are to prevent early rebleeding and cerebral ischemia from arterial spasm. Nimodipine, a calcium channel blocking agent, is effective in reducing the incidence of spasm and should be administered as quickly as possible (Allen et al, 1983). Nimodipine is not presently commercially available in the United States, but other calcium channel blocking agents are probably effective and should be tried.

Surgical clipping and excision of the aneurysm is the definitive treatment. Early surgery is recommended in conscious patients in order to prevent rebleeding. Six months' survival in patients who are conscious at time of admission is approximately 86 percent. In contrast, six months' survival is only 20 percent among patients who are comatose on admission.

ARTERIOVENOUS MALFORMATIONS

Arteriovenous malformations account for almost 9 percent of subarachnoid hemorrhage at all ages, but comprise a considerably larger share of subarachnoid hemorrhage in childhood. Approximately 0.14 percent of the population has an arteriovenous malformation. A familial occurrence has not been documented. Two types of malformations are described. The first arises from an abnormal communication between primitive choroidal arteries and veins. Such malformations are in the midline and give rise to the vein of Galen malformation, malformations involving the choroid plexus, and shunts between cerebellar arteries and the straight sinus. The other type arises between superficial arteries and veins and results in an arteriovenous malformation within the parenchyma of the cerebral hemisphere. The vessels of the scalp, skull, and dura are interconnected, causing anastomotic channels between the extracranial and intracranial circulations to remain patent. Approximately 90 percent of arteriovenous malformations are supratentorial and 10 percent are infratentorial.

Deep Midline Malformations

Deep midline malformations, especially those involving the great vein of Galen, generally become symptomatic during infancy.

Clinical Features. Large midline arteriovenous malformations produce a hemodynamic stress in the newborn because of the large quantities of blood shunted from the arterial to the venous systems (Luessenhop, 1984). The heart enlarges in an effort to keep up with the demands of the shunt, but high-output failure ensues. Such newborns often first come to the attention of a pediatric cardiologist with a suspicion of congenital heart disease. The intracranial malformation is then diagnosed serendipitously during cardiac catheterization.

When the hemodynamic stress is not severe and cardiac compensation is possible, the onset of symptoms is delayed until infancy or early childhood. In such children, the malformation becomes manifest by direct compression of the tegmentum and aqueduct, causing obstructive hydrocephalus. Onset of symptoms is usually before age five and always before age ten. The lateral ventricles enlarge, causing headache, lethargy, and vomiting. In infants, there is enlargement of the head and bulging of the fontanelle.

Small, deep midline malformations become manifest because of spontaneous bleeding. The peak onset is after age twenty, but may be as early as age five. Small malformations are more likely to bleed than are large ones. In two thirds of cases, the hemorrhage is into the parenchyma of the brain and in one third into the subarachnoid space. Because bleeding is often from the venous rather than the arterial side of the malformation, the onset of symptoms is not as catastrophic as with arterial aneurysms. The evolution of symptoms may be over several hours and there is not a characteristic clinical syndrome. Most patients describe sudden onset of severe headache, neck stiffness, and vomiting. Fever is frequently associated. Focal neurologic

deficits depend upon the location of the malformation and may include hemiparesis, sensory disturbances, and oculomotor palsies. Many patients recover completely from the first hemorrhage; the risk of recurrent hemorrhage is 6 percent in the first year and 2 percent each year afterwards (Graf et al, 1983).

Diagnosis. Most arteriovenous malformations are easily visualized on CT with contrast enhancement. CT demonstrates the degree of ventricular enlargement as well. However, the development of a therapeutic plan requires four-vessel arteriography in order to fully demonstrate all arterial and venous channels.

Treatment. Complete surgical resection is the optimal goal of therapy, but is difficult to accomplish when dealing with deep midline malformations. Such lesions are usually managed by a combination of embolization and surgical ligation of large feeding arteries. The goal is to reduce the volume of the malformation sufficiently to relieve high-output cardiac failure or hydrocephalus. Frequently, hydrocephalus must be shunted because hemorrhage in and around the third ventricle and aqueduct has caused irrevocable damage. Proton beam therapy to induce endothelial proliferation with narrowing of the vessel walls is another alternative for inoperable malformations (Kjellberg et al, 1983).

Supratentorial Malformations

Clinical Features. Among children with arteriovenous malformations in and around the cerebral hemispheres, half will present with intracranial hemorrhage and half with seizures. Recurrent vascular headache may precede the onset of hemorrhage and seizures or may develop concurrently. Headaches are usually unilateral, but may not occur consistently on the same side. In some patients, the headaches have a migraine quality: scintillating scotoma and unilateral throbbing pain. The incidence of such migraine-like headaches in patients with arteriovenous malformations does not appear to be greater than in the population at large. It is likely that the malformation provokes a migraine attack in people who are genetically predisposed (Mohr, 1984).

Most patients who have seizures will have at least one focal seizure; however, among all seizures associated with arteriovenous malformations, half are focal and half are generalized. No specific location of the malformation has a higher incidence of seizures. However, superficial malformations, especially in the centroparietal region, are associated with the highest incidence of hemorrhage. Hemorrhage may be only subarachnoid or may dissect into the brain parenchyma.

Diagnosis. Contrasted CT provides excellent visualization of the malformation in most children. Four-vessel arteriography is required to define all arterial and venous channels.

Treatment. The options for management of supratentorial and infratentorial malformations are the same and include surgical excision, embolization, and proton beam therapy. Superficial malformations are more accessible for direct surgical excision than those deep in the midline. In considering these three modalities of treatment, alone or in combination, one must balance the decision to do something against the decision to do nothing based on the likelihood of further bleeding and the morbidity of intervention.

■ Infectious Disorders

Infections of the brain and meninges produce increased intracranial pressure by causing cerebral edema, by obstructing the flow and reabsorption of cerebrospinal fluid, and by impairing venous outflow. Symptoms and signs of increased intracranial pressure are frequently the initial manifestations in bacterial and fungal infections and may also be the initial manifestation of viral encephalitis. However, viral infections are more likely to present with seizures, personality change, or decreased consciousness and therefore are discussed in Chapter 2.

BACTERIAL MENINGITIS

The offending organism and the clinical features of bacterial meningitis vary with age (Table 4.7). Therefore, it is useful to discuss the syndromes of bacterial meningitis by age group: the newborn, infancy and early childhood, and school age.

Meningitis in the Newborn

Meningitis occurs in 1 per 2,500 live births and accounts for up to 4 percent of all neonatal deaths. It is always a consequence of septicemia and target organs other than brain are infected. The two risk factors that correlate best with sepsis and meningitis are low birth weight and maternal infection.

Table 4.7 MOST COMMON ORGANISMS RESPONSIBLE FOR BACTERIAL MENINGITIS

Newborn
  Group B streptococcus
  Escherichia coli
  Other enterobacteriaceae
  Listeria monocytogenes
Infancy and preschool
  Haemophilus influenzae
  Streptococcus pneumoniae
  Neisseria meningitides
  Mycobacterium tuberculosis
School age
  Streptococcus pneumoniae
  Neisseria meningitides
  Mycobacterium tuberculosis

An early onset and late onset pattern of meningitis have been identified in the newborn. In early onset meningitis, the infection is acquired at the time of delivery and responsible organisms are almost always *Escherichia coli* or group B streptococcus. The child becomes symptomatic during the first week, and the mortality rate is 20 to 50 percent. In late-onset meningitis, the infection is postnatal and symptoms may begin as early as the fourth day post partum but usually begin after the first week. Newborns requiring intensive care are specifically at risk for late onset meningitis because infection is introduced by instrumentation. The responsible organisms are not only *E. coli* and group B streptococcus, but also *Staphylococcus*, *Pseudomonas*, and *Klebsiella*. Mortality rate is 10 to 20 percent.

Clinical Features. Fetuses infected in utero or during delivery may experience respiratory distress and shock within the first twenty-four hours. Other features that may be associated with septicemia include hyperthermia, hypothermia, jaundice, hepatomegaly, lethargy, anorexia, and vomiting (Klein and Marcy, 1983).

In meningitis of late onset, the clinical manifestations are variable. Initial symptoms are usually nonspecific and include lethargy, disturbed feeding, and irritability. As the meningitis worsens, hyperthermia is present in 61 percent, respiratory distress or apnea in 54 percent, and seizures in 40 percent. Bulging of the fontanelle occurs in only 28 percent and nuchal rigidity in 15 percent. Shock is the usual cause of death.

Diagnosis. The diagnosis of septicemia and meningitis in the newborn is often difficult to establish on the basis of symptoms and signs. Lumbar puncture must be prompted by the first suspicion of septicemia. Even in the absence of infection, the cerebrospinal fluid of high-risk newborns contains an average of 8.4 leukocytes/mm^3 with a range of 0 to 32 (Sarff et al, 1976). Sixty percent are polymorphonuclear leukocytes. The protein concentration has a mean value of 90 mg/dl (0.9 g/L), with a range from 20 to 170 mg/dl (0.2 to 1.7 g/L). In newborns with meningitis, the leukocyte count is usually in the thousands and protein concentration may vary from less than 30 mg/dl (0.3 g/L) to more than 1,000 mg/dl (10 g/L). A Gram-stained smear of cerebrospinal fluid provides identification of an organism in less than half of affected newborns. Even when the smear is positive, identification may be inaccurate.

Treatment. Treatment is initiated with the first suspicion of sepsis. Laboratory confirmation is not required. The choice of initial antibiotic coverage differs from hospital to hospital, but usually includes ampicillin and either gentamicin or cefotaxime (Bell, 1985). All antibiotics are administered intravenously in divided doses (Table 4.8). If an organism is identified on culture, specific therapy is initiated.

E. coli is best treated with ampicillin and cefotaxime, group B streptococcus with penicillin or ampicillin, and *Klebsiella pneumoniae* with cefotaxime and an aminoglycoside. *Pseudomonas* is difficult to eradicate, and combined intravenous and intrathecal therapy may be required. Carbenicillin and gentamicin are preferred for intravenous use.

Neonatal meningitis is treated for at least two weeks beyond the time the cerebrospinal fluid becomes sterile. Two days after antibiotic therapy is discontinued, the cerebrospinal fluid should be cultured again. If the culture is positive, a second course of therapy is indicated.

Citrobacter diversus infections often result in a hemorrhagic necrosis of the brain with liquefaction of the cerebral white matter and abscess formation (Foreman et al, 1984). These abscesses are readily identified on CT. Surgical drainage is generally not indicated and could cause further damage to the overlying preserved cortex.

Table 4.8 ANTIBIOTIC DOSAGE FOR NEWBORNS

Ampicillin	150–200 mg/kg/day IV (q8h)
Carbenicillin	300 mg/kg/day IV (q8h)
Cefotaxime	100–150 mg/kg/day IV (q8H)
Gentamicin	
<1 week	5 mg/kg/day IV (q12h)
>1 week	7.5 mg/kg/day IV (q8h)
Penicillin G	250,000–400,000 units/kg/day IV (q8h)

Although the overall mortality rate for bacterial meningitis is less than 50 percent, significant neurologic sequelae are immediately evident in 50 percent of survivors. The more common sequelae include mental and motor disabilities, hydrocephalus, convulsive disorders, deafness, and visual loss. Even in the presence of a normal head circumference, follow-up CT is essential to exclude completely underlying hydrocephalus.

Meningitis in Infants and Young Children

From six weeks until three months of age, group B streptococcus remains a leading cause of meningitis and *E. coli* becomes less common. Other important organisms are *Streptococcus pneumoniae*, *Listeria monocytogenes*, and *Salmonella*. *Haemophilus influenzae* first makes an appearance at this time and becomes the predominant organism, along with *S. pneumoniae* and *Neisseria meningitides*, up to age five.

Clinical Features. In infants and young children, meningitis is usually characterized by fever, irritability, and neck stiffness. A bulging fontanelle is noted in young infants. Headache, vomiting, and lethargy are the initial manifestations after the fontanelle has closed. Seizures generally occur during the first twenty-four hours and may be the presenting event. Once seizures have occurred, there is a declining state of consciousness. Seizures can be focal or generalized and may be difficult to control. The overall incidence of seizures in children with meningitis is 30 percent, but the rate is higher with *H. influenzae*.

Examination reveals a sick and irritable child who resists being touched or moved. Ophthalmoscopic examination is usually normal or demonstrates only minimal papilledema. Focal neurologic signs are unusual except in tuberculous meningitis or when abscess formation has occurred.

The rapidity with which neurologic function declines is probably dependent upon the severity of cerebral edema and cerebral vasculitis. Death may ensue from brainstem compression due to transtentorial herniation. Peripheral vascular collapse can result from brainstem herniation, from endotoxic shock, or from adrenal failure. Sixty percent of children with meningococcemia will have a characteristic petechial or hemorrhagic rash. The rash, though generalized, is most prominent below the waist.

Neck stiffness, characterized by limited mobility and pain on attempted flexion of the head, is caused by meningeal irritation. Other signs of meningeal irritation are those of Kernig and Brudzinski. Both are tested with the patient supine. The *Kernig sign* is marked by pain and resistance to extending the knee with the leg flexed at the hip, the *Brudzinski sign* by spontaneous flexion at the hips when the neck is passively flexed. These signs of meningeal irritation can be noted in subarachnoid hemorrhage as well as in infectious meningitis.

Diagnosis. Lumbar puncture and examination of the cerebrospinal fluid are essential for the diagnosis of bacterial meningitis. However, since bacterial meningitis is often associated with septicemia, cultures of the blood, urine, and nasopharynx are indicated as well. The peripheral white blood count, especially immature granulocytes, is usually increased. Peripheral leukocytosis is much more common in bacterial than in viral infections, but cannot be used as an absolute method to rule out viral meningitis. Platelet count is important because some infections are associated with thrombocytopenia. Blood glucose concentration must be measured concurrently in order to properly evaluate the cerebrospinal fluid concentration of glucose. Serum electrolytes, especially sodium, should be measured as well. Inappropriate antidiuretic hormone secretion is present in the majority of patients with acute bacterial meningitis (Kaplan and Feigen, 1978). A tuberculin skin test should be administered to every child at risk for tuberculous meningitis.

Lumbar puncture must be performed as quickly as possible when there is any suspicion of bacterial meningitis. Generalized increased intracranial pressure is always part of acute bacterial meningitis and is not a contraindication to lumbar puncture. Information to be derived from the procedure includes opening and closing pressures, appearance, white blood cell count with differential, red blood cell count, concentration of glucose and protein, Gram stain, and culture. The characteristic findings are increased pressure, a cloudy appearance, a cellular response of several thousand polymorphonuclear leukocytes, a reduction in the concentration of glucose to less than half of that in the plasma, and an elevated concentration of protein. However, the classic findings of bacterial meningitis may vary with the organism, the timing of the lumbar puncture, the prior use of antibiotics, and the immunocompetence of the host.

Treatment. Ampicillin and chloramphenicol are generally administered to all infants and children younger than five years of age in whom bacterial meningitis is suspected prior to identi-fication of the offending organism. These two antibiotics cover the three organisms that account for the majority of cases (see Table 4.7). Cefuroxime is now considered equally as effective as ampicillin and chloramphenicol in the initial treatment of meningitis and is an acceptable alternative (Eichenwald, 1987). Gram stain identification is useful, but can be misleading, and the final choice of antibiotic therapy should await the results of culture and antibiotic sensitivity.

There are several exceptions to the choice of ampicillin and chloramphenicol for the initial treatment of bacterial meningitis. Meningitis in children with a ventricular shunt in place is usually caused by a staphylococcal species, and nafcillin may be added to the ampicillin and chloramphenicol combination or given alone if gram-positive cocci are present on smear. Meningitis secondary to chronic sinusitis or dental infection is frequently caused by anaerobic and aerobic organisms. Penicillin G and chloramphenicol are therefore a reasonable choice for initial therapy, although cefotaxime may be needed for some gram-negative organisms not covered by chloramphenicol. Meningitis following trauma is usually caused by *S. pneumoniae*, whereas meningitis following neurosurgical procedures may be due to either streptococcal or staphylococcal organisms. Gram-negative organisms may be responsible as well, and a combination of penicillin G and cefotaxime is recommended.

Once a specific organism is identified, a specific antibiotic or combination of antibiotics is then chosen (Table 4.9).

The outcome for infants and children with bacterial meningitis depends upon the infecting organism and the speed with which appropriate antibiotic therapy is initiated. Ten percent of children will have persistent bilateral or unilateral hearing loss following bacterial meningitis (Dodge et al, 1984). The incidence is 31 percent following infection with *S. pneumoniae* and 6 percent with *H. influenzae*. Hearing loss occurs early and is probably not related to the choice of antibiotic.

Table 4.9 ANTIBIOTIC DOSAGES FOR CHILDREN

Ampicillin	300–400 mg/kg/day IV (q4h)
Cefotaxime	150 mg/kg/day IV (q4h)
Chloramphenicol	75–100 mg/kg/day p.o. or IV (q6h)
Nafcillin	200 mg/kg/day (q4h)
Penicillin G	250,000 units/kg/day IV (q4h)

Meningitis in Older Children

H. influenzae is rarely a cause of bacterial meningitis in school-aged children. *S. pneumoniae* and *N. meningitides* are the major pathogens in the United States, whereas *Mycobacterium tuberculosis* is an important cause of meningitis in Third World countries. The signs and symptoms of bacterial meningitis in school-aged children do not differ substantially from those encountered in preschool children, except that the child is better able to describe the discomfort of meningismus and early diagnosis is more likely. Penicillin G is the treatment of choice for *S. pneumoniae* or *N. meningitides*.

Tuberculous Meningitis

Worldwide, tuberculosis remains a leading causes of morbidity and death in children. In the United States, it represents less than 5 percent of all bacterial meningitis in children but occurs with higher frequency among subpopulations with poor sanitation. Children are infected by inhalation of the organism from adults. Pulmonary tuberculosis occurs first and is then disseminated to other organs within the first six months of primary pulmonary infection.

Clinical Features. The peak incidence of tuberculous meningitis is between six months and two years of age. Onset of symptoms tends to be more insidious than with other bacterial meningitides, but sometimes progresses in a fulminating fashion. Most often, fever develops first and the child then becomes listless and irritable. Irritability may be caused in part by headache, which is a constant feature. Vomiting and abdominal pain are sometimes associated. Headache and vomiting increase in frequency and severity and are accompanied by signs of meningismus during the second week after onset of fever. Seizures may occur early, but more often occur after meningismus is established. The state of consciousness declines progressively and focal neurologic deficits are noted. Most common are cranial neuropathies and hemipareses. Papilledema occurs relatively early in the course. Without treatment, death is invariable within three to five weeks from onset.

Diagnosis. Tuberculosis must be considered in any child with a household contact. General use of tuberculin skin testing in children is critical to early detection. Once a child's skin test is positive, isoniazid therapy is initiated even if the child is asymptomatic.

In the early stages, children with tuberculous meningitis may manifest only fever. The peripheral white blood count is generally elevated between 10,000 and 20,000/cu mm. Hyponatremia and hypochloremia are frequently present secondary to inappropriate secretion of antidiuretic hormone. The cerebrospinal fluid is usually cloudy and increased in pressure. The leukocyte count in the cerebrospinal fluid may range from 10 to 250 cells/cu mm and rarely exceeds 500. Lymphocytes predominate. The concentration of glucose declines throughout the course of the illness and is generally less than 35 mg/dl (1.8 mmol/L). Conversely, the concentration of protein increases steadily and is usually greater than 100 mg/dl (1 g/L).

Smears of cerebrospinal fluid stained by acid-fast technique generally demonstrate the bacillus. Recovery of the organism from the cerebrospinal fluid is not always successful even using guinea pig inoculation.

Treatment. The prognosis for survival and for neurologic recovery is enhanced by early treatment. Once a child becomes comatose, complete neurologic recovery is unlikely. Mortality rates of 20 percent are recorded even when treatment is initiated early.

The drugs currently recommended for treatment of tuberculous meningitis include isoniazid, 20 mg/kg/day orally up to 500 mg/day; streptomycin, 20 mg/kg/day IM up to 1 g/day; and rifampin, 15 mg/kg/day orally up to 600 mg/day. Streptomycin and rifampin are continued for eight weeks after clinical and laboratory improvement have been established. Isoniazid is continued for two years.

The use of corticosteroids to reduce inflammation has been contested. Some believe it is useful, while others fear it may impair the immune response and worsen the disease. In children who present with advanced tuberculous meningitis and in whom intracranial pressure is greatly increased because of cerebral edema and hydrocephalus, corticosteroids should be used to reduce cerebral edema.

Communicating hydrocephalus is a common complication of tuberculous meningitis because of impaired reabsorption of cerebrospinal fluid. The size of the ventricles must be assessed by CT at periodic intervals whenever there is unexplained deterioration of mental function. Before the infection is brought under control, communicating hydrocephalus may be treated by repeated lumbar punctures and acetazolamide. In many cases, obstructive hydrocephalus will later develop and these children will require a surgical shunt.

Brain Abscess

Predisposing factors to pyogenic brain abscess in children include congenital heart disease, ear and sinus infection, head injuries, and cystic fibrosis (Fischer et al, 1981). Brain abscesses in the newborn are almost always the result of meningitis due to *C. diversus* and other species of Enterobacteriaceae. Pyogenic abscesses in children younger than five months of age but beyond the neonatal period are uncommon and most often occur in children with hydrocephalus and shunt infection. The organisms most often responsible are species of Staphylococcus.

After five months of age, congenital heart disease accounts for half of all cases of pyogenic brain abscess. Abscess caused by chronic ear infection is now uncommon in the United States, but remains a frequent problem in less developed countries (Yang, 1981). The infecting organisms are diverse, and many abscesses contain a mixed flora. Coagulase-positive *S. aureus* and anaerobic streptococcus are the organisms most frequently recovered. In up to 20 percent of cases, no organism can be recovered.

Clinical Features. The clinical features of brain abscess, like any space-occupying lesion, depend upon the age of the child and the location of the mass. Prior to the actual encapsulation of the abscess, there is a period of cerebritis characterized by fever, headache, and lethargy. Seizures may occur as well, but in the absence of seizures the initial symptoms may not be sufficiently severe to arouse suspicion of cerebral infection. If the period of cerebritis is not diagnosed, the initial clinical manifestations are not different from other mass lesions. In infants, there is abnormal head growth, a bulging fontanelle, and failure to thrive. Seizures are sometimes present. In older children, signs of increased intracranial pressure develop and there is evidence of focal neurologic dysfunction. Fever is present in only 60 percent of cases, and meningeal irritation is relatively uncommon. Therefore, it is frequently difficult by clinical features alone to separate pyogenic brain abscess from other mass lesions such as brain tumor. Eighty percent of abscesses are in the cerebral hemispheres. Hemiparesis, hemianopia, and seizures are the usual clinical features. Cerebellar abscess most often occurs secondary to chronic otitis and is manifest by nystagmus and ataxia.

Diagnosis. The combination of headache and papilledema, with or without focal neurologic dysfunction, suggests the possibility of a mass lesion and leads to CT. Most abscesses appear as an area of decreased density surrounded by a rim of intense enhancement referred to as a "ring lesion." This ring lesion, though characteristic, is not diagnostic. Malignant brain tumors may have a similar appearance (Fig. 4.8). Ring enhancement occurs during the late stages of cerebritis just before capsule formation has occurred. After the capsule forms, the diameter of the ring decreases in size and the center becomes more hypodense. Multiple abscesses may be present.

Treatment. The development of CT has altered the management of cerebral abscess. Previously, surgical drainage was initiated as soon as abscess formation was identified. Now there is a tendency to treat even encapsulated abscesses medically and to follow the progress with serial scans (Berg et al, 1978).

The initial step in treatment is to reduce brain swelling by the use of corticosteroids. An intravenous antibiotic regimen is then initiated that generally includes a penicillinase-resistant penicillin such as methicillin, 300 mg/kg/day, and chloramphenicol, 100 mg/kg/day. This combination is selected for its effectiveness against *Staphylococcus* and mixed gram-negative organisms. If an organism can be identified by culture of spinal fluid or blood, then more spe-

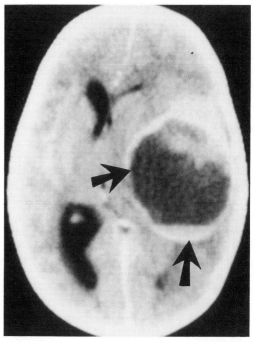

Figure 4.8 Ring enhancement surrounding a malignant tumor. A large cavity with a mural nodule is surrounded by a ring of contrast enhancement (arrows). The mass is producing falx herniation.

cific antibiotic therapy is selected. In general, penicillin-G is preferable to ampicillin if penicillin-sensitive organisms are recovered.

If medical therapy does not resolve the abscess, surgical drainage is necessary. Even in such cases, prolonged medical therapy prior to surgery increases the success of total excision.

Subdural and Epidural Empyema

Meningitis in infants and sinusitis in older children are the most common predisposing factors causing infection in the subdural space. The subdural space is sterile in children with bacterial meningitis, but can become contaminated by organisms if subdural tap is performed before the subarachnoid space is sterilized with antibiotics or by secondary thrombophlebitis of perforating cerebral veins. In older children, subdural and epidural abscesses are usually caused by penetrating head injuries or chronic mastoiditis.

Infections of the subdural space are difficult to contain and may extend over an entire hemisphere.

Clinical Features. Subdural empyema produces increased intracranial pressure because of mass effect, cerebral edema, and vasculitis. Vasculitis leads to thrombosis of cortical veins resulting in focal neurologic dysfunction as well as increased intracranial pressure. Children with subdural infections are very sick. There are headache, fever, vomiting, seizures, and states of decreasing consciousness. Unilateral and alternating hemipareses are common. Papilledema is a constant feature in children who are comatose.

Diagnosis. Subdural empyema should be suspected in children with meningitis whose condition declines after an initial period of recovery or in children who continue to have increased intracranial pressure of uncertain cause. Examination of the cerebrospinal fluid may not be helpful and sometimes is normal. The usual abnormality is a mixed cellular response, generally less than 100 cells/cu mm, with a lymphocytic predominance. The concentration of glucose is normal, and the concentration of protein is only mildly elevated.

CT is particularly helpful in demonstrating a subdural or epidural abscess. The infected collection appears as a lens-shaped mass of increased lucency just beneath the skull. A shift of midline structures is generally present.

In infants, abscess can be reached by subdural puncture and the organism identified. Subdural puncture can also be used to drain much of the abscess.

Treatment. The child with subdural or epidural empyema must be treated with corticosteroids for increased intracranial pressure, antibiotics to eradicate the organisms, and anticonvulsants for seizures. Surgical drainage of subdural empyema had been considered an absolute necessity; it now appears that many can be treated medically, using CT to monitor progress (Leys et al, 1986).

FUNGAL INFECTIONS

Fungi exist in two forms: molds and yeast. Molds are filamentous and divided into segments by hyphae. Yeast are unicellular organisms surrounded by a thick cell wall and sometimes a capsule. Several fungi exist as yeast forms in tissue, but are filamentous when grown in culture. Such fungi are said to be dymorphic or dyphasic. The common fungal pathogens are listed in Table 4.10.

Fungal infections of the central nervous system may result in an acute, subacute, or chronic meningitis; solitary or multiple abscesses; and granulomas (Bell, 1981). Fungal infections of the nervous system are most common in children who are immunosuppressed, especially those with leukemia or acidosis. Fungal infections also occur in children who are immunocompetent. *Cryptococcus neoformans* and *Coccidioides immitis* are the leading causes of fungal meningitis in immunocompetent children.

Cryptococcal Meningitis

C. neoformans is carried by birds, especially pigeons, and is widely disseminated in soil. Human infection is acquired by inhalation. The organism is disseminated widely in the blood, but has a predilection for the central nervous system. It is an important cause of subacute and chronic meningoencephalitis.

Table 4.10   COMMON FUNGAL PATHOGENS

Yeast forms
Cryptococcus neoformans
Candida species
Dimorphic forms
Histoplasma capsulatum
Blastomyces dermatitidis
Coccidioides immitis
Mold forms
Aspergillus species

Clinical Features. Cryptococcal meningitis is uncommon before age ten and perhaps only 10 percent of cases occur before age twenty. Males are affected more often than females. Most children with cryptococcal meningitis are immunologically competent.

Onset of symptoms is usually insidious; chronic headache is the major feature. The headache waxes and wanes, but eventually becomes continuous and associated with nausea, vomiting, and lethargy. Body temperature may remain normal, especially in older children and adults, but younger children often have low-grade fever. Personality and behavioral changes are relatively common. The child becomes moody, listless, and sometimes frankly psychotic. Increased intracranial pressure is characterized by blurred vision, diplopia, and papilledema. Seizures and focal neurologic dysfunction are not early features, but are signs of vasculitis, hydrocephalus, and granuloma formation.

Diagnosis. The diagnosis of cryptococcal meningitis is often missed even when suspected. The cerebrospinal fluid may be normal, but most often demonstrates an increased opening pressure and a lymphocytic leukocytosis that generally averages fewer than 100 cells/cu mm. The concentration of protein is almost always elevated, generally greater than 100 mg/dl (1 g/L), and the concentration of glucose is usually less than 40 mg/dl (2 mmol/L). Rapid diagnosis is possible if the fungus can be demonstrated in cerebrospinal fluid by the India ink technique. It is the only encapsulated fungus to invade the central nervous system and has a characteristic appearance on smear. However, the organism is not usually present in the lumbar subarachnoid space and must be obtained from cerebrospinal fluid at the base of the brain. This can be achieved either by removing very large volumes of cerebrospinal fluid by lumbar puncture or by cisternal puncture.

Ease of diagnosis has been greatly improved by the development of a latex agglutination test that reacts to the polysaccharide capsule of the organism. The test is reasonably accurate, but false-negative results occur and serologic studies do not replace the actual demonstration of the organism. The latex agglutination technique can also be performed on the cerebrospinal fluid and titers of 1:8 or greater are considered significant and support the diagnosis of cryptococcal meningitis.

Treatment. Amphotericin B is the drug of choice for the treatment of cryptococcal menin-

gitis (Bell, 1981). It is given intravenously diluted with 5 percent dextrose and water in a drug concentration no greater than 1 mg per 10 ml of fluid. Nephrotoxicity is the limiting factor in achieving desirable blood levels. The intravenous regimen is generally the same for all fungal infections of the nervous system and is summarized in Table 4.11. The total dose varies with the response and the side effects, but is usually in the range of 1,500 to 2,000 mg/1.7 meter square of body surface.

The toxic effects include chills, fever, nausea, and vomiting. Anemia and nephrotoxicity must be monitored with frequent blood counts and urinalyses. Renal impairment is manifested by the appearance of cells or casts in the urine, elevated blood urea nitrogen, and decreased creatinine clearance. When renal impairment occurs, the drug must be discontinued and then restarted at a lower dose.

Patients who do not tolerate amphotericin can be treated with 5-fluorocystosine or miconazole. 5-fluorocystosine is rarely effective alone, but must be used in combination with low-dose amphotericin B. It is given orally at a dose of 100 to 150 mg/kg/day in four divided doses. The intravenous dose of miconazole is 30 mg/kg/day in three divided doses over a 30-minute period of infusion.

Seriously ill patients, treated very late in the course of the disease, should also be treated intrathecally with amphotericin B and miconazole.

The efficacy of therapy can be followed by demonstrating a decline of the agglutination titer in the cerebrospinal fluid. Periodic CT is necessary to monitor for the development of hydrocephalus.

Coccidioidomycosis

C. immitis is endemic in the San Joaquin Valley of California and all southwestern states. Infection is by inhalation; almost 90 percent of individuals become infected within ten years of moving into an endemic area. Only 40 percent

Table 4.11 DOSAGE SCHEDULE
FOR AMPHOTERICIN B

Initial Dose
Mild cases, 0.1 mg/kg/day
Severe cases, 0.25 mg/kg/day
Daily IV infusions over 4–6 hours
Maintenance
Up to 0.6 mg/kg/day as tolerated

of patients become symptomatic; the other 60 percent are identified only by positive skin test.

Clinical Features. Following respiratory infection, there is malaise, fever, cough, myalgia, and chest pain. The pulmonary infection is self-limited. Dissemination of the fungus from the lung to other organs occurs in only 1 per 400 individuals. However, the dissemination rate is considerably higher in infants than in older children and adults.

Coccidioidal meningitis is almost always caused by hematogenous spread from lung to meninges, but sometimes occurs by direct extension following infection of the skull. Symptoms of meningitis develop two to four weeks after the onset of respiratory symptoms. The major features are headache, apathy, and confusion. These symptoms may persist for weeks or months without concurrent seizures, meningismus, or focal neurologic disturbances. If the meningitis is allowed to become chronic, hydrocephalus eventually develops because the basilar meningitis prevents reabsorption of cerebrospinal fluid.

Diagnosis. Coccidioidal meningitis should be suspected in patients living in endemic areas when headache develops following an acute respiratory infection. Skin hypersensitivity among individuals living in an endemic area is not helpful, since a large percentage of the population is exposed and has a positive skin test. The cerebrospinal fluid generally demonstrates increased pressure and a lymphocytic cellular response of 50 to 500 cells/cu mm. Eosinophils are frequently present as well. The concentration of protein ranges from 100 to 500 mg/dl (1 to 5 g/L), and the concentration of glucose is less than 35 mg/dl (1.8 mmol/L). The diagnosis is confirmed by isolation of the fungus, but this is often difficult to accomplish. Complement-fixing antibodies appear in the blood and in the cerebrospinal fluid. A positive serologic test in the cerebrospinal fluid is diagnostic, but false-negative results are possible.

Treatment. Amphotericin B is the drug of choice for coccidioidal meningitis. It must be administered both intravenously (Table 4.11) and intrathecally. The initial intrathecal dose is 0.1 mg for the first three injections and then increased to 0.25 to 0.5 mg three or four times each week. Treatment must be prolonged, and some would recommend weekly intrathecal injections indefinitely. Adverse reactions to intrathecal administration include aseptic meningitis and pain in the back and legs.

Intravenous and intrathecal administration of miconazole may be used in patients unable to tolerate high doses of amphotericin B. Ketoconazole, a new synthetic antifungal agent, has excellent activity against *C. immitis* in culture, but penetrates the cerebrospinal fluid poorly and is not recommended for systemic therapy of coccidioidal meningitis.

Candidal Meningoencephalitis

Candida is a common inhabitant of the mouth, vagina, and intestinal tract. Ordinarily, it causes no symptoms; however, it can multiply and become an important pathogen in children who are immunosuppressed, taking multiple antibiotics, suffering from debilitating diseases, and are being treated with long-term vascular catheters. The most common sites of infection are mouth (thrush), skin, and vagina. Candidal meningitis is almost unheard of in normal, nonhospitalized children.

Clinical Features. *Candida* reaches the brain and other organs by vascular dissemination. The brain is less often involved than other organs, and the prominent manifestations of candidal sepsis include fever, lethargy, and vomiting. Hepatosplenomegaly and arthritis may be present.

Cerebral involvement can be in the form of meningitis, abscess formation, or both. When there is meningoencephalitis, the clinical manifestations are fever, vomiting, meningismus, papilledema, and seizures leading to states of decreased consciousness. In some individuals, a single large cerebral abscess forms that presents as focal neurologic dysfunction and papilledema (Black, 1970).

Diagnosis. Cerebral candidiasis should be suspected in children with risk factors for disseminated disease who have unexplained fever. The organism can be isolated from blood, joint effusion fluid, or cerebrospinal fluid. When meningitis is present, a predominantly neutrophilic response is present in the cerebrospinal fluid associated with a protein concentration, which is generally 100 mg/dl (1 g/L). The concentration of glucose is only slightly reduced. Children who have a candidal abscess rather than meningitis are likely to have normal or near-normal cerebrospinal fluid. Instead, a mass lesion resembling a pyogenic abscess or tumor is demonstrated on CT.

Treatment. When candidal infections develop in children because of indwelling vascular catheters, the catheter must be removed. Amphotericin B and 5-fluorocytosine are used together and thought to have a synergistic effect. Dosages are the same as for other fungal infections, and the drugs should be administered for six to twelve weeks, depending upon the efficacy of therapy and presence of adverse reactions.

Other Fungal Infections

Histoplasmosis is endemic in the central United States and causes pulmonary infection. Miliary spread is unusual. Neurologic histoplasmosis may take the form of leptomeningitis, focal abscess, or multiple granulomas. Blastomycosis is primarily a disease of North America. It reaches the brain by hematogenous spread from the lungs and produces multiple abscesses that give the appearance of metastatic disease on CT. Cellular response in the cerebrospinal fluid is markedly increased when fungi produce meningitis and may be normal or only mildly increased when there is abscess formation. Amphotericin B is the mainstay of therapy for all fungal infections; myconazole is used in combination with amphotericin B against *Histoplasma capsulatum*.

■ Benign Intracranial Hypertension
(Pseudotumor Cerebri)

The term pseudotumor cerebri is used to characterize increased intracranial pressure in the absence of mass lesion or hydrocephalus. The syndrome may have an identifiable, specific, underlying cause or may be idiopathic. A specific cause can usually be found in children younger than six years of age, while most idiopathic cases occur after age eleven. Between ages six and eleven, half of cases are idiopathic and half are symptomatic (Couch et al, 1985).

Some causes of pseudotumor are listed in Table 4.12. A cause-and-effect relationship has not been established in all of these conditions. The most frequent causes are otitis media, head trauma, the use of certain drugs and vitamins, and feeding following malnutrition.

Idiopathic pseudotumor cerebri is primarily a disorder of the second and third decades. Females are more often affected than males and tend to be obese. Brain volume is enlarged because of increased cerebral blood volume or cerebral edema, or both. In addition, reabsorption of cerebrospinal fluid is impaired, but hydrocephalus does not occur (Gjerris et al, 1985).

Table 4.12 SECONDARY PSEUDOTUMOR CEREBRI

Drugs
1. Corticosteroid withdrawal
2. Nalidixic acid
3. Oral contraceptives
4. Tetracycline
5. Vitamin A

Systemic Disorders
1. Guillain-Barré syndrome
2. Iron deficiency anemia
3. Leukemia
4. Polycythemia vera
5. Protein malnutrition
6. Systemic lupus erythematosus

Head Trauma

Infections
1. Otitis media
2. Sinusitis

Metabolic
1. Adrenal insufficiency
2. Diabetic ketoacidosis (treatment)
3. Galactosemia
4. Hyperadrenalism
5. Hyperthyroidism
6. Hypoparathyroidism
7. Menarche
8. Pregnancy

Clinical Features. The presenting symptom is generally headache. An abducens nerve palsy may be present as well, and papilledema is almost invariable. Some children have nausea and vomiting, but most are not acutely ill and mentation is normal.

Neurologic examination is otherwise unremarkable, and there are no signs of focal neurologic dysfunction. The major concern is for vision. If left untreated, some children will have progressive papilledema and optic atrophy. Loss of vision may be rapid and severe (Baker et al, 1985). Early diagnosis and treatment are therefore essential to preserve vision.

Diagnosis. Pseudotumor cerebri is a diagnosis of exclusion. In a child who presents with headache and papilledema, an enhanced CT scan must be done to exclude a mass lesion or hydrocephalus. In children with pseudotumor cerebri, the ventricles are usually small and the normal sulcal markings may be obliterated by the increased cerebral volume.

Underlying causes of pseudotumor cerebri must be excluded by careful history and physical examination. Ordinarily, these are easily identified.

Treatment. A single lumbar puncture, with the closing pressure reduced to half of the opening pressure, is sufficient to reverse the process in most cases. The mechanism by which this is effective is unknown, but it seems that a transitory change in the cerebrospinal fluid dynamics is sufficient to allow the pressure to readjust.

It is commonplace for children with pseudotumor cerebri to be treated with acetazolamide, 10 mg/kg/day, following the initial lumbar puncture. It is not clear whether or not this is an important addition to lumbar puncture. If symptoms return, lumbar puncture should be repeated on subsequent days. Serial lumbar punctures are rarely needed.

Occasionally, children continue to have increased intracranial pressure despite the use of lumbar puncture and acetazolamide. In such children, studies should be repeated to look for a cause other than idiopathic pseudotumor cerebri. If none is found and intracranial pressure remains high, lumboperitoneal shunt may be needed.

References

1. Allan WC, Dransfield DA, Tito AM: Ventricular dilation following periventricular-intraventricular hemorrhage: Outcome at age 1 year. Pediatrics 73:158, 1984.
2. Allen GS, Ahn HS, Preziosi TJ, et al: Cerebral arterial spasm—A controlled trial of nimodipine in patients with subarachnoid hemorrhage. N Engl J Med 308:619, 1983.
3. Allen JC: Childhood brain tumors: Current status of clinical trials in newly diagnosed and recurrent disease. Pediatr Clin North Am 32:633, 1985.
4. Ashwal S, Hinshaw DB Jr, Bedros A: CNS primitive neuroectodermal tumors of childhood. Med Pediatr Oncol 12:180, 1984.
5. Aucoin PJ, Kotilainen HR, Gantz NM, et al: Intracranial pressure monitors. Epidemiologic study of risk factors and infections. Am J Med 80:369, 1986.
6. Baker RS, Carter D, Hendrick B, et al: Visual loss of pseudotumor cerebri of childhood. Arch Ophthalmol 103:1681, 1985.
7. Bell WE: Treatment of fungal infections of the central nervous system. Ann Neurol 9:417, 1981.
8. Bell WE: Current therapy of acute bacterial meningitis in children: Part I. Pediatr Neurol 1:5, 1985.
9. Bell WE: Current therapy of acute bacterial meningitis in children: Part II. Pediatr Neurol 1:201, 1985.
10. Berg B, Franklin G, Cuneo R, et al: Nonsurgical cure of brain abscess: Early diagnosis and follow-up with computerized tomography. Ann Neurol 3:474, 1978.
11. Black JT: Cerebral candidiasis: case report of cerebral abscess secondary to Candida albicans, and review of the literature. J Neurol Neurosurg Psychiatry 33:864, 1970.
12. Cohen ME, Duffner PK: Ependymomas. In Cohen ME, Duffner PK, eds. Brain Tumors in Children. Raven Press, New York, 1984, p 136.
13. Couch R, Camfield PR, Tibbles JAR: The changing picture of pseudotumor cerebri in children. Can J Neurol Sci 12:48, 1985.
14. Cutler RWP, Spertell RB: Cerebrospinal fluid: A selective review. Ann Neurol 11:1, 1982.
15. Dodge PR, Hallowell D, Reigin RD, et al: Prospective evaluation of hearing impairment as a sequela of acute bacterial meningitis. N Engl J Med 311:869, 1984.
16. Dohrmann GJ, Farwell JR, Flannery JT: Ependymomas and ependymoblastomas in children. J Neurosurg 45:273, 1976.
17. Duffner PK, Cohen ME, Myers MH, et al: Survival of children with brain tumors: SEER program, 1973–1980. Neurology 36:597, 1986.
18. Eichenwald HF: Bacterial meningitis: is there "best" antimicrobial therapy? Eur J Pediatr 146:216, 1987.
19. Emery JR, Peabody JL: Head position affects intracranial pressure in newborn infants. J Pediatr 103:950, 1983.
20. Fenichel GM, Webster DL, Wong WKT: Intracranial hemorrhage in the term newborn. Arch Neurol 41:30, 1984.
21. Fischer EG, McLennan JE, Suzuki Y: Cerebral abscess in children. Am J Dis Child 135:746, 1981.
22. Fishman RA: Cerebrospinal Fluid in Disease of the Nervous System. WB Saunders Co, Philadelphia, 1980.
23. Foreman SD, Smith EE, Ryan NJ, et al: Neonatal citrobacter meningitis: Pathogenesis of cerebral abscess formation. Ann Neurol 16:655, 1984.
24. Gjerris F, Sorensen PS, Vorstrup S, et al: Intracranial pressure, conductance to cerebrospinal fluid outflow, and cerebral blood flow in patients with benign intracranial hypertension (pseudotumor cerebri). Ann Neurol 17:158, 1985.
25. Graf CJ, Perret GE, Torner JC: Bleeding from cerebral arteriovenous malformation as part of their natural history. J Neurosurg 58:331, 1983.
26. Graus F, Walker RW, Allen JC: Brain metastases in children. J Pediatr 103:558, 1983.
27. Guidetti B, Spallone A: The surgical treatment of choroid plexus papillomas. The result of 27 years experience. Neurosurg Rev 4:129, 1981.
28. Harsh GR, Edwards MSB, Wilson CB: Intracranial arachnoid cysts in children. J Neurosurg 64:835, 1986.
29. Hill A, Perlman J, Volpe JJ: Relationship of pneumothorax to occurrence of intraventricular hemorrhage in the premature newborn. Pediatrics 69:144, 1982.
30. Hill A, Volpe JJ: Normal pressure hydrocephalus in the newborn. Pediatrics 68:623, 1981.
31. Kaplan SL, Feigin RD: The syndrome of inappropriate secretion of antidiuretic hormone in children with bacterial meningitis. J Pediatr 92:758, 1978.
32. Kassell NF, Torner JC: The international cooperative study on timing of aneurysm surgery—An update. Stroke 15:566, 1984.
33. Kjellberg RN, Hanamura T, Davis KR, et al: Bragg-peak proton-beam therapy for arteriovenous malformations of the brain. N Engl J Med 309:269, 1983.
34. Klein JO, Marcy SM: Bacterial sepsis and meningitis. In Remington JS, Klein JO, eds. Infectious Diseases of the Fetus and Newborn Infant. 2nd edition. WB Saunders Co, Philadelphia, 1983.
35. Kreusser KL, Tarby TJ, Kovnar E, et al: Serial lumbar punctures for at least temporary amelioration of neonatal posthemorrhagic hydrocephalus. Pediatrics 75:719, 1985.
36. Kuban KCK, Leviton A, Krishnamorthy KS, et al:

Neonatal intracranial hemorrhage in preterm infants. Pediatrics 65:30, 1980.

37. Lazzara A, Ahmann P, Dykes F, et al: Clinical predictability of intraventricular hemorrhage in preterm infants. Pediatrics 65:30, 1980.

38. Leys D, Destee A, Petit H, et al: Management of subdural intracranial empyemas should not always require surgery. J Neurol Neurosurg Psychiatry 49:635, 1986.

39. Luessenhop AJ: Natural history of cerebral arteriovenous malformations. In Wilson CB, Stein BM, eds. Intracranial Arteriovenous Malformations. Williams & Wilkins, Baltimore, 1984, p 12.

40. McCarton-Daum C, Danziger A, Ruff H, et al: Periventricular low density as a predictor of neurobehavioral outcome in very low-birthweight infants. Dev Med Child Neurol 25:559, 1983.

41. McMenamin JB, Shackleford GD, Volpe JJ: Outcome of neonatal intraventricular hemorrhage with periventricular echodense lesions. Ann Neurol 15:285, 1984.

42. Miller JD: Intracranial pressure monitoring. Arch Neurol 42:1191, 1985.

43. Miller JD, Bobo H, Kapp JP: Inaccurate pressure readings for subarachonid bolts. Neurosurgery 19:253, 1986.

44. Mohr JP: Neurological manifestations and factors related to therapeutic decisions. In Wilson CB, Stein BM, eds. Intracranial Arteriovenous Malformations. Williams & Wilkins, Baltimore, 1984, p 1.

45. Naidich TP, McLone DG, Radkowski MA: Intracranial arachnoid cysts. Pediatr Neurosci 12:112, 1986.

46. Packer RJ, Sutton LN, Rosenstock JG, et al: Pineal region tumors of childhood. Pediatrics 74:97, 1984.

47. Palma L, Russo A, Mercuri S: Cystic cerebral astrocytomas in infancy and childhood: Long-term results. Child's Brain 10:79, 1983.

48. Ropper AH: In favor of intracranial pressure monitoring and aggressive therapy in neurologic practice. Arch Neurol 42:1194, 1985.

49. Sarff LD, Platt LH, McCracken GH, Jr: Cerebrospinal fluid evaluation in neonates: A comparison of high risk infants with and without meningitis. J Pediatr 88:473, 1976.

50. Scher MS, Wright FA, Lockman LA, et al: Intraventricular hemorrhage in the fullterm neonate. Arch Neurol 39:769, 1982.

51. Schulte FJ: Intracranial tumors in childhood—concepts of treatment and prognosis. Neuropediatria 15:3, 1984.

52. Schulte FJ, Herrmann HD, Muller D, et al: Pineal region tumors of childhood. Eur J Pediatr 146:233, 1987.

53. Shinnar S, Gammon K, Bergman EW Jr, et al: Management of hydrocephalus in infancy: Use of acetazolamide and furosemide to avoid cerebrospinal fluid shunts. J Pediatr 107:31, 1985.

54. Speer ME, Blifeld C, Rudolph AJ, et al: Intraventricular hemorrhage and vitamin E in the very-low-birth-weight infant: Evidence for efficacy of early intramuscular vitamin E administration. Pediatrics 74:1107, 1984.

55. Steer CR: Barbiturate therapy in the management of cerebral ischemia. Dev Med Child Neurol 24:219, 1982.

56. Volpe JJ, Pasternak JF, Allen WC: Ventricular dilatations preceding rapid head growth following neonatal intracranial hemorrhage. Am J Dis Child 131:1212, 1977.

57. Weibers DO, Whisnant JP, O'Fallon WM: The natural history of unruptured intracranial aneurysms. N Engl J Med 304:696, 1981.

58. Weisberg LA: Cerebral computed tomography in the diagnosis of supratentorial astrocytoma. Comput Tomogr 4:87, 1980.

59. Welch K: The intracranial pressure in infants. J Neurosurg 52:693, 1980.

60. Williamson WD, Desmond MM, Wilson GS, et al: Survival of low-birthweight infants with neonatal intraventricular hemorrhage: Outcome in the preschool years. Am J Dis Child 137:1181, 1983.

61. Yang S-Y: Brain abscess: a review of 400 cases. J Neurosurg 55:794, 1981.

5 Psychomotor Retardation and Regression

The differential diagnosis of psychomotor retardation (developmental delay) is quite different than that of psychomotor regression. Slow progress in the attainment of developmental milestones may be secondary to either a static (Table 5.1) or a progressive encephalopathy (Table 5.2). In contrast, the loss of developmental milestones previously attained is always evidence of a progressive disease of the nervous system. In the differential diagnosis of progressive diseases of the nervous system, those with onset during infancy are somewhat different from those with onset during childhood (see Tables 5.2 and 5.3).

■ Developmental Delay

Delayed achievement of developmental milestones is one of the more common problems evaluated by child neurologists. In the approach to the problem, there are two important questions to be asked: (1) Is delay restricted to specific areas of development or global? (2) Is there only developmental delay, or is there also developmental regression?

The second question is often difficult to answer in young infants. Even in static encephalopathies, new symptoms such as involuntary movements and seizures may occur. Many progressive diseases of the nervous system can present with delayed acquisition of milestones without other neurologic deficits. However, once it is clear that milestones previously achieved have been lost or that focal neurologic deficits are evolving, a progressive disease of the nervous system must be considered.

The Denver Developmental Screening Test (DDST) is an efficient and reliable method for assessing development in the doctor's office. It rapidly assesses four different components of development: personal-social, fine motor adaptive, language, and gross motor. The results can be amplified by several different psychometric tests, but the DDST in combination with neurologic assessment provides sufficient information to initiate further diagnostic studies.

LANGUAGE DELAY

Normal infants and children have a remarkable facility for acquiring language. Children exposed to two languages simultaneously will ordinarily learn both languages. Vocalization of vowels occurs in the first month, and laughing and squealing are well established by five months. At six months, infants begin articulating consonants, usually M, D, and B. These are translated by parents to mean "mama," "dada," and bottle or baby, although this is certainly not

Table 5.1. DIAGNOSIS OF DEVELOPMENT DELAY: NO REGRESSION

Predominant Speech Delay
1. Hearing loss
2. Infantile autism
3. Histidinemia

Predominant Motor Delay
1. Hypotonic infant (see Chapter 6)
2. Ataxia (see Chapter 10)
3. Hemiplegia (see Chapter 11)
4. Paraplegia (see Chapter 12)

Global Delay
1. Chromosomal disturbances
2. Cerebral malformations
3. Intrauterine infection
4. Perinatal disorders
5. Progressive encephalopathies (see Table 5.2)

118

Table 5.2 PROGRESSIVE ENCEPHALOPATHY:
ONSET BEFORE AGE TWO

Hypothyroidism

Aminoacidurias
1. Phenylketonuria
2. Homocystinuria
3. Histidinemia
4. Maple syrup urine disease
   a. Intermediate form
   b. Thiamine-responsive form

Disorders of Lysosomal Enzymes
1. Mucopolysaccharidoses
   a. Type I (Hurler)
   b. Type II (Sanfilippo)
2. Mucolipidoses
   a. Type II (I-cell)
   b. Type IV
3. Disorders of glycoprotein degradation
   a. Mannosidosis I
   b. Fucosidoses I and II
   c. Sialidosis II (infantile form)
4. Sphingomyelin lipidosis (Niemann-Pick type A)
5. Glucosylceramide lipidosis (Gaucher I)
6. Globoid cell leukodystrophy (Krabbe)
7. Sulfatide lipidoses (metachromatic leukodystrophy)
8. GM$_1$ gangliosidosis, I and II
9. GM$_2$ gangliosidosis (Tay-Sachs, Sandhoff)

Disorders of Mitochondrial Enzymes
1. Subacute necrotizing encephalomyelopathy (Leigh)
2. Progressive infantile poliodystrophy (Alper)
3. Trichopoliodystrophy (Menkes)
4. Mitochondrial myopathy, encephalopathy, lactic acidosis, stroke (see Chapter 11)

Other Known Enzyme Deficiencies
1. Galactosemia-transferase deficiency
2. Lesch-Nyhan disease

Neurocutaneous Syndromes
1. Tuberous sclerosis
2. Neurofibromatosis
3. Chédiak-Higashi syndrome

Genetic and Idiopathic Disorders of Gray Matter
1. Infantile neuroaxonal dystrophy
2. Rett syndrome
3. Infantile ceroid lipofuscinosis (Santavuori)

Genetic Disorders of White Matter
1. Alexander disease
2. Pelizaeus-Merzbacher disease
3. Spongy degeneration of infancy (Canaven)
4. Neonatal adrenoleukodystrophy (see Chapter 6)

Progressive Hydrocephalus

AIDS Dementia (see Chapter 2)

before it can be encoded. By two years of age, children have learned to combine at least two words, understand more than 250 words, and follow many simple verbal directions.

Hearing Loss

The major cause of isolated delay in speech development is hearing loss. Hearing loss also may occur concomitantly with global developmental retardation. Examples of the latter are rubella embryopathy, cytomegalic inclusion disease, neonatal meningitis, kernicterus, and several genetic disorders. Hearing loss need not be profound, and it can be quite insidious, yet still produce delayed speech development. Consider the high-frequency hearing loss inherent to telephone conversation; it prevents the clear distinction of many consonants that we learn to fill in through experience. Infants do not have this experience.

Hearing loss should be suspected and tested by formal audiometry in any infant with isolated delay in speech development. Crude testing in the office by slamming objects and ringing bells is an inadequate approach to diagnosis. Hearing loss should be suspected in children with global retardation caused by disorders ordinarily associated with hearing loss or in retarded children who fail to imitate sounds. Other clues to hearing loss in children include excessive use of gesture

Table 5.3 PROGRESSIVE ENCEPHALOPATHY:
ONSET AFTER AGE TWO

Disorders of Lysosomal Enzymes
1. Mucopolysaccharidoses types II, III, and VII
2. Disorders of glycoprotein degradation
   a. Mannosidosis II
   b. Aspartylglycosaminuria
3. Sphingomyelin lipidosis (Niemann-Pick type C)
4. Glucosylceramide lipidosis (Gaucher III)
5. Late-onset globoid cell leukodystrophy (Krabbe)
6. Juvenile sulfatide lipidosis

Genetic Disorders of Gray Matter
1. Ceroid lipofuscinosis
   a. Late infantile (Bielschowsky-Jansky)
   b. Juvenile
2. Huntington disease
3. Mitochondrial disorders
4. Xeroderma pigmentosum

Genetic Disorders of White Matter
1. Adrenoleukodystrophy
2. Cerebrotendinous xanthomatosis
3. Alexander disease

Infectious Diseases
1. Subacute sclerosing panencephalitis
2. Chronic rubella encephalopathy
3. AIDS dementia (see Chapter 2)

the intention of the infant. These first attempts at vowels and consonants are automatic and sometimes occur even in deaf children. In the months that follow, the infant imitates many speech sounds, babbles and coos, and finally learns the specific use of mama and dada by one year of age. Receptive skills are always more highly developed than expressive skills because it is necessary to decode language

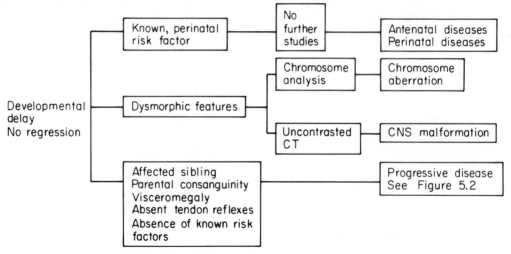

Figure 5.1 Evaluation of infants with developmental delay but with no evidence of psychomotor regression.

and intent and staring at the lips of people who are talking.

Infantile Autism

Infantile autism was originally described as a form of psychosis secondary to abnormal mother-child bonding. It is now generally regarded as an organic brain disease with several possible causes.

Clinical Features. Clinical features include failure of language development and severe impairment of interpersonal relationships with onset at birth or during infancy (Herskowitz and Rosman, 1982). Failure of language development is more likely to bring such infants to medical attention than is impairment of interpersonal relationships. Such infants show no affection to their parents or other care providers, but treat people as if they were inanimate objects. Other behavioral disturbances, sometimes associated, are a morbid preoccupation with spinning objects, stereotyped behavior such as rocking and spinning, and relative insensitivity to pain.

Diagnosis. This is a clinical diagnosis and cannot be confirmed by laboratory tests.

Treatment. Some aspects of the severely aberrant behavior can be improved by behavior modification techniques. However, despite the best program of treatment, these children function in a moderate to severe retarded range, albeit with some individuals having islands of normal ability (idiot savant).

Histidinemia

Histidinemia is a rare inborn error of metabolism with an incidence similar to that of phenylketonuria (one per 15,000 live births). The disorder is due to deficiency of the enzyme histidase, which catalyzes the conversion of histidine to urocanic acid. The defect is ordinarily transmitted by autosomal recessive inheritance, but also may be transmitted as an autosomal dominant trait (LaDu, 1978).

Clinical Features. Affected children are normal at birth. The common presenting symptom is delayed speech development, which may be secondary to short auditory memory span. Hearing is normal. Approximately one half of children have only a speech defect and are otherwise intellectually normal. The other half have some evidence of mild to moderate retardation (see Table 5.2). Several associated physical findings have been reported in individual children, none of which are consistent among all cases.

Diagnosis. Ferric chloride can be used for rapid screening. The presence of imidazole pyruvic acid in urine produces an effervescent blue color. Definitive diagnosis requires an elevated concentration of histidine in blood and urine.

Treatment. Treatment is not available. Diet therapy has no effect on eventual outcome.

DELAYED MOTOR DEVELOPMENT

Infants with delayed gross motor development, but normal language and personal social

Table 5.4 CLINICAL INDICATIONS FOR
CHROMOSOME ANALYSIS*

Head and Neck
1. Occipital scalp defect
2. Small or low-set ears
3. Mongoloid slant (non-Oriental)
4. Microphthalmia
5. Hypertelorism or hypotelorism
6. High nasal bridge
7. Small or fish mouth
8. Small mandible
9. Webbed neck

Limbs
1. Low-set thumb
2. Overlapping fingers
3. Abnormal dermatoglyphics
4. Rocker-bottom feet
5. Polydactyly

Genitourinary
1. Polycystic kidney
2. Ambiguous genitalia

*Modified from Jones KL, Jones MC: A clinical approach to the dysmorphic child. In Emery AEH, Rimoin DL, eds. Principles and Practice of Medical Genetics. Churchill Livingstone, New York, 1983, p 152.

skills are often hypotonic and may have a neuromuscular disease (see Chapter 6). Isolated delay in motor function may also be caused by ataxia (see Chapter 10), mild hemiplegia (see Chapter 11), and mild paraplegia (see Chapter 12). Many such children have a mild form of cerebral palsy, sufficient to delay the achievement of motor milestones, but not severe enough to cause a recognizable disturbance of cognitive function during infancy. Mild disturbances in cognitive function are more often detected when the child enters school.

GLOBAL DEVELOPMENTAL DELAY

Most infants with global developmental delay have a static encephalopathy, usually as a result of antenatal or perinatal disturbances. However, a small percentage of infants with developmental delay and no evidence of regression will prove to have an underlying genetic disease. An exhaustive search to determine an underlying etiology in every infant who is developing slowly, but has no evidence of developmental regression, has a poor cost-benefit ratio. Factors that increase the likelihood of finding a progressive disease are summarized in Figure 5.1.

Chromosomal Disturbances

Abnormalities in chromosome structure or number are the single most common cause of

severe mental retardation, but still comprise only a third of the total. Abnormalities of autosomal chromosomes are always associated with infantile hypotonia (see Chapter 6). In addition, there are usually multiple minor abnormalities of the face and limbs, which in themselves are not abnormal but assume diagnostic significance in combination. Clinical features that suggest chromosomal aberrations are summarized in Table 5.4, and the major chromosome syndromes are presented in Table 5.5.

With one exception, all chromosomal aberrations causing developmental retardation are readily diagnosed by standard culture techniques. *Fragile-X syndrome*, identified by a secondary constriction located in band XQ27, requires specialized techniques that must be requested beforehand (Opitz, 1984). The defect is transmitted as an X-linked recessive trait occurring in approximately one per 1,000 males. The phenotype includes a long face in which the forehead is prominent, the midface hypoplastic, and the chin enlarged. Other abnormalities include a high-arched palate, thick lips with the lower one protruding, large malformed ears, and testicular enlargement in 80 percent of postpubertal men. Affected males are moder-

Table 5.5 SELECTED AUTOSOMAL
SYNDROMES*†

5 p monosomy	Characteristic "cri du chat" cry Moonlike face Hypertelorism Microcephaly
10 p trisomy	Dolichocephaly "Turtle's beak" Osteoarticular anomalies
Partial 12 p monosomy	Microcephaly Narrow forehead Pointed nose Micrognathia
18 trisomy	Pointed ears Micrognathia Occipital protuberance Narrow pelvis Rocker-bottom feet
21 trisomy	Hypotonia Round flat (mongoloid) facies Brushfield spots Flat nape of neck

*Modified from DeGrouchy J, Turleau J: Autosomal disorders. In Emery AEH, Rimoin DL, eds. Principles and Practice of Medical Genetics. Volume 1. Churchill Livingstone, New York, 1983, p 15.
†Growth retardation and mental retardation are features of all autosomal chromosome disorders.

ately retarded, and up to one third of carrier females are mildly retarded.

The phenotype is not sufficiently expressed in infancy to alert physicians, but special culture techniques should be requested whenever there is a pattern of X-linked mental retardation.

Cerebral Malformations

Approximately 3 percent of all children have at least one major malformation that "seriously interferes with viability or physical well-being" (Kalter and Warkany, 1983). The etiologic factors responsible for these malformations have been identified in no more than 20 percent of cases. Many intrauterine diseases cause destructive changes in the developing brain that result in organ malformation. The exposure of an embryo to infectious or toxic agents during the first weeks after conception could disorganize the delicate sequencing of neural development at a time when the brain is incapable of generating a cellular response. Alcohol, lead, prescription drugs, and substances of abuse have all been implicated in the production of cerebral malformations. However, a cause-and-effect relationship is difficult to establish in many cases, and even if all possibilities are accepted as proven, toxic exposure would account for less than 3 percent of all malformations.

Cerebral malformations should be suspected in any child who is dysmorphic or who has malformations of other organs or any abnormality of head size and shape (see Chapter 18). In such children, an uncontrasted computerized tomographic (CT) scan may be helpful in identifying a major malformation.

Intrauterine Infections

The three most commonly identified intrauterine infections are toxoplasmosis, cytomegalic inclusion disease, and rubella embryopathy. Three percent of all newborns demonstrate elevated concentrations of immunoglobulin (IgM) in cord blood, but only in 20 percent of these can the elevated concentration be accounted for by known infectious agents (Sever et al, 1979). It is likely, as demonstrated in animal models, that maternal viral infections early in pregnancy may cause malformations of the embryo without leaving traditional pathologic evidence of viral infection.

Toxoplasmosis

Toxoplasma gondii is a protozoon that is estimated to infect one per 1,000 live births in the United States each year. The symptoms of toxoplasmosis infection of the mother are usually so mild as to go unnoticed. Transplacental transmission of toxoplasmosis is possible only if primary maternal infection occurs during pregnancy (Remington and Desmonts, 1983). During the last trimester, the rate of placental transmission is highest, but fetuses who are infected are least likely to be symptomatic. During the first trimester, the transmission rate is lowest, but fetuses who are infected have the most serious sequelae.

Clinical Features. Twenty-five percent of infected newborns have multisystem involvement (fever, rash, hepatosplenomegaly, jaundice, and thrombocytopenia) at birth. Neurologic dysfunction is manifested by seizures, altered states of consciousness, and increased intracranial pressure. The triad of hydrocephalus, chorioretinitis, and intracranial calcification is the hallmark of congenital toxoplasmosis in older children. Eight percent of infected newborns, asymptomatic at birth, will later show neurologic sequelae, of which psychomotor retardation is a prominent feature.

Diagnosis. The most reliable serologic test in the newborn for the diagnosis of congenital toxoplasmosis is the demonstration of IgM-indirect fluorescent antibody to toxoplasma in the umbilical cord blood. In older children, the diagnosis requires not only serologic evidence of prior infection but also compatible clinical features.

Treatment. In newborns with clinical evidence of toxoplasmosis, pyrimethamine (Daraprim), 0.5 mg/kg, and sulfadiazine, 25 mg/kg, are administered orally every twelve hours for twenty-one days. Because pyrimethamine is a folic acid antagonist, folic acid, 0.1 mg/kg/day, is given as well. Peripheral platelet count must be monitored regularly (Remington and Desmonts, 1983). Prednisone, 1 to 2 mg/kg/day, should be added to the therapy in newborns with high concentrations of cerebrospinal fluid protein or chorioretinitis. The twenty-one day course of pyrimethamine and sulfadiazine is repeated every three or four months during the first year.

Cytomegalic Inclusion Disease

The cytomegalovirus is a member of the herpes group and produces chronic infection characterized by long periods of latency punctuated by intervals of reactivation. It is transmitted by adults during sexual activity and produces a silent infection of the cervix. Pregnancy may cause reactivation of maternal infection, and cytomegalovirus can be cultured from the urine in 1 to 2 percent of all live births in the United States. Fortunately, fewer than 0.05 percent of newborns with viruria have symptoms of cytomegalic inclusion disease.

Clinical Features. Cytomegalic inclusion disease is difficult to differentiate from other intrauterine infections on the basis of clinical examination alone. The typical clinical presentation includes skin rash, hepatosplenomegaly, jaundice, chorioretinitis, and microcephaly with cerebral calcification. Cytomegalic inclusion disease can also present as microcephaly without evidence of systemic infection (Hanshaw et al, 1976).

Diagnosis. Isolation of cytomegalovirus from the urine or cerebrospinal fluid indicates active infection in the newborn. In infants with developmental delay and microcephaly, the diagnosis of cytomegalic inclusion disease is made by serologic demonstration of prior infection and a consistent pattern of intracranial calcification.

Treatment. Arabinosides suppress viruria in 50 percent of patients, but do not influence outcome. Acyclovir is being assessed in several centers. The benefit of any therapy is difficult to evaluate. Brain damage is considerable and probably complete at the time of birth. Damage to other organs is self-limited.

Rubella Embryopathy

Clinical Features. This multisystem disease is characterized by intrauterine growth retardation, cataracts and chorioretinitis, congenital heart disease, sensorineural deafness, hepatosplenomegaly, jaundice, anemia, thrombocytopenia, and rash (Desmond et al, 1967). Neurologic dysfunction is manifested by lethargy, hypotonia, and seizures. Seizures may be delayed in onset until three months of age.

Diagnosis. Rubella embryopathy should not be considered a cause of psychomotor retardation unless there are other signs and symptoms of rubella infection in the newborn.

Treatment. Treatment is not available for active infection. Fortunately, this disorder has almost disappeared since the introduction of routine immunization of children.

Perinatal Disorders

Perinatal infection, asphyxia, and trauma are the major perinatal events that result in psycho-motor retardation (see Chapter 1). The important infectious diseases are bacterial meningitis (see Chapter 4) and herpes encephalitis (see Chapter 1). Although the overall mortality rate for bacterial meningitis is now less than 50 percent, significant neurologic sequelae are noted almost immediately in 50 percent of survivors. The most common sequelae are mental and motor disabilities, hydrocephalus, epilepsy, deafness, and visual loss. Psychomotor retardation may be the only or the most prominent sequelae. Progressive mental deterioration can occur if meningitis causes a secondary hydrocephalus.

■ Progressive Encephalopathies of Infancy

There are three questions to be answered from the history and physical examination before laboratory diagnosis is initiated:

1. Are symptoms and signs referable only to the nervous system, or is there evidence of multiorgan involvement, i.e., hepatosplenomegaly (Fig. 5.2)?

2. If the disease is limited to the nervous system, are peripheral nerves involved as well? An early sign of peripheral neuropathy in infancy is loss of the Achilles tendon reflex. More advanced neuropathy is manifested by distal weakness and hypotonia, and subclinical neuropathy is manifested by electrophysiologic studies (see Chapters 6, 7, and 9).

3. Does the disease process affect primarily the gray matter or the white matter? Early features of gray matter disease are personality change, seizures, and dementia. White matter disease is characterized by focal neurologic deficits and blindness. Whether the process begins in the gray matter or the white matter, eventually there will be clinical features of dysfunction in both. In primary diseases of gray matter, the EEG is usually abnormal early in the course of disease and is sometimes characteristic. Cortical atrophy can be demonstrated by CT scan, and if the brainstem is involved, brainstem auditory evoked responses may be abnormal. Magnetic resonance imaging (MRI) demonstrates cerebral demyelination with remarkable clarity (Fig. 5.3). Visual evoked responses and motor conduction velocities are useful in documenting demyelination, even subclinical, in the optic and peripheral nerves, respectively.

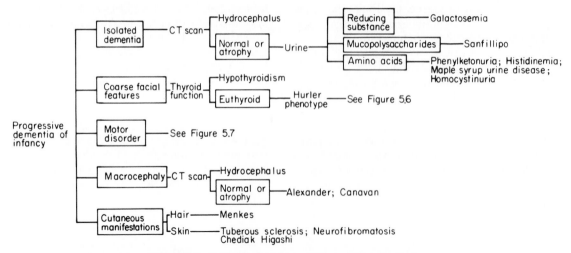

Figure 5.2 Evaluation of infants with progressive dementia.

HYPOTHYROIDISM

Congenital hypothyroidism secondary to thyroid dysgenesis occurs in one per 4,000 live births. The etiology is unknown, but the occasional familial occurrence in siblings has suggested either a genetic basis or an underlying maternal factor. Early diagnosis and treatment are imperative to ensure a favorable outcome.

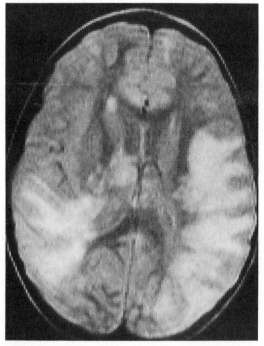

Figure 5.3 Krabbe disease. Magnetic resonance image demonstrates extensive demyelination of cerebral hemispheres.

Fortunately, newborn screening has become universal in the United States and virtually all cases are detected by this method.

Clinical Features. Affected individuals are usually asymptomatic at birth. Clinical features evolve insidiously during the first weeks post partum, and their significance is not always appreciated. Frequently, the gestation lasts for more than forty-two weeks and birth weight is greater than 4 kg (Smith et al, 1975). Early clinical features include (1) a widely open posterior fontanelle, (2) constipation, (3) jaundice, (4) poor temperature control, and (5) umbilical hernia. The tongue is sometimes large and makes feeding difficult. Edema of the eyes, hands, and feet may be present at birth but is often not recognized in early infancy.

Diagnosis. Radiographs of the long bones demonstrate delayed maturation, and radiographs of the skull demonstrate excessive numbers of wormian bones. A definitive diagnosis relies upon the demonstration of low serum concentrations of thyroxine (T_4) and high serum concentrations of thyroid-stimulating hormone (TSH).

Treatment. Once a diagnosis of congenital hypothyroidism is established, treatment is initiated with 25 to 50 μg of sodium-1-thyroxine daily. Early treatment allows normal mental development. The ultimate intelligence of the hypothyroid infant declines progressively with each month of delay.

AMINOACIDURIAS

Disorders of amino acid metabolism produce symptoms of gray matter dysfunction initially

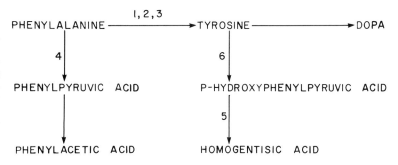

Figure 5.4 Phenylalanine metabolism. *1,* Phenylalanine hydroxylase. *2,* Dihydropteridine reductase. *3,* Tetrahydrobiopterin. *4,* Phenylalanine transaminase. *5, p*-Hydroxyphenylpyruvic acid. *6,* Tyrosine transaminase. (Reprinted from Fenichel GM: Neonatal Neurology. Churchill Livingstone, New York, 1985.)

(mental retardation, seizures), but have a profound affect upon myelination as well.

Phenylketonuria

Phenylketonuria is a disorder of phenylalanine metabolism secondary to partial or total deficiency of the hepatic enzyme phenylalanine hydroxylase (Guttler, 1984; Scriver and Clow, 1980). The deficiency is transmitted by autosomal recessive inheritance and occurs in approximately one per 16,000 live births. Because phenylalanine cannot be adequately hydroxylated to tyrosine, phenylalanine accumulates and is transaminated to phenylpyruvic acid (Fig. 5.4). Phenylpyruvic acid is oxidized to phenylacetic acid, which is excreted in the urine and causes a musty odor.

Clinical Features. Affected children are normal at birth and would not be detected in the absence of compulsory mass screening. The screening test detects hyperphenylalaninemia, which is not synonymous with phenylketonuria (Table 5.6). A precise determination of blood

Table 5.6 DIFFERENTIAL DIAGNOSIS OF HYPERPHENYLALANINEMIA

Classic Phenylketonuria
Complete hydroxylase deficiency (0–6%)

Benign Variants
Partial hydroxylase deficiency (6–30%)
Transitory hydroxylase deficiency
Phenylalanine transaminase deficiency
Other

Malignant Variants
Dihydropteridine reductase deficiency
Tetrahydrobiopterin synthesis deficiency

Tyrosinemia
Transitory tyrosinemia
Tyrosinosis

Liver Disease
Galactose-1-phosphate uridyl transferase deficiency

phenylalanine and tyrosine concentrations must be performed in every newborn detected by the screening test in order to differentiate classic phenylketonuria from other conditions. In newborns with classic phenylketonuria, hyperphenylalaninemia develops forty-eight to seventy-two hours after initiation of a milk feed. Blood phenylalanine concentrations are 20 mg/dl (1200 μmol/L) or greater, and serum tyrosine levels are less than 5 mg/dl (275 μmol/L). When blood phenylalanine concentrations reach 15 mg/dl (900 μmol/L), phenylalanine spills over in the urine and the addition of ferric chloride solution (five to ten drops of FeCl to 1 ml of urine) produces a green color.

Untreated infants appear normal during the first months, but there may be a musty odor of the skin as a result of phenylacetic acid in the sweat. Developmental delay is sometimes manifested by the third month and always before the end of the first year. By the beginning of the second year, developmental regression is evident. Behavioral disturbances characterized by hyperactivity and aggressiveness are commonplace; focal neurologic deficits are unusual. Approximately 25 percent of affected infants have seizures. Some have infantile spasms and hypsarrhythmia; others have tonic-clonic seizures. A frequent feature of infants with phenylketonuria is blond hair, pale skin, and blue eyes owing to diminished pigment production. Eczema is common. These skin changes are the only non-neurologic manifestations of phenylketonuria.

Diagnosis. Benign variants of phenylketonuria are generally characterized by blood phenylalanine levels of less than 25 mg/dl (1500 μmol/L), frequently less than 15 mg/dl (900 μmol/L) and a normal concentration of tyrosine. The malignant forms of phenylketonuria are secondary to disturbances in tetrahydrobiopterin. Seizures are the initial symptom and are followed by mental retardation and motor deficits.

Transitory tyrosinemia is estimated to occur in 2 percent of term newborns and in 25 percent of prematures. It is caused by a transitory deficiency of the enzyme p-hydroxyphenylpyruvic acid. It is a benign condition and can be distinguished from phenylketonuria because the blood concentrations of tyrosine and phenylalanine are both elevated.

Treatment. All experts agree that a phenylalanine-restricted diet should be started immediately in all newborns with a blood phenylalanine concentration of 30 mg/dl (1800 μmol/L) or greater; some would start diet therapy at a concentration of 20 mg/dl (1200 μmol/L). After three months of therapy, a three day challenge of phenylalanine, 180 mg/kg/day, is indicated to distinguish mild variants from classic phenylketonuria. Children with phenylketonuria have a blood phenylalanine concentration of 20 mg/dl (1200 μmol/L) or greater and need to be continued on restricted diets. Those with a blood concentration lower than 20 mg/dl (1200 μmol/L) probably have a benign variant and do not require further dietary restriction of phenylalanine. The present goal of therapy is to maintain blood phenylalanine concentrations between 5 and 10 mg/dl (300 to 600 μmol/L). Diet therapy should be maintained indefinitely; discontinuation may lead to intellectual deterioration (Seashore et al, 1985).

Tetrahydrobiopterin is a cofactor for the enzymes phenylalanine hydroxylase, tyrosine hydroxylase, and tryptophan hydroxylase. Deficiency of tetrahydrobiopterin can be due to defective recycling or defective synthesis. In infants with cofactor deficiency, a diet restricted in phenylalanine reduces the blood phenylalanine concentration, but does not prevent neurologic deterioration. For these children, tetrahydrobiopterin administration is the therapy of choice (Hoganson et al, 1984).

Homocystinuria

Homocystinuria can be caused by three different genetic defects. The defect associated with mental retardation is almost complete deficiency of the enzyme cystathionine-β-synthase (Fig. 5.5). Transmission is by autosomal recessive inheritance. Heterozygotes have partial deficiencies. Cystathionine-β-synthase catalyzes the condensation of serine and homocysteine to form cystathionine. When the enzyme is deficient, the concentrations of homocysteine, homocystine, and methionine in the blood and urine are elevated. It is hypermethioninemia that is detected in newborn screening programs.

Clinical Features. Affected individuals appear normal at birth. Global developmental delay is usually the first clinical manifestation, and intelligence will decline progressively with age in untreated children. Most eventually function in the mildly retarded range, but at least 20 percent have normal intelligence (Mudd and Levy, 1983). Thromboembolism affecting large arteries, small arteries, and veins is a life-threatening complication of homocystinuria. Emboli may occur in infancy or be delayed until adult life. Occlusion of the coronary or carotid arteries can lead to sudden death or severe neurologic handicap. Thromboembolism is the first clue to diagnosis in 15 percent of cases (Mudd et al, 1985). Dislocation of the lens, an almost constant feature of homocystinuria, typically occurs between the ages of two and ten, but may be delayed until adult life. Ninety-seven percent of all patients have lens dislocation by age forty. Osteoporosis is a constant feature in older children. The spine is affected first and most severely, resulting in scoliosis and sometimes vertebral collapse. Many children are tall and thin and have a Marfan syndrome habitus. This habitus does not develop until middle or late

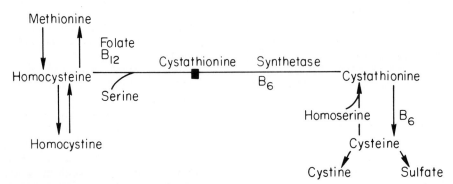

Figure 5.5 Metabolic disturbance in homocystinuria. Absence of cystathionine synthetase blocks the metabolism of homocysteine, causing the accumulation of homocystine and methionine.

childhood and serves as a clue to diagnosis in fewer than 40 percent of cases.

The diagnosis should be suspected in any infant with isolated and unexplained developmental delay, because disease-specific features need not appear until later in childhood. The presence of either thromboembolism or lens dislocation strongly suggests homocystinuria.

Diagnosis. Rapid screening is available by adding 1 ml of a 5 percent aqueous solution of sodium cyanide to 1 ml of urine. After waiting five minutes at room temperature, add three to five drops of a 5 percent aqueous solution of sodium nitroprusside. If homocystine is present in the urine, the solution will turn a deep red color. Definitive diagnosis is made by demonstrating a deficiency of cystathionine-β-synthase either in the liver or in cultured fibroblasts.

Treatment. The administration of pyridoxine, 500 to 1,000 mg/day, is effective in reducing or eliminating the biochemical abnormalities in a third of patients. An equal number are not pyridoxine-responsive, and the remainder have an intermediate response. Folate must be given concomitantly. Most patients who respond to pyridoxine probably have a low level or mutant form of cystathionine-β-synthase activity that is enhanced by the addition of cofactor.

The most widely used dietary treatment for homocystinuria is methionine restriction and cystine supplementation. When initiated in the newborn, mental retardation is prevented and the incidence of lens dislocation may be decreased. Information is not yet available to assess the efficacy of diet in preventing thromboembolic events or osteoporosis. Newborns who are pyridoxine-responsive should be treated both with methionine restriction and pyridoxine.

Maple Syrup Urine Disease (Mild)

The three major branched-chain amino acids are leucine, isoleucine, and valine. In the course of their metabolism, they are first transaminated to alpha-ketoacids and then further catabolized by oxidative decarboxylation (Fig. 5.5). Deficiency of the enzyme branched-chain ketoacid dehydrogenase, which is responsible for oxidative decarboxylation, is associated with at least three different phenotypes: classic, intermittent, and mild maple syrup urine disease. The classic and intermittent forms are characterized by acute encephalopathies with ketoacidosis (see Chapters 1 and 10). The mild form presents as progressive mental retardation without ketoaci-

dosis (Kodama et al, 1976). The amounts of dehydrogenase enzyme activity in the mild and intermittent forms are approximately the same (5 to 40 percent), whereas activity in the classic form is 0 to 2 percent. Phenotypic difference between the mild and intermittent forms may be related to protein intake. Some infants with the mild form are thiamine-responsive. The enzyme defect in these cases may be unique.

Clinical Features. Infants with mild maple syrup urine disease are normal at birth, slow in achieving milestones, and hyperactive. They generally function in the moderately retarded range of intelligence. Physical development is normal except for coarse, brittle hair. The urine may have the odor of maple syrup. Acute mental changes, seizures, and focal neurologic deficits do not occur.

Diagnosis. Preliminary screening is accomplished by demonstrating either a yellow precipitate when 0.2 ml of a 0.5 percent solution of 2,4-dinitrophenylhydrazine in 2N hydrochloride, or a navy blue color when five to ten drops of a 5 to 10 percent solution of ferric chloride are added to 1 ml of urine. Definitive diagnosis requires the demonstration of branched-chain ketoacids and amino acids in the blood and urine.

Treatment. All infants with mild maple syrup urine disease should be put on a protein-restricted diet. In addition, a trial of 100 mg/day of thiamine is given to determine whether the biochemical error is thiamine-responsive. If 100 mg is not effective, then daily dosages up to 1 g of thiamine should be tried before the condition is designated as thiamine-refractory (Pueschel et al, 1979).

DISORDERS OF LYSOSOMAL ENZYMES

Lysosomes are cytoplasmic vesicles containing enzymes that degrade the products of cellular catabolism. When lysosomal enzymes are deficient, abnormal storage of materials occurs. One or several organs may be affected. Mental retardation and regression are features of many lysosomal storage diseases. In some—such as acid lipase deficiency (Wolman disease) and ceramide deficiency (Farber lipogranulomatosis)—mental retardation occurs, but is neither a prominent nor a presenting feature. Such disorders are omitted from the discussion.

Mucopolysaccharidoses

Type I (Hurler Syndrome)

The Hurler syndrome results from absence of the lysosomal hydrolase α-L-iduronidase. The defect is transmitted by autosomal recessive inheritance. Dermatan sulfate and heparan sulfate cannot be fully degraded and appear in the urine. Mucopolysaccharides are stored in the cornea, collagen, and leptomeninges. In addition, gangliosides are stored in cortical neurons.

Clinical Features. Affected children are normal during the first year. In the second year, first there is arrest of development and then slow regression. Motor dysfunction affects the corticospinal tracts and the peripheral nerves. A distinctive "Hurler phenotype" evolves (Table 5.7). Clouding of the cornea is present in all cases, sometimes causing complete blindness. Facial features become coarse, there is progressive hepatosplenomegaly, umbilical hernia, and skeletal deformities that produce dwarfism, kyphoscoliosis, and limited movement of the joints. The skeletal deformities, termed dysostosis multiplex, produce characteristic radiographic features: hypoplasia of the lateral clavicle, rounding and sometimes hypoplasia of the thoracolumbar vertebral bodies, flaring of the pelvis with hypoplasia of the acetabula, broadening of the ribs, and widening of the diaphyses of long bones. The skull loses its convolutional markings, the sella turcia is enlarged, and the orbits shallow. Communicating hydrocephalus may result from thickening of the leptomeninges. Death usually occurs by age ten.

Diagnosis. The diagnosis is suggested by the physical and radiographic appearance, the presence of vacuolated lymphocytes, and mucopolysacchariduria. A simple screening test is the appearance of a metachromatic spot when a drop of urine is placed on paper impregnated with toluidine blue. Definitive diagnosis requires the demonstration of enzyme deficiency in leukocytes or cultured fibroblasts.

Treatment. Treatment is not available.

Table 5.7   THE HURLER PHENOTYPE

Abdominal hernia
Coarse facial features
Corneal opacity
Deafness
Dysostosis multiplex
Mental retardation
Stiff joints
Visceromegaly

Mucopolysaccharidosis III

The type III disorder is distinct from other mucopolysaccharidoses because only heparan sulfate is stored in viscera and appears in the urine. Gangliosides are stored in neurons. Four different, but related, enzyme deficiencies have been implicated. All are transmitted by autosomal recessive inheritance.

Clinical Features. The Hurler phenotype is not prominent, but hepatomegaly is present in two thirds of cases. Dwarfism does not occur. The major feature is neurologic deterioration characterized by delayed motor development beginning towards the end of the second year, followed by an interval of arrested mental development, and progressive dementia. Hyperactivity and sleep disorders are relatively common between the ages of two and four. Most affected children are severely retarded by age eleven and dead before age twenty. However, considerable variability exists and Sanfillipo disease should be considered even when the onset of mental regression occurs after age five.

Diagnosis. The diagnosis should be suspected in infants and children with progressive psychomotor regression and a positive screening test for mucopolysacchariduria. The presence of heparan sulfate, but not dermatan sulfate, in the urine is presumptive evidence of the disease. Specific diagnosis requires the demonstration of enzyme deficiency in cultured fibroblasts.

Treatment. Treatment is not available.

Mucolipidoses

Mucolipidosis II (I-Cell Disease)

Mucolipidosis type II is caused by partial or complete deficiency of several acid hydrolases. It resembles Hurler syndrome, except that symptoms appear earlier, the neurologic deterioration is more rapid, and mucopolysacchariduria is not present.

Clinical Features. Affected newborns are small for dates and may have hyperplastic gums. Coarsening of facial features and limitation of joint movements occur within the first months. The complete Hurler phenotype is present within the first year, except that corneal opacification is a less constant feature. Death usually occurs before age five from congestive heart failure.

Diagnosis. I-cell disease should be considered in infants with Hurler phenotype and a negative screening test for mucopolysacchariduria (Fig. 5.6). Definitive diagnosis requires the demon-

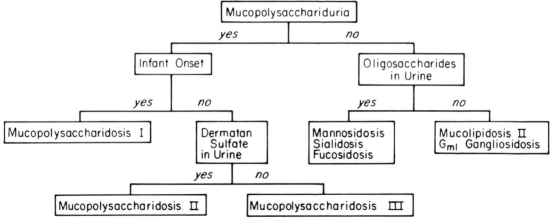

Figure 5.6 Evaluation of infants with a Hurler phenotype.

stration of enzyme deficiency in cultured fibroblasts.

Treatment. Treatment is not available.

Mucolipidosis IV

Type IV mucolipidosis is transmitted by autosomal recessive inheritance in Ashkenazi Jews. The suspected defect is deficiency of the enzyme ganglioside sialidase. Gangliosides, phospholipids, and acidic mucopolysaccharides accumulate in many tissues.

Clinical Features. Age at onset is during infancy. Developmental delay and visual impairment due to corneal clouding and retinal degeneration are the major features (Amir et al, in press). Mental retardation is profound. There are no typical facial features, skeletal abnormalities, or visceromegaly. Longevity of affected children has not been established.

Diagnosis. Mucolipidosis IV should be suspected in Jewish children with psychomotor delay or regression and corneal clouding. The electroretinogram usually shows a reduction in amplitude or absent. Diagnosis is confirmed by the demonstration of ganglioside storage in cultured fibroblasts.

Treatment. Corneal transplant may be useful to restore vision, but treatment is not available for the mental deterioration.

Fucosidoses I and II

This rare disorder is caused by deficiency of the lysosomal enzyme α-fucosidase. Two clinical types are recognized, both present during infancy. Type II is more slowly progressive and allows longer survival.

Clinical Features. The onset of psychomotor retardation and regression is three to eighteen months in type I and one to two years in type II. In both types a Hurler phenotype (Table 5.7) develops, except that corneal opacities are not present and skeletal abnormalities are restricted to the spine. Infants with fucosidosis type II survive to early adult life. An additional distinctive feature is that type I patients experience increased sweating while type II patients have anhydrosis and angiokeratoma.

Diagnosis. The diagnosis is suspected in infants with a Hurler phenotype but absent mucopolysacchariduria (Fig. 5.6). Vacuolated lymphocytes are present in the peripheral blood. Demonstration of fucosidase deficiency in leukocytes or fibroblasts provides definitive diagnosis.

Treatment. Treatment is not available.

Sialidosis II

Type II sialidosis is a rare disorder caused by a deficiency of the glycoprotein-specific α-neuraminidase (sialidase). Three different clinical syndromes have been described: a *congenital* form (I) with hydrops fetalis, an *infantile* form (II) with Hurler phenotype, and a *juvenile* form (III) characterized only by myoclonus and a cherry-red spot of the macula (Table 5.8).

Clinical Features. Infants, by appearance, are first thought to have a mucopolysaccharidosis. Towards the end of the first decade, ataxia, myoclonus, and seizures develop, sometimes associated with a cherry-red spot of the macula. Mental retardation is present, but progressive dementia is not a feature.

Table 5.8 LYSOSOMAL ENZYME DISORDERS WITH A CHERRY-RED SPOT

Cherry-red spot–myoclonus (see Chapter 1)
Farber lipogranulomatosis
GM_1 gangliosidosis
GM_2 gangliosidosis
Metachromatic leukodystrophy
Niemann-Pick disease
Sialidosis III

Diagnosis. Vacuolated lymphocytes are present in the peripheral blood and the urine contains oligosaccharides. Definitive diagnosis requires demonstration of the enzyme deficiency in cultured fibroblasts.

Treatment. Treatment is not available.

Niemann-Pick Disease, Type A

Caused by a deficiency in the enzyme sphingomyelinase, type A Niemann-Pick disease is transmitted by autosomal recessive inheritance. Several phenotypes affecting children and adults are described.

Clinical Features. The acute infantile form presents during the first months of life with feeding difficulty, failure to thrive, and hepato-

megaly. Splenomegaly occurs later and is not prominent. A cherry-red spot is present in 50 percent of cases (Table 5.8). Psychomotor regression, characterized by postural hypotonia and loss of reactivity to the environment, occurs during the first year but may be overlooked because of the child's failure to thrive. With time, there is continued emaciation, a tendency for opisthotonos, exaggerated tendon reflexes, and blindness. Seizures are uncommon.

Diagnosis. The diagnosis is suggested by the clinical course (Fig. 5.7). Vacuolated histiocytes are present in the bone marrow and vacuolated lymphocytes in the peripheral blood. Definitive diagnosis requires the demonstration of sphingomyelinase deficiency in leukocytes or cultured fibroblasts.

Treatment. Treatment is not available.

Glucosylceramide Lipidosis
(Gaucher Disease II)

Type II Gaucher disease, caused by a deficiency of the enzyme glucocerebrosidase, is transmitted by autosomal recessive inheritance. The most common form of the disease (type I) does not affect the nervous system. Type II is

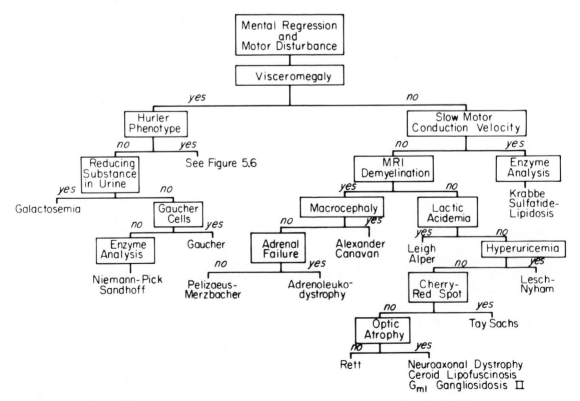

Figure 5.7 Evaluation of infants with progressive mental regression and motor disturbances.

an acute and devastating disorder of infants affecting the brain and viscera. Type III is characterized by neurovisceral storage as well, but the onset is in childhood and the course slow.

Clinical Features. Infants with Gaucher disease type II usually have symptoms of neurovisceral dysfunction before six months of age and frequently before three months of age. The initial symptoms are motor regression and cranial nerve dysfunction. Children are first hypotonic and then spastic. Head retraction is an early and characteristic sign that probably is due to meningeal irritation. Difficulties in sucking and swallowing, trismus, and oculomotor palsies are typical. Mental deterioration is rapid, but seizures are uncommon. Splenomegaly is more prominent than hepatomegaly, and jaundice is not expected. Hypersplenism results in anemia, thrombocytopenia, and leukopenia. Death usually occurs during the first year and always by the second.

Diagnosis. The presence of Gaucher cells in the reticuloendothelial system is diagnostic. These cells are altered macrophages measuring 20 to 100 μm. The cytoplasm has the appearance of wrinkled tissue paper, and the nucleus is eccentric. The cells are best identified from bone marrow aspirate stained by periodic acid–Schiff reaction. Heterozygotes can be identified by a partial decrease in enzyme activity in leukocytes. However, a reliable method for prenatal diagnosis has not been established.

Treatment. Efforts to treat the disease by enzyme replacement are still experimental. Splenectomy may improve the hematologic abnormalities, but does not provide long-term relief of symptoms.

Globoid Cell Leukodystrophy
(Krabbe Disease)

Krabbe disease is a rapidly progressive demyelinating disorder of infants caused by deficient activity of the enzyme galactocerebroside-β-galactosidase. The defect is transmitted by autosomal recessive inheritance.

Clinical Features. The median age of onset is four months with a range of one to seven months (Hagberg, 1984). Initial symptoms are irritability and hyperreactivity to stimuli. This is followed by progressive hypertonicity in the skeletal muscles. Unexplained low-grade fever is common. Psychomotor development arrests and then regresses. Within two to four months, the infant is in a permanent position of opisthotonos and has lost all previously achieved mile-

stones. Tendon reflexes become hypoactive and disappear. Startle myoclonus and seizures develop. The infant becomes blind, and by one year 90 percent are either dead or in a chronic vegetative state.

Several variant forms of globoid leukodystrophy are described with different clinical features: infantile spasm syndrome (see Chapter 1), focal neurologic deficits (see Chapters 10 and 11), and polyneuropathy (see Chapter 7). The juvenile form is discussed later in this chapter.

Diagnosis. Magnetic resonance imaging demonstrates diffuse demyelination of the cerebral hemispheres. Motor nerve conduction velocity of peripheral nerves is usually prolonged, and the protein content of cerebrospinal fluid is elevated (Fig. 5.7). Definitive diagnosis requires the demonstration of deficient activity of galactocerebroside-β-galactosidase in leukocytes or cultured fibroblasts.

Treatment. Treatment is not available.

Sulfatide Lipidoses
(Metachromatic Leukodystrophy)

Metachromatic leukodystrophy is a disorder of central and peripheral myelin metabolism due to deficient activity of the enzyme arylsulfatase A. It is transmitted by autosomal recessive inheritance. Several different clinical presentations are recognized (Kolodny and Moser, 1978). Because peripheral neuropathy is a prominent feature of the late infantile form of metachromatic leukodystrophy, the condition is discussed in Chapter 7 (Flaccid Limb Weakness in Childhood).

Clinical Features. The onset of symptoms is ordinarily in the second year, but many affected infants have a history of slow achievement of motor milestones during the first year. Flaccid weakness of the legs and areflexia are usually caused by peripheral neuropathy. These "peripheral" symptoms persist for three to twelve months before there is evidence of cerebral degeneration. The prominent cerebral symptoms are mental regression, dysarthria, optic atrophy, and ataxia. At this stage, the disease becomes rapidly progressive and within a few months the child is quadriplegic and in a vegetative state.

Diagnosis. Metachromatic leukodystrophy should be suspected in any child with mental regression and a peripheral neuropathy. The protein content of the cerebrospinal fluid is invariably elevated and motor nerve conduction velocities are always slow. Definitive diagnosis requires demonstration of deficient activity of arylsulfatase A in peripheral lymphocytes, cultured fibroblasts, or serum.

Treatment. Treatment is not available, but prenatal diagnosis can be accomplished by determining the activity of arylsulfatase A in cultured amniotic fluid cells.

GM₁ Gangliosidosis I, II

GM₁ gangliosidosis is caused by deficiency of the lysosomal enzyme β-galactosidase. Ganglioside GM₁ is stored in the brain and viscera. The disease is transmitted by autosomal recessive inheritance. An early (I) and late (II) infantile form are recognized.

GM₁ Gangliosidosis I

Difficulty in feeding and failure to thrive are noted shortly after birth. Edema of the limbs may be present as well. Psychomotor development is first slow and then regresses. Affected newborns are poorly responsive, hypotonic, and hypoactive. The Hurler phenotype is present (Table 5.7), except that the cornea is clear and a cherry-red spot of the macula is present in 50 percent of patients (Table 5.8). Symptoms are rapidly progressive, and many infants die within one year. Those who survive the first year are in a vegetative state.

Diagnosis. Infantile GM₁ gangliosidosis can be distinguished from Hurler syndrome by the absence of mucopolysacchariduria and the presence of a cherry-red spot. Definitive diagnosis requires demonstration of the enzyme deficiency in leukocytes, cultured fibroblasts, or serum.

Treatment. Treatment is not available.

GM₁ Gangliosidosis II

Clinical Features. Affected infants are normal during the first year, and symptoms of motor incoordination then develop. Ataxia, dysarthria, and strabismus are the initial manifestations. These are followed by mental regression, lethargy, spasticity, and seizures. The Hurler phenotype is not present: corneal clouding and hepatosplenomegaly do not occur, and skeletal radiographs demonstrate only mild beaking of vertebral bodies and metacarpal bones.

Diagnosis. Diagnosis requires demonstration of the deficient enzyme in leukocytes, cultured fibroblasts, or serum.

Treatment. Treatment is not available.

GM₂ Gangliosidosis

There are two forms of GM₂ gangliosidoses: Tay-Sachs disease and Sandhoff disease. Both are transmitted by autosomal recessive inheritance. Tay-Sachs disease is due to deficiency of the enzyme hexosaminidase A. Gene frequency is 1:30 in Ashkenazi Jews and 1:300 in gentiles. The central nervous system is the only affected organ. Sandhoff disease is a rare disorder with neurovisceral storage, described in non-Jewish children, resulting from deficiency of both hexosaminidase A and B. Juvenile forms of Tay-Sachs and Sandhoff disease have been described as well (Johnson, 1981).

Tay-Sachs Disease

Clinical Features. The onset of symptoms is between three and six months. An abnormal startle reaction (Moro reflex) to noise or light is characteristically the first symptom. Motor regression begins between four and six months. The infant may be brought for medical attention because of either delayed achievement of motor milestones or loss of milestones previously attained. A cherry-red spot of the macula is present in almost every patient, but is not specific for Tay-Sachs disease and can be seen in several storage diseases and in central retinal artery occlusion (Table 5.8) (Kivlin et al, 1985). The cherry-red spot develops as retinal ganglion cells in the parafoveal region accumulate stored material, swell, and burst. The red color of the normal fundus can then be seen. Optic atrophy and blindness follow.

By one year of age, the infant is severely retarded, unresponsive, and spastic. During the second year, the head enlarges in size and seizures develop. Most children die by five years of age.

Diagnosis. The diagnosis should be strongly suspected in any Jewish child with psychomotor retardation and a cherry-red spot of the macula. Definitive diagnosis requires the demonstration of deficient activity of hexosaminidase A in white blood cells or serum. Heterozygotes can be detected by the same assay. Prenatal diagnosis is possible by amniocentesis.

Treatment. Treatment is not available.

Sandhoff Disease

The clinical features and course of Sandhoff disease are identical to those of Tay-Sachs disease. The only difference is that organs other than the central nervous system are sometimes involved. Moderate hepatosplenomegaly may be present, and occasionally patients have bony deformities similar to infantile GM_1 gangliosidosis.

Diagnosis. The disease should be suspected in every non-Jewish infant with a Tay-Sachs phenotype. Peripheral lymphocytes are not vacuolated, but foamy histocytes may be present in the bone marrow. Diagnosis is accomplished by demonstrating hexosaminidase deficiency in leukocytes, cultured fibroblasts, or serum. Prenatal diagnosis is available by the detection of N-acetylglucosaminyl-oligosaccharides in amniotic fluid (Warner et al, 1986).

Treatment. Treatment is not available.

DISORDERS OF PYRUVATE METABOLISM AND MITOCHONDRIAL ENZYMES

Subacute Necrotizing Encephalomyelopathy (Leigh Disease)

Leigh disease is a progressive poliodystrophy primarily affecting neurons of the brainstem, thalamus, basal ganglia, and cerebellum. The pathology is similar to Wernicke encephalopathy, but the mammillary bodies are spared. It is likely that the pathologic features can be caused by more than one enzyme deficiency in pyruvate metabolism (Prick et al, 1981a; Willems et al, 1977). Most cases are transmitted by autosomal recessive inheritance, but X-linked inheritance occurs as well (Livingstone et al, 1984).

Clinical Features. The age at onset is during the first year in 60 percent, during the second year in 20 percent, and after infancy in 20 percent. Children who have symptoms in early infancy tend to experience a steadily progressive course with severe disability and death. The initial symptoms are some combination of developmental delay, failure to thrive due to poor feeding or vomiting, hypotonia, and seizures. Symptoms are made worse by intercurrent infection or ingestion of a heavy carbohydrate meal. Three typical, but not constant, features during infancy are respiratory disturbances, abnormal ocular motility, and hypotonia. Respiratory disturbances are at first episodic and can be characterized by Cheyne-Stokes breathing, ataxic breathing, or central hyperventilation. Respiratory distress is the usual cause of death. Ocular motility dysfunction varies from nystagmus to ophthalmoplegia. Hypotonia results from

a combination of peripheral neuropathy and disturbed cerebellar function.

Children with onset of symptoms during the second year have similar symptoms, but the course is less rapidly progressive and symptoms more intermittent with exacerbations at time of infection.

Diagnosis. Blood concentrations of lactate and pyruvate are usually elevated and rise even higher at the time of clinical exacerbation. Lesions in the brainstem and around the third ventricle may be visualized on CT and MRI, and the interpeak latency of waves V-III is prolonged on brainstem auditory evoked response. Motor nerve conduction velocities are usually slowed. When peripheral neuropathy is present, the protein content of the cerebrospinal fluid is elevated. Studies should be undertaken to search for disturbances in pyruvate utilization: deficiencies in pyruvate decarboxylase, multiple carboxylases, pyruvate dehydrogenase, or respiratory chain enzymes. Muscle biopsy specimens have been useful for enzyme analysis in several patients.

Treatment. Patients with disorders of pyruvate utilization are less likely to have acute exacerbations of illness on a carbohydrate-restricted diet. Calories should be provided primarily as lipid. Large doses of thiamine are helpful in some patients.

Oral acetazolamide has been useful in the treatment of cases transmitted by X-linked recessive inheritance (Evans et al, 1978). The mechanism of action is unknown. It is not clear whether acetazolamide is effective in cases transmitted by autosomal recessive inheritance as well.

Progressive Infantile Poliodystrophy (Alper Disease)

Alper disease was described originally as a progressive degeneration of cerebral gray matter and probably encompassed several different disease processes. Familial cases of progressive infantile poliodystrophy associated with mitochondrial myopathy led to studies of pyruvate utilization (Shapira et al, 1975; Hart et al, 1977). Deficiencies in pyruvate carboxylase activity and respiratory chain function have been identified (Prick et al, 1981b).

Clinical Features. The onset of symptoms is either during infancy or childhood. Symptoms with infantile onset tend to be sporadic in occurrence and are characterized first by delay in the achievement of developmental milestones and then by seizures. The seizures are either myoclonic or tonic-clonic. Status epilepticus can be the first manifestation of the seizure diathesis. Prolonged seizures are sometimes followed by transient hemiplegia. Psychomotor regression becomes evident and blindness may occur.

Diagnosis. Definitive diagnosis is accomplished only by postmortem examination. However, an elevated blood concentration of lactate should be a clue to disturbed pyruvate utilization and should suggest investigation of mitochondrial enzymes in liver and skeletal muscle. A carbohydrate load in the form of an oral glucose tolerance test raises the blood lactate concentration two or three times normal and worsens symptoms.

Treatment. It is reasonable to recommend a low-carbohydrate diet for children with disorders of pyruvate utilization. However, no specific treatment has proved to be effective in Alper disease.

Kinky Hair Disease
(Menkes Syndrome)

Menkes syndrome is believed to be a primary defect in intestinal transport of copper. The symptoms are attributed to a secondary deficiency of copper-dependent enzymes, especially cytochrome-c-oxidase. Some patients demonstrate enzyme deficiency in muscle, brain, and liver mitochondria (French et al, 1972); others show decreased copper concentration only in the brain (Nooijen et al, 1981).

Clinical Features. The initial symptoms usually develop in the first three months. Symptom development is first arrested and then regresses. The infant becomes lethargic and less reactive. Myoclonic seizures, provoked by stimulation, are an early and almost constant feature. By the end of the first year, the infant is in a chronic vegetative state and most will die before eighteen months.

The appearance of the scalp hair and eyebrows is almost pathognomonic. The hair is sparse, poorly pigmented, and wiry in texture. The shaft breaks easily and forms short stubble (kinky hair). Radiographs of the long bones suggest osteogenesis imperfecta. Other facial abnormalities include abnormal fullness of the cheeks, a high-arched palate, and micrognathia. Fullness of the cheeks also occurs in cerebrohepatorenal syndrome (see Chapter 6) in which mitochondrial abnormalities are present as well.

Diagnosis. In infants with clinical features of Menkes disease, the diagnosis can be established by the microscopic appearance of the hair shaft and by the demonstration of decreased plasma concentrations of copper.

Treatment. Administration of copper has no effect on the course of disease. Treatment is not available.

OTHER KNOWN ENZYME DEFICIENCIES

Galactosemia: Transferase Deficiency

Three separate inborn errors of lactose metabolism are known to produce galactosemia in the newborn, but only galactose-1-phosphate uridyl transferase deficiency produces mental retardation. The defect is transmitted by autosomal recessive inheritance.

Clinical Features. Affected newborns appear normal at birth, but have already begun to develop cataracts. The initial symptoms are provoked by the first milk feeding and include failure to thrive, vomiting, diarrhea, jaundice, and hepatomegaly. During this time, some newborns have clinical features of increased intracranial pressure, probably due to cerebral edema. The combination of a tense fontanelle and vomiting suggests a primary intracranial disturbance and can delay the diagnosis and treatment of the metabolic error.

Diagnosis. Galactosemia should be considered in any newborn with vomiting and hepatomegaly, especially when cataracts are associated. The best time to test the urine for reducing substances (Clinitest tablets) is after feeding. Specific tests for glucose (Testape, Clinistix) are negative. Most cases of galactosemia in newborns are now detected by routine screening tests.

Treatment. Symptoms are reversible by providing a lactose-free diet. However, eventual intellectual outcome is optimized when diet therapy is initiated early (Fishler et al, 1980).

Unfortunately, a subset of children with galactosemia exist who develop mental retardation even when diet therapy is adequate (Lo et al, 1984). The achievement of developmental milestones is delayed during the first year and by age five, intellectual function is moderately retarded. After age five, truncal ataxia develops and progresses in severity. Associated with ataxia is a coarse resting tremor of the limbs. Cataracts and hepatomegaly are not present because of the restricted diet. The enzyme deficiency in children who deteriorate neurologically does not appear different from that in those who respond favorably to lactose-free diets.

Lesch-Nyhan Disease

Lesch-Nyhan disease is caused by a deficiency of the enzyme hypoxanthine guanine-phosphoribosyltransferase. It is transmitted by X-linked inheritance.

Clinical Features. Affected newborns appear normal at birth, except for mild hypotonia (Watts et al, 1982). Delayed motor development and poor head control are present during the first three months. This is followed by progressive limb rigidity and torticollis or retrocollis. The progression of neurologic disturbance is insidious, and many affected patients are thought to have cerebral palsy. During the second year, facial grimacing, corticospinal tract dysfunction, and involuntary movements (usually chorea, but sometimes athetosis) develop.

It is not until after age two, and sometimes considerably later, that affected children begin biting their fingers, lips, and cheeks. Compulsive self-mutilation is characteristic, but not invariable, and causes severe disfigurement. It is often necessary to wrap the hands or to remove teeth in order to prevent further harm. In addition to self-directed aggressive behavior, aggressive behavior towards caretakers may be present as well. Mental retardation is constant, but of variable severity. Intelligence is difficult to evaluate because of behavioral and motor disturbances.

Diagnosis. Uric acid concentrations are increased in the blood and urine. Indeed, some parents note a reddish discoloration of diapers caused by uric acid. Definitive diagnosis requires the demonstration that hypoxanthine-guanine-phosphoribosyltransferase activity is absent in erythrocytes or cultured fibroblasts.

Treatment. Allopurinol decreases the urine concentration of uric acid and prevents the development of nephropathy. However, treatment is not available to prevent progressive degeneration of the nervous system.

NEUROCUTANEOUS SYNDROMES

Tuberous Sclerosis

Tuberous sclerosis is transmitted by autosomal dominant inheritance, and there is considerable variation in its phenotypic expression.

Clinical Features. The most common initial symptom of neurologic dysfunction during in-

fancy is seizures, especially infantile spasms (see Chapter 1). Some infants have evidence of developmental delay before the onset of seizures. The delay is often insufficient to prompt medical consultation. Most children with tuberous sclerosis who are mentally retarded will eventually have seizures.

Diagnosis. Tuberous sclerosis should be suspected in infants with developmental delay when hypopigmented areas are present in the skin. These areas may be oval or leaf-shaped and are scattered on the trunk or limbs. Depigmented areas are readily delineated by illumination with a Wood's light.

In late infancy and early childhood, café-au-lait spots develop and an isolated raised plaque in the skin over the lower back or buttocks (shagreen patch) may be present as well. During childhood, adenoma sebaceum (actually angiokeratomas) appear on the face, usually in a butterfly distribution. Other organ involvement includes retinal tumors, rhabdomyoma of the heart, renal tumors, and cysts of the kidney, bone, and lung. Seizures and mental retardation are due to disturbed histogenesis of the brain. Neurons are decreased in number and astrocytes are large and bizarre in shape. Glial tumors are common in the subependymal region and may cause obstructive hydrocephalus.

Treatment. Anticonvulsants are helpful in reducing seizure frequency, but rarely provide complete control. The mental retardation is not reversible. Genetic counseling is an important aspect of patient management. Although the disease is transmitted by autosomal dominant inheritance, gene expression is so variable that neither parent may appear affected. Sporadic cases were thought to be common. However, 25 percent of parents without personal or family history of tuberous sclerosis are shown to be affected by careful history and physical examination, including Wood's light examination of the skin, funduscopic examination, renal ultrasound, and cranial CT (Cassidy et al, 1983).

Neurofibromatosis

Neurofibromatosis is divided into central and peripheral types (Kanter et al, 1980). Both are transmitted by autosomal dominant inheritance and have marked variation in expression. Central neurofibromatosis is characterized by bilateral acoustic neuroma beginning at about twenty years of age.

Clinical Features. Peripheral neurofibromatosis is believed to be the most common single-gene disorder affecting the nervous system. Mild cases are characterized by café-au-lait spots and subcutaneous neurofibromas. Axillary freckles are particularly common.

Patients with severe cases have developmental and neoplastic disorders of the nervous system. No more than 10 percent of patients with neurofibromatosis are retarded. Those who are retarded are more likely to present with seizures than developmental delay. Nevertheless, neurofibromatosis should be suspected in any infant with psychomotor retardation and café-au-lait spots.

Diagnosis. Five café-au-lait spots greater than 1.5 cm in diameter are considered diagnostic, but more than two are suggestive of neurofibromatosis. Approximately 25 percent of cases are new mutations (Miller and Hall, 1978). Among the other 75 percent, the mother is twice as likely as the father to be the affected parent when the disease begins early and is more severe.

Treatment. Management is primarily symptomatic: (1) anticonvulsant drugs for seizures, (2) surgery for accessible tumors, and (3) orthopedic procedures for bony deformities. Treatment is not available for the mental retardation.

Chédiak-Higashi Syndrome

This is a rare disorder transmitted by autosomal recessive inheritance.

Clinical Features. Affected children are born with deficient pigment of the skin and hair. Areas of skin depigmentation form bizarre patterns that resemble giant fingerprints. Recurrent infections are prominent during infancy.

Neurologic symptoms evolve during the first two years. These include developmental retardation, seizures, and severe peripheral neuropathy. Symptoms of autonomic dysfunction, increased perspiration and failure to produce overflow tears, are common and may suggest dysautonomia.

Diagnosis. This is primarily a clinical diagnosis based upon the combination of neurologic dysfunction and pigmentary changes. Examination of peripheral blood smear is confirmatory. The nuclei of polymorphonuclear leukocytes are pyknotic and their cytoplasm contains large oval and fusiform granules that stain for myeloperoxidase.

Treatment. Treatment is not available.

IDIOPATHIC DISORDERS OF GRAY MATTER

Infantile Neuroaxonal Dystrophy

This is a disorder of axon terminals transmitted by autosomal recessive inheritance. It shares many pathologic features with Hallervorden-Spatz disease (see Chapter 14), and some believe it is an infantile form (Defendini et al, 1973).

Clinical Features. Affected children usually develop normally during the first year, but never walk independently. Towards the end of the first year, motor regression is evidenced by clumsiness and frequent falling. The infant is first hypotonic and hyporeflexic. Muscle atrophy may be present as well. At this stage, a peripheral neuropathy is suspected, but motor nerve conduction velocity and the protein content of the cerebrospinal fluid are normal.

After the initial phase of hypotonia, symptoms of cerebral degeneration become prominent. Increasing spastic quadriparesis, optic atrophy, involuntary movements, and mental regression are evident. By two years of age, most children are severely handicapped and death usually occurs by age eight.

Diagnosis. A definitive diagnosis requires postmortem examination of the brain. The characteristic findings are large eosinophilic spheroids, caused by axonal swelling, throughout the gray matter.

Treatment. Treatment is not available.

Rett Syndrome

Rett syndrome occurs only in girls. All cases are sporadic, and there are no known instances of consanguinity (Hagberg et al, 1983). A fragile site at the Xp22 chromosome (Wahlstrom, 1985) and a viral etiology (Chu et al, 1986) have been suggested.

Clinical Features. Affected girls are normal during the first year. Beginning usually at twelve months, but as early as five months and as late as eighteen months, there is developmental arrest. Within a few months, rapid developmental regression occurs characterized by loss of language skills, decreased use of the hands, and autistic behavior. Head growth arrests with eventual microcephaly. Dementia is usually severe. Although affected girls are unable to sustain interest in the environment, stimulation produces an exaggerated, stereotyped reaction consisting of jerking movements of the trunk and limbs with episodes of disorganized breathing and apnea, followed by hyperpnea (Glaze et al, 1987). During these episodes there may be circumoral cyanosis and diffuse perspiration. Similar episodes may also occur without stimulation, but not during sleep. Such episodes are frequently interpreted as seizures, although it is not clear that they are epileptic in nature. Typical tonic-clonic seizures, partial complex seizures, or myoclonic seizures occur in most children between the ages of two and four (Al-Mateen et al, 1986).

A characteristic feature of the syndrome is loss of purposeful hand movements before the age of three. They are replaced by stereotyped activity that looks like hand ringing or washing. Repetitive blows to the face are another form of stereotyped hand movement.

The initial rapid progression is followed by a continued slower progression of neurologic deterioration. Spastic paraparesis and quadriparesis are frequent endpoints.

Diagnosis. Diagnosis is based entirely upon the clinical features. Laboratory tests are not helpful. It was originally believed that affected girls had hyperammonemia, but this has not been substantiated in subsequent reports.

Treatment. Seizures respond to standard anticonvulsant drugs, but treatment is not available for the underlying disease.

Neuronal Ceroid Lipofuscinosis (Santavuori Disease)

In this group of genetic disorders, lipopigment is deposited in neurons and some visceral tissues. These disorders are usually classified by age at onset and rapidity of progression. The more common types occur after age two (see "Progressive Encephalopathies of Childhood" later in this chapter). The *early infantile type* (Santavuori disease) occurs primarily in Finnish people and is believed transmitted by autosomal recessive inheritance.

Clinical Features. Age at onset is usually the second year, but may be the first. Visual impairment and myoclonus are initial features. Rapid deterioration, characterized by psychomotor regression, hypotonia, ataxia, and hyperkinesia, follows. Seizures are not prominent.

Total blindness develops between the ages of two and three. The macula has degenerated and has a brownish color, the optic disk is atrophic, and the peripheral retina is hypopigmented.

Diagnosis. Antemortem diagnosis can be es-

tablished by ultrastructure studies of leukocytes, skin, or conjunctiva. Fifteen to 21 percent of lymphocytes or monocytes contain granular, osmiophilic membrane-bound cytoplasmic inclusions (Baumann and Markesbery, 1982). Skin and conjunctival biopsies reveal similar granular inclusions in endothelial and neuronal cells (Arsenio-Nunes et al, 1981).

Treatment. Seizures and myoclonus should be treated with a combination of valproic acid, clonazepam, and phenobarbital (see Chapter 1). Treatment is not available for the underlying metabolic error.

GENETIC DISORDERS OF WHITE MATTER

Alexander Disease

This is a rare disorder thought to be a disease of astrocytes (Borrett and Becker, 1985). All cases are sporadic, and a genetic basis is only suspected. Rosenthal fibers are the hallmark of disease. These are rod-shaped or round bodies that stain red with hematoxylin and eosin and black with myelin. They appear as small granules within the cytoplasm of astrocytes. Rosenthal fibers are scattered diffusely in the cerebral cortex and the white matter, but have a predilection for the subpial, subependymal, and perivascular regions.

Clinical Features. Rosenthal fibers are pathologic features of three clinical syndromes. First and most common is the *infantile form,* which affects primarily males. The onset may be anytime from birth to early childhood. These infants demonstrate arrest and regression of psychomotor development and enlargement of the head owing to megalencephaly, spasticity, and seizures. Optic atrophy does not occur. CT scans and cerebrospinal fluid examinations are normal. Death usually occurs by the second or third year.

The *juvenile form* presents with bulbar symptoms, and the *adult form* has a course that suggests multiple sclerosis.

Diagnosis. Definitive diagnosis relies entirely upon the demonstration of Rosenthal fibers by postmortem examination. However, the disease can be suspected in infants with evidence of progressive leukodystrophy and macrocephaly.

Treatment. Treatment is not available.

Pelizaeus-Merzbacher Disease

This demyelinating encephalopathy is transmitted by X-linked recessive inheritance and is thought to be caused by defective biosynthesis of proteolipid protein (Koeppen et al, 1987). Two major clinical syndromes are recognized, one with onset in the newborn and the other during early infancy (Seitleberger, 1970).

Clinical Features. The first symptoms of the neonatal form suggest spasmus nutans (see Chapter 15). There is intermittent nodding movement of the head and pendular nystagmus. Chorea or athetosis develops, psychomotor development is arrested by the third month, and regression follows. Limb movements become ataxic and tone spastic, first in the legs and then the arms. Optic atrophy and seizures are a late occurrence. Death occurs by five to seven years of age.

When the onset of disease is at the end of the first month or later, the symptoms are the same as in the neonatal form, but the course is more prolonged and survival to adult life is relatively common.

Diagnosis. Magnetic resonance imaging has not been reported in regard to this disease, but would be expected to demonstrate demyelination of the hemispheres. For a definitive diagnosis, postmortem examination is required. Both cerebral and cerebellar atrophy are present because of diffuse demyelination in which patches of normal myelin remain. Nerve cells and axons appear normal. When survival is prolonged, there is complete absence of myelin in the cerebral hemispheres.

Treatment. Treatment is not available.

Spongy Degeneration of Infancy (Canavan)

This disorder affects primarily Jewish children and is transmitted by autosomal recessive inheritance.

Clinical Features. Psychomotor arrest and regression occur during the first six months post partum. Clinical manifestations include decreased awareness of the environment, difficulty in feeding, irritability, and hypotonia. The initial flaccidity is eventually replaced by spasticity. A characteristic posture with leg extension, arm flexion, and head retraction is assumed, especially when the child is stimulated. Macrocephaly is noted by six months of age. The head continues to enlarge throughout infancy and reaches a plateau by the third year. Optic atrophy leading to blindness is noted between six and ten months.

Diagnosis. To make a definitive diagnosis, postmortem examination is needed. MRI has

not been reported in regard to this disease, but should demonstrate cerebral demyelination. Demyelination of peripheral nerves does not occur, and the cerebrospinal fluid is normal.

Treatment. Treatment is not available.

PROGRESSIVE HYDROCEPHALUS

Clinical Features. Progressive dilation of the ventricular system may be a consequence of congenital malformations, infectious diseases, intracranial hemorrhage, or connatal tumors. Whatever the cause, the clinical features of increasing intracranial pressure are very much the same. Head circumference enlarges; the anterior fontanelle feels full; and the child becomes lethargic, has difficulty feeding, and vomits. Ataxia and a spastic gait are common.

Diagnosis. Progressive hydrocephalus is often insidious in prematures with intraventricular hemorrhage, especially when there is delayed progression after initial arrest (Volpe, 1977). Hydrocephalus should always be suspected in newborns and infants with excessive head growth; the diagnosis is readily confirmed by CT.

Treatment. Ventriculoperitoneal shunt is the usual procedure to relieve hydrocephalus in newborns and small infants with primary dilation of the lateral ventricles (see Chapter 18).

■ Progressive Encephalopathies of Childhood (Onset after Age 2)

DISORDERS OF LYSOSOMAL ENZYMES

Mucopolysaccharidoses

The mucopolysaccharidoses result from deficiencies of enzymes involved in the catabolism of dermatan sulfate, heparan sulfate, or keratan sulfate. There are at least seven different major types of mucopolysaccharidoses. Four of these affect the nervous system and produce mental retardation: types I, II, III, and VII. Types I and III have their onset in infancy and have been discussed in the prior section. Types II and VII ordinarily have their onset in childhood following two or more years of normal development (Fig. 5.8).

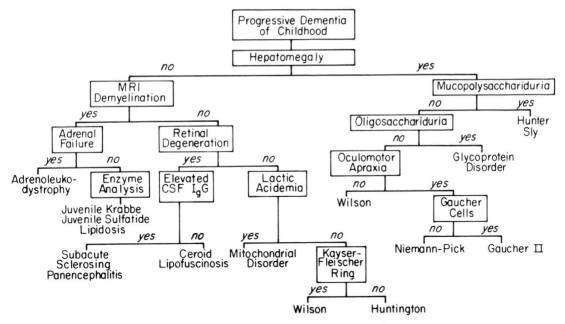

Figure 5.8 Evaluation of children with progressive dementia.

Mucopolysaccharidosis II
(Hunter Syndrome)

Clinical Features. Patients with the Hunter syndrome have a Hurler phenotype (see Table 5.7), but lack corneal clouding. This syndrome is distinguished further from other mucopolysaccharidoses because transmission is by X-linked recessive inheritance. A rare subtype is transmitted by autosomal recessive inheritance. Iduronate sulfatase is the deficient enzyme; dermatan and heparan sulfate are stored in the viscera and appear in the urine.

The Hurler phenotype may develop rapidly or evolve slowly during childhood and may not be recognized until the second decade or later. A prominent feature is the appearance of a nodular ivory-colored lesion of the back, usually around the shoulders and upper arms. Mental regression, due to neuronal storage of gangliosides, is slowly progressive, but many patients come to attention because of chronic hydrocephalus. Affected children survive into adult life. The accumulation of storage materials in collagen causes the entrapment of peripheral nerves, especially the median and ulnar.

Diagnosis. Diagnosis is suggested by the presence of mucopolysacchariduria with equal excretion of dermatan and heparan sulfate. Definitive diagnosis requires the demonstration of enzyme deficiency in cultured fibroblasts or serum. Prenatal diagnosis is accomplished by determining idoronate sulfatase activity in amniotic fluid.

Treatment. Nerve entrapment and hydrocephalus can be relieved by appropriate surgical procedures. Treatment is not available for the underlying storage disease.

Mucopolysaccharidosis VII
(Sly Disease)

This is a rare disorder due to deficiency of the enzyme β-glucuronidase. It is transmitted by autosomal recessive inheritance.

Clinical Features. There is an incomplete Hurler phenotype with hepatosplenomegaly, inguinal hernias, and dysostosis multiplex as the major features (Bernsen et al, 1987). Corneal clouding does not occur, and the face, though unusual, is not typical of the Hurler phenotype. Psychomotor retardation develops after age two, but is not a constant feature.

Diagnosis. Both dermatan and heparan sulfate are present in the urine, producing a positive screening test for mucopolysacchariduria. Specific diagnosis requires the demonstration of β-glucuronidase deficiency in leukocytes or cultured fibroblasts.

Treatment. Treatment is not available.

Disorders of Glycoprotein Degradation

Mannosidosis II

Clinical Features. The later-onset juvenile-adult form of mannosidosis is characterized by normal early development followed by mental regression during childhood or adolescence. Dysostosis multiplex is not a prominent feature, but deafness is constant.

Diagnosis. Vacuolated lymphocytes are present in peripheral blood. The urine contains oligosaccharides, but not mucopolysaccharides. Definitive diagnosis requires demonstration of deficient activity of B-mannosidase in cultured fibroblasts.

Treatment. Treatment is not available.

Aspartylglycosaminuria

This is a very rare condition that occurs primarily in Finland. There is a deficiency of the enzyme N-aspartyl-β-glucosaminidase. The defect is transmitted by autosomal recessive inheritance.

Clinical Features. Affected individuals are healthy in early infancy, but later experience recurrent infection, diarrhea, and inguinal hernia. During early childhood, coarsening of facial features takes place and hepatomegaly occasionally develops. Lens opacities occur after age ten. Speech may be delayed, but mental development is otherwise normal until age five. Afterwards, there is a slowly progressive regression of mental and motor skills, resulting in severe retardation and generalized weakness.

Diagnosis. Vacuolated lymphocytes are present in the peripheral blood of most patients, and a mild form of dysostosis multiplex is demonstrated radiographically. The urine is negative for mucopolysaccharides and positive for oligosaccharides. For a definitive diagnosis, the demonstration of enzyme deficiency in leukocytes or cultured fibroblasts is necessary.

Treatment. Treatment is not available.

Sphingomyelin Lipidosis
(Niemann-Pick Disease, Type C)

The chronic neuronopathic form is similar to the acute infantile form, except that onset is usually after age two, progression is slower, and there is not a specific racial predilection. As in other forms of Niemann-Pick disease, sphingomyelinase is the deficient enzyme. The defect is transmitted by autosomal recessive inheritance.

Clinical Features. The onset of neurologic deterioration is between two and eight years. Important features are mental regression, cerebellar ataxia, seizures, and an apraxia of vertical gaze. The eyes move well reflexly, but not voluntarily. Oculomotor apraxia in children is caused by only a limited number of disorders (see Chapter 15). Abnormalities in other organs are limited to mild splenomegaly and the presence of storage cells in the bone marrow. The course is characterized by progressive psychomotor retardation and seizures. Most children die before fifteen years of age.

Diagnosis. Examination of bone marrow reveals two unusual storage cells. One is large and vacuolated, the other is smaller. Both contain dark granular material. Definitive diagnosis requires demonstration of sphingomyelinase deficiency in leukocytes or cultured fibroblasts. Heterozygote detection and prenatal diagnosis is possible.

Treatment. Treatment is not available.

Glucosylceramide Lipidosis
(Gaucher Disease, Type III)

The late onset type of Gaucher disease, like other types, is caused by deficiency of the enzyme glucocerebrosidase and transmitted by autosomal recessive inheritance.

Clinical Features. Age at onset ranges from early childhood to adult life. Hepatosplenomegaly usually precedes neurologic deterioration. The most common neurologic manifestations are seizures and mental regression (Nishimura and Barranger, 1980). Mental regression varies from mild memory loss to severe dementia. In many patients, myoclonus and myoclonic seizures develop. Some combination of spasticity, ataxia, and cranial nerve dysfunction may be present as well. Vertical oculomotor apraxia, as described in Niemann-Pick disease, may occur in late onset Gaucher disease as well.

Diagnosis. Gaucher cells are present in the bone marrow and are virtually diagnostic. Confirmation requires the demonstration of deficient glucocerebrosidase activity in hepatocytes or leukocytes.

Treatment. Treatment is not available.

Late-Onset Globoid Leukodystrophy (Krabbe Disease)

This disorder is caused by deficiency of the enzyme galactosylceramide β-galactosidase and is transmitted by autosomal recessive inheritance. The severity of enzyme deficiency and of neuropathology is similar in the late onset and infantile cases (Crome et al, 1973).

Clinical Features. Neurologic deterioration usually begins between the ages of two and six, but may start as early as the second year. The major features are mental regression, cortical blindness, and generalized or unilateral spasticity (Loonen et al, 1985). The disease more often presents as progressive spasticity than dementia. Unlike the infantile form, peripheral neuropathy does not occur and the protein content of the cerebrospinal fluid is normal. The course is one of progressive neurologic deterioration resulting in a vegetative state.

Diagnosis. Magnetic resonance imaging demonstrates diffuse demyelination of the cerebral hemispheres. Definitive diagnosis requires demonstration of enzyme deficiency in leukocytes or cultured fibroblasts.

Treatment. Treatment is not available.

Juvenile Sulfatide Lipidosis
(Metachromatic Leukodystrophy)

The juvenile form of sulfatide lipidosis, like the infantile form, is caused by a deficiency of the enzyme arylsulfatase A and transmitted by autosomal recessive inheritance. The percentage of residual arylsulfatase A activity is the same in the infantile and juvenile forms and the reason for the phenotypic difference remains unexplained.

Clinical Features. The onset of symptoms is generally between five and ten years, but may be delayed to adolescence or as early as late infancy. Those with early onset of the juvenile form are clinically different from the infantile form despite the age overlap. Clinical symptoms of peripheral neuropathy do not occur, progression is slow, and the protein content of the cerebrospinal fluid is normal (Haltia et al, 1980).

Mental regression, speech disturbances, and clumsiness of gait are the prominent initial features. The dementia is slowly progressive over a period of three to five years, but sometimes progresses rapidly to a vegetative state (Kolodny et al, 1979). There may be a delay of several years between the onset of dementia and the appearance of other neurologic disturbances. In some, ataxia is an early and prominent manifestation. In all affected children, a spastic quadriplegia eventually develops and most will have convulsions. Death usually occurs during the second decade.

Diagnosis. The juvenile form can overlap in

age with a late-onset form that usually presents with psychosis or dementia (Alves et al, 1986).

Magnetic resonance imaging demonstrates demyelination in the cerebral hemispheres. Motor nerve conduction velocities may be normal early in the course. Definitive diagnosis requires demonstration of arylsulfatase A deficiency in leukocytes or cultured fibroblasts.

Treatment. Treatment is not available.

GENETIC DISORDERS OF GRAY MATTER

Ceroid Lipofuscinosis

Several disorders characterized by dementia and blindness are now considered to be forms of ceroid lipofuscinoses. When these disorders were first described, different eponymic designations were used depending upon age at onset. The common pathologic feature is the accumulation of autofluorescent lipopigments, ceroid and lipofuscin, within the brain, retina, and some visceral tissues. Childhood cases are thought to be transmitted by autosomal recessive inheritance, but some adult cases are transmitted as an autosomal dominant trait.

An early infantile form was described in the previous section. In addition, there is an infantile or childhood form (Bielschowsky-Jansky), a juvenile form (Spielmeyer-Vogt-Sjögren), and several adult forms.

Late Infantile Type
(Bielschowsky-Jansky)

Clinical Features. Age at onset is two to four years. Seizures rather than blindness are the initial feature. The seizures are myoclonic, akinetic, and tonic-clonic in character and are usually refractory to anticonvulsant drugs. Severe ataxia develops, owing in part to seizures and in part to motor system deterioration. This is followed by myoclonus, involuntary movements, and dementia. Dementia sometimes precedes the first seizure.

Ophthalmoscopic examination is abnormal prior to visual symptoms and reveals attenuation of vessels, early optic atrophy, and pigmentary degeneration of the macula. The loss of motor, mental, and visual function is relentlessly progressive, and within a period of months the child is in a chronic vegetative state.

Diagnosis. Antemortem diagnosis is accomplished by skin and conjunctival biopsy (Arsenio-Nunes et al, 1981). Curvilinear inclusions are observed by electron microscopy within the cytoplasm of endothelial and neuronal cells. In addition, azurophilic granules are present in neutrophilic leukocytes stained by the Giemsa method.

Treatment. Seizures are difficult to control, but may respond in part to a combination of valproic acid, clonazepam, and phenobarbital (see Chapter 1). Treatment is not available for the underlying metabolic error.

Juvenile Type (Spielmeyer-Vogt-Sjögren Disease)

Clinical Features. The mean age at onset is six years with a range from four to nine. Unlike patients with the late infantile type, these children frequently present because of decreasing visual acuity. Ophthalmoscopic examination reveals attenuation of retinal vessels, a patchy retinal atrophy that resembles retinitis pigmentosa, mild optic atrophy, and a granular discoloration of the macula that may have a "bull's-eye" appearance with a dull red spot in the center.

The dementia is characterized by declining school performance and behavioral disturbances. Delusions and hallucinations are common. Blindness and dementia are the only symptoms for many years. Late in the course, speech becomes slurred and Parkinson-like rigidity develops. Myoclonic jerks and tonic-clonic seizures begin some years after onset, but are not usually severe. Death usually occurs within fifteen years of onset.

Diagnosis. Antemortem diagnosis is reasonably certain by the characteristic retinal changes and confirmed by skin and conjunctival biopsy. Fingerprint bodies are present in the cytoplasm of several cell types (Arsenio-Nunes et al, 1981). The electroretinogram demonstrates depressed or absent retinal potentials early in the course. Leukocytes in the peripheral blood are frequently abnormal. Translucent vacuoles are present in lymphocytes and azurophilic granules in neutrophils.

Treatment. Treatment is not available for the underlying metabolic defect. Seizures usually respond to standard anticonvulsant drugs.

Huntington Disease

This chronic degenerative disease of the nervous system is transmitted by autosomal dominant inheritance, and it is believed that all cases are traceable to a single family. There are no new mutations.

Clinical Features. The ordinary age of onset is between the ages of thirty-five and fifty-five, but the onset may be as early as four years. When Huntington disease begins in childhood, the father is the affected parent in 90 percent of cases (Myers et al, 1983). Extrachromosomal organelles, such as mitochondria, are inherited exclusively from the mother and may modify the expression of the gene.

Chorea, a cardinal feature in adults, is uncommon in early childhood. The initial manifestations are progressive dementia, rigidity, and seizures. Declining school performance brings the child to medical attention. The course in children is relentlessly progressive with rapid deterioration of mental and motor function and early death.

Diagnosis. Diagnosis requires evidence of disease in one of the parents. Atrophy of the caudate nucleus and the cerebral cortex are characteristic CT features.

Treatment. Although chorea may be diminished by the use of haloperidol, no treatment is available for the dementia.

Mitochondrial Encephalomyopathies

The mitochondrial encephalomyopathies encompass a diverse group of disorders with defects in oxidative metabolism. Three such disorders are described in the section on progressive encephalopathies of infancy. Later onset mitochondrial disorders generally present as progressive external ophthalmoplegia or myopathy. However, dementia and seizures may be the prominent features in some families (Hart et al, 1977). Genetic transmission is ordinarily by autosomal recessive inheritance.

Clinical Features. The clinical features are similar to those of progressive infantile poliodystrophy, except that the onset of dementia is delayed until age six or later. Preceding the dementia there may be years of intermittent vomiting, lethargy, and headaches. Generalized tonic-clonic convulsions can precede the onset of dementia or at least bring the child, who is already demonstrating poor school performance, to medical attention. The subsequent course is variable and probably depends upon the underlying defect in mitochondrial metabolism. In many children, a myopathy will develop; in others, spasticity and blindness develop.

Diagnosis. Many children with mitochondrial enzyme defects have an increased blood concentration of lactate. However, the blood lactate concentration may vary with diet and a glucose-lactate tolerance test is useful as a screening test for disturbances in mitochondrial function. An ordinary glucose tolerance test is administered except that blood for lactate as well as glucose concentrations are measured at the same times. Lactate levels do not rise significantly in normal children, but rise two or three times the upper limit of normal in children with defective mitochondrial metabolism. In addition, the elevated concentration of glucose is slow in returning to normal.

When myopathy is present in addition to dementia, muscle biopsy usually demonstrates ragged red fibers (see Fig. 7.7).

Treatment. Children with defects in mitochondrial enzymes should be placed on a low-carbohydrate, high-fat diet. While this does not cure the underlying defect, it helps to relieve symptoms caused by lactic acidosis. No other treatment is available.

Xeroderma Pigmentosum

This is a genetic disorder characterized by defective desoxyribonucleic acid (DNA) repair. Ten genetic subtypes have been defined. Group A is the most common form and is associated with neurologic deterioration (Mimaki et al, 1986).

Clinical Features. In affected children, a photosensitive dermatitis develops during the first year; in many cases skin cancer will develop as well. Progressive psychomotor retardation and poor head growth leading to microcephaly are noted after age three. After age seven, sensorineural hearing loss and spinocerebellar degeneration may be noted. Approximately one third of patients are short in stature.

Diagnosis. The skin rash suggests the diagnosis, which is confirmed by the demonstration of abnormal DNA repair in cultured fibroblasts. The EEG is frequently abnormal and demonstrates epileptiform activity. Delayed motor and sensory conduction may be demonstrated by electromyography (EMG).

Treatment. Treatment is not available.

DISEASES OF WHITE MATTER

Adrenoleukodystrophy

Adrenoleukodystrophy is a progressive demyelination of the central nervous system associated with adrenal cortical failure. It is transmitted by X-linked inheritance. The precise enzyme defect has not been established, but all affected persons accumulate very-long-chain fatty acids, particularly hexacosanoate, in tissues and plasma. Many cases previously designated as Schilder's disease were probably the juvenile form of adrenoleukodystrophy.

Clinical Features. There is considerable variation in clinical expression. Neurologic deterioration precedes clinical evidence of adrenal insufficiency in 85 percent of cases (Moser and Moser, 1984). Melanoderma may be the only feature of adrenal disease and then in only isolated areas of the skin and mucosal surfaces. In rare instances, when adrenal failure is early and prominent, the subsequent neurologic manifestations may be attributed to adrenal failure and not recognized as a coexisting problem.

The onset of neurologic manifestations can occur anytime during childhood and may even be delayed until adult life. Most affected boys are five to ten years of age. The first symptoms are usually an alteration in behavior ranging from a withdrawn state to aggressive outbursts. Poor school performance follows invariably and may lead parents to seek psychologic services. Neurologic deterioration is then relentlessly progressive and includes disturbances of gait and coordination, loss of vision and hearing, and ultimate deterioration to a vegetative state. Seizures are a late manifestation.

Diagnosis. The protein concentration of cerebrospinal fluid is generally increased. CT reveals hypodensities near the trigones of the lateral ventricles with contrast enhancement around the edges. MRI is more sensitive than CT, and T2-weighted images demonstrate high signal intensity in the periventricular white matter even when symptoms are minimal (Huckman et al, 1986). Adrenal insufficiency may be documented in asymptomatic children by demonstrating a subnormal response to stimulation by adrenocorticotropic hormone (ACTH). However, up to 15 percent may have a normal response and definitive diagnosis requires a plasma assay of very-long-chain fatty acids. The assay also permits identification of carrier females and the prenatal diagnosis of affected fetuses by measuring long-chain fatty acid concentrations in amniocytes.

Treatment. Corticosteroids reverse clinical symptoms of adrenal insufficiency, but treatment is not available for the neurologic deterioration.

Cerebrotendinous Xanthomatosis

This is a rare disorder transmitted as an autosomal recessive trait. An enzyme deficiency causes a block in bile acid synthesis, resulting in the storage of sterols in all tissues, but especially the central nervous system (Salen et al, 1986).

Clinical Features. Dementia begins in early childhood, but is insidious in its progression so that affected children seem mildly retarded rather than actively deteriorating. By age fifteen, cataracts are present and tendinous xanthoma begin to form. They are small at first and may go unnoticed until adult life. Progressive spasticity and ataxia develop during adolescence, and the patient becomes incapacitated in early adult life. A demyelinating neuropathy may be present as well (Argov et al, 1986). Speech and swallowing are impaired and death occurs from brainstem dysfunction or myocardial infarction.

Diagnosis. The triad of cataracts, tendon xanthoma, and progressive neurologic deterioration is diagnostic, but not expressed completely until late in the course. Definitive diagnosis requires the demonstration of increased concentrations of cholestanol in plasma or xanthomas.

Treatment. Chenodeoxycholic acid, administered orally 750 mg/day, decreases cholestanol plasma and tissue concentrations by expanding the deficient bile pool. Improvement in neurologic function occurs.

INFECTIOUS DISEASES

Infectious diseases are an uncommon cause of progressive dementia in childhood. Tuberculosis and several fungal species may produce a chronic meningitis characterized by personality change and some decline in higher intellectual function. *Cryptococcus* is especially notorious for its long indolent course. However, the major features of these infections are fever and headache. Chronic meningitis is not a serious consideration in the differential diagnosis of isolated psychomotor regression.

In contrast, chronic viral infections, especially HIV (see Chapter 2), may at times produce a clinical picture similar to many genetic disorders in which dementia is a prominent feature.

Subacute Sclerosing Panencephalitis (SSPE)

This is a form of chronic measles encephalitis that was at one time endemic in several parts of the world, but has almost disappeared in countries that require routine measles immunization. In a nonimmunized population, the average age of onset is eight years. As a rule, children with SSPE have experienced natural infection with the rubeola virus at an early age, half before age two. A concomitant infection with a second virus at the time of initial exposure to measles and immunosuppression are additional risk factors for developing SSPE. In the United States, incidence rates were highest in rural areas, especially in the southeastern states and the Ohio River valley.

Clinical Features. The first symptoms of disease are personality change and declining school performance. Personality change may be aggressive behavior or withdrawal. Psychologic rather than medical services may be sought at this time. However, retinal examination during this early stage already demonstrates pigmentary changes in the macula. Generalized seizures, usually myoclonic, develop next. An EEG at this time is characteristic and demonstrates periodic bursts of spike-wave complexes (approximately every 5 to 7 seconds) occurring synchronously with the myoclonic jerk. After the onset of seizures, there is rapid neurologic deterioration characterized by spasticity, dementia, and involuntary movements. Within a period of one to six years from the onset of symptoms, the child is in a chronic vegetative state.

Diagnosis. The diagnosis can be suspected from the clinical course and characteristic EEG. Confirmation requires demonstration of an elevated antibody titer against rubeola, usually associated with elevated gamma globulin concentrations, in the cerebrospinal fluid. The cerebrospinal fluid is otherwise normal. Plasma rubeola antibody titers are also markedly elevated.

Treatment. No drug is effective in treating the disease, but prevention is available by measles immunization.

Progressive Rubella Panencephalitis

Clinical Features. This disorder is usually limited to children who have had congenital rubella infection (Townsend et al, 1975) but can occur after postnatal rubella as well (Wolinsky et al, 1976). These children may have cataracts, cardiac abnormalities, and other stigmata of congenital rubella, but may have no evidence of neurologic dysfunction. Then, usually during adolescence, progressive neurologic deterioration occurs that is similar clinically and pathologically to subacute sclerosing panencephalitis.

Diagnosis. The rubella antibody titer in the cerebrospinal fluid is greatly elevated.

Treatment. Treatment is not available.

References

1. Al-Mateen M, Philippart M, Shields WD: Rett syndrome. A commonly overlooked progressive encephalopathy in girls. Am J Dis Child 140:761, 1986.
2. Alves D, Pires MM, Guimaraes A, et al: Four cases of late onset metachromatic leucodystrophy in a family: clinical, biochemical and neuropathological studies. J Neurol Neurosurg Psychiatry 49:1417, 1986.
3. Amir N, Zlotogora J, Bach G: Mucolipidosis type IV: Clinical spectrum and natural history. Pediatrics (in press).
4. Argov Z, Soffer D, Eisenberg S, et al: Chronic demyelinating peripheral neuropathy in cerebrotendinous xanthomatosis. Ann Neurol 29:89, 1986.
5. Arsenio-Nunes ML, Goutieres F, Aicardi J: An ultramicroscopic study of skin and conjunctival biopsies in chronic neurological disorders of childhood. Ann Neurol 9:163, 1981.
6. Baumann RJ, Markesbery WR: Santavuori disease: Diagnosis by leukocyte ultrastructure. Neurology 32:1277, 1982.
7. Beaudet AL: Disorders of glycoprotein degradation: mannosidosis, fucosidoses, sialidosis, and aspartylglycosaminuria. In Stanbury JB, Wyngaarden JB, Fredrickson DS, eds: The Metabolic Basis of Inherited Disease. 4th edition. McGraw-Hill Book Co, New York, 1978, p 788.
7a. Bernsen PLJA, Wevers RA, Gabreels FJM, et al: Phenotypic expression in mucopolysaccharidosis VII. J Neurol Neurosurg Psychiatry 50:699, 1987.
8. Borrett D, Becker LE: Alexander's disease. A disease of astrocytes. Brain 108:367, 1985.
9. Cassidy SB, Pagon RA, Pepin M, et al: Family studies in tuberous sclerosis. JAMA 249:1302, 1983.
10. Chu AB, Nerurkar LS, Witzel N, et al: Reye's syndrome: Salicylate metabolism, viral antibody levels, and other factors in surviving patients and unaffected family members. Am J Dis Child 140:1009, 1986.
11. Crome L, Hanefeld F, Patrick D, et al: Late onset globoid cell leukodystrophy. Brain 96:841, 1973.
12. Defendini R, Markesbery WR, Mastri AR, et al: Hallervorden-Spatz disease and infantile neuroaxonal dystrophy. Ultrastructural observations, anatomical pathology and nosology. J Neurol Sci 20:7, 1973.
13. de Grouchy J, Turleau J: Autosomal disorders. In Emery AEH, Rimoin DL, eds: Principles and Practice of Medical Genetics. Volume 1. Churchill Livingstone, New York, 1983, p 15.
14. Desmond MM, Wilson GS, Melnick JL, et al: Congenital rubella encephalitis. J Pediatr 71:311, 1967.
15. Evans OB, Kilroy AW, Fenichel GM: Acetazolamide in the treatment of pyruvate dysmetabolism syndromes. Arch Neurol 35:302, 1978.
16. Fishler K, Koch R, Donnell GN, et al: Developmental aspects of galactosemia from infancy to childhood. Clin Pediatr 19:38, 1980.
17. French JH, Sherard ES, Lubell H et al: Trichopoliodystrophy. I. Report of a case and biochemical studies. Arch Neurol 26:229, 1972.
18. Glaze DG, Frost JD Jr, Zoghibi HY, et al: Rett's syndrome: Characterization of respiratory patterns and sleep. Ann Neurol 21:377, 1987.
19. Güttler F: Phenylketonuria: 50 years since Folling's discovery and still expanding our clinical and biochemical knowledge. Acta Pediatr Scand 73:705, 1984.
20. Haas JE, Johnson ESJ, Farrell DJ: Neonatal-onset adrenoleukodystrophy in a girl. Ann Neurol 12:449, 1982.
21. Hagberg B: Krabbe's disease: Clinical presentation of neurological variants. Neuropediatria 15:11, 1984.
22. Hagberg B, Aicardi J, Dias K, et al: A progressive syndrome of autism, dementia, ataxia, and loss of purposeful hand use in girls: Rett's syndrome: report of 35 cases. Ann Neurol 14:471, 1983.
23. Haltia T, Palo J, Haltia M, et al: Juvenile metachromatic leukodystrophy. Clinical, biochemical, and neuropathological studies in nine new cases. Arch Neurol 37:42, 1980.
24. Hanshaw JB, Scheiner AP, Moxley AW, et al: CNS effects of silent cytomegalovirus infection. N Engl J Med 295:468, 1976.
25. Hart ZH, Chang C-H, Perrin EVD, et al: Familial poliodystrophy, mitochondrial myopathy, and lactate acidemia. Arch Neurol 34:180, 1977.
26. Herskowitz J, Rosman NP: Autism, schizophrenia, and other psychoses. In Pediatrics, Neurology, and Psychiatry: Common Ground. Macmillan Publishing Co, New York, 1982, p 65.
27. Hoganson G, Berlow S, Kaufman S, et al: Biopterin synthesis defects: Problems in diagnosis. Pediatrics 74:1004, 1984.
28. Huckman MS, Wong PWK, Sullivan T, et al: Magnetic resonance imaging compared with computed tomography in adrenoleukodystrophy. Am J Dis Child 140:1001, 1986.
29. Johnson WG: The clinical spectrum of hexosaminidase deficiency diseases. Neurology 31:1453, 1981.
30. Jones KL, Jones MC: A clinical approach to the dysmorphic child. In Emery AEH, Rimoin DL, eds: Principles and Practice of Medical Genetics. Churchill Livingstone, New York, 1983, p 152.
31. Kalter H, Warkany J: Congenital malformations: Etiologic factors and their role in prevention. N Engl J Med 308:424, 1983.
32. Kanter WR, Eldridge R, Fabricant R, et al: Central neurofibromatosis with bilateral acoustic neuroma: Genetic, clinical and biochemical distinctions from peripheral neurofibromatosis. Neurology 30:851, 1980.
33. Kivlin JD, Sanborn GE, Myers GG: The cherry-red spot in Tay-Sachs and other storage diseases. Ann Neurol 17:356, 1985.
34. Kodama S, Seki A, Hanabusa M, et al: Mild variant of maple syrup urine disease. Eur J Pediatr 124:31, 1976.
35. Koeppen AH, Ronca NA, Greenfield EA, et al: Defective biosynthesis of proteolipid in Pelizaeus-Merzbacher disease. Ann Neurol 21:159, 1987.
36. Kolodny EH, Moser HW: Sulfate lipidoses: metachromatic leucodystrophy. In Stanbury JB, Wyngaarden JB, Fredrickson DS, eds: The Metabolic Basis of Inherited Disease. 4th edition. McGraw-Hill Book Co, New York, 1978, p 881.
37. Kolodny EH, Srinivasa R, Spielvogel C, et al: Genetic heterogeneity in aryl sulfatase A (ASA) deficiency. Neurology 29:576, 1979.
38. LaDu BN: Histinemia. In Stanbury JB, Wyngaarden JB, Fredrickson DS, eds: The Metabolic Basis of Inherited Disease. 4th edition. McGraw-Hill Book Co, New York, 1978, p 317.
39. Livingstone IR, Gardner-Medwin D, Pennington RJT: Familial intermittent ataxia with possible X-linked recessive inheritance. J Neurol Sci 64:89, 1984.
40. Lo W, Packman S, Nash S, et al: Curious neurologic sequelae in galactosemia. Pediatrics 73:309, 1984.
41. Loonen MCB, Van Diggelen HC, Janse HC, et al: Late-onset globoid cell leucodystrophy (Krabbe's disease). Clinical and genetic delineation of two forms and their relation to the early-infantile form. Neuropediatria 16:137, 1985.

42. Miller M, Hall JG: Possible maternal effect on severity of neurofibromatosis. Lancet 2:1071, 1978.

43. Mimaki T, Itoh N, Abe J, et al: Neurological manifestations in xeroderma pigmentosum. Ann Neurol 20:70, 1986.

44. Moser HW, Moser AE: Adrenoleukodystrophy: Survey of 303 cases: Biochemistry, diagnosis, and therapy. Ann Neurol 16:628, 1984.

45. Mudd SH, Levy HL: Disorders of transulfuration. In Stanbury JB, Wyngaarden JB, Fredrickson DS, eds: The Metabolic Basis of Inherited Disease. 5th edition. McGraw-Hill Book Co, New York, 1983, p 522.

46. Mudd SH, Skouby F, Levy HL, et al: The natural history of homocystinuria due to cystathionine-β-synthase deficiency. Am J Hum Genet 37:1, 1985.

47. Myers RH, Goldman D, Bird ED, et al: Maternal transmission in Huntington's disease. Lancet 1:208, 1983.

48. Nishimura RN, Barranger JA: Neurologic complications of Gaucher's disease, type 3. Arch Neurol 37:92, 1980.

49. Nooijen JL, DeGroot CJ, VanDenHamer CJA, et al: Trace element studies in three patients and a fetus with Menkes' disease. Effect of copper therapy. Pediatr Res 15:284, 1981.

50. Opitz JM: X-linked Mental Retardation. Alan R. Liss Inc, New York, 1984.

51. Prick M, Gabreels F, Renier W, et al: Pyruvate dehydrogenase deficiency restricted to brain. Neurology 31:398, 1981a.

52. Prick MJJ, Gabreels FJM, Renier WO, et al: Progressive infantile poliodystrophy. Association with disturbed pyruvate oxidation in muscle and liver. Arch Neurol 38:767, 1981b.

53. Pueschel SM, Bresnan MJ, Shih VE, et al: Thiamine-responsive intermittent branched chain ketoaciduria. J Pediatr 94:629, 1979.

54. Remington JS, Desmonts G: Toxoplasmoses. In Remington JS, Klein JO, eds: Infectious Diseases of the Fetus and Newborn Infant. 2nd edition. WB Saunders Co, Philadelphia, 1983, p 144.

55. Salen G, Shefer S, Berginer VM: Familial diseases with storage of sterols other than cholesterol: Cerebrotendinous xanthomatosis and sitosterolemia with xanthomatosis. In Stanbury JB, Wyngaarden JB, Fredrickson DS, eds: The Metabolic Basis of Inherited Disease. 5th edition. McGraw-Hill Book Co, New York, 1983, p 713.

56. Seashore MR, Friedman E, Novelly RA, et al: Loss of intellectual function in children with phenylketonuria after relaxation of dietary phenylalanine restriction. Pediatrics 75:226, 1985.

57. Seitelberger F: Pelizaeus-Merzbacher disease. In Vinken PJ, Bruyn GW (eds): Handbook of Clinical Neurology. Volume 10. North Holland Publ Co, Amsterdam, 1970, p 150.

58. Scriver CR, Clow CL: Phenylketonuria: Epitome of human biochemical genetics. N Engl J Med 303:1336 and 1394, 1980.

59. Sever JL, Larsen JW Jr, Grossman JH III: Handbook of Perinatal Infections. Little, Brown & Co, Boston, 1979.

60. Shapira Y, Cederbaum SD, Cancilla PA, et al: Familial poliodystrophy, mitochondrial myopathy, and lactate acidemia. Neurology 25:614, 1975.

61. Smith DW, Klein AM, Henderson JR, et al: Congenital hypothyroidism—signs and symptoms in the newborn period. J Pediatr 87:958, 1975.

62. Townsend JJ, Baringer JR, Wolinsky JS, et al: Progressive rubella panencephalitis. Late onset after congenital rubella. N Engl J Med 292:990, 1975.

63. Volpe JJ, Pasternak Jf, Allen WC: Ventricular dilatation preceding rapid head growth following neonatal intracranial hemorrhage. Am J Dis Child 131:1212, 1977.

64. Wahlstrom J: Genetic implications of Rett syndrome. Brain Dev 7:573, 1985.

65. Warner TG, Turner MW, Toone JR, et al: Prenatal diagnosis of infantile GM₂ gangliosidosis type II (Sandhoff disease) by detection of N-acetylglucosaminyl-oligosaccharides in amniotic fluid with high-performance liquid chromatography. Prenat Diagn 6:393, 1986.

66. Watts RWE, Spellacy E, Gibbs DA: Clinical, postmortem, biochemical and therapeutic observations on the Lesch-Nyhan syndrome with particular reference to the neurological manifestations. Q J Med 201:43, 1982.

67. Willems JL, Monnens LAH, Trijbels JMF, et al: Leigh's encephalomyopathy in a patient with cytochrome c oxidase deficiency in muscle tissue. Pediatrics 60:850, 1977.

68. Wolinsky JS, Berg BO, and Maitland CJ: Progressive rubella panencephalitis. Arch Neurol 33:722, 1976.

6 The Hypotonic Infant

■ Definitions

Tone is the resistance of muscle to stretch. Two kinds of tone are measured clinically: phasic and postural.

Phasic tone is a rapid brief contraction to a high intensity stretch. It is examined by testing the tendon reflexes. When a hammer strikes the patella tendon, the quadriceps muscles is stretched and the spindle apparatus, sensing the stretch, sends an impulse through the sensory nerve to the spinal cord. This information is transmitted to the alpha motor neuron and the quadriceps muscle contracts (monosynaptic reflex).

Postural tone is a prolonged contraction to a low-intensity stretch. Gravity is the stimulus that provokes a steady, low-amplitude stretch on antigravity muscles. They respond with prolonged contraction. When postural tone is depressed, the infant is less able to maintain the body and limbs against gravity and is hypotonic.

The maintenance of normal tone requires an intact central and peripheral nervous system. Therefore, it is not surprising that hypotonia is a common symptom of neurologic dysfunction and is encountered in diseases of the brain, spinal cord, nerves, and muscles (Table 6.1). One anterior horn cell and all the muscle fibers that it innervates make up a *motor unit*. A primary disorder of the anterior horn cell body is a *neuronopathy,* of the axon or its myelin covering is a *neuropathy,* and of the muscle fiber is a *myopathy.* In infancy and childhood, diseases of the brain are far more common than diseases of the motor unit. The term *cerebral hypotonia* is used to encompass all causes of postural hypotonia due to cerebral disease or defect.

■ The Appearance of Hypotonia

When lying in the supine position, all hypotonic infants look very much the same without regard to the underlying cause or the localization of abnormality within the nervous system (Fig. 6.1). There is a paucity of spontaneous movement, the legs are fully abducted with the lateral surface of the thighs against the examining table, and the arms lie either extended at the sides of the body or flexed at the elbow with the hands beside the head. Pectus excavatum is present when there is long-standing weakness in the muscles of the chest wall. Infants who lie motionless eventually develop flattening of the occiput and loss of hair on the portion of the scalp that is in constant contact with the crib sheet. When the infant is placed in a sitting posture, the heads falls forward, the shoulders droop, and the limbs hang limply.

Newborns who are hypotonic in utero may be born with either dislocation of the hips, arthrogryposis, or both. Dislocation of the hip is a common feature of intrauterine hypotonia because the formation of a normal hip joint requires the forceful contraction of muscles to pull the head of the femur into the acetabulum. Arthrogryposis varies in severity from clubfoot, the most common manifestation, to symmetric flexion deformities of all limb joints. Joint contractures are believed to be a nonspecific consequence of intrauterine immobilization. However, among the several disorders that equally decrease fetal movement, some regularly produce arthrogryposis and others never do. The differential diagnosis of arthrogryposis is summarized in Table 6.2. Those conditions due to abnormality in the fetal brain or motor unit are

147

Table 6.1 DIFFERENTIAL DIAGNOSIS OF INFANTILE HYPOTONIA

Cerebral Hypotonia
1. Chromosome disorders
   a. Trisomy
   b. Prader-Willi syndrome
2. Chronic nonprogressive encephalopathy
   a. Cerebral malformation
   b. Perinatal distress
   c. Postnatal disorders
3. Peroxisomal disorders
   a. Cerebrohepatorenal syndrome (Zellweger)
   b. Neonatal adrenoleukodystrophy
4. Other metabolic defects
   a. Acid maltase deficiency
   b. Infantile GM_1 gangliosidosis
5. Other genetic defects
   a. Familial dysautonomia
   b. Cohen syndrome
   c. Oculocerebrorenal syndrome (Lowe)
6. "Benign" congenital hypotonia

Neonatal Spinal Cord Injury
1. Breech presentation
2. Cephalic presentation

Motor Neuron Disorders
1. Spinal muscular atrophies
   a. Acute infantile
   b. Chronic infantile
   c. Infantile neuronal degeneration
   d. Neurogenic arthrogryposis
   e. Incontinentia pigmenti
2. Polyneuropathies
   a. Congenital hypomyelinating neuropathy
   b. Chronic inflammatory demyelinating polyneuropathy
   c. Hereditary motor-sensory neuropathies

Disorders of Neuromuscular Transmission
1. Infantile botulism
2. Myasthenia gravis
   a. Juvenile myasthenia
   b. Transitory neonatal myasthenia
   c. Familial infantile myasthenia

Fiber Type Disproportion Myopathies
1. Congenital fiber type disproportion myopathy
2. Myotubular (centronuclear) myopathy
   a. Acute
   b. Chronic
3. Nemaline (rod) myopathy
4. Central core disease

Muscular Dystrophies
1. Congenital muscular dystrophy
   a. Fukuyama type
   b. Leukodystrophy
   c. Cerebro-ocular dystrophy
2. Myotonic dystrophy

Metabolic Myopathies
1. Acid maltase deficiency
2. Cytochrome-c-oxidase deficiency
3. Carnitine deficiency
4. Phosphofructokinase deficiency
5. Phosphorylase deficiency

Infantile Myositis

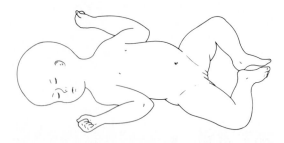

Figure 6.1 Illustration of hypotonia, with the infant at rest. The thighs are fully abducted (frog-leg), and the arms lie in a flaccid position beside the head. (Reprinted with permission of Fenichel GM: Neonatal Neurology. Churchill Livingstone, New York, 1985.)

also part of the differential diagnosis of infantile hypotonia.

The tone of infants who appear hypotonic at rest can be further evaluated by the traction response, by vertical suspension, and by horizontal suspension.

THE TRACTION RESPONSE

The traction response is the most sensitive measure of postural tone and can be tested in prematures within the confines of an isolette. The response is initiated by grasping the hands and pulling the infant to a sitting position. In a normal infant, the head lifts from the surface immediately with the body. When the sitting position is attained, the head is held erect in the midline. During traction, the examiner should feel the infant pulling back against traction and observe flexion at the elbow, knee, and ankle

Table 6.2 DIFFERENTIAL DIAGNOSIS OF ARTHROGRYPOSIS

Nonfetal causes
Fetal, non-nervous system causes
Cerebral malformations
Chromosomal disorders
Cerebrohepatorenal syndrome
Motor unit disorders
   Congenital cervical spine atrophy
   Congenital fiber type disproportion myopathy
   Congenital muscular dystrophy
   Familial infantile myasthenia
   Infantile neuronal degeneration
   Myotonic dystrophy
   Neurogenic arthrogryposis
   Phosphofructokinase deficiency
   Transitory neonatal myasthenia

(Fig. 6.2). A traction response is not present in prematures of less than 33 weeks' gestation. After 33 weeks, there is considerable head lag but the neck flexors consistently respond to traction by lifting the head. At term, only minimal head lag is present; when the sitting posture is attained, the head may continue to lag or may become erect momentarily and then fall forward.

The presence of more than minimal head lag and failure to counter traction by flexion of the limbs are abnormal and indicate hypotonia.

VERTICAL SUSPENSION

The examiner places both hands in the infant's axillae and without grasping the thorax lifts straight up. The muscles of the shoulders should be strong enough to press down against the examiner's hands and allow the infant to suspend vertically without falling through. While the infant is in vertical suspension, the head is held erect in the midline and the legs are kept flexed at the knee, hip, and ankle. When the hypotonic infant is suspended vertically, the head falls forward, the legs dangle, and there is a tendency to slip through the examiner's hands because of weakness in the muscles of the shoulder.

HORIZONTAL SUSPENSION

When suspended horizontally, a normal infant keeps the head erect, maintains the back straight, and demonstrates flexion at the elbow,

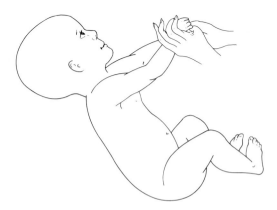

Figure 6.2 Normal traction response. The lift of the head is almost parallel to the lift of the body, and there is flexion in all limb joints. (Reprinted with permission of Fenichel GM: Neonatal Neurology. Churchill Livingstone, New York, 1985.)

Table 6.3 COMBINED CEREBRAL AND MOTOR UNIT HYPOTONIA

Acid maltase deficiency
Familial dysautonomia
Infantile neuronal degeneration
Lipid storage diseases
Mitochondrial disorders
Neonatal myotonic dystrophy
Perinatal asphyxia secondary to motor unit disease

hip, knee, and ankle. A healthy term newborn makes intermittent efforts to maintain the head erect, the back straight, and the limbs flexed against gravity. Hypotonic newborns and infants drape over the examiner's hands with the head and legs hanging limply.

■ Approach to Diagnosis

The first step in diagnosis is to determine whether the site of pathology is cerebral, spinal, or motor unit. More than one site may be involved (Table 6.3). The brain and the peripheral nerves are concomitantly involved in some lipid storage diseases, mitochondrial disorders with a deficiency of respiratory chain enzymes, and familial dysautonomia. Both brain and skeletal muscles are abnormal in acid maltase deficiency and neonatal myotonic dystrophy. Several motor unit disorders produce sufficient hypotonia at birth to impair respiration and produce perinatal asphyxia (Table 6.4). Such infants will have cerebral hypotonia as well. Finally, newborns with spinal cord injuries are frequently the product of long, difficult deliveries in which brachial plexus injuries and depressed cerebral function from asphyxia are present as well.

CLUES TO THE DIAGNOSIS OF CEREBRAL HYPOTONIA

Most newborns with cerebral hypotonia do not pose a diagnostic dilemma and are usually

Table 6.4 MOTOR UNIT DISORDERS WITH PERINATAL RESPIRATORY DISTRESS

Acute infantile spinal muscular atrophy
Congenital hypomyelinating neuropathy
Familial infantile myasthenia
Myotonic dystrophy
Neurogenic arthrogryposis
X-linked myotubular myopathy

identified by history and physical examination. There are many clues to the diagnosis of cerebral hypotonia (Table 6.5), but most important is the presence of other abnormal brain functions: states of decreased consciousness and seizures. Cerebral malformation is the likely explanation for hypotonia in an infant with dysmorphic features or with malformations in other organs.

A tightly fisted hand in which the thumb is constantly enclosed by the other fingers and does not open spontaneously (fisting), and adduction of the thigh so that the legs are crossed when the infant is suspended vertically (scissoring) are considered precursors of spasticity and indicate cerebral dysfunction. Postural reflexes may be elicited in newborns and infants with cerebral hypotonia even when there is a paucity of spontaneous movement. In some acute encephalopathies, and especially in metabolic disorders, the Moro reflex may be exaggerated. The tonic neck reflex is an important indicator of cerebral abnormality if the responses are excessive, obligatory, and persist beyond six months of age. When hemispheric damage is severe but the brainstem is intact, turning the head produces full extension of both ipsilateral limbs and tight flexion on the contralateral side. An obligatory reflex is one in which these postures are maintained for as long as the head is kept rotated. Tendon reflexes are generally normal or brisk, and clonus may be present as well.

CLUES TO MOTOR UNIT DISORDERS

Disorders of the motor unit are not associated with malformations of other organs except for joint deformities and the maldevelopment of bony structures. The face sometimes looks dysmorphic when facial muscles are weak or when the jaw is underdeveloped.

Tendon reflexes are absent or depressed. Total loss of reflexes in muscles with residual movement is more likely caused by neuropathy than myopathy, whereas diminished reflexes consistent with the degree of weakness is more

Table 6.5 CLUES TO CEREBRAL HYPOTONIA

Abnormalities of other brain function
Dysmorphic features
Malformations of other organs
Fisting of the hands
Scissoring on vertical suspension
Movement through postural reflexes
Normal or brisk tendon reflexes

Table 6.6 CLUES TO MOTOR UNIT DISORDERS

No abnormalities of other organs
Absent or depressed tendon reflexes
Muscle atrophy
Fasciculations
Failure of movement on postural reflexes

often encountered in myopathy than in neuropathy (Table 6.6). Muscle atrophy suggests motor unit disease, but does not exclude cerebral hypotonia. Failure of growth and even atrophy can be considerable in brain damaged infants. The combination of atrophy and fasciculations is strong evidence for denervation. However, the observation of fasciculations in newborns and infants is often restricted to the tongue and it is difficult, if not impossible, to distinguish fasciculations from normal random movements of the tongue unless atrophy is present.

Postural reflexes, such as the tonic-neck and positive supporting reaction, cannot be superimposed upon weak muscles. The motor unit is the final common pathway of tone; limbs that will not move voluntarily cannot be moved reflexly.

■ Cerebral Hypotonia

Hypotonia is a feature of almost every cerebral disorder in newborns and infants. This section will not deal with those conditions in which the major presenting symptoms are states of decreased consciousness, seizures, and progressive psychomotor retardation. Rather, the discussion is limited to those conditions in which hypotonia is so prominent a feature that the examining physician may consider the possibility of motor unit disease.

CHROMOSOME DISORDERS

The study of human chromosome morphology began only thirty years ago. Numerical rearrangements were discovered first and structural rearrangements later. The development of staining techniques that produce unique banding patterns for each chromosome greatly improved the ability to identify structural rearrangements. Despite considerable syndrome diversity, common characteristics of autosomal chromosome aberrations in the newborn are dysmorphic features of the hands and face and profound hypotonia. For this reason, chromosome studies are indicated in any hypotonic newborn with dysmorphic features of the hands and face, with or without other organ malformation (Table 6.7).

Prader-Willi Syndrome

The Prader-Willi syndrome is characterized by hypotonia, hypogonadism, mental retardation, and obesity. The majority of children with this syndrome have a deletion and translocation of a segment of chromosome 15 between proximal band 15Q11 and distal band 15Q13. The abnormal chromosome is contributed by the father. A 15/15 translocation is usual, but translocations to other autosomes and to the Y chromosome may occur (Berry et al, 1981; Butler and Palmer, 1983).

Clinical Features. Decreased fetal activity is recorded in 75 percent of pregnancies and associated with a 10 percent incidence of congenital hip dislocation and a 6 percent incidence of clubfoot. At birth, the hypotonia is profound and tendon reflexes are either absent or greatly depressed. Feeding problems are invariable, and prolonged nasogastric tube feeding is common (Table 6.8). Cryptorchidism is present in 84 percent and hypogenitalism in 100 percent.

Both the hypotonia and feeding difficulty persist throughout early infancy and are later replaced by relatively normal muscle tone and insatiable hunger. Developmental milestones are delayed, and mental retardation is a constant feature. Minor abnormalities that become more obvious during infancy include a narrow bifrontal diameter of the skull, strabismus, almond-shaped eyes, enamel hypoplasia, and small hands and feet. During childhood, obesity is the rule. The combination of obesity and minor abnormalities of the face and limbs produces a "family resemblance" among children with this syndrome.

Diagnosis. The combination of hypotonia, difficulty feeding, and cryptorchidism in the new-

Table 6.7 HYPOTONIA AND DYSMORPHIC FEATURES

Cerebral dysgenesis
Cerebrohepatorenal syndrome
Chromosomal aberrations
Cohen syndrome
Fiber type disproportion myopathies
Neonatal adrenoleukodystrophy
Neonatal myotonic dystrophy
Prader-Willi syndrome

Table 6.8 DIFFICULTY OF FEEDING IN THE ALERT NEWBORN

Cohen syndrome
Familial dysautonomia
Familial infantile myasthenia
Hypoplasia of bulbar motor nuclei (see Chapter 17)
Infantile neuronal degeneration
Neurogenic arthrogryposis
Myophosphorylase deficiency
Myotonic dystrophy
Prader-Willi syndrome
Transitory neonatal myasthenia

born always warrants chromosome analysis with special reference to chromosome 15. Other studies are not helpful, and if chromosomes are not studied, diagnosis is delayed until the development of obesity.

Treatment. Specific treatment is not available.

CHRONIC NONPROGRESSIVE ENCEPHALOPATHY

Cerebral dysgenesis may be due to known or unknown noxious environmental agents, chromosomal disorders, or genetic defects. In the absence of an acute encephalopathy, hypotonia may be the only symptom at birth or during early infancy. Hypotonia is usually worse at birth and tends to get better with time. Cerebral dysgenesis should be suspected when hypotonia is coupled with malformations in other organs or abnormalities in head size and shape. Uncontrasted computerized tomography (CT) or magnetic resonance imaging (MRI) of the head is advisable when cerebral malformation is suspected. The identification of a major cerebral malformation provides useful information not only for prognosis but also on the feasibility of aggressive therapy to correct malformations in other organs.

Brain injuries occur in the perinatal period and less commonly throughout infancy secondary to anoxia, hemorrhage, infection, and trauma. The sudden onset of hypotonia in a previously well newborn or infant, with or without signs of encephalopathy, should always suggest a cerebral cause. The premature who demonstrates a decline in spontaneous movement and tone may have an intraventricular hemorrhage. Hypotonia is an early feature of meningitis in term and premature newborns. During the acute phase, tendon reflexes may be diminished or absent.

PEROXISOMAL DISORDERS

Peroxisomes are subcellular organelles that participate in the catabolism of very-long-chain fatty acids, the synthesis of plasmalogens and bile acids, and the catabolism of pipecolic acid, dicarboxylic acid, and phytanic acid (Schutgens et al, 1986). Peroxide is generated in the course of several oxidation reactions and catabolized by the enzyme catalase. The chemical abnormalities usually associated with peroxisomal defects include elevated concentrations of very-long-chain fatty acids in tissue and plasma, secretion of abnormal bile acid precursors, hyperpipecolic acidemia and aciduria, and decreased concentrations of tissue plasmalogens.

Cerebrohepatorenal Syndrome (Zellweger)

Cerebrohepatorenal syndrome is probably transmitted by autosomal recessive inheritance. Biochemical and anatomic abnormalities have been reported, but the basic defect is still unknown. The biochemical disturbances include nonspecific aminoaciduria, increased serum levels of iron and copper, alterations in bile acid synthesis, pipecolic acidemia, and the accumulation of very-long-chain fatty acids in ocular tissue (Arneson et al, 1982). The important anatomic abnormalities are an absence of peroxisomes and abnormal mitochondria in brain, liver, and skeletal muscle (Sarnat et al, 1983).

Clinical Features. Affected newborns have severe hypotonia, arthrogryposis, and dysmorphic features. The arthrogryposis is characterized by limited extension of the fingers (camptodactyly) and flexion deformities of the knee and ankle. Suck and cry are weak, and tendon reflexes diminished or absent. Characteristic craniofacial abnormalities include a pear-shaped head owing to a high forehead and an unusual fullness of the cheeks, widened sutures, micrognathia, a high-arched palate, flattening of the bridge of the nose, and hypertelorism. Abnormalities of other organs include biliary cirrhosis, polycystic kidneys, retinal degeneration, and cerebral malformation.

Generalized seizures have their onset anytime during infancy. Death usually occurs during infancy from aspiration, gastrointestinal bleeding, or liver failure.

Diagnosis. Clinical diagnosis can be made on the basis of specific organ involvement. In addition, muscle biopsy reveals large aggregates of mitochondria and increased lipid in subsarcolemmal intermyofibrillary spaces. Liver biopsy demonstrates biliary dysgenesis and iron storage. This disorder differs from neonatal adrenoleukodystrophy, not only by the dysmorphic features and lack of adrenal atrophy but also by the storage of both saturated and unsaturated very-long-chain fatty acids (Kelley et al, 1986).

Treatment. Treatment is not available.

Neonatal Adrenoleukodystrophy

The neonatal form of adrenoleukodystrophy is transmitted by autosomal recessive inheritance. The childhood form, discussed in Chapter 5, is transmitted by X-linked inheritance.

Clinical Features. In some newborns with adrenoleukodystrophy, there is phenotypic resemblance to the cerebrohepatorenal syndrome.

The initial clinical features are hypotonia and failure to thrive. Tendon reflexes are present and often brisk. Abnormal facial features, hepatomegaly, and retinitis pigmentosa are constant features (Aubourg et al, 1986). Progressive neurologic deterioration ensues and is characterized by convulsions, blindness, psychomotor retardation, and spasticity. The adrenal glands are hypoplastic, but symptoms of adrenal failure are not present. Death usually occurs during early childhood.

Diagnosis. The diagnosis is established by demonstrating poor adrenal function and increased plasma concentrations of very-long-chain fatty acids in the serum. Increased concentrations of phytanic acid and trihydroxycoprostanic acid may be present as well.

Treatment. Dietary treatment and plasma exchange are being tested for efficacy in the childhood form and may be beneficial in newborns as well (Moser et al, 1984).

OTHER METABOLIC DEFECTS

It is unusual for inborn errors of metabolism, other than peroxisomal disorders, to be seen with hypotonia alone. There are, however, two disorders presenting in the newborn or early infancy that sometimes are exceptions to the rule: acid maltase deficiency and generalized GM_1 gangliosidosis. Acid maltase deficiency, the more common of the two, produces a severe myopathy and is discussed with other metabolic myopathies. Generalized GM_1 gangliosidosis is discussed in Chapter 5.

OTHER GENETIC DEFECTS

Familial Dysautonomia

Familial dysautonomia, the Riley-Day syndrome, was originally described as a genetic disorder transmitted by autosomal recessive inheritance in Ashkenzai Jews. Similar clinical syndromes also occur in non-Jewish infants; these are often sporadic and the mode of inheritance is not clear.

Clinical Features. In the newborn, the important clinical features are meconium aspiration, poor or no suck reflex, and hypotonia (Axelrod et al, 1987). Hypotonia is caused by disturbances in the brain, the dorsal root ganglia, and the peripheral nerves. Tendon reflexes are hypoactive or absent. The feeding difficulty is unique to familial dysautonomia and provides a clue to diagnosis. Sucking and swallowing are normal separately but cannot be coordinated for effective feeding. Other clinical features that may be noted either in the newborn or later in infancy include pallor, temperature instability, absent fungiform papillae of the tongue, diarrhea and abdominal distention, poor weight gain, lethargy, episodes of irritability, absent corneal reflexes, a labile blood pressure, and failure to produce overflow tears.

Diagnosis. Diagnosis should be suspected from the constellation of clinical symptoms and can be confirmed by the pilocarpine or histamine tests. The instillation of one drop of 0.0625 percent pilocarpine solution into the conjunctival sac has no effect on a normal pupil, but causes immediate pupillary constriction in infants with dysautonomia. This is an example of denervation hypersensitivity. An intradermal injection of 0.1 ml of histamine sulfate (one per 10,000) produces an erythematous wheal followed by a painful flare that extends more than 5 cm and lasts for over an hour in normal children. In infants with dysautonomia, the same injection produces a wheal 2 to 3 cm in diameter with a sharp red border, but the axon flare, an axon reflex, is lacking.

Treatment. Treatment is symptomatic. Bethanechol (Urecholine), 1 to 2 mg/kg/day orally, is thought to be helpful. Its use is based on the observation that injections of acetylcholine produce a transient relief of some symptoms. Longevity has increased because of improved symptomatic treatment.

Cohen Syndrome

The Cohen syndrome is believed to be transmitted by autosomal recessive inheritance. No specific metabolic defect has been identified (Balestrazzi et al, 1980).

Clinical Features. The important clinical manifestations in the newborn are hypotonia, feeding difficulty, and dysmorphic features. Hypotonia varies from minimal to profound and generally persists throughout infancy. Associated dysmorphic features are an antimongoloid slant of the eyes, micrognathia, a high-arched palate, narrow hands and feet, cubitus valgus, genua valga, hypoextensibility of the elbows and proximal interphalangeal joints, simian creases, and shortening of the metacarpals and metatarsals (Kousseff, 1981). Tone improves during infancy, and the feeding difficulty ends. Older children are obese, small of stature, late in the onset of puberty, and severely retarded.

Diagnosis. This syndrome is readily confused with the Prader-Willi syndrome. Diagnosis requires recognition of the constellation of clinical features. Chromosome analysis is normal, and other laboratory tests are not informative.

Treatment. Treatment is not available.

Oculocerebrorenal Syndrome (Lowe Syndrome)

Oculocerebrorenal syndrome is transmitted by X-linked recessive inheritance. Partial expression in the form of minor lenticular opacities is seen in female carriers. The primary abnormality of this disease has not been established, but a mitochondrial disorder causing multiple organ dysfunction is likely (Gobernado et al, 1984; Wisniewski et al, 1984).

Clinical Features. The important features at birth are hypotonia and hyporeflexia associated with congenital cataracts and glaucoma. The combination of congenital cataracts and hypotonia in newborns and young infants is only seen in oculocerebrorenal syndrome, rubella syndrome, Down syndrome, and neonatal myotonic dystrophy. Other features that appear later in infancy are mental retardation and a disorder of the renal tubules resulting in metabolic acidosis, proteinuria aminoaciduria, and defective acidification of the urine. Most infants fail to thrive and die. Survivors are mentally retarded and blind.

Diagnosis. Diagnosis depends upon recognition of the clinical constellation.

Treatment. Treatment is not available.

BENIGN CONGENITAL HYPOTONIA

The term benign congenital hypotonia is retrospective and refers to infants who are hypotonic at birth or shortly thereafter and then develop normal tone. It surely encompasses many different pathologic processes affecting either the brain, the motor unit, or both. A large subset of such children probably have cerebral hypotonia. An increased incidence of mental retardation, learning disabilities, and other sequelae of cerebral abnormality is evident later in life, despite the recovery of normal muscle tone.

■ Spinal Cord Injury

Only in the newborn does spinal cord injury enter the differential diagnosis of hypotonia. Injuries to the cervical spinal cord occur almost exclusively during vaginal delivery; approximately 75 percent are associated with breech presentation and 25 percent with cephalic presentation. Because the injuries always occur on a background of a difficult and prolonged delivery, states of decreased consciousness are common and hypotonia may be falsely attributed to asphyxia or cerebral trauma (Painter and Bergman, 1982). However, the presence of impaired sphincter function and loss of sensation below the midchest should suggest myelopathy.

INJURIES IN BREECH PRESENTATION

Traction injuries to the lower cervical and upper thoracic regions of the cord occur almost exclusively in newborns in whom the angle of extension of the fetal head exceeds 90 percent. Indeed, the risk of spinal cord injury to a fetus in breech position whose head is hyperextended is greater than 70 percent. In such cases, delivery should always be by cesarean section. The tractional forces applied to the extended head are sufficient not only to stretch the cord but actually to herniate the brainstem through the foramen magnum. In addition, the hyperextended position compromises the vertebral arteries as they enter the skull.

The spectrum of pathologic findings varies from edema of the cord without loss of anatomic continuity to massive hemorrhage (epidural, subdural, and intramedullary), which is most pronounced in the lower cervical and upper thoracic segments but may extend the entire length of the cord. Concurrent hemorrhage in the posterior fossa and laceration of the cerebellum may be present as well.

Clinical Features. Mild tractional injuries, in which there is edema of the cord but not intraparenchymal hemorrhage or loss of anatomic continuity, produce little or no clinical manifestations. The major feature is hypotonia, which may be falsely attributed to asphyxia.

Severed tractional injuries are accompanied by hemorrhage into the posterior fossa. Such newborns are unconscious and atonic at birth. There is flaccid quadriplegia with diaphragmatic breathing. Most will not survive the neonatal period. Injuries restricted to the low cervical and high thoracic segments produce near-normal strength in the biceps and weakness of the triceps. The result is flexion of the arms at the elbows and flaccid paraplegia. Spontaneous movement and tendon reflexes in the legs are absent, but foot withdrawal from pinprick may occur as a spinal reflex. The bladder is distended, and there is dribbling of urine. Sensory levels are difficult to detect, but may be deduced by the absence of sweating below the injury.

Diagnosis. Radiographs of the vertebrae are normal, as bony displacement does not occur. Magnetic resonance imaging is diagnostic to demonstrate intraspinal edema and hemorrhage.

Newborns who are unconscious are generally thought to have intracerebral hemorrhage or asphyxia (see Chapter 2), and the diagnosis of spinal cord injury may not be considered until consciousness is regained and the typical motor deficits observed. Even then, a neuromuscular disorder may be considered. The disturbance in bladder function and the development of progressive spastic paraplegia alert the physician to the correct diagnosis.

Treatment. The treatment of spinal cord traction injuries of the newborn is the same as the management of cord injuries in older children (see Chapter 12).

INJURIES IN CERVICAL PRESENTATION

These are high cervical cord injuries caused by twisting of the neck during midforceps rotation when the trunk fails to rotate with the head. The risk is greatest when there is absence of amniotic fluid because of delay from time of membrane rupture to application of forceps. The spectrum of injury varies from intraparenchymal hemorrhage to complete transection. Transection usually occurs at the level of a fractured odontoid process with altantoaxial dislocation.

Clinical Features. Newborns are flaccid and fail to breathe spontaneously. Those with milder injuries may develop shallow, labored respirations, but all require assisted ventilation at birth. Most are unconscious at birth owing to edema in the brainstem. When consciousness is regained, eye movements, sucking, and the withdrawal reflex are the only movements observed. Tendon reflexes are at first absent, but later become exaggerated if the child survives. The bladder becomes distended, and there is overflow incontinence. Priapism may be present as well. Sensation is difficult to assess because the withdrawal reflex is present.

Death generally occurs in the first week from sepsis or respiratory complications. Some children have survived for several years.

Diagnosis. Most children with high cervical cord injuries are thought to have neuromuscular disorders, especially infantile spinal muscular atrophy, because the limbs are flaccid but the eye movements are normal. An electromyogram (EMG) of the limbs should exclude that possibility. Radiographs of the cervical vertebrae are usually normal; odontoid fracture with atlanto-axial dislocation occurs in the minority of patients. Magnetic resonance imaging is useful in demonstrating the spinal cord injury.

Treatment. Newborns with high cervical cord injuries are intubated and provided with respiratory assistance before the diagnosis is established. Further management is the same as for other spinal cord transection syndromes (see Chapter 12).

■ Motor Unit Disorders

EVALUATION OF MOTOR UNIT DISORDERS

In the diagnosis of infants with cerebral hypotonia, the choice of laboratory tests varies considerably from one disease entity to another. This is not the case with motor unit hypotonia. A battery of tests are available that readily define the anatomy and etiology of pathologic processes affecting the motor unit (Table 6.9). The sequence in which they are done is important.

Serum Creatine Kinase

Increased serum concentrations of creatine kinase (CK) are a reflection of skeletal or cardiac muscle necrosis. Blood should be drawn for CK

Table 6.9 EVALUATION OF MOTOR UNIT DISORDERS

Serum creatine kinase
Electrodiagnosis
  Electromyography
  Nerve conduction studies
  Repetitive stimulation
Muscle biopsy
Nerve biopsy
Tensilon test

determination prior to the performance of EMG or muscle biopsy, as either procedure will elevate the serum CK concentration. Laboratory reference values of normal serum CK concentration are usually based upon findings from nonambulatory patients. Normal values tend to be higher in an ambulatory population. The total concentration of CK and its isoenzymes increases significantly with acidosis. Levels as high as 1,000 IU/L may be recorded in severely asphyxiated newborns, but even normal newborns have a higher than normal concentration during the first twenty-four hours post partum (Warburton et al, 1981). A normal CK level in a hypotonic infant is strong evidence against a rapidly progressive myopathy, but it does not exclude fiber type disproportion myopathies and some metabolic myopathies. Conversely, a mild elevation in the concentration of CK is sometimes encountered in rapidly progressive neuronopathies (spinal muscular atrophy).

Electrodiagnosis

The EMG is extremely useful in the diagnosis of infantile hypotonia when it is performed by an experienced physician. It enables one to predict the final diagnosis in 82 percent of infants younger than three months of age with hypotonia of motor unit origin. Fewer than 5 percent of hypotonic infants with a normal EMG will have an abnormal muscle biopsy (Packer et al, 1982). The needle portion of the study helps to distinguish myopathic from neuropathic processes. Myopathies are generally characterized by the appearance of brief, small-amplitude, polyphasic potentials (BSAPPs). Neuropathies are characterized by the presence of denervation potentials at rest (fibrillations, fasciculations, sharp waves) and motor unit potentials that are large in size, prolonged in duration, and polyphasic in shape. Studies of nerve conduction velocity are useful in distinguishing axonal from demyelinating neuropathies; demyelinating neuropathies cause greater slowing of conduction velocity. Repetitive nerve stimulation studies demonstrate disturbances in neuromuscular transmission.

Muscle Biopsy

Muscle biopsy should not be undertaken unless the tissue can be processed by histochemical techniques. The muscle selected for biopsy should be weak, but still capable of moving. When there is symmetric weakness, the muscles of one limb should be studied by EMG and the muscles of the other limb reserved for biopsy. Adequate tissue can be obtained either by needle or by open biopsy, depending upon the physician's preference.

Histochemistry is essential for the complete evaluation of muscle histology because special techniques are needed to demonstrate fiber types and storage materials. Human skeletal muscle can be arbitrarily divided into two fiber types on the basis of the intensity of reaction to myosin adenosine triphosphatase (ATPase) at pH 9.4. Type I fibers react weakly to ATPase, are characterized by oxidative metabolism, and serve a tonic function. Type II fibers react intensely to ATPase, utilize glycolytic metabolism, and serve a phasic function. Type I and II fibers are generally equal in number and distributed in a checkerboard pattern. Disorders may be characterized by abnormalities in fiber type number, fiber type size, or both.

The important storage materials identified in skeletal muscle are glycogen and lipid. In most storage disorders, vacuoles are present in the fibers that contain the abnormal material. The vacuoles are seen with light microscopy, and the specific material is identified by its histochemical reaction.

Nerve Biopsy

Sural nerve biopsy is indicated only in patients with electrodiagnostic evidence of sural neuropathy. Nerve biopsy is useful in differentiating axonal from demyelinating neuropathies and can be diagnostic in demonstrating storage material by use of histochemical techniques.

The Tensilon Test

Edrophonium chloride (Tensilon) is a rapidly acting anticholinesterase that produces a temporary reversal of weakness in patients with myasthenia. Before Tensilon is administered, a specific affected muscle should be selected for observation (ptosis, oculomotor paresis, facial weakness). Rare patients are supersensitive to Tensilon and may stop breathing because of depolarization of endplates or an abnormal vagal response. Equipment for mechanical ventilation should always be available when the test is performed. In newborns, a subcutaneous injection of 0.15 mg/kg produces a response within 10 minutes. In infants, the drug is given intravenously at a dose of 0.2 mg/kg and reverses weakness within one minute.

SPINAL MUSCULAR ATROPHIES

Spinal muscular atrophies are a heterogeneous group of disorders, usually genetic in origin, characterized by the degeneration of anterior horn cells in the spinal cord and motor nuclei of the brainstem (neurononopathy). The onset of symptoms is at any age from the newborn to adult life. Some spinal muscular atrophies are marked by a generalized distribution of weakness, and others affect specific muscle groups. Those in which onset occurs in infancy have generalized weakness and present as infantile hypotonia. Infantile spinal muscular atrophy (Werdnig-Hoffman disease) is one of the more common disorders of the motor unit causing infantile hypotonia.

Two clinical syndromes of infantile spinal muscular atrophy, both transmitted by autosomal inheritance, can be distinguished. One is an acute fulminating form with onset at birth or within the first six months, and the other is a chronic form with onset after three months of age. Both the acute and chronic forms were once thought to be the variable expression of the same genetic defect. They are now considered to be genetically distinct with a consistent course of disease within individual kinships (Pearn et al, 1973).

Acute Infantile Spinal Muscular Atrophy

Clinical Features. Neuronal degeneration begins in utero, and deficient fetal movement is noted in one third of pregnancies (Pearn, 1973). Such newborns have a generalized weakness affecting proximal more than distal muscles, hypotonia, and areflexia. At rest, the characteristic posture of hypotonia is assumed. Paradoxical respirations are observed because intercostal paralysis and thoracic collapse occur before diaphragmatic movement is impaired. Despite intrauterine hypotonia, arthrogryposis is not present. Neurogenic arthrogryposis was believed to be a manifestation of infantile spinal muscular atrophy; it is now believed to be a distinct entity and is described separately in this chapter.

Newborns who are hypotonic in utero and weak at birth may have difficulty in adapting to extrauterine life and experience postnatal asphyxia and encephalopathy. The majority are able to breathe adequately at first and appear alert despite the generalized weakness because facial expression is relatively preserved and extraocular movement is normal.

When the onset of weakness is in infancy, the decline in strength can be sudden or decremental. At times, there is the appearance of improvement because of normal cerebral development, but the progression of weakness is relentless. Atrophy and fasciculations may be observed in the tongue. After the gag reflex is lost, feeding becomes difficult and death results from aspiration and pneumonia. When weakness is present at birth, death occurs by six months of age. Infants with later onset of symptoms may survive to one year.

Diagnosis. The diagnosis is readily established by laboratory investigation. Serum concentration of CK is ordinarily normal, but may be mildly elevated in infants with rapidly progressive weakness. EMG studies demonstrate fibrillations and fasciculations at rest and an increased mean amplitude of motor unit potentials. Motor nerve conduction velocities may be slowed, but are usually normal (Moosa and Dubowitz, 1976). The histopathologic findings in muscle are diagnostic. Routine histologic stains demonstrate groups of small fibers adjacent to groups of fibers that are normal or hypertrophied in size. The diagnostic features of acute infantile spinal muscular atrophy are revealed by the myosin ATPase reaction. All hypertrophied fibers are type I. Fibers of medium and small size are a mixture of types I and II (Fig. 6.3). The normal checkerboard arrangement of fiber types is replaced by type grouping; a sign of reinnervation in which large numbers of fibers of the same type are contiguous.

Treatment. Treatment is not available for this disorder, nor is there a method for prenatal diagnosis.

Chronic Infantile Spinal Muscular Atrophy

Clinical Features. The chronic form of infantile spinal muscular atrophy has its onset after

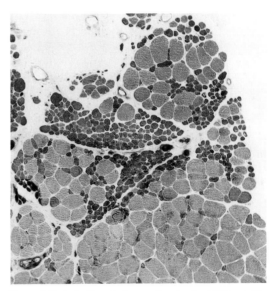

Figure 6.3 Infantile spinal muscular atrophy (ATPase). The normal checkerboard pattern is lost. Groups of large type I fibers (light shade) are adjacent to groups of small type II fibers (dark shade). (Reprinted with permission of Fenichel GM: Neonatal Neurology. Churchill Livingstone, New York, 1985.)

three months of age. Therefore, when the onset of weakness is between three and six months, it is not possible at the time of presentation to predict whether the course of illness will be acute or chronic. Initial weakness is usually symmetric and affects the proximal muscles of the legs, the arms, or all limbs. Pelvic weakness is more frequent than shoulder weakness as an initial symptom. Distal muscles are affected little or not at all during early infancy. Tendon reflexes of weak muscles are depressed or unobtainable. Facial muscles are not affected early in the course, and extraocular muscles are spared completely.

The course during infancy is one of slowly progressive weakness that is not life-threatening. In some children, the progression of weakness ceases and stabilizes for many years. Eventually, slow progression of weakness resumes. Improvement never occurs, and even during periods of stabilization the EMG continues to demonstrate fibrillations and fasciculations.

During childhood, there is a tendency for contractures to develop. Pseudohypertrophy of the calves and gluteal muscles is common and may suggest Duchenne muscular dystrophy. As the plantar flexor muscles become progressively weaker, the foot everts into an equinovarus posture. Death results from respiratory insufficiency. The mean age of survival is thirty years.

Diagnosis. The serum concentration of CK is normal. EMG findings are identical to those described for the acute infantile form. Muscle biopsy demonstrates groups of small fibers adjacent to fibers of normal size. Type grouping is usually present, but type I fiber hypertrophy is not.

Treatment. Although there is no treatment for the underlying disease, physical therapy and other rehabilitative measures may prevent contractures and maintain function.

Infantile Neuronal Degeneration

Clinical Features. Fourteen infants have been reported in which the typical features of infantile spinal muscular atrophy are combined with degenerative changes in the cerebellum, thalamus, and peripheral sensory nerves (Steiman et al, 1980). The disorder is thought to be transmitted as an autosomal recessive trait because of three families with two or more affected siblings. All have presented with hypotonia and areflexia, and one had arthrogryposis as well. The hypotonia is primarily due to denervation, but probably has a cerebral component. In half of cases, initial symptoms appeared at birth; in the other half, they appeared during early infancy. Dyspnea, weak cry, and difficulty in feeding are prominent features in the newborn, all of whom die within five months. The symptoms are the same when the onset is delayed until early infancy, but survivals beyond two years of age are recorded.

Diagnosis. Infantile neuronal degeneration can be differentiated from infantile spinal muscular atrophy by electrophysiologic studies. Motor nerve conduction velocities are slow, and sensory nerve responses are absent or reduced.

Treatment. Treatment is not available.

Neurogenic Arthrogryposis

The term neurogenic arthrogryposis was originally used to denote the association of arthrogryposis with infantile spinal muscular atrophy. Most cases are sporadic. Transmission by autosomal recessive inheritance is documented in some families, but the recent demonstration of neurogenic arthrogryposis in only one of identical twins suggests that some sporadic cases may not be genetic in origin (Sul et al, 1982). Transmission by autosomal dominant inheritance has been described in two kindreds. The clinical and pathologic features in these families distinguish them from the sporadic cases and from those transmitted by autosomal recessive inheritance.

Clinical Features. In neurogenic arthrogryposis, the most active phase of disease is in utero. Severely affected newborns have respiratory and feeding difficulties, and some will die of aspiration. The less severely affected survive and experience little or no progression of their weakness. Indeed, the respiratory and feeding difficulties tend to get better with time.

Contractures are present in both proximal and distal joints. Micrognathia and a high-arched palate may be associated, and a pattern of facial anomalies is present in some newborns that suggests trisomy 18.

Diagnosis. The diagnosis is suspected in newborns with arthrogryposis in whom the serum concentration of CK is normal and the EMG is compatible with a neuropathic process. Muscle histology reveals the typical pattern of denervation and reinnervation. However, myopathic features may be present as well: increased collagen and adipose tissue, structural derangements in medium-sized fibers, and fibrosis of the muscle spindle capsule.

Treatment. The joint deformities respond to physical therapy, and an intensive program of rehabilitation should be initiated as quickly after birth as possible.

Incontinentia Pigmenti

Incontinentia pigmenti usually presents with neonatal seizures and is described fully in Chapter 1. It is characterized by the combination of typical skin lesions and cerebral malformations. Occasional cases are reported in which identical skin lesions are associated with progressive anterior horn cell degeneration (Larsen et al, 1987).

POLYNEUROPATHIES

Polyneuropathies are uncommon in childhood and even more uncommon during infancy. Table 6.10 lists those polyneuropathies that have their onset during infancy. They are divided into those that primarily affect the myelin (demyelinating) and those that primarily affect the axon (axonal). In the newborn and infant, the term demyelinating also includes disorders in which myelin has failed to form (hypomyelinating). Only congenital hypomyelinating neuropathy regularly presents in a hypotonic infant.

Table 6.10 POLYNEUROPATHIES WITH
POSSIBLE ONSET IN INFANCY

Demyelinating
  Congenital hypomyelinating neuropathy
  Metachromatic leukodystrophy (see Chapter 5)
  Globoid cell leukodystrophy (see Chapter 5)
  Postinfectious polyradiculoneuropathy (see Chapter 7)
  Chronic inflammatory demyelinating polyneuropathy
  Hereditary motor-sensory neuropathy I (see Chapter 7)
  Hereditary motor-sensory neuropathy III (see Chapter 7)
Axonal
  Familial dysautonomia
  Subacute necrotizing encephalopathy (see Chapters 5 and 10)
  Hereditary motor-sensory neuropathy II (see Chapter 7)
  Infantile neuronal degeneration
  Idiopathic with encephalopathy (see Chapter 7)

However, chronic inflammatory demyelinating polyneuropathy may sometimes have a neonatal onset. The distinction is important because the latter is steroid-responsive. The initial symptom in the other conditions is more likely to be a progressive gait disturbance or psychomotor retardation. A complete discussion of the clinical approach to neuropathy is found in Chapter 7.

Congenital Hypomyelinating Neuropathy

The term congenital hypomyelinating neuropathy may encompass several different disorders with similar clinical and pathologic manifestations (Guzzetta et al, 1982; Kennedy et al, 1977; Ulrich et al, 1981). Most cases have been sporadic, and while it has been reported in cousins and in siblings of both sexes, autosomal recessive inheritance has not been established. Indeed, autosomal dominant inheritance has been suggested in some families because of minor abnormalities in parents: pes cavus, scoliosis, and slow conduction velocities.

Clinical Features. The symptoms and signs in the newborn are indistinguishable from acute infantile spinal muscular atrophy. There is progressive flaccid weakness and atrophy of the skeletal muscles, a bulbar palsy that spares extraocular motility, and areflexia. Respiratory insufficiency causes death during infancy.

Some children are not identified as abnormal until late infancy when they fail to meet motor milestones (Harati and Butler, 1985). Examination reveals diffuse weakness, distal atrophy, and areflexia. The progression of weakness is slow and not life-threatening during childhood. Sensation remains intact. These late-onset cases may be demyelinating rather than hypomyelinating neuropathies.

Peripheral nerves enlarge and may become palpable when there is prolonged survival.

Diagnosis. The serum concentration of CK is normal, EMG is consistent with denervation, and motor nerve conduction velocities are extremely slow, usually less than 10 meters/second. The protein concentration of the cerebrospinal fluid is markedly elevated in almost every case. Muscle biopsy reveals groups of atrophic fibers adjacent to groups of normal fibers, without fiber hypertrophy.

Definitive antemortem diagnosis is established by sural nerve biopsy, which reveals naked axons without evidence of myelin formation. There is no evidence of inflammation or lipid storage. However, it is impossible to completely eliminate the possibility of chronic inflammatory demyelinating neuropathy by laboratory investigation.

Treatment. Treatment is not available for congenital hypomyelinating neuropathy, but every case should be given a trial of corticosteroids to determine whether the neuropathy is responsive.

Chronic Inflammatory Demyelinating Polyneuropathy

Clinical Features. The onset of symptoms may be at birth or anytime during infancy. Motor delay or generalized weakness are the initial features. Either proximal or distal muscles can be more severely affected. Tendon reflexes are absent. Nerves become enlarged and are palpable (Sladky et al, 1986).

Diagnosis. The protein content of the cerebrospinal fluid is elevated, and motor nerve conduction velocities are markedly slow. Sural nerve biopsy shows changes of chronic demyelination with multifocal endoneurial edema and a mononuclear cell infiltrate.

Treatment. All patients become stronger within four weeks of starting oral prednisone, 2 mg/kg/day. Following the initial response, the children should be maintained on long-term alternate day therapy at doses ranging from 0.3 to 1 mg/kg.

DISORDERS OF NEUROMUSCULAR TRANSMISSION

Infantile Botulism

Human botulism ordinarily results from eating food contaminated by preformed exotoxin of the organism *Clostridium botulinum*. The exotoxin produces a cholinergic blockade of skeletal muscle and end organs innervated by autonomic nerves by preventing the release of acetylcholine. Infantile botulism is an age-limited disorder in which *C. botulinum* is ingested, colonizes the intestinal tract, and produces toxin in situ (Arnon et al, 1977).

Clinical Features. The clinical spectrum of infantile botulism includes (1) asymptomatic carriers of organisms, (2) mild hypotonia and failure to thrive, (3) severe, progressive, life-threatening paralysis, (4) and sudden infant death (Thompson et al, 1980). Infected infants are between two and twenty-six weeks of age and usually live in a dusty environment adjacent to constructional or agricultural soil disruption. There is a distinct seasonal incidence between March and October. Most infants experience a prodromal syndrome of constipation and poor feeding. Progressive bulbar and skeletal muscle weakness and loss of tendon reflexes develop four to five days later. Typical features on examination include diffuse hypotonia, ptosis, dysphagia, weak cry, and dilated pupils that react sluggishly to light. The syndrome suggests either postinfectious polyradiculoneuropathy (Guillain-Barré syndrome, infantile spinal muscular atrophy, or generalized myasthenia gravis). Clinical differential of infantile botulism from Guillain-Barré syndrome is difficult, and some reports of Guillain-Barré syndrome during infancy may actually have infantile botulism. Infantile botulism differs from infantile spinal muscular atrophy by the early appearance of facial and pharyngeal weakness, the presence of ptosis and dilated pupils, and the occurrence of severe constipation. Infants with generalized myasthenia do not have dilated pupils, absent reflexes, or severe constipation.

Diagnosis. Electrophysiologic studies provide the first clue to diagnosis. Repetitive stimulation between 20 and 50 Hz reverses the presynaptic block and produces an incremental increase in the size of the motor unit potentials in 90 percent of cases (Cornblath et al, 1983). The EMG demonstrates short-duration, low-amplitude motor unit potentials. The diagnosis is confirmed by the isolation of organism from the stool.

Treatment. Infantile botulism is a self-limited disease generally lasting two to six weeks. The use of antitoxin and antibiotics does not influence its course. Indeed, gentamicin, an agent that produces presynaptic neuromuscular blockade, may worsen the condition. Intensive care is required throughout the period of profound hypotonia, and many infants require ventilator support. Sudden apnea and death are a constant danger.

Juvenile Myasthenia

The term juvenile myasthenia denotes cases of myasthenia gravis in children that are similar in clinical form and autoimmune basis to myasthenia gravis in adults (Fenichel, 1978). In most cases, a circulating globulin can be demonstrated that binds to the acetylcholine receptor protein (AChRP) and functionally decreases the number of motor endplates available for binding by acetylcholine.

Clinical Features. The onset of symptoms is always after age six months and usually after two years. The initial symptoms in infants, as in older children and adults, are usually ptosis and diplopia. In some infants, there is generalized weakness and respiratory insufficiency may develop. Muscle atrophy is not present, and tendon reflexes are present even in weak muscles.

Diagnosis. Juvenile myasthenia is readily distinguished from genetic myasthenic syndromes (congenital myasthenia and familial infantile myasthenia) because symptoms are not present at birth. Diagnosis relies upon a positive response to intravenous Tensilon, 0.2 mg/kg. Increased serum concentrations of AChRP antibody are ordinarily present in infants with generalized juvenile myasthenia, but not in infants with only ocular involvement, or with genetic myasthenia (Seybold and Lindstrom, 1981).

Treatment. Infants with mild myasthenia, especially those with only ocular involvement, should be treated with anticholinesterase medication. The choices are neostigmine, 0.5 mg/kg orally every four hours, or pyridostigmine, 2 mg/kg orally every four hours. Both drugs are started at these low dosages and slowly increased as tolerated. The major adverse side effect is diarrhea. Infants with severe generalized myasthenia and high serum concentrations of antibody should undergo thymectomy. Following thymectomy, oral prednisone, 2 mg/kg every other day, is started and the dose reduced by 10 percent each month until the lowest dose is reached that prevents return of symptoms.

Transitory Neonatal Myasthenia

A transitory myasthenic syndrome is observed in 10 to 15 percent of offspring of myasthenic mothers. Affected and unaffected newborns have the same high concentration of AChRP antibody as their mothers (Donaldson et al, 1981; Lefvert and Osterman, 1983; Ohta et al, 1981). Passive transfer of antibody from mother to fetus clearly occurs, but does not fully explain the development of symptoms in only a small percentage of newborns. It is believed that symptomatic newborns synthesize antibody de novo because the antibody in affected newborns is a different idiotype than the antibody in the mothers and that the half-life of antibody in affected newborns is four to eight times longer than in unaffected newborns.

Clinical Features. Difficulty feeding and generalized hypotonia are the major clinical features. Affected children are eager to feed, but sucking fatigues quickly and prevents adequate nutrition. The onset of symptoms is usually within hours of birth, but can be delayed until the third day. Some newborns have had intrauterine hypotonia and are born with arthrogryposis. Weakness of cry and facial expression is present in 50 percent, but limitation of extraocular movement and ptosis is present in only 15 percent. Respiratory insufficiency is uncommon. Weakness becomes progressively worse in the first few days and then improves. The mean duration of symptoms is eighteen days with a range of five days to two months. Recovery is complete, and transitory neonatal myasthenia does not develop into myasthenia later in life.

Diagnosis. The diagnosis of transitory neonatal myasthenia is accomplished by demonstrating high serum concentrations of AChRP antibody in the newborn and temporary reversal of weakness by the subcutaneous injection of 0.15 mg/kg of Tensilon.

Treatment. Newborns with severe generalized weakness and respiratory distress should be treated with exchange transfusion. For those who are less impaired, an intramuscular injection of 0.1 neostigmine methylsulfate prior to feeding provides sufficient improvement in sucking and swallowing to allow adequate nutrition. The dose is progressively reduced as symptoms remit. Neostigmine may also be administered through a nasogastric tube at a dose ten times the parenteral level.

Familial Infantile Myasthenia

Two genetic forms of myasthenia are recognized in the newborn: congenital myasthenia gravis and familial infantile myasthenia. Both may be caused by several different defects in neuromuscular transmission. Congenital myasthenia presents as ophthalmoparesis and ptosis without generalized hypotonia and is discussed in Chapter 15. Familial infantile myasthenia is characterized by generalized hypotonia, severe and repeated bouts of respiratory insufficiency, and feeding difficulty (Albers et al, 1984; Robertson et al, 1980). The mothers do not have myasthenia gravis, but the frequent occurrence of this disorder in siblings suggests autosomal recessive inheritance.

Clinical Features. All newborns with familial infantile myasthenia are severely hypotonic at birth, and many require mechanical ventilation (Smit and Barth, 1980). Arthrogryposis may be present as well. Although facial and skeletal muscles are weak, extraocular motility is usually normal. Within weeks, the infants become stronger and can be extubated. However, episodes of weakness and life-threatening apnea occur repeatedly throughout infancy and childhood, sometimes even into adult life (Gieron and Korthals, 1985).

Diagnosis. The diagnosis is established by the subcutaneous injection of Tensilon, 0.15 mg/kg, which reverses the weakness and the respiratory distress within ten minutes of injection. Further confirmation, if needed, can be accomplished by the demonstration of a decrement in the amplitude of successive motor unit potentials with repetitive nerve stimulation. The serum concentration of AChRP antibodies is not elevated.

Treatment. Long-term treatment with neostigmine or pyridostigmine is needed to prevent sudden episodes of apnea at the time of intercurrent illness. Treatment should be continued throughout childhood. Because there is no evidence for an immunopathy (Vincent et al, 1981), there is no rational basis for thymectomy or immunosuppressive therapy.

FIBER TYPE DISPROPORTION MYOPATHIES

Several "congenital myopathies" have been described that present as neonatal hypotonia and are diagnosed only by muscle biopsy. The common feature is that type I fibers are greater in number, but smaller in size, than type II fibers (Fig. 6.4). This fiber type predominance, in the absence of fiber degeneration, has led to the notion that fiber type disproportion myopathies are not primary diseases of muscle, but are

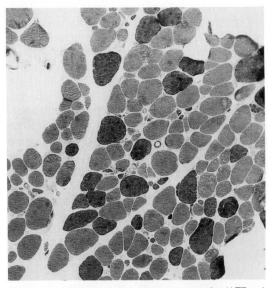

Figure 6.4 Fiber type disproportion myopathy (ATPase). Type I fibers (light shade) are more numerous than type II fibers (dark shade). Type II fibers are generally larger in diameter than type I fibers. (Reprinted with permission of Fenichel GM: Neonatal Neurology. Churchill Livingstone, New York, 1985.)

actually developmental abnormalities of innervation (Elder et al, 1983). In some patients, fiber type disproportion is the only histologic abnormality and this finding is referred to as *congenital fiber type disproportion myopathy*. In others, a unique histologic feature is present for which the condition is named. The fiber type disproportion myopathies with unique histologic features are myotubular myopathy, nemaline myopathy, and central core disease.

Congenital Fiber Type Disproportion Myopathy

The congenital fiber type disproportion myopathies are a heterogeneous group of diseases that share a similar pattern of muscle histology. The presenting feature of all such disease is infantile hypotonia (Curless, 1977; Sulaiman et al, 1983). Both sexes are equally involved. Most cases are sporadic. Some are clearly transmitted by autosomal dominant inheritance, and others are familial, but without a definite pattern of genetic transmission. Despite the label "congenital," an identical pattern of fiber type disproportion may be present in patients who are asymptomatic at birth and develop weakness during childhood.

Clinical Features. In newborns, weakness may be mild or so severe as to cause respiratory

insufficiency. Many have experienced intrauterine hypotonia and demonstrate congenital hip dislocation, dysmorphic features, and joint contractures. Proximal muscles are weaker than distal muscles. Facial weakness, ptosis, and disturbances of ocular motility may be present as well. In infants with axial weakness, kyphoscoliosis often develops during childhood. Tendon reflexes are depressed or absent. Intellectual function is normal.

Weakness is most severe during the first two years and then either improves or becomes relatively stable.

Diagnosis. Muscle biopsy demonstration of type I fiber predominance and hypotrophy is essential for diagnosis. Other laboratory studies are not helpful. The serum concentration of CK may be slightly elevated or normal, and the EMG may be consistent with a neuropathic process, a myopathic process, or both. Nerve conduction velocities are normal.

Treatment. Physical therapy should be initiated immediately, not only to relieve existing contractures but also to prevent new contractures from developing.

Myotubular (Centronuclear) Myopathy

Several different clinical syndromes are included under this title. Some are clearly transmitted by X-linked inheritance, others by autosomal dominant inheritance, and still others are sporadic and possibly transmitted by autosomal recessive inheritance (Kinoshite et al, 1975; Meyers et al, 1974; Pavone et al, 1980). The common histologic feature on muscle biopsy is an appearance that suggests the persistence of fetal myotubes (Sarnat et al, 1981).

Acute Myotubular Myopathy

Clinical Features. This form is transmitted by X-linked inheritance and presents in the newborn with generalized hypotonia and respiratory distress. Decreased fetal movement during pregnancy and polyhydramnios are common. Sucking, swallowing, and tendon reflexes are depressed or absent. Ptosis, and sometimes complete ophthalmoplegia, may be present. Repeated episodes of apnea, asphyxia, and pneumonia usually lead to death during the neonatal period or in early infancy.

Diagnosis. The serum concentration of creatine kinase is normal. The EMG may suggest a neuropathic process, a myopathic process, or both. Muscle biopsy reveals type I fiber predominance and hypotrophy, the presence of many internal nuclei, and a central area of increased oxidative enzyme and decreased myosin ATPase activity.

Treatment. No treatment is available for this disorder, nor is there a method for prenatal diagnosis.

Chronic Myotubular Myopathy

Clinical Features. These are cases that may be transmitted by either autosomal dominant or autosomal recessive inheritance. Some patients present with hypotonia at birth, others come to attention because of delayed motor development. Limb weakness may be predominantly proximal or distal. The axial and neck flexor muscles are weak as well. Ptosis, but not ophthalmoplegia, is sometimes present at birth. During infancy there is slowly progressive ophthalmoplegia, loss of facial expression, continuing weakness of limb muscles, and loss of tendon reflexes. Many affected patients have convulsions and mental deficiency.

Diagnosis. The serum concentration of CK is normal, and the EMG is abnormal but not diagnostic. Muscle biopsy is essential for diagnosis and identical to the acute form.

Treatment. Treatment is not available, nor is there a method for prenatal diagnosis.

Nemaline (Rod) Myopathy

Nemaline myopathy is probably transmitted by autosomal dominant inheritance (Kondo and Yuasa, 1980). Penetrance is variable, and affected parents may be asymptomatic.

Clinical Features. Hypotonia is usually mild, but can be so severe as to cause immediate respiratory insufficiency and neonatal death (Norton et al, 1983). Affected newborns often appear normal, and attention is not sought until infancy because of delayed achievement of motor milestones. The infant is hypotonic with greater weakness in proximal than distal muscles. Weakness of facial muscles causes a dysmorphic appearance in which the face appears long and narrow and the palate high and arched. Axial weakness is present as well and leads to scoliosis. Weakness is not progressive and tends to stabilize, albeit with some residual handicap.

Diagnosis. The concentration of serum CK is either normal or only mildly elevated. The EMG may be normal, and when abnormal it is not diagnostic. Muscle biopsy is essential for diag-

nosis (Fulthorpe et al, 1969). Multiple, small, rod-like particles, thought to be structural protein, are present within most, if not all, muscle fibers (Fig. 6.5). Similar rod-like structures are also seen as a nonspecific histologic feature in some inflammatory myopathies, but only in nemaline myopathy is type I fiber predominance associated.

Treatment. Treatment is not available, nor is there a method for prenatal diagnosis. Asymptomatic affected parents can sometimes be detected by muscle biopsy; rod bodies and fiber type predominance are present.

Central Core Disease

Central core disease is a rare but distinct genetic entity transmitted by autosomal dominant inheritance (Byrne et al, 1982).

Clinical Features. Mild hypotonia is noted immediately after birth or during the first month. Congenital dislocation of the hips is relatively common. Weakness is greater in proximal than in distal limb muscles. Tendon reflexes of weak muscles are depressed or absent. Extraocular motility, facial expression, and swallowing are normal. Some children become progressively weaker, have motor impairment, and develop kyphoscoliosis. In others, weakness remains mild and never causes disability.

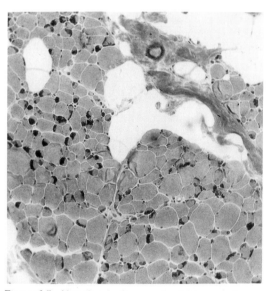

Figure 6.5 Nemaline (rod) myopathy (trichrome). A spectrum of fiber sizes is present. The small fibers are all type I and contain rod-like bodies in a subsarcolemmal position. (Reprinted with permission of Fenichel GM: Neonatal Neurology. Churchill Livingstone, New York, 1985.)

Diagnosis. The serum concentration of CK is normal, and the EMG may be normal as well. More frequently, the EMG suggests a myopathic process. Diagnosis depends upon muscle biopsy. Sharply demarcated cores of closely packed myofibrils undergoing varying degrees of degeneration are present in the center of all type I fibers. Because of the tight packing of myofibrils, the cores are deficient in sarcoplasmic reticulum, glycogen, and mitochondria.

Treatment. Treatment is not available, nor is there a method for prenatal diagnosis.

MUSCULAR DYSTROPHIES

Congenital Muscular Dystrophy

Congenital muscular dystrophy is not a single nosologic entity, but rather a collection of conditions in which muscular dystrophy is present at birth (Echenne et al, 1986; McMenamin et al, 1982a). Most cases are sporadic, but some involve affected siblings or parental consanguinity, suggesting autosomal recessive inheritance.

Clinical Features. Among the many reports of congenital muscular dystrophy, there is one subgroup that is more homogeneous than others. The clinical features include (1) generalized hypotonia and weakness, which may involve facial muscles but spare extraocular motility; (2) fixed joint deformities, of which clubfoot and torticollis are particularly common; (3) absent or diminished tendon reflexes; and (4) normal intelligence (Lazaro et al, 1979). The most progressive and active phase of muscle degenera-

tion occurs in utero. Postnatally, the weakness may remain stationary or may continue to progress, but there is always a tendency for more contractures to develop.

Diagnosis. The serum concentration of CK may be normal or elevated in the newborn and tends to decline with age; however, it does not correlate with the severity of weakness. Occasionally, elevated serum concentrations of CK can be demonstrated in siblings or parents. The EMG is consistent with a myopathic process.

Muscle histologic appearance is characteristic. There is variation in fiber size with occasional central nucleation, extensive fibrosis and proliferation of adipose tissue, fibers undergoing regeneration and degeneration, and thickening of the muscle spindle capsule (Fig. 6.6).

Treatment. Physical therapy is important to prevent further contractures. Antenatal diagnosis is not available.

Fukuyama Type

A clinical syndrome of congenital muscular dystrophy associated with cerebral dysplasia has been described in Japanese newborns (McMenamin et al, 1982b). It is the second most prevalent form of muscular dystrophy in Japan, but is rare in Japanese or non-Japanese children born in other parts of the world. Autosomal recessive inheritance is suspected.

Clinical Features. Affected newborns have arthrogryposis; hypotonia; generalized weakness, including that of the face; and depressed or absent tendon reflexes. In addition to mus-

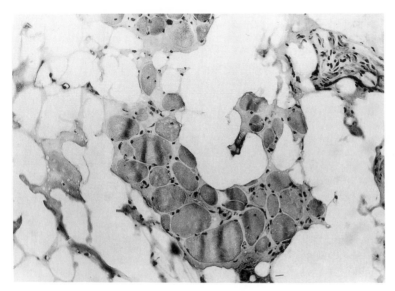

Figure 6.6 Congenital muscular dystrophy (trichrome). Proliferation of adipose tissue is excessive and out of proportion to the degree of muscle fiber degeneration. (Reprinted with permission of Fenichel GM: Neonatal Neurology. Churchill Livingstone, New York, 1985.)

cular abnormalities, there are microcephaly, mental retardation and seizures.

Diagnosis. The serum concentration of CK is generally elevated and the EMG myopathic. Muscle biopsy demonstrates excessive proliferation of adipose tissue and collagen out of proportion to the degree of fiber degeneration. Typical CT abnormalities are dilation of the cerebral ventricles and subarachnoid space, and lucency of cortical white matter.

Treatment. No treatment is available for this disorder, nor is there a method for prenatal diagnosis.

Leukodystrophy

The combination of congenital muscular dystrophy and demyelination of the cerebral hemispheres has been described in caucasian children (Egger et al, 1983). Several sibling pairs have been reported, thus suggesting autosomal recessive inheritance.

Clinical Features. Affected newborns are hypotonic, and some have arthrogryposis as well. Feeding disturbances and apnea may be associated. Tendon reflexes are diminished or absent. Intelligence is normal at first, but progressive dementia and epilepsy occur during childhood.

Diagnosis. The serum concentration of CK is elevated, and the EMG is consistent with a myopathic process. Nerve conduction velocity is normal. The EEG may demonstrate epileptiform activity. CT or MRI is necessary for antemortem diagnosis and demonstrates abnormalities in the cerebral white matter. Some children with normal intelligence also have neuroimaging evidence of leukodystrophy, and it is difficult to separate such cases into distinct subgroups.

Treatment. No treatment is available for this disorder, nor is there a method for prenatal diagnosis.

Cerebro-ocular Dysplasia

Cerebro-ocular dysplasia is characterized by the combination of congenital muscular dystrophy and ocular anomolies. Mild to severe cerebral malformations may be associated (Echenne et al, 1986).

Clinical Features. Hypotonia and arthrogryposis are present at birth. Hydrocephalus is almost a constant feature. Several different cerebral malformations may be associated: abnormal gyral patterns, heterotopias, hypomyelination, and agenesis of tracts. Ocular abnormalities

include corneal clouding, cataract, retinal dysplasia or detachment, and optic nerve hypoplasia.

Diagnosis. All newborns with muscular dystrophy and eye-brain abnormalities, no matter how mild any one element may be, should be considered to have this syndrome.

Treatment. No treatment is available for this disorder, nor is there a method for prenatal diagnosis.

Myotonic Dystrophy

Myotonic dystrophy is a multisystem disorder transmitted by autosomal dominant inheritance. Ordinarily, symptoms begin in young adult life and include weakness of the face and distal limb muscles, cataracts, multiple endocrinopathies, frontal baldness in males, and myotonia. Myotonia is a disturbance of the muscle membrane that prevents normal relaxation after contraction.

Clinical Features. A neonatal form of myotonic dystrophy sometimes occurs in the offspring of affected mothers. It has been suggested that an abnormal factor is present in the mother's serum that crosses the placenta and affects only genetically predisposed fetuses (Harper and Dyken, 1972). Women with myotonic dystrophy become weaker and have greater myotonia during pregnancy (Sarnat et al, 1976). Polyhydramnios is common. Labor is prolonged because of inadequate uterine contraction, and forceps assistance is frequently needed. Severely affected newborns have inadequate diaphragmatic and intercostal muscle function and are incapable of spontaneous respiration. In the absence of prompt intubation and mechanical ventilation, many will die immediately after birth. The newborn's precarious ventilatory reserve is further complicated by perinatal asphyxia as a consequence of the prolonged and difficult delivery.

Prominent clinical features in the newborn include (1) facial diplegia, in which the mouth is oddly shaped so that the upper lip forms an inverted V; (2) generalized muscular hypotonia; (3) joint deformities ranging from bilateral clubfoot to generalized arthrogryposis; and (4) gastrointestinal dysfunction, including choking, regurgitation, aspiration, swallowing difficulties, and gastroparesis. The distribution of limb weakness in the newborn is more proximal than distal. Tendon reflexes are usually absent in weak muscles. Myotonia is not evident by percussion and may not be demonstrable on EMG. Cardiomyopathy is a contributing cause of early neonatal deaths. Congenital cataract has been reported only once. Long-term prognosis is poor, and all affected children are mentally and physically handicapped.

Diagnosis. The diagnosis of myotonic dystrophy in the newborn requires the diagnosis of myotonic dystrophy in the mother. She is likely to have many clinical features of disease. If myotonia is not present on examination, it should be demonstrated by EMG. It is characterized by the repetitive firing of very-short-duration potentials that decline in frequency and amplitude.

Muscle biopsy of affected infants reveals an apparent maturational arrest that may be confused with myotubular myopathy (Sarnat and Silbert, 1976). Changes are most profound in muscles surrounding a fixed joint. The fibers are small and round, contain many internal nuclei, and are not completely filled with myofibrils (myotubes). Unlike myotubular myopathy, neonatal myotonic dystrophy demonstrates type II rather than type I fiber predominance.

Treatment. The immediate treatment is intubation and mechanical ventilation. Fixed joints respond to physical therapy and casting. Gastroparesis may be alleviated by metoclopramide therapy (Bodensteiner and Greenow, 1984).

METABOLIC MYOPATHIES

Acid Maltase Deficiency (Pompe Disease)

Acid maltase is a lysosomal enzyme, present in all tissues, that hydrolyzes maltose and other branches of glycogen to yield glucose. It has no function in maintaining blood glucose concentrations. Three distinct clinical forms of deficiency are recognized: infantile, childhood (see Chapter 7), and adult. All are transmitted by autosomal recessive inheritance (Loonen et al, 1981).

Clinical Features. The onset of the infantile form may be immediately after birth, but is more usual during the second month. Profound generalized hypotonia without atrophy and congestive heart failure are the initial symptoms. Hypotonia is the result of glycogen storage in the brain, spinal cord, and skeletal muscles causing mixed signs of cerebral and motor unit dysfunction: decreased awareness and depressed tendon reflexes. The mixed signs may be confusing, but the presence of cardiomegaly is almost diagnostic (see also carnitine deficiency). The electrocardiogram (EKG) is abnormal and demon-

strates short PR intervals and high QRS complexes on all leads. Most patients are dead by one year of age from cardiac failure.

Diagnosis. Diagnosis is established by muscle biopsy. Large vacuoles containing glycogen are observed in muscle fibers. Definitive diagnosis requires the demonstration of deficient acid maltase activity in fibroblasts or other tissues.

Treatment. A high-protein diet has been found helpful in childhood form of the disease, but has not yet proved useful in the infantile form.

Cytochrome-c-Oxidase Deficiency

The electron transfer chain and oxidative phosphorylation are the principal sources of adenosine triphosphate (ATP) synthesis. Deficiencies of mitochondrial enzymes comprising the electron transfer chain in skeletal muscle may present as hypotonia in the newborn or infant and as exercise intolerance in older children (see Chapter 8). The defect in infantile hypotonia is usually a deficiency of complex IV (cytochrome-c-oxidase) (Heiman-Patterson et al, 1978). Deficiencies in other complexes may be associated (Sengers et al, 1984). Most cases are sporadic, and a specific genetic pattern of transmission has not been established. Two affected children had siblings with early infant death. Another had an affected second cousin.

Clinical Features. Clinical features vary with the number of enzyme deficiencies, the percentage reduction in enzyme activity, and the presence of mitochondrial enzyme deficiencies in organs other than muscle. The typical syndrome is characterized by profound generalized weakness, causing difficulty feeding and early respiratory failure and death, severe lactic acidosis, and the DeToni-Franconi-Debré syndrome (glycosuria, proteinuria, phosphaturia, and generalized aminoaciduria). Onset is anytime within the first six months. Ptosis, ophthalmoplegia, and macroglossia may be present as well. Newborns with multiple enzyme deficiencies in multiple organs die within six months.

A reversible cytochrome-c-oxidase deficiency has been reported in three newborns (Zeviani et al, 1987). The early features are indistinguishable from those associated with progressive fatal cases, but a spontaneous increase in cytochrome-c-oxidase activity occurs during infancy associated with increased strength.

Diagnosis. A deficiency of respiratory chain enzymes should be suspected in any hypotonic infant with lactic acidosis. The serum concentration of CK is elevated, but the EMG may be normal. Muscle biopsy reveals vacuoles, mainly in type I fibers, with abnormal glycogen and lipid accumulations. Mitochondria are large in size, increased in number, and abnormal in structure (ragged-red fibers).

Treatment. No effective treatment is available for the multiorgan enzyme deficiency. However, supportive care should be provided for newborns with cytochrome-*c*-oxidase deficiency of muscle, since the enzyme deficiency may be transitory.

Carnitine Deficiency

Carnitine is an essential cofactor in the transfer of long-chain fatty acids across the inner mitochondrial membrane. Deficiencies of carnitine may occur as primary genetic defects or secondary to other disorders (see Table 2.5). Primary muscle carnitine deficiency usually presents in older children as progressive proximal weakness (see Chapter 7). The defect may be transmitted by autosomal dominant inheritance with variable penetrance; reduced levels of carnitine are present in the skeletal muscle of an asymptomatic parent.

Clinical Features. There is one report of an infant with muscle carnitine deficiency (Hart et al, 1978). The mother reported diminished movements during pregnancy, and the child seemed limp at birth. Early motor milestones were achieved at the appropriate time, but walking was delayed. Congestive heart failure developed at twenty-three months. There was mild generalized hypotonia, and tendon reflexes were normal. During the next seven months, progressive muscular weakness developed, tendon reflexes were lost, and death occurred following cardiac arrest.

Diagnosis. Primary muscle carnitine deficiency should be suspected in hypotonic infants with cardiomegaly. The other disorder that causes this combination is acid maltase deficiency. Muscle biopsy reveals vacuoles primarily in type I muscle. The vacuoles stain for lipid, but not for glycogen. The presence of both lipid and glycogen storage should suggest a deficiency in one of the respiratory chain enzymes. Such deficiencies may produce secondary carnitine deficiency in muscle. Definitive diagnosis requires a demonstration of reduced levels of carnitine in muscle but normal concentrations in serum.

Treatment. Several patients with primary muscle carnitine deficiency, including the infant described above, have been treated with L-carnitine. The results in other children have been variable. Nevertheless, a trial of L-carnitine, 100 mg/kg/day in three divided doses, is recommended in all cases of primary muscle carnitine deficiency.

Phosphofructokinase Deficiency

The usual presentation of muscle phosphofructokinase deficiency is cramps on exercise and myoglobinuria (see Chapter 8). Symptoms usually begin in childhood, and patients are otherwise asymptomatic. A neonatal form of phosphofructokinase deficiency has been reported in four children (Serviedi et al, 1986). The defect is transmitted by autosomal recessive inheritance and presents as infantile hypotonia.

Clinical Features. The onset of symptoms is at birth. Hypotonia, weakness, respiratory deficiency, and joint deformities are present. The tendon reflexes are diminished or absent. Cerebral and corneal abnormalities may be present. Death occurs during infancy or early childhood.

Diagnosis. The serum concentration of CK is normal. The EMG, at least late in the disease, is consistent with a myopathic process. Muscle biopsy is critical for diagnosis. Light microscopy reveals only nonspecific myopathy, but electron microscopy demonstrates an abnormal accumulation of subsarcolemmal and intramyofibrillary glycogen. Large cytoplasmic vacuoles, as in acid maltase deficiency, are not present. Phosphofructokinase activity is absent in skeletal muscle but present in red blood cells and fibroblasts.

Treatment. Treatment is not available for this disorder.

Phosphorylase Deficiency

Myophosphorylase deficiency (McArdle disease) is typically characterized by exercise intolerance in young adults and progressive myopathy in middle life (see Chapter 8). A neonatal form of variable severity is now recognized (Cornelio et al, 1983; DiMauro and Hartlage, 1978). It is reported in siblings and probably transmitted, as in later-onset cases, by autosomal recessive inheritance. Indeed, the enzyme deficiency appears identical at all ages and the reason for clinical heterogeneity is not understood.

Clinical Features. Newborns with myophosphorylase deficiency have difficulty with sucking and swallowing immediately post partum or shortly thereafter. In some, weakness is so profound as to produce immediate respiratory insufficiency. In others, weakness is progressive over several months or years. The child appears alert and has normal cranial nerve function. The tongue and the heart are not affected. Tendon reflexes are depressed or absent.

Diagnosis. The serum concentration of CK is elevated, and the EMG is abnormal, showing features of both neuropathy and myopathy. Muscle biopsy is diagnostic. Fibers vary in size from atrophic to normal and contain peripheral vacuoles that react intensely for glycogen. The glycogen concentration of muscle is greatly elevated, and phosphorylase activity cannot be detected.

Treatment. A high-protein diet is useful in older patients with phosphorylase deficiency, but has not yet been tried in newborns.

■ Infantile Myositis

There have been only eleven case reports of infantile myositis; three were newborns. It is unlikely that these represent a single nosologic entity (Roddy et al, 1986; Thompson, 1982).

Clinical Features. Affected newborns have difficulty breathing immediately after birth and require resuscitation or intubation. In others, the onset of symptoms is two to twelve months of age. Infants are hypotonic and have diminished or absent tendon reflexes.

Diagnosis. The serum concentration of CK is markedly elevated, and the EMG is consistent with myopathy. Muscle biopsy reveals diffuse inflammation and considerable proliferation of connective tissue. Muscle fiber degeneration may be seen as well.

Treatment. A trial of prednisone is appropriate in infants with inflammatory myopathy. High doses of prednisone, 2 mg/kg/day, are initiated, changed to alternate-day doses after one week and then rapidly tapered over three to six months, depending upon response.

References

1. Albers JW, Faulkner JA, Dorovini-Zis K, et al: Abnormal neuromuscular transmission in an infantile myasthenic syndrome. Ann Neurol 16:28, 1984.
2. Arneson DW, Tipton RE, Ward JC: Hyperpipecolic acidemia: Occurrence in an infant with clinical findings of the cerebrohepatorenal (Zellweger) syndrome. Arch Neurol 39:713, 1982.
3. Arnon SS, Midura TF, Clay SA, et al: Infant botulism: Epidemiological clinical and laboratory aspects. JAMA 237:1946, 1977.
4. Aubourg P, Scotto J, Rocchiccioli F, et al: Neonatal adrenoleukodystrophy. J Neurol Neurosurg Psychiatry 49:77, 1986.
5. Axelrod FB, Porges RF, Sein ME: Neonatal recognition of familial dysautonomia. J Pediatr 110:946, 1987.
6. Balestrazzi P, Corrini L, Villani G, et al: The Cohen syndrome: Clinical and endocrinological studies of two new cases. J Med Genet 17:430, 1980.
7. Berry AC, Whittingham AJ, Neville BGR: Chromosome 15 in floppy infants. Arch Dis Child 56:882, 1981.
8. Bodensteiner JB, Greenow JE: Gastroparesis in neonatal myotonic dystrophy. Muscle Nerve 7:486, 1984.
9. Butler MG, Palmer CG: Parental origin of chromosome 15 deletion in Prader-Willi syndrome. Lancet 1:1285, 1983.
10. Byrne E, Blumbergs PC, Hallpike JF: Central core disease: Study of a family with five affected generations. J Neurol Sci 53:77, 1982.
11. Cornblath DR, Sladky JT, Sumner AJ: Clinical electrophysiology of infantile botulism. Muscle Nerve 6:448, 1983.
12. Cornelio F, Bresolin N, DiMauro S, et al: Congenital myopathy due to phosphorylase deficiency. Neurology 33:1383, 1983.
13. Curless RG, Nelson MB: Congenital fiber type disproportion in identical twins. Ann Neurol 2:455, 1977.
14. DiMauro S, Hartlage P: Fatal infantile form of muscle phosphorylase deficiency. Neurology 28:1124, 1978.
15. Donaldson JO, Penn AS, Lisak PP, et al: Antiacetylcholine receptor antibody in neonatal myasthenia gravis. Am J Dis Child 135:222, 1981.
16. Echenne B, Arthuis M, Billard C, et al: Congenital muscular dystrophy and cerebral CT scan abnormalities. Results of a collaborative study of the Société de Neurologie Infantile. J Neurol Sci 75:7, 1986.
17. Egger J, Kendall BE, Erdohazi M, et al: Involvement of the central nervous system in congenital muscular dystrophies. Dev Med Child Neurol 25:32, 1983.
18. Elder GB, Dean D, McComas AJ, et al: Infantile centronuclear myopathy: Evidence suggesting incomplete innervation. J Neurol Sci 60:79, 1983.
19. Fenichel GM: Clinical syndromes of myasthenia in infancy and childhood: A review. Arch Neurol 35:97, 1978.
20. Fulthorpe JJ, Gardner-Medwin D, Hudgson P, et al: Nemaline myopathy: A histological and ultrastructural study of skeletal muscle from a case presenting with infantile hypotonia. Neurology 19:735, 1969.
21. Gieron MA, Korthals JK: Familial infantile myasthenia: Report of three patients with follow-up to adulthood. Arch Neurol 42:143, 1985.
22. Gobernado JM, Lousa M, Gimemo A, et al: Mitochondrial defects in Lowe's oculocerebrorenal syndrome. Arch Neurol 41:208, 1984.
23. Guzzetta F, Ferriere G, Lyon G: Congenital hypomyelination polyneuropathy. Pathological findings compared with polyneuropathies starting later in life. Brain 105:395, 1982.
24. Harati Y, Butler IJ: Congenital hypomyelinating neuropathy. J Neurol Neurosurg Psychiatry 48:1269, 1985.
25. Harper PS, Dyken PR: Early-onset dystrophia myotonica: Evidence supporting a maternal environmental factor. Lancet 2:53, 1972.
26. Hart ZH, Chang CH, DiMauro S, et al: Muscle carnitine deficiency and fatal cardiomyopathy. Neurology 28:147, 1978.
27. Heiman-Patterson TD, Bonilla E, DiMauro S, et al: Cytochrome-c-oxidase deficiency in a floppy infant. Neurology 28:147, 1978.

28. Kelley RI, Datta NS, Dobyns WB, et al: Neonatal adrenoleukodystrophy: New cases, biochemical studies, and differentiation from Zellweger and related peroxisomal polydystrophy syndromes. Am J Med Genet 23:869, 1986.
29. Kennedy R, Sung JH, Berry JF: A case of congenital hypomyelination neuropathy. Arch Neurol 34:337, 1977.
30. Kinoshite M, Satoyoshi E, Matsuo N: "Myotubular myopathy" and "Type I fiber atrophy" in a family. J Neurol Sci 26:575, 1975.
31. Kondo K, Yuasa T: Genetics of congenital nemaline myopathy. Muscle Nerve 3:308, 1980.
32. Kousseff BG: Cohen syndrome: Further delineation and inheritance. Am J Med Genet 9:25, 1981.
33. Larsen R, Ashwal S, Peckham N: Incontinentia pigmenti: Association with anterior horn cell degeneration. Neurology 37:446, 1987.
34. Lazaro RP, Fenichel GM, Kilroy AW: Congenital muscular dystrophy: Case reports and reappraisal. Muscle Nerve 2:349, 1979.
35. Lefvert AK, Osterman PO: Newborn infants to myasthenic mothers: A clinical study and an investigation of acetylcholine receptor antibodies in 17 children. Neurology 33:133, 1983.
36. Loonen MCB, Busch HFM, Koster JF, et al: A family with different clinical forms of acid maltase deficiency (glycogenosis type II): Biochemical and genetic studies. Neurology 31:1209, 1981.
37. McMenamin JB, Becker LE, Murphy EG: Congenital muscular dystrophy: A clinicopathologic report of 24 cases. J Pediatr 100:692, 1982a.
38. McMenamin JB, Becker LE, Murphy EG: Fukuyama-type congenital muscular dystrophy. J Pediatr 101:580, 1982b.
39. Meyers KR, Golomb HM, Hansen JL, et al: Familial neuromuscular disease with "myotubes." Clin Genet 5:327, 1974.
40. Moosa A, Dubowitz V: Motor nerve conduction velocity in spinal muscular atrophy in childhood. Arch Dis Child 51:974, 1976.
41. Moser HW, Moser AE, Singh I, et al: Adrenoleukodystrophy: Survey of 303 cases: Biochemistry, diagnosis, and therapy. Ann Neurol 16:628, 1984.
42. Norton P, Ellison P, Sulaiman AR, et al: Nemaline myopathy in the neonate. Neurology 33:351, 1983.
43. Ohta M, Matsubarba F, Hayashi K, et al: Acetylcholine receptor antibodies in infants of mothers with myasthenia gravis. Neurology 31:1019, 1981.
44. Packer RJ, Brown MJ, Berman PH: The diagnostic value of electromyography in infantile hypotonia. Am J Dis Child 136:1057, 1982.
45. Painter MJ, Bergman I: Obstetrical trauma to the neonatal central and peripheral nervous system. Semin Perinatol 6:89, 1982.
46. Pavone L, Mollica F, Grasso A, et al: Familial centronuclear myopathy. Acta Neurol Scand 62:33, 1980.
47. Pearn JH: Fetal movements and Werdnig-Hoffmann disease. J Neurol Sci 18:373, 1973.
48. Pearn JH, Carter CO, Wilson J: The genetic identity of acute infantile spinal muscular atrophy. Brain 96:463, 1973.
49. Robertson WC Jr, Chun RWM, Kornguth SE: Familial infantile myasthenia. Arch Neurol 37:117, 1980.
50. Roddy SM, Ashwal S, Peckham N, et al: Infantile myositis: A case diagnosed in the neonatal period. Pediatr Neurol 2:241, 1986.
51. Sarnat HB, O'Connor T, Byrne PA: Clinical effects of myotonic dystrophy on pregnancy and the neonate. Arch Neurol 33:459, 1976.
52. Sarnat HB, Machin G, Darwish HZ, et al: Mitochondrial myopathy of cerebro-hepato-renal (Zellweger) syndrome. Can J Neurol Sci 10:170, 1983.
53. Sarnat HB, Roth SI, Jimenez JF: Neonatal myotubular myopathy: Neuropathy and failure of postnatal maturation of fetal muscle. Can J Neurol Sci 8:313, 1981.
54. Sarnat HB, Silbert SW: Maturational arrest of fetal muscle in neonatal myotonic dystrophy. Arch Neurol 33:466, 1976.
55. Schutgens RBH, Heymans HSA, Wanders RJA, et al: Peroxisomal disorders: A newly recognized group of genetic diseases. Eur J Pediatr 144:430, 1986.
56. Sengers RCA, Trijbees JMF, Bakkeren JAJM, et al: Deficiency of cytochrome b and aa₃ in muscle from an infant with cytochrome oxidase deficiency. Eur J Pediatr 141:178, 1984.
57. Servidei S, Bonilla E, Diedrich RG, et al: Fatal infantile form of muscle phosphofructokinase deficiency. Neurology 36:1465, 1986.
58. Seybold ME, Lindstrom JM: Myasthenia gravis in infancy. Neurology 31:476, 1981.
59. Sladky JT, Brown MJ, Berman PH: Chronic inflammatory demyelinating polyneuropathy of infancy: A corticosteroid-responsive disorder. Ann Neurol 20:76, 1986.
60. Smit LME, Barth PG: Arthrogryposis multiplex congenita due to congenital myasthenia. Dev Med Child Neurol 22:371, 1980.
61. Steiman GS, Rorke LB, Brown MJ: Infantile neuronal degeneration masquerading as Werdnig-Hoffmann disease. Ann Neurol 8:317, 1980.
62. Sul YC, Mrak RE, Evans OB, et al: Neurogenic arthrogryposis in one identical twin. Arch Neurol 39:717, 1982.
63. Sulaiman A, Swick HM, Kindu D: Congenital fiber type disproportion with unusual clinico-pathologic manifestations. J Neurol Neurosurg Psychiatry 46:175, 1983.
64. Thompson CE: Infantile myositis. Dev Med Child Neurol 24:307, 1982.
65. Thompson JA, Glasgow LA, Warpinski JR, et al: Infant botulism: Clinical spectrum and epidemiology. Pediatrics 66:936, 1980.
66. Ulrich J, Hirt H-R, Kleihues P, et al: Connatal polyneuropathy: A case with proliferated microfilaments in Schwann cells. Acta Neuropathol 55:39, 1981.
67. Vincent A, Cull-Candy SG, Newsom-Davis J, et al: Congenital myasthenia: Endplate acetylcholine receptors and electrophysiology in five cases. Muscle Nerve 4:316, 1981.
68. Warburton D, Singer DB, Oh W: Effects of acidosis on the activity of creatine phosphokinase and its isoenzymes in the serum of newborn infants. Pediatrics 68:195, 1981.
69. Wisniewski KE, Kieras FJ, French JH, et al: Ultrastructural, neurological and glycosaminol05ly abnormalities in Loew's syndrome. Ann Neurol 16:40, 1984.
70. Zevianai M, Peterson P, Servidei E, et al: Benign reversible muscle cytochrome c oxidase deficiency: A second case. Neurology 37:64, 1987.

7 Flaccid Limb Weakness in Childhood

This chapter deals with presenting complaints of chronic progressive or acute flaccid weakness of the limbs. The differential diagnosis is primarily limited to disorders of the motor unit. Flaccid weakness of the legs may be an initial feature of disturbances in the lumbosacral region, but other symptoms of spinal cord dysfunction are usually present as well. In children with flaccid weakness of the legs in whom the arms are fully spared, reference should be made to the differential diagnosis in Chapter 12. Cerebral disorders may cause flaccid weakness, but dementia (see Chapter 5) or seizures (see Chapter 1) are usually present concomitantly.

■ Symptoms and Signs of Neuromuscular Disease

THE PRESENTING COMPLAINT

Limb weakness in children is almost always noted first in the legs and then the arms (Table 7.1). There are two reasons for this: (1) many neuromuscular disorders affect the legs before the arms, and (2) symptoms of mild leg weakness are more obvious than those of mild arm weakness. In young children with neuromuscular disease, delayed development of motor skills may be an initial complaint or a prominent feature of the past history. If the degree of motor delay is marginal and other developmental skills are normal, the delay is easily rationalized by parents and grandparents, e.g., "I do everything for him," or "his father was also a slow baby."

Older children are frequently referred because they are unable to keep up with peers. Schoolteachers are especially adroit at identifying children in this category. These children may be thought to tire easily or have a systemic disorder.

Those in whom exercise intolerance is due to persistent weakness are discussed in this chapter. A second group, who are normal when not exercising but "run out of energy" or have muscle cramps when exercised, probably have an underlying metabolic myopathy; these patients are discussed in Chapter 8.

An abnormal gait is often the presenting symptom for either proximal or distal leg weakness. With proximal weakness, the pelvis is not stabilized and waddles from side to side as the child walks. Running is especially difficult and accentuates the hip waddle.

Toe-walking is commonly encountered in Duchenne dystrophy because the pelvis is thrust forward to shift the center of gravity and the gastrocnemius muscle is replaced by collagen and fat. Toe-walking is seen also in upper motor neuron disorders that cause spasticity. There should be little difficulty in distinguishing flaccid from spastic muscles by palpation. In addition, dystrophy is associated with hyporeflexia and spasticity with hyperreflexia.

Children with footdrop tend to lift the knee high in the air in order for the foot to clear the ground. The weak foot then comes down with a slapping motion (steppage gait).

Frequent falling is an early complaint when there is distal weakness, especially weakness of the evertors and dorsiflexors of the foot, and is a later feature with proximal weakness. Falling is first noted when the child is walking on uneven surfaces. The child is thought to be clumsy, but after a while parents realize that the child is "tripping on nothing at all." One parent remarked that the child could "trip on a blade of grass."

Adolescents and adults, but usually not children with weakness, complain of specific disabilities. A young woman with proximal weakness

Table 7.1 SYMPTOMS OF
NEUROMUSCULAR DISEASE

Slow motor development
Easy fatigability
Frequent falls
Abnormal gait
  Waddle
  Toe-walking
  Steppage
Specific disability
  Arm elevation
  Hand grip
  Rising from floor
  Climbing stairs

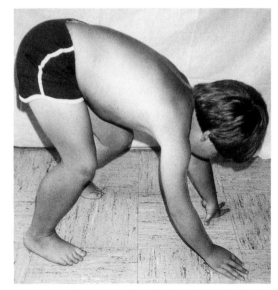

Figure 7.1 Gower sign. The child rises from the floor by pushing off with the hands to overcome proximal pelvic weakness.

may have difficulty keeping her arms elevated to groom her hair or rotate the shoulder in order to get into and out of garments that have a zipper or hook in the back. Weakness in hand muscles is frequently spotted by teachers who become upset with the child's handwriting. Adolescents may notice difficulty in unscrewing jar tops or working with tools. Teachers report to parents when children are slower than classmates in climbing stairs, getting up from the floor, and skipping and jumping. A specific complaint may be reported to the physician, but more likely the problem is presented as being "unable to keep up with the other children."

When there is weakness in the limbs, there may be weakness in the muscles of the head and neck as well. Questions should be asked specifically about double vision, drooping of eyelids, difficulty chewing and swallowing, loss of facial expression and facial strength (whistling, sucking, chewing, blowing), and the clarity and tone of speech. Weakness of neck muscles is frequently brought to attention while riding in a car. When there is sudden acceleration or deceleration, the neck muscles are unable to stabilize the head, which snaps backward or forward.

PHYSICAL FINDINGS

The physician should begin the examination by watching the child sit, stand, and walk. Have the child sit on the floor and then rise without using the hands to push off in order to test the strength of proximal leg muscles. When pelvic muscles are weak, the child is unable to rise from the floor without using the hand for assistance (Fig. 7.1). With greater weakness, the hands are used to climb up the legs (Gower sign). After observing gait, have the child stand

and walk first on toes and then on heels (Table 7.2).

During this period of observation and again during muscle strength testing, it is important to determine the presence of atrophy or hypertrophy. Wasting of muscles around the shoulder is easily seen because bony prominences stand out even further. Wasting of hand muscles causes flattening of the thenar and hypothenar eminences. Wasting of the quadriceps muscles causes a tapering appearance to the thigh that is exaggerated when the patient is asked to tense the thigh by straightening the knee. Atrophy of the anterior tibial and peroneal muscles gives the anterior border of the tibia a sharp appearance, and atrophy of the gastrocnemius muscle diminishes the normal contour of the calf.

Table 7.2 SIGNS OF
NEUROMUSCULAR DISEASE

Observation
  Functional ability
  Atrophy and hypertrophy
  Fasciculations
Palpation
  Tenderness
  Muscle texture
Examination
  Strength
  Tendon reflexes
  Myotonia
  Joint contractures

Table 7.3 PROGRESSIVE
PROXIMAL WEAKNESS

1. Spinal cord disorders (Chapter 12)
2. Juvenile spinal muscular atrophy
   a. Autosomal recessive
   b. Autosomal dominant
   c. Hexosaminidase A deficiency
3. Limb-girdle myasthenia
   a. Familial
   b. Sporadic
4. Muscular dystrophies
   a. Duchenne/Becker
   b. Limb-girdle
   c. Facioscapulohumeral syndrome
5. Inflammatory myopathies
   a. Dermatomyositis
   b. Polymyositis
6. Metabolic myopathies
   a. Acid maltase deficiency
   b. Other carbohydrate myopathies
      1. Myophosphorylase deficiency (see Chapter 8)
      2. Debrancher enzyme deficiency (see Chapter 8)
   c. Muscle carnitine deficiency
   d. Other lipid myopathies
   e. Mitochondrial myopathies
7. Endocrine myopathies
   a. Thyroid
   b. Parathyroid
   c. Adrenal cortex

As individual muscles are examined for strength, they should also be palpated for texture and tenderness. The texture of normal muscle is quite different from the flabby texture of denervated muscle and the rubbery consistency of dystrophic muscle infiltrated with collagen and fat. Tenderness generally suggests an inflammatory process.

Loss of tendon reflexes occurs early in denervation, especially if there is sensory neuropathy, but tends to parallel the degree of weakness in myopathy. Tendon reflexes are usually normal in patients with myasthenia gravis even during times of weakness and may be normal in met-

abolic myopathies between episodes of recurrent weakness.

Myotonia, a disturbance in muscle relaxation following contraction, is described in the section on myotonic dystrophy.

■ Progressive Proximal Weakness

Progressive proximal weakness in childhood is most often due to myopathy, usually a muscular dystrophy (Table 7.3). Juvenile spinal muscular atrophy is the only chronic denervating disease in which weakness is more proximal than distal. It is readily distinguished from myopathic disorders by electromyography (EMG) and muscle biopsy. Limb-girdle myasthenia is extremely uncommon, but it is an important consideration because specific treatment is available (Table 7.4).

SPINAL MUSCULAR ATROPHIES

The juvenile form of spinal muscular atrophy (Wohlfart-Kugelberg-Welander disease) was initially thought to be genetically distinct from infantile spinal muscular atrophy (see Chapter 6). Later, reports of chronic and arrested forms of infantile spinal muscular atrophy and the occurrence of infantile and juvenile onset cases in siblings supported the conclusion that infantile and juvenile types with autosomal recessive inheritance are genetically homogeneous; however, if heterogeneous, they cannot be distinguished by phenotype (Bundey and Lovelace, 1975; Pearn et al, 1978a). The only distinction possible at this time is between an autosomal recessive and an autosomal dominant form. The prevalence of juvenile spinal muscular atrophy

Table 7.4 DISTINGUISHING FEATURES IN PROXIMAL WEAKNESS

Diagnostic Tool	Neuronopathy *Tendon Reflex Absent*	Myopathy *Tendon Reflex Depressed or Absent*	Myasthenia *Tendon Reflex Normal*
Electromyography	Fasciculations; denervation potentials; high-amplitude, long-duration, polyphasic motor units	Brief, small-amplitude polyphasic motor units	Normal
Nerve conduction studies	Normal or mildly slow	Normal	Abnormal repetitive stimulation
Creatine kinase	Normal or mildly elevated	Elevated	Normal
Muscle biopsy	Group atrophy; group typing	Fiber necrosis; fatty replacement; excessive collagen	Normal

in England is 1.2 per 100,000, an incidence of one in 24,100 live births (Pearn, 1978a). The overwhelming majority of these are transmitted by autosomal recessive inheritance.

Autosomal Recessive Type

Fetal movements are reported as normal, and the child is normal at birth. The onset of weakness is between ages one and three years in 95 percent of children. Onset in the other 5 percent may be any time during childhood or adolescence (Hausmanowa-Petrusewicz et al, 1979). The age at onset does not necessarily predict the degree of eventual disability. Although both sexes are affected, males are affected more severely than females.

Clinical Features. The initial symptom is usually a disturbance of gait caused by proximal leg weakness. Calf hypertrophy may be present as well and suggests the erroneous diagnosis of Duchenne muscular dystrophy. The disease progresses very slowly, sometimes in a stepwise fashion, and often appears to be arrested. The progression of weakness may be either to the distal muscles of the legs or the proximal muscles of the arms. The hands are affected last. Some weakness of the facial muscles may be present, but extraocular motility is almost always spared. Indeed, ophthalmoplegia is so uncommon that such cases may prove to be genetically distinct. Tendon reflexes of weak muscles are absent or greatly diminished.

In some children, the arms are more profoundly affected than the legs, and these children are likely to have facial weakness as well. Within the same kindred, some children may have predominant leg weakness whereas their siblings have predominant arm weakness.

It is impossible to predict eventual disability at the onset of symptoms. Some children become handicapped quickly, whereas others continue walking into adult life. The pattern of progression in other family members provides a clue to prognosis, but cannot be counted upon to predict the future in any specific patient.

Diagnosis. The serum concentration of creatine kinase may be two to four times the upper limit of normal. Elevated concentrations of creatine kinase correlate directly with the duration of illness.

The most helpful investigations are the EMG and nerve conduction studies. Sensory nerve conduction is always normal, but motor nerve conduction velocity is occasionally prolonged late in the course. Needle EMG examination displays spontaneous discharges (fasciculations, fibrillations, and positive sharp waves) in about half of patients. With exertion, motor unit potentials are consistently of large amplitude and often polyphasic, prolonged in duration, and reduced in number.

Muscle biopsy results reveal a pattern of denervation similar to that observed in infantile spinal muscular atrophy. Groups of atrophic fibers are adjacent to groups of fibers that are normal or hypertrophied in size. Hypertrophied fibers are always type I. In children with chronic denervation, "myopathic" changes may be seen as well. Because of sampling error, occasional biopsy specimens demonstrate only myopathic features. Therefore, confirmation by muscle biopsy is not essential if the EMG is clearly consistent with a spinal muscular atrophy.

Treatment. Proper management of children with spinal muscular atrophy increases longevity and decreases disability. The goals are to maintain function and prevent contractures. Children who quickly take to a wheelchair will develop disuse atrophy and scoliosis. Dietary counseling is usually needed to prevent obesity, which only causes greater strain on weakened muscles. The prevention of contractures usually requires range of motion exercise and the early use of splints, especially at night.

Families should be provided with genetic counseling. Antenatal diagnosis is not available.

Autosomal Dominant Type

There is both a juvenile and an adult-onset proximal spinal muscular atrophy transmitted by autosomal dominant inheritance. The juvenile and adult types are genetically distinct, and there is complete concordance for age of onset within families. Among the juvenile cases, more than 90 percent have their onset before the age of five years and 100 percent before the age of ten (Pearn, 1978b). It would be impossible to distinguish a new dominant mutation from the autosomal recessive form.

Clinical Features. The pattern of weakness in the autosomal dominant type is somewhat more generalized than in the autosomal recessive type, but proximal muscles are still affected more severely than distal muscles. Symptoms progress slowly, and some patients report no worsening of weakness after adolescence. Most patients are ambulatory and function well into middle and late adult life. Bulbar weakness is unusual and is mild when present. Extraocular muscles are not affected. Tendon reflexes are depressed or absent in weak muscles. Joint contractures are uncommon.

Diagnosis. The serum concentration of creatine kinase is normal or only mildly elevated. The EMG is diagnostic, as in the autosomal recessive type. Muscle biopsy provides further confirmation of diagnosis.

Treatment. Treatment is the same for both the dominant and recessive forms. Genetic counseling should stress the complete penetrance of the phenotype. Antenatal diagnosis is not available. When family history is negative, genetic counseling is difficult, but autosomal dominant inheritance should be considered if age at onset is after three years.

GM₂ Gangliosidosis

The typical clinical expression of hexosaminidase A deficiency is Tay-Sachs disease (see Chapter 5). Several phenotypic variants of the enzyme deficiency are described with onset throughout childhood and adult life. All are transmitted by autosomal recessive inheritance. Most, but not all, of these patients are of Ashkenazi Jewish origin. A juvenile onset type occurs in which the initial manifestations mimic juvenile spinal muscular atrophy (Parnes et al, 1985).

Clinical Features. Weakness, wasting, and cramps of the proximal leg muscles begin after infancy and frequently not until adolescence. This is followed by distal leg weakness, proximal and distal arm weakness, and tremor. After motor neuron dysfunction is established, signs of cerebral degeneration (personality change, intermittent psychosis, dementia) become evident (Mantovani et al, 1985; Parnes et al, 1985).

Examination reveals a mixture of upper and lower motor neuron signs. The macula is usually normal, and the cranial nerves are intact, with the exception of atrophy and fasciculations in the tongue. Fasciculations may be present in the limbs as well. Tendon reflexes may be absent or exaggerated, depending upon the relative severity of upper and lower motor neuron dysfunction. Plantar responses are sometimes extensor and sometimes flexor. Tremor, but not dysmetria, is present in the outstretched arms, and sensation is intact.

In some patients cerebral dysfunction never develops and only motor neuron disease is present; adults are reported with only dementia and psychosis. The course is variable and compatible with prolonged survival.

Diagnosis. The serum concentration of creatine kinase is normal or only mildly elevated. Motor and sensory nerve conduction velocities are normal, but needle EMG demonstrates neuropathic motor units. Autonomic neurons obtained by intestinal biopsy are distended by Sudan black–B positive material and are indistinguishable from those in Tay-Sachs disease.

Definitive diagnosis requires the demonstration of severely deficient or absent hexosaminidase A activity in leukocytes or cultural fibroblasts.

Treatment. Treatment is not available. Heterozygote detection is possible because enzyme activity is partially deficient. Prenatal diagnosis is available as well.

LIMB-GIRDLE MYASTHENIA

Several patients who show electrophysiologic or pharmacologic evidence of myasthenia have been described with proximal weakness and sometimes wasting. In many such patients, the weakness responds to standard treatment for myasthenia gravis. Limb-girdle myasthenia may have a genetic basis, or it can be caused by acquired autoimmune myasthenia gravis.

Familial Limb-Girdle Myasthenia

This term encompasses three families in which two or more siblings have been affected with a similar disorder (DiMauro et al, 1985; Johns et al, 1973; McQuillen, 1966).

Clinical Features. In two of the families, the children at ages thirteen and fourteen developed progressive proximal weakness which then remained stationary. In the third family, mild, nonprogressive proximal weakness was present from infancy. Ocular motility, facial expression, and bulbar function were spared, and tendon reflexes were present in every case. Members of the family, in whom weakness had started in infancy, were not evaluated until adult life. At that time, a cardiomyopathy was present as well.

Diagnosis. Limb weakness responds to the intravenous injection of 10 mg of edrophonium chloride (Tensilon). Repetitive stimulation studies demonstrate a decremental response that can be reversed by the injection of Tensilon or other anticholinesterase medication. The EMG suggests a myopathy because polyphasic action potentials of short duration are present. Muscle biopsies were performed during adolescence in two siblings and the results were normal. In the other two families, muscle biopsy specimens during adult life revealed tubular aggregates, sometimes in association with peripheral vesicles arising from the sarcoplasmic reticulum (Dobkin and Verity, 1978). These morphologic changes need not distinguish these families from ones with normal histologic appearance, as the patients with tubular aggregates were twenty to forty years older than the others. Biopsy specimens from the family with weakness beginning at birth also demonstrated type I atrophy (or hypotrophy), suggesting fiber type disproportion myopathy (see Chapter 6).

The serum concentration of antibody to acetylcholine receptor protein was investigated in only one family and was normal.

Treatment. Limb weakness in patients with familial limb-girdle myasthenia responds to treatment with anticholinesterase medication (see next section for doses). Thymectomy and immunosuppressive therapy are not indicated because there is no evidence of an abnormal immune state. However, one patient who showed only a moderate response to anticholinesterase medication appeared to improve when corticosteroids were added to the therapy.

Sporadic Limb-Girdle Myasthenia

Clinical Features. Myasthenia gravis may begin in children as a progressive proximal weakness affecting primarily the limb-girdle musculature and sparing ocular motility (Fenichel, 1978). Weakness need not fluctuate with exercise. Muscles of facial expression may be affected, although other bulbar function is spared. Tendon reflexes can be hypoactive, but are usually present. The clinical manifestations suggest limb-girdle dystrophy or polymyositis.

Diagnosis. A normal serum concentration of creatine kinase should alert the physician to the possibility of myasthenia gravis. Intravenous injection of Tensilon, 10 mg, reverses the weakness immediately (see Chapter 6). Repetitive nerve stimulation produces a decremental response. The EMG is usually normal, but sometimes demonstrates an increase in polyphasic units. The serum concentration of antibody to acetylcholine receptor protein is usually elevated in children with generalized myasthenia. However, a normal titer does not exclude the diagnosis.

Treatment. Children with generalized myasthenia may be given a trial of anticholinesterase therapy. The initial dose of neostigmine is 0.5 mg/kg every four hours in children younger than five years of age and 0.25 mg/kg in older children, not to exceed 15 mg per dose. The equivalent dose of pyridostigmine is four times the dose of neostigmine. After the efficacy and side effects are ascertained, the dose should be slowly increased as needed. Side effects are referable to cholinergic excess, e.g., salivation or diarrhea.

Most children with generalized myasthenia require thymectomy followed immediately by high-dose corticosteroid therapy. Corticosteroids are initiated at a dose of 2 mg/kg/daily, not to exceed 100 mg, for a week and then changed to an alternate-day schedule. The dose is then decreased monthly by 10 percent until a maintenance dose of approximately 20 percent of the initial dose is attained.

MUSCULAR DYSTROPHIES

The dystrophies are a group of genetic myopathies that are distinguished by mode of transmission, age of onset, and pattern of weakness (Table 7.5).

Duchenne/Becker Muscular Dystrophy

Duchenne and Becker muscular dystrophy are both transmitted by X-linked inheritance. Becker dystrophy, which tends to be later in onset and slower in progression, was once thought to be a distinct genetic entity. It is now believed that the Duchenne and Becker forms of muscular dystrophy are variable phenotypic expressions of the same gene defect located on the short arm of the X chromosome. They are discussed here as a single entity. Duchenne dystrophy is worldwide in distribution with a mean incidence of one case per 4,425 male live births (Moser, 1984). There have been countless hypotheses to explain the pathophysiology of muscle destruction in this disease; recent evidence suggests an absence of the structural protein nebulin (Zeviani et al, 1987).

Clinical Features. Most children with Duchenne muscular dystrophy present with gait disturbance prior to age five and frequently prior to age three. Toe-walking and frequent falling are typical initial complaints. Some delay in achieving motor milestones is often elicited in retrospect. Early symptoms are insidious and likely to be dismissed by both parents and physicians. Children may not be brought to medical attention until proximal weakness is sufficiently severe to cause difficulty in rising from the floor and an obvious waddling gait. At this stage, mild proximal weakness is present in pelvic muscles and Gower's sign (Fig. 7–1) is present. The calf muscles are large and rubbery in texture (Fig. 7–2). The Achilles tendon is shortened, and the heels do not quite touch the floor. Tendon reflexes may still be present at the ankle and knee, but are difficult to obtain.

The decline in motor strength is linear throughout childhood (Brooke et al, 1983). Between the ages of three and six, however, most children show some functional improvement because of cerebral maturation. Children of the same age may vary widely in the severity of weakness. Most maintain their ability to walk and climb stairs until age eight. Between ages three and eight, there is progressive contracture of the Achilles tendon and the iliotibial band, increased lordosis, a more pronounced waddling gait, and increased toe walking. Gait is more precarious, and increased falling is reported. Tendon reflexes at the knees and ankles are lost, and proximal weakness develops in the arms.

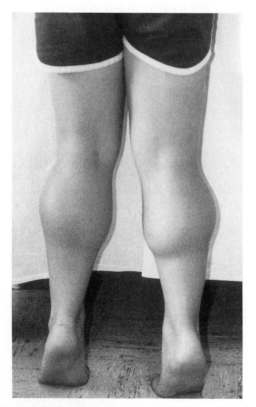

Figure 7.2 Enlarged calf muscles in Duchenne muscular dystrophy. Enlarged calves may also be seen in other neuromuscular disorders.

After age eight, functional ability declines rapidly because of increasing muscle weakness and contractures. By nine years, some children require a wheelchair, but most can remain ambulatory until age twelve and may continue to stand in braces until age sixteen.

Clinical variability among children of the same age continues throughout the course of the illness. The functional ability of ten-year-olds varies from wheelchair confinement to climbing stairs without difficulty. Some fifteen-year-olds will walk unassisted. Those with onset of weakness after age five or with ability to walk after age fifteen are generally considered to have Becker muscular dystrophy. However, some children with onset before age five will continue walking after age fifteen and some with onset after age five may be wheelchair-confined before age fifteen. Therefore, accurate prognosis is difficult at the time of initial presentation.

Children confined to wheelchairs tend to develop scoliosis and deterioration of pulmonary function. Symptoms of nocturnal hypoventilation begin when vital capacity declines to less than 20 percent of predicted normal. There are frequent awakenings and fear of sleep.

The immediate cause of death is not always clear, but respiratory insufficiency is a contributing factor in almost every case. Arrhythmia secondary to cardiomyopathy can be documented in some boys. In others with chronic hypoxia, intercurrent infection or aspiration produces respiratory arrest. Most children die at home without medical monitoring or postmortem examination.

Diagnosis. The initial laboratory tests of value in the diagnosis of Duchenne muscular dystrophy are serum enzymes, EMG studies, and muscle biopsy. Before age five, the serum concentration of creatine kinase should be ten times the upper limit of normal. The concentration then declines with age at an approximate rate of 20 percent per year.

The EMG is consistent with a myopathy and ordinarily demonstrates small polyphasic potentials and increased early recruitment of motor units. Fibrillations and positive sharp waves may be present at rest. Muscle biopsy is important to exclude other conditions, such as acid maltase deficiency, which may mimic Duchenne muscular dystrophy. The biopsy specimen demonstrates fibers undergoing degeneration, large fibers that stain intensely, and considerable replacement of muscle by fat and collagen tissues (Fig. 7.3).

Treatment. Although Duchenne muscular dystrophy is not curable, it is treatable. Recent

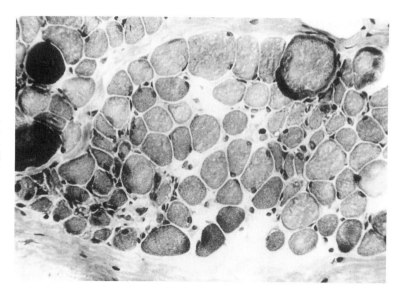

Figure 7.3 Muscle biopsy in Duchenne muscular dystrophy (trichrome). Considerable fiber degeneration, proliferation of collagen, and fatty replacement of muscle are present.

evidence indicates that prednisone may provide a temporary increase in strength and function (Brooke et al, 1987), but its long-term value is still unproven.

Four factors that contribute to disability are (1) weakness, (2) contractures, (3) disuse, and (4) depression. Treatment goals are to maintain function, prevent contractures, and provide psychologic support not only for the child but also for the family. The debilitating effect of inactivity is frequently overlooked. Disuse impairs muscle strength, decreases cardiovascular endurance, and promotes contractures (Vignos, 1983). Therefore, *every* effort should be made to keep children standing and walking as long as possible.

Once the diagnosis is established, parents should be instructed on passive stretching exercises to prevent contractures of the Achilles tendon, the iliotibial band, and flexors of the hip. If the foot remains in plantar flexion while the child sleeps, a lightweight plastic ankle-foot orthodesis should be provided to maintain the foot in a neutral position. When walking becomes precarious, triple release surgery is performed to release contractures of the hip flexors, iliotibial band, and Achilles tendon through tiny stab wounds. Long-leg casts are immediately applied, and the child is at least standing and possibly walking the day after surgery. Standing or walking is then maintained through the use of long-leg braces. The likelihood of scoliosis is reduced if the child can be kept standing for several hours each day. External appliances have not proved useful to prevent scoliosis, but the recent development of a surgical technique

to wire the lamina together may prove effective in preventing scoliosis without the need for long-term immobilization.

After age twelve, electrocardiography (EKG) and chest radiographs should be performed yearly. If the resting pulse is greater than 100 and the heart is enlarged, prophylactic digitalis may prove useful.

Symptomatic nocturnal hypoventilation may be treated with overnight mouth intermittent positive pressure (Bach et al, 1987). Respiratory assistance may be useful also during the daytime at times of respiratory infection.

Carrier detection has traditionally been performed by determining the serum concentration of creatine kinase. The best technique is to determine the average of three serum creatine kinase concentrations done one month apart. The average concentration is elevated in only 35 percent of obligate carriers if one allows a false-positive rate of less than 2.5 percent (Griggs et al, 1985). However, since creatine kinase falls with age, the rate of carrier detection using this technique will be highest in the first two decades. Indeed, during the first decade, the accuracy of picking up the carrier state may be as high as 75 percent in the sisters of affected boys.

Occasional female carriers of Duchenne muscular dystrophy have manifested weakness. The weakness is usually mild, proximal in distribution, sometimes asymmetric, and either slowly progressive or stationary (Olson and Fenichel, 1982).

The major hope for accurate carrier detection is by linkage analysis using restriction fragment length polymorphism. Although this technique is useful only in selected families, it may be effective for prenatal diagnosis as well.

Limb-Girdle Muscular Dystrophy

The term limb-girdle dystrophy is used to describe cases of proximal muscle weakness beginning in the second or third decade and progressing slowly to severe disability after twenty years. Both sexes are affected equally, and although most cases are sporadic in occurrence, autosomal recessive inheritance is suspected. Limb-girdle muscular dystrophy is not a single genetic entity. Indeed, many recently described myopathies that are due to inborn errors in metabolism had been categorized previously as limb-girdle dystrophy before a specific enzyme defect had been identified.

Clinical Features. Patients with slowly progressive symmetric proximal weakness, with or without facial involvement, and diminished or absent tendon reflexes should be considered to have limb-girdle dystrophy if other specific entities can be excluded. Either the pelvic or shoulder girdle muscles can be affected first.

The most common problem in differential diagnosis is between limb-girdle and Becker muscular dystrophy. Enlargement of the calves may occur in both disorders, but is much more prominent in Becker muscular dystrophy. The distinction between these two dystrophies is important for accurate genetic counseling. In addition to Duchenne/Becker muscular dystrophy, other conditions to be considered in the differential diagnosis include juvenile spinal muscular atrophy, acid maltase deficiency, endocrine myopathies, and polymyositis.

Diagnosis. The serum concentration of creatine kinase is elevated, but not to the same extent seen in early Duchenne muscular dystrophy. The EMG is consistent with a myopathy: brief, small-amplitude, polyphasic potentials. Muscle histology varies with the stage of disease. The earliest changes are variation in fiber size and increase in internal nuclei. Later, fiber splitting and an uneven distribution of mitochondria produce a "moth-eaten appearance" when histochemical reactions for oxidative enzymes are applied. Both fiber types are affected equally (Fig. 7.4).

Treatment. The treatment goals in limb-girdle muscular dystrophy are the same as those for Duchenne muscular dystrophy. The only difference is that contractures are not as serious a problem.

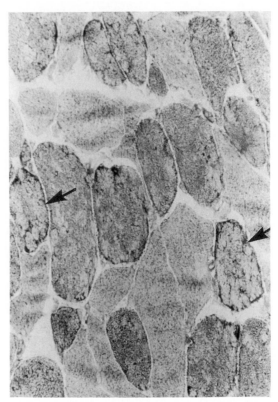

Figure 7.4 Moth-eaten appearance in limb-girdle dystrophy (DPNH). The usual lace-like appearance of the mitochondria is replaced by mitochondrial clumping.

Facioscapulohumeral Syndrome

Progressive facioscapulohumeral weakness was originally considered a muscular dystrophy with autosomal dominant inheritance. Later, similar patterns of weakness were described secondary to spinal muscular atrophy and polymyositis. It is now recognized that patients with genetic facioscapulohumeral weakness may have histologic evidence of myopathy, neuropathy, and inflammation. Therefore, the term facioscapulohumeral syndrome is presently used to designate this entity, which, although predominantly a dystrophy, has elements of denervation as well. The genetic defect has complete penetrance but variable expression.

Clinical Features. The usual onset of weakness is in the second decade, but may begin as early as infancy (Bailey et al, 1986). Initial involvement is usually in the shoulder girdle with subsequent spread to the face, but the reverse also occurs. The progression of weakness is insidious and diagnosis is often delayed. Family history may be denied, because affected family members are unaware they have a problem.

Patients are eventually aware of a change in facial expression. Late in the course, speech becomes indistinct and leg muscles are sometimes involved. Anterior tibial weakness is most prominent, but proximal weakness may occur as well. In patients with only minimal facial weakness, the combination of proximal weakness in the arms and distal weakness in the legs may suggest a scapuloperoneal syndrome.

The course of facioscapulohumeral syndrome is ordinarily benign; most patients do not become disabled, and life expectancy is normal. An exception is the infantile form (Bailey et al, 1986). Facial weakness and ptosis are noted as early as the first year and are followed by progressive proximal weakness of the arms and legs. The rapidity of progression mimics Duchenne muscular dystrophy; death occurs during adolescence. The course in affected parents is not unusual, and the reason for early onset is unknown.

Facioscapulohumeral syndrome has been described in association with Coats syndrome: retinal telangiectasia, exudation, and detachment. Hearing loss and mental retardation may be present as well (Taylor et al, 1982; Wulff et al, 1982).

Diagnosis. The serum concentration of creatine kinase can be normal or increased to five times normal. The EMG may show denervation potentials, myopathic motor units, or both. Histologic changes in many limb muscles are minimal; the supraspinatus yields the highest abnormal return (Bodensteiner and Schochet, 1986). Occasional fibers are noted undergoing degeneration, small angulated denervated fibers may be seen, and inflammatory cells can be present as well.

Treatment. Treatment is not available for weakness. The retina should be carefully examined for Coats syndrome. Retinal telangiectasia can be treated by coagulation and blindness prevented.

INFLAMMATORY MYOPATHIES

The inflammatory myopathies are a heterogeneous group of disorders that together make up the most common form of acquired muscle disease. The incidence rate for hospital diagnosis of polymyositis is five cases per million population per year. These occur in a bimodal age distribution with the childhood mode composing 21 percent of the total. The trough between the two distribution curves is between fifteen and twenty-four years.

The leading hypotheses concerning the pathophysiology of inflammatory myopathy are viral infection and immunopathy. The two are not mutually exclusive because viral infection may occur on the background of an abnormal immune state and immune-mediated destruction of tissue may be generated by a viral infection (Whitaker, 1982). Acute infectious myositis is dealt with in the section on acute generalized weakness (Table 7.5). Idiopathic dermatomyositis and polymyositis are discussed in this section.

Dermatomyositis

Dermatomyositis is a systemic angiopathy in which the process of vascular occlusion and infarction accounts for all pathologic changes observed in muscle, connective tissue, skin, gastrointestinal tract, and small nerves. More than 30 percent of adults with dermatomyositis have an underlying malignancy, but cancer is not a factor in children. The childhood form of dermatomyositis is a relatively homogeneous disease that probably has a single etiology.

Clinical Features. Peak incidence is generally between the ages of five and ten years, but an onset as early as four months has been reported. The presentation of illness may be insidious or fulminating. An insidious onset is characterized by fever, fatigue, and anorexia in the absence

Table 7.5 THE MUSCULAR DYSTROPHIES

	Genetic Type	Age at Onset (Years)	Age at Disability (Years)	Pattern of Weakness
Duchenne	X-linked	0–5	10–15	Proximal
Becker	X-linked	5–15	15–25	Proximal
Limb-girdle	Autosomal	10–30	20–40	Proximal
Facioscapulohumeral	Autosomal dominant	10–30	30–50	Proximal arm, face
Myotonic	Autosomal	10–30	30–50	Distal limbs, face
Scapuloperoneal	Autosomal dominant	20–30	30–50	Proximal arm and distal leg
	Autosomal recessive	0–10	5–15	
Emery-Dreifuss	X-linked	5–15	25–50	Proximal arm and distal leg

of rash or weakness. These symptoms may persist for weeks or months and suggest an underlying infection. In most children, dermatitis precedes myositis. The characteristic rash is marked by an erythematous discoloration and edema of the upper eyelids that spreads to involve the entire periorbital and malar regions. Erythema and edema of the extensor surfaces overlying the joints of the knuckles, elbows, and knees develop later. With time, the skin appears atrophic and scaly.

The myopathy is characterized by proximal weakness, stiffness, and pain, which are most severe in the shoulder and pelvic girdles. Weakness generalizes and flexion contractures develop rapidly and produce joint deformities. Tendon reflexes become increasingly difficult to obtain and are finally absent.

Calcinosis of subcutaneous tissue, especially under discolored areas of skin, occurs in 60 percent of children. When severe, it produces an armor-like appearance, *calcinosis universalis,* on radiographs. Some children may have only minor skin and muscle symptoms and present instead with stiffness.

Gastrointestinal tract infarction is a leading cause of death. Ulcerations may extend the length of the bowel and are sometimes preceded by pneumatosis intestinalis as the vasculitis allows the submucosal dissection of intraluminal bowel gas. Recent accounts indicate a mortality rate of less than 5 percent (Bowyer et al, 1982).

Diagnosis. The combination of fever, rash, myalgia, and weakness is compelling evidence for the diagnosis of dermatomyositis. The serum concentration of creatine kinase is usually elevated early in the course. The EMG is always abnormal at the time of active myositis. The major features are increased insertional activity, fibrillations, and positive sharp waves at rest, and brief, small-amplitude polyphasic potentials with contraction. The diagnostic feature on muscle biopsy is perifascicular atrophy (Fig. 7.5). Capillary necrosis usually starts at the periphery of the muscle fascicle and causes ischemia in the adjacent muscle fibers. The most profound atrophy occurs in fascicular borders that face large connective tissue septa. Type I and type II fibers are affected equally.

Treatment. The inflammatory process is thought to be active for approximately two years. Corticosteroids are generally accepted as effective in suppressing the inflammatory response and providing symptomatic relief, without curing the underlying disease. The best results are obtained when corticosteroids are

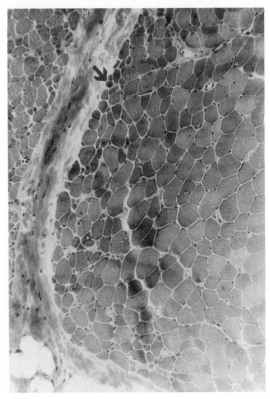

Figure 7.5 Perifascicular atrophy in childhood dermatomyositis (trichrome). The muscle fibers at the edge of each fascicle are atrophied.

started early in high doses and are maintained for long periods of time (Henriksson and Sandstedt, 1982).

Prednisone is initiated at a dose of 2 mg/kg/day. The response follows a predictable pattern. Temperature returns to normal within forty-eight hours. Serum concentrations of creatine kinase return to normal by the second week and there is simultaneous evidence of increasing muscle strength. When this occurs, the same dose of prednisone should be given on alternate days in order to reduce the frequency and severity of corticosteroid-induced side effects. Both alternate-day and everyday therapy are equally effective if the doses are large and the treatment is maintained. As muscle strength increases, the dose of alternate-day prednisone is tapered at a rate of 10 mg per month in children taking more than 50 mg every other day until an alternate-day dose of 50 mg is attained. Further reductions are then at a rate of 5 mg per month. In most children, the maintenance dose needed for normal muscle strength and normal serum concentrations of creatine kinase is 10 to 25 mg every other day. The response of the skin rash to prednisone is variable: in some children, the rash heals completely; in most, there will be some permanent scar of the disease.

Although most children demonstrate a dramatic improvement and seem normal in three months, prednisone must be continued for a full two years. If treatment is discontinued prematurely, relapse is invariable. Children treated intermittently are more likely to develop calcinosis and contractures. Indeed, corticosteroids are useful in the treatment of calcinosis universalis. In addition to prednisone, a well-structured program of physical therapy is needed to prevent contractures.

Eighty percent of children with dermatomyositis have a favorable outcome if high-dose prednisone is started within four months of the onset of symptoms. Those children who do not demonstrate an immediate response to high-dose prednisone should be started on oral methotrexate, 10 to 20 mg/m^2, given twice weekly. Regular monitoring of liver function and white blood cell count is required. If these measures fail, plasmapheresis is a reasonable alternative.

It is generally believed that once the disease becomes inactive, reactivation is unlikely. However, late progression or recurrence may occur and should be treated with an additional one year course of corticosteroids.

Polymyositis

Polymyositis without evidence of other target organ involvement is uncommon prior to puberty. Several infants with polymyositis have been reported, some affected from birth (see Chapter 6). Children with systemic lupus erythematosus may present with myalgia and arthralgia, but generally do not have muscle weakness at onset. Skin, joint, and systemic manifestations are usually well established prior to the onset of myopathy. Polymyositis in adolescence is similar to the disorder in adult life, with the exception that malignancy is not a causative factor.

Clinical Features. Polymyositis presents as a symmetric proximal weakness that begins insidiously and progresses to moderate handicap within weeks to months. Prolonged periods of stability or even remission may occur that suggest the diagnosis of limb-girdle muscular dystrophy because of the slow progress. Tendon reflexes are present early in the course and become hypoactive as muscle bulk is lost. Cardiorespiratory complications are not as frequent in childhood as in adult polymyositis.

Diagnosis. The serum concentration of creatine kinase is not invariably elevated, but the EMG is almost always abnormal and typically demonstrates both myopathic and neuropathic features. Several different patterns of abnormality are present on muscle biopsy and perivascular inflammation need not be present. Instead, features of myopathy, denervation, or both may be observed (Mastaglia and Ojeda, 1985).

Treatment. The same treatment schedule suggested for childhood dermatomyositis should be used for children with polymyositis. Unfortunately, the response to corticosteroids is far less predictable in polymyositis than in dermatomyositis. Children who do not respond to corticosteroids should be treated with methotrexate.

METABOLIC MYOPATHIES

Juvenile Acid Maltase Deficiency

The initial symptoms of acid maltase deficiency may occur in infancy, childhood, or adult life. The enzyme defect appears to be the same, no matter the age of onset, and different ages of onset may occur within the same family (Angelini and Engel, 1972; Loonen et al, 1981). The defect is always transmitted by autosomal recessive inheritance. It is not clear why the age of onset varies so widely.

Clinical Features. Infants with acid maltase deficiency have glycogen storage in both skeletal and cardiac muscle. Death occurs during infancy due to cardiac failure (see Chapter 6).

In the childhood form, only skeletal muscle is involved and the main clinical feature is slowly progressive proximal limb weakness. Tendon reflexes are hypoactive or unobtainable. Occasionally, children have mild hypertrophy of the calves simulating Duchenne muscular dystrophy. The course of illness is one of steady progression leading to disability and respiratory insufficiency by the end of the second decade. The later the onset of symptoms, the longer and more benign the course.

Diagnosis. The diagnosis of acid maltase deficiency depends upon the demonstration of glycogen storage on muscle biopsy and the absence of acid maltase in muscle or fibroblasts. There are some children with evidence of lysosomal glycogen storage disease in whom acid maltase deficiency cannot be demonstrated (Riggs et al, 1983). These children have a somewhat different clinical syndrome, characterized not only by proximal muscle weakness but also by cardiomyopathy, intellectual impairment, and possible liver involvement. The enzyme deficiency is uncertain.

Treatment. Treatment is not available.

Other Carbohydrate Myopathies

McArdle disease and debrancher enzyme deficiency may sometimes present as slowly progressive proximal weakness and must at least be considered in the differential diagnosis. The usual presentation, however, is exercise intolerance, and for this reason these disorders are discussed in Chapter 7.

Muscle Carnitine Deficiency

Carnitine is an essential cofactor in the transfer of long-chain fatty acids across the inner mitochondrial membrane and for the conversion of acyl-coenzyme A to acetyl coenzyme A (Rebouche and Engel, 1983; Stumpf et al, 1985). Carnitine deficiency states occur in newborns receiving total parenteral alimentation, secondary to several disorders of intermediary metabolism, and as a primary genetic disease. Primary carnitine deficiency is transmitted by autosomal recessive inheritance. Clinical manifestations may be restricted to skeletal muscle or may cause systemic symptoms resembling Reye syndrome (see Chapter 2). Initially, muscle and systemic carnitine deficiency were believed to be separate entities distinguished by the presence of normal or reduced levels of serum carnitine, respectively. This distinction does not hold true for all cases.

Clinical Features. The major clinical feature of muscle carnitine deficiency is progressive proximal weakness, affecting the legs before and more severely than the arms, with onset in childhood. Occasional patients have cardiomyopathy as well. The cardiomyopathy is not manifested clinically, but is recognized on EKG and echocardiography.

Diagnosis. The serum concentration of creatine kinase is elevated. The EMG may suggest a neuropathic process early in the course and then may become consistent with myopathy. A muscle biopsy specimen reveals fiber necrosis with lipid storage and a reduced carnitine content.

Treatment. Dietary therapy with L-carnitine is effective and safe. Diarrhea is the major side effect. The usual dose is 100 mg/kg/day in three or four divided doses.

Other Lipid Myopathies

Patients have been reported with progressive proximal weakness during childhood, lipid storage in muscle, and normal carnitine content. Such patients have in common a disturbance of mitochondrial fatty acid oxidation. In some, there are obvious morphologic abnormalities of mitochondria (Askansas et al, 1985); in others, only biochemical abnormalities can be identified (Carroll et al, 1986). These disorders are genetically heterogeneous and difficult to separate from the mitochondrial myopathies.

Clinical Features. Progressive proximal weakness begins anytime from early childhood to adolescence. The legs are affected first and then the arms. Exercise intolerance is noted, and in some cases the ingestion of fatty foods leads to nausea and vomiting. The pattern and progression of weakness may simulate Duchenne muscular dystrophy even to the presence of calf hypertrophy. Limb weakness is steadily progressive, and cardiomyopathy may develop as well.

Diagnosis. The serum concentration of creatine kinase is markedly elevated. The EMG is abnormal and consistent with a myopathic process. Muscle biopsy is critical to diagnosis. Type I muscle fibers contain fatty droplets. Carnitine and carnitine palmityltransferase levels are normal.

Treatment. Propranolol has been found beneficial in improving strength in some patients (Martyn et al, 1981). The mechanism of action is unknown. Patients with fat intolerance may show improvement on a diet free of long-chain fatty acids.

Mitochondrial Myopathies

Mitochondrial (respiratory chain) myopathies are a heterogeneous group of disorders characterized by the presence of morphologic mitochondrial abnormalities in muscle. These morphologic abnormalities are a compensatory mechanism secondary to disturbances in enzyme systems leading to adenosine triphosphate (ATP) production.

Clinical Features. The age at onset varies from birth to adult life, but is before age twenty in 60 percent of cases. Three clinical syndromes are described: (1) progressive external ophthalmoplegia and exercise intolerance (see Chapter 8); (2) exercise intolerance alone (see Chapter 8); and (3) encephalopathy, myopathy, and lactic acidosis (DiMauro et al, 1985; Petty et al, 1986). Occasionally, mitochondrial myopathies present as progressive proximal limb weakness. Those that present in this manner are not genetically homogeneous. More often than not, the myopathy is associated with abnormalities in other systems, such as cardiomyopathy, renal tubular disturbances, and stroke-like episodes (McLeod et al, 1975).

Diagnosis. The concentration of serum creatine kinase is frequently normal, and the EMG is not diagnostic. Diagnosis depends upon muscle biopsy results. The characteristic feature by light microscopy is the appearance of ragged red fibers (Fig. 7.6). In these fibers, there is an increase in the size and number of mitochondria that are often concentrated beneath the sarcolemma. When the trichrome stain is applied, the clumped mitochondria stain red and give the fiber a ragged appearance.

In vitro studies of mitochondrial metabolism localize deficiencies to complex I or complex III of the mitochondrial respiratory chain, but a typical clinical picture is not associated with each complex disturbance.

Treatment. Treatment is not available, and trials of thiamine, menadione, or ubiquinone have been disappointing.

ENDOCRINE MYOPATHIES

Progressive proximal limb weakness may occur in patients with hyperthyroidism and hypothyroidism, hyperparathyroidism and hypoparathyroidism, and hyperadrenalism and hypoadrenalism.

Clinical Features. In general, patients with endocrine myopathy have systemic signs of endocrine disease prior to the onset of weakness, but some may present with weakness as the initial feature. This is especially true in patients with primary or secondary hypoparathyroidism and in thyroid disorders. Weakness is much more prominent in the legs than the arms. Tendon reflexes, even in weak muscles, are normal or diminished, but generally not absent.

Diagnosis. The serum concentration of creatine kinase is typically normal. The EMG is not diagnostic; it may be normal, myopathic, or neuropathic. Many endocrinopathies produce neuropathy as well as myopathy. In Cushing disease and in hyperparathyroidism, muscle histologic studies reveal type II fiber atrophy. Other conditions demonstrate nonspecific myopathic changes that vary with the severity of endocrinopathy.

Treatment. In all endocrine myopathies, weakness is reversed by treating the underlying endocrinopathy.

■ Progressive Distal Weakness

Progressive distal weakness in childhood is most often due to neuropathy (see Table 7.4). Among the slowly progressive neuropathies of childhood, hereditary disorders are far more frequent than acquired disorders. The only common acquired neuropathy is postinfectious polyradiculoneuropathy (Guillain-Barré syndrome) and weakness evolves rapidly (Table 7.6).

DIAGNOSIS IN NEUROPATHY

The typical presentation of neuropathy in children is progressive symmetric distal weakness affecting initially the legs and then the arms. When sensation is disturbed, there are dysesthesias consisting of tingling, "pins and needles," or burning sensations of the feet. The weakness and sensory loss move from distal to proximal in a glove-and-stocking distribution. Tendon reflexes are lost early in the course of disease, especially when sensory fibers are affected.

An important first step in diagnosis is to determine the primary site of pathology: cell body (anterior horn cell), nerve axon, or myelin. This is accomplished by electrodiagnosis (Table 7.7). In primary disorders of the cell body (*neuronop-*

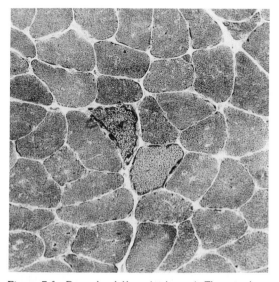

Figure 7.6 Ragged-red fibers (trichrome). The mitochondria are enlarged and stain intensely with hematoxylin.

Table 7.6 PROGRESSIVE DISTAL WEAKNESS

Spinal Cord Disorders (see Chapter 12)

Spinal Muscular Atrophy

Hereditary Motor Sensory Neuropathy (HMSN)
1. HSMN I: Charcot-Marie-Tooth
2. HMSN II: Neuronal Charcot-Marie-Tooth
3. HMSN III: Déjérine-Sottas
4. HMSN IV: Refsum

Other Genetic Neuropathies
1. Sulfatide lipidoses: metachromatic leukodystrophy
2. Other leukodystrophies
3. Disorders of pyruvate metabolism
4. Familial amyloid neuropathy (see Chapter 9)

Neuropathies with Systemic Diseases
1. Drugs
2. Toxins
3. Uremia
4. Systemic vasculitis

Idiopathic Neuropathy
1. Chronic demyelinating neuropathy
2. Chronic axonal neuropathy

Myopathies
1. Myotonic dystrophy
2. Hereditary distal myopathies

Scapulo(humeral)peroneal
1. Neuronopathy
2. Emery-Dreifuss syndrome
3. With dementia

athy), an EMG of resting muscle demonstrates fibrillations and fasciculations. With voluntary contraction, the number of motor unit potentials is reduced but the amplitude is normal or increased as a result of collateral reinnervation. Motor conduction nerve velocity is normal or only slightly diminished, and the amplitude of sensory action potential is normal. In *axonopathies*, there are fibrillations at rest and a reduced number of motor unit potentials that are normal or increased in amplitude. High-amplitude potentials may be polyphasic. Motor nerve con-

Table 7.7 ELECTRODIAGNOSIS
IN NEUROPATHY

	Neuron-opathy	Axonal	Demyeli-nating
Fasciculations	+ + +	+ + +	+
Denervation potentials	+ + +	+ + +	+
Reduced number of motor units	+ + +	+ + +	0
High-amplitude potentials	+ + +	+ + +	0
Slow motor velocity	0	+	+ + +
Reduced sensory potentials	0	+	+ + +

duction velocity is normal or mildly reduced, and the amplitude of sensory action potentials may be reduced as well. *Demyelinating* neuropathies are characterized by marked slowing of motor conduction velocity and reduced amplitude of sensory evoked potentials. The EMG may be normal early in the course of disease.

SPINAL MUSCULAR ATROPHY

The distal form of spinal muscular atrophy is genetically heterogeneous. The trait may be transmitted by autosomal dominant or recessive inheritance. Severe and mild forms exist for each type of inheritance that may be genetically distinct (Harding and Thomas, 1980; Pearn et al, 1978b).

Clinical Features. The disease usually presents with weakness and wasting in the anterior compartment of the legs associated with pes cavus deformities of the feet. Tendon reflexes may be preserved. The clinical picture is indistinguishable from hereditary motor sensory neuropathy I. In the severe autosomal recessive form, weakness progresses to involve the proximal muscles of the legs and sometimes the hands. Weakness in the arms varies from family to family with concordance among individual kindreds. Approximately 25 percent of patients have scoliosis.

Occasional families are described in which weakness begins in the hands and is either confined to the arms (Lander et al, 1976) or affects the legs later and less severely (Meadows and Marsden, 1969). When the arms are affected exclusively and predominantly, the mode of transmission is autosomal dominant inheritance.

The onset of distal spinal muscular atrophies is always before age twenty. With the exception of the severe autosomal recessive form, the prognosis is generally good. Progression of weakness is slow and sometimes appears to arrest. The distinction between mild and severe autosomal recessive forms is possible only when other family members are affected. The course of disease runs true within each family.

Diagnosis. Electrodiagnosis is critical to distinguish these disorders from peripheral neuropathies. Motor nerve conduction velocity is normal despite total denervation of the small muscles of the foot. Sensory evoked potentials are also normal. The serum concentration of creatine kinase is ordinarily normal, but may be mildly elevated. Muscle biopsy results demonstrate nonspecific changes of denervation, and the sural nerve is normal.

Treatment. Treatment is not available, nor is there a method for antenatal diagnosis.

HEREDITARY MOTOR SENSORY NEUROPATHY

The term hereditary motor sensory neuropathy (HSMN) is used to encompass several different genetic neuropathies that previously had been known by a variety of eponyms. Almost one half of idiopathic polyneuropathies will be found to belong to this group when detailed family histories are taken and other family members are examined (Dyck et al, 1981).

HSMN I: Charcot-Marie-Tooth Disease

This is a dominantly inherited hypertrophic neuropathy with prominent peroneal atrophy. The Roussy-Lévy syndrome is also included in this classification. Variability in clinical expression is considerable, and personal examination, including electrodiagnosis, may be needed to demonstrate the phenotype in parents.

Clinical Features. The initial symptoms are either foot deformities or gait disturbances, usually beginning in the second decade or later but sometimes in early infancy (Vanasse and Dubowitz, 1981). Dysesthesias are never an early symptom, although some patients, because of foot deformity, may complain of pain resulting from pressure from shoes. Pes cavus is typical, and hammertoes may be present as well. These deformities are caused by weakness of the intrinsic foot muscles and result in foreshortening of the foot and elevation of the arch. The initial gait disturbance is usually described as clumsiness, especially in running.

HSMN I is not a severe disorder in childhood. Examination reveals pes cavus, weakness of the peroneal muscles, and diminished reactivity of the Achilles tendon reflex (Hagberg and Lyon, 1981). With time, the anterior tibial as well as the peroneal muscles become weak, producing foot drop. The gastrocnemius and soleus muscles may be involved as well. Eventually, weakness may spread to the proximal muscles of the legs and the distal muscles of the arms. Scoliosis is present in only a minority of patients. Cramps with exercise and fasciculations are present in weak muscles. Sensation is generally normal.

Enlargement of peripheral nerves occurs in adults, but not in children. The enlargement is caused by repeated episodes of demyelination and remyelination.

Diagnosis. Diagnosis relies upon a characteristic clinical picture and positive family history. Motor nerve conduction velocities are less than 50 percent of normal in affected individuals. The cerebrospinal fluid protein content is usually normal in children, but may be elevated in adults. Muscle histologic appearance reveals nonspecific changes of denervation; myopathic changes may be present as well in older individuals. "Onion bulb" formation is noted in peripheral nerves that have undergone repeated episodes of demyelination and remyelination but is not pathognomonic.

Treatment. No specific treatment is available, but proper foot care may minimize discomfort and maximize function. Shoes should be roomy and soft to prevent rubbing against bony prominences. Footwear that is molded to the shape of the foot may be especially useful. When foot drop is present, a lightweight plastic ankle-foot orthodesis that fits into the patient's own shoe may be helpful not only in lifting the foot but also in preventing turning and injury of the ankle.

HMSN II: Charcot-Marie-Tooth Disease, Neuronal Type

This disorder is transmitted by autosomal dominant inheritance and clinically resembles HMSN I, except that symptoms are considerably milder. The pathologic process is primarily axonal rather than demyelinating; as a consequence, motor nerve conduction velocities are either normal or only mildly prolonged (Berciano et al, 1986).

Clinical Features. The peak age at onset is during the second decade. Cases with onset in early childhood may be genetically distinct and transmitted by autosomal recessive inheritance (Ouvrier et al, 1981).

Distal weakness begins in the legs and can be asymmetric. The hands are affected later. Tendon reflexes are generally absent at the ankle, but may be preserved at the knee and elbow. Distal sensory loss is present in most children. In some, all modalities are affected; others experience loss of pain or vibration and position sense. Progression of symptoms is slow, and disability does not occur until middle adult life.

Diagnosis. The cerebrospinal fluid protein content is normal, as is the serum concentration of creatine kinase. Motor conduction velocity is 60 percent or more of normal. The EMG demonstrates a denervation pattern in affected muscles.

Treatment. Specific treatment is not available.

HMSN III: Déjérine-Sottas Disease

This is a demyelinating and remyelinating neuropathy transmitted by autosomal recessive inheritance. Many cases are sporadic. Parental consanguinity is a factor in many families. However, the heterozygote parent has no evidence of neuropathy either by clinical examination or by electrodiagnosis (Dyck, 1984).

Clinical Features. Slow motor development and hypotonia are frequently present during the first year. Weakness begins distally in the limbs and progresses to involve the proximal muscles by the second decade. Sensory ataxia is present in all patients (Ouvrier et al, 1987). Clubfoot and scoliosis are associated findings. Distal sensory loss of all modalities is readily demonstrated on examination. Tendon reflexes are absent. Peripheral nerves enlarge, and the great auricular, the median, and the ulnar nerves are frequently palpable. Associated findings in some patients include miosis, sluggish pupillary responses to light, nystagmus, and choreiform movements of the fingers.

Diagnosis. The cerebrospinal fluid protein content is generally elevated in proportion to the severity of weakness. Motor nerve conduction velocities are markedly prolonged, and sensory potentials are reduced in amplitude. Sural nerve biopsy demonstrates massive interstitial hypertrophy and marked onion bulb formation. These typical findings are not pathognomonic and are seen in HMSN I as well. There is sufficient overlap in the clinical, electrodiagnostic, and pathologic features of HMSN I and HMSN III that the two disorders are differentiated primarily by their mode of genetic transmission (Hagberg and Lyon, 1981).

Treatment. A metabolic abnormality of lipid metabolism has been suggested, but never established. Treatment is not available.

HMSN IV: Refsum's Disease

Refsum's disease is an inborn error of phytanic acid metabolism reported mainly from Scandinavia, Great Britain, Germany, and France. Autosomal recessive transmission is suspected because of a high incidence of consanguinity in affected families and no evidence of disease in parents (Refsum, 1984). In fibroblasts

derived from homozygotes, the rate of phytanic acid oxidation is 3 percent of control samples; in heterozygotes the rate is 50 percent.

Clinical Features. Age at onset varies from the first to the third decade, but is sometimes difficult to date because initial symptoms are insidious. The cardinal clinical manifestations are retinitis pigmentosa, chronic or recurrent polyneuropathy, and cerebellar ataxia. Retinitis pigmentosa is a constant finding and is indispensable for diagnosis. Night blindness is often the first symptom. The neuropathy is hypertrophic, symmetric, and distal, affecting both motor and sensory fibers. Vibration and position sense are more diminished than are pain and temperature. Tendon reflexes become progressively hyporesponsive and are finally lost. The ataxia may be of cerebellar origin; nystagmus and intention tremor are sometimes present but could be caused by sensory neuropathy. Other symptoms include progressive loss of hearing, cataracts, cardiomyopathy, ichthyosis, and pes cavus.

The course is variable; there may be steady progression, long periods of stability, or remissions and exacerbations. Sudden death from cardiac arrhythmia may occur as a consequence of cardiomyopathy.

Diagnosis. The protein content of the cerebrospinal fluid is always elevated in the range of 100 to 700 mg/dl (1 to 7 g/L). Motor and sensory nerve conduction velocities are markedly reduced. The EMG is consistent with denervation. Electroretinography demonstrates a severe abnormality of the photoreceptors of the retina involving both rods and cones. Definitive diagnosis requires demonstration of reduced oxidation of phytanic acid in cultured fibroblasts. Antenatal diagnosis is accomplished by measuring phytanic acid oxidation in amniotic cells.

Treatment. Phytanic acid is not produced endogenously and must be derived completely from diet. Exacerbations of disease correlate well with blood levels of phytanic acid. Treatment is available by a combination of diet and plasma exchange (Gibberd et al, 1979). This has proved successful in preventing progression of symptoms and in reversing symptoms already present.

OTHER GENETIC NEUROPATHIES

Sulfatide Lipidosis: Metachromatic Leukodystrophy

This is an inherited disorder of myelin metabolism due to defective activity of the enzyme arylsulfatase A. It is transmitted by autosomal recessive inheritance. Three forms are recognized: late infantile, juvenile, and adult. The late infantile form is the most common of the three. Juvenile and adult onset cases affect primarily the brain and are difficult to distinguish from each other. All three forms are thought to be genetically distinct (Martin et al, 1982). Only the late infantile form is discussed in this section.

Clinical Features. After a period of normal development, gait disturbances develop, usually by age two, but can be delayed until age four. Initial examination reveals distal weakness of the feet with loss of the Achilles tendon reflex. There is progression of weakness to all limbs, resulting in generalized hypotonia and hyporeflexia. Later, brain function deteriorates with development of dementia, spasticity, and blindness.

Diagnosis. The protein content of the cerebrospinal fluid is elevated, and motor nerve conduction velocities are reduced at the time of initial leg weakness. The diagnosis is confirmed by demonstrating the absence of arylsulfatase A in white blood cells.

Treatment. Treatment is not available, but prenatal diagnosis is possible by analysis of arylsulfatase A in amniocytes.

Other Leukodystrophies

Peripheral neuropathy occurs in *globoid cell leukodystrophy* (Krabbe disease), but is not as prominent a feature as in metachromatic leukodystrophy. The disorder presents in infancy with psychomotor retardation and irritability rather than flaccid weakness (see Chapter 5). Tendon reflexes may be absent or hyperactive, and motor nerve conduction velocity is reduced in half of cases. Cerebrospinal fluid protein concentration is always elevated.

Cockayne's syndrome is characterized by progeria, small stature, ataxia, retinitis pigmentosa, deafness, and mental retardation. A primary segmental demyelinating neuropathy may be present as well, but is not an initial symptom (Ohnishi et al, 1987). The neuropathy is manifest by hyporeflexia and reduced motor nerve conduction velocity.

Other disorders of lipid metabolism in which demyelinating neuropathy is present, but not an important feature, include Niemann-Pick disease, Gaucher disease, and Farber disease.

Disorders of Pyruvate Metabolism

Deficiencies of enzymes comprising the pyruvate dehydrogenase complex and pyruvate carboxylase have been recognized. The resulting clinical syndromes vary with the specific enzyme and the percentage of enzyme deficiency. Common manifestations among the several disorders of pyruvate metabolism include lactic acidosis, ataxia, hypotonia, ophthalmoplegia, mental retardation, and peripheral neuropathy. Symptoms may be either progressive or recurrent. Peripheral neuropathy is frequently demonstrated by electrodiagnosis, but is not prominent on clinical examination. This group of disorders is discussed in Chapter 10.

Familial Amyloid Neuropathy

All familial amyloid neuropathies are transmitted by autosomal dominant inheritance (Cohen and Rubinow, 1984).

Clinical Features. Peripheral neuropathy, affecting both the somatic and autonomic nervous systems, is the cardinal manifestation of primary familial amyloidosis. Other organ involvement sometimes occurs, but not to the same degree encountered in secondary amyloidosis. Potential sites of amyloid deposition include kidney, heart, gastrointestinal tract, liver, and skin.

The onset of symptoms may be anytime from the second to the sixth decades. The initial symptoms are sensory. (Sensory symptoms are described in Chapter 9.) Autonomic dysfunction follows and is manifested by dysfunction of gastrointestinal motility, hypotension, and cardiac arrhythmia. Weakness, wasting, fasciculations, and loss of tendon reflexes occur later in the course of disease. Ocular abnormalities are common and may include scalloping of the pupillary margin, delayed reaction to light, visual floaters, and blindness. The progress is slow but relentless, leading to disability and death within fifteen years from onset of symptoms.

Among some kindreds with familial amyloid neuropathy, the hands are affected before the feet and patients present with a carpal tunnel syndrome: pain, paresthesias, and numbness in the medial nerve distribution. Symptoms of autonomic dysfunction follow, but the legs are unaffected.

Diagnosis. The protein content of the cerebrospinal fluid is normal or only mildly increased. Motor nerve conduction velocities are generally reduced, and nerve biopsy results demonstrate the presence of amyloid when special stains are applied.

Treatment. Treatment is not available.

NEUROPATHIES WITH SYSTEMIC DISEASE

Drugs

Several drugs that are used widely in children, such as chloramphenicol and phenytoin, are capable of producing a polyneuropathy. However, the neuropathy is usually subclinical and is manifested only by electrodiagnosis or loss of Achilles tendon reflex. Three drugs that produce clinical evidence of motor and sensory neuropathy are vincristine, nitrofurantoin, and isoniazid (Evans, 1979).

Vincristine

Clinical Features. Neuropathy is an expected complication of vincristine therapy (Casey et al, 1973). The Achilles tendon reflex is lost first; later, other tendon reflexes become less reactive and may be lost. The first symptoms are paresthesias, often starting in the fingers rather than the feet, and then progressing to mild loss of superficial sensation, but not position sense. Weakness follows sensory loss and is evidenced by clumsiness in the hands and cramps in the feet. Distal muscles are affected more than proximal muscles and extensors more than flexors. Weakness may progress rapidly with loss of ambulation in a few weeks. The initial weakness may be asymmetric and suggests mononeuropathy multiplex.

Diagnosis. Electrodiagnostic studies are consistent with axonal neuropathy; fibrillations and fasciculations are seen on the EMG, but motor nerve conduction velocity is normal.

Treatment. The neuropathy is dose-related and usually resolves one to three months after the drug is discontinued.

Isoniazid

Clinical Features. The initial symptoms are numbness and paresthesias of the fingers and toes. If therapy is continued, superficial sensation is diminished in a glove-and-stocking pattern. Distal limb weakness follows and is associated with tenderness of the muscles and burning dysesthesias. The Achilles tendon reflex is diminished or absent.

Diagnosis. Isoniazid neuropathy should be suspected in any child who develops a neuropathy while taking the drug.

Treatment. Isoniazid interferes with pyridoxine metabolism and produces neuropathy by causing a pyridoxine deficiency state. The administration of pyridoxine along with isoniazid prevents neuropathy without interfering with antituberculous activity. The longer that symptoms are allowed to progress, the longer the time until recovery. Although pyridoxine is able to prevent the development of neuropathy, it has little effect on the speed of recovery once neuropathy is established.

Nitrofurantoin

Clinical Features. Nitrofurantoin neuropathy most often occurs in patients with impaired renal function. High blood concentrations of the drug produce an axonal neuropathy. The initial symptoms are usually paresthesias, followed within a few days or weeks by glove-and-stocking sensory loss and weakness of distal muscles. Occasionally, pure motor neuropathy may be present.

Diagnosis. Nitrofurantoin neuropathy should be suspected in any child with neuropathy taking the drug. It may be difficult to distinguish from uremic neuropathy.

Treatment. Recovery is usually complete when the drug is stopped. Occasional patients have gone on to complete paralysis and death despite discontinuation of nitrofurantoin.

Toxins

Several heavy metals, inorganic chemicals, and insecticides are reported to produce polyneuropathies in children (Evans, 1979). In adults, heavy metal poisoning is generally caused by industrial exposure, agricultural exposure, or attempted homicide. Small children who have a single accidental ingestion are more likely to present with acute symptoms of systemic disease or central nervous system dysfunction and not with a slowly progressive neuropathy. At times, progressive distal weakness may be observed as a presenting sign in older children who are addicted to sniffing glue or gasoline. Yet, even in these cases, there are usually symptoms of central nervous system dysfunction as well.

Uremia

Some degree of neuropathy occurs at one time or another in many children being treated by long-term periodic hemodialysis. In most series, uremic neuropathy is more common in males than females but the reason for the sex bias is not clear.

Clinical Features. The earliest symptoms may be muscle cramps in the hands and feet, burning feet, or restless legs. Loss of the Achilles tendon reflex can be demonstrated at the onset. Following the initial sensory symptoms, there is progression to a severe distal, symmetric, mixed motor, and sensory polyneuropathy affecting the legs more than the arms. The rate of progression is variable and may be fulminating or may evolve over several months.

A small proportion of uremic patients develop a pure motor neuropathy (McGonigle et al, 1985). Symptoms begin after hemodialysis is started and may be initiated by septicemia. There is rapid progression of distal weakness in all limbs that does not respond to dialysis but may be reversed by renal transplant.

Diagnosis. Demyelination occurs out of proportion to axonal changes. Therefore, the determination of motor nerve conduction velocity is used widely to monitor the severity of neuropathy. Slow conduction velocities are present even before clinical symptoms occur. There is a high degree of correlation between reductions in creatine clearance and slowing of the conduction velocity.

Treatment. Early neuropathy can be reversed by dialysis. Patients with severe neuropathy rarely recover fully despite adequate treatment.

Systemic Vasculitis and Vasculopathy

Polyneuropathy and mononeuropathy multiplex are relatively common neurologic complications of vasculitis in adults but not in children. Children with lupus erythematosus are generally sicker than adults, but peripheral neuropathy is not a prominent feature of their disease (Coleman et al, 1977). When neuropathy is present, it is not an initial feature.

IDIOPATHIC NEUROPATHY

Chronic Demyelinating Neuropathy

Acquired demyelinating neuropathies are categorized into acute and chronic forms. The acute form is called *Guillain-Barré syndrome* and is described in the section that follows (Table 7.8). The chronic form is referred to by several titles: the two most commonly used are *chronic inflammatory demyelinating polyradiculoneuropathy* and *chronic relapsing dysimmune polyneuropathy*. The acute and chronic forms may be

Table 7.8 ACUTE GENERALIZED WEAKNESS

Infectious disorders
Enterovirus infections
Guillain-Barré syndrome
Acute infectious myositis
Neuromuscular blockade
Tick paralysis
Myasthenia gravis
Botulism
Periodic paralysis
Hypokalemic
Hyperkalemic
Normokalemic
Acute intermittent porphyria

difficult to distinguish from each other at the onset of symptoms, but are identified by their subsequent course.

It is generally believed that the chronic demyelinating neuropathies, like the Guillain-Barré syndrome, are immune mediated. However, while a clear relationship exists between the Guillain-Barré syndrome and a preceding viral infection, the provocative stimulus for chronic demyelinating neuropathies is unknown.

Clinical Features. Chronic demyelinating neuropathy affects adults more often than children, but may be present even at birth (see Chapter 6). The usual presenting symptoms are both weakness and paresthesias in the distal portions of the limbs; only rarely is there only motor or only sensory involvement. The course may be steadily progressive, stepwise, or characterized by recurrent episodes of acute polyradiculoneuropathy with only partial or complete recovery between episodes. Whichever the course, there is some evidence of progression for at least six months and sometimes several years. There must not be evidence of a positive family history of a similar disorder, other organ involvement, or abnormal storage of material in nerves.

Diagnosis. The protein content of the cerebrospinal fluid is always elevated, and a small number of mononuclear cells may be present as well. Motor nerve conduction velocity is slow (Dalakas and Engel, 1981).

Acquired demyelinating neuropathies in children can be differentiated from familial demyelinating neuropathies by electrodiagnosis. Acquired neuropathies demonstrate a multifocal disturbance of conduction velocity, whereas in hereditary disorders there is uniform slowing of conduction throughout the entire length of the nerve (Miller et al, 1985).

Treatment. Prednisone is considered the treatment of choice (Dyck et al, 1982). A relapsing course may occur spontaneously or may be related to the intermittent use of prednisone. Patients who respond to prednisone frequently relapse when prednisone is withdrawn. Therapy should be initiated with relatively high doses of prednisone, 2 mg/kg/day, not to exceed 100 mg and then changed to alternate-day therapy. Because of the relapsing nature of the disease, it is wise to maintain low-dose corticosteroid therapy for several years.

Chronic Axonal Neuropathy

Clinical Features. Most axonal neuropathies are either hereditary or toxic. Glue sniffing is an example of a toxic cause. Occasionally, children are encountered with a progressive axonal neuropathy for which no etiology can be determined. Most often, the initial symptom is progressive weakness of the feet, with or without sensory findings. Parents and siblings should be studied by electrodiagnosis to be certain that they are not involved (Dyck et al, 1981).

Giant axonal neuropathy is a clinically distinct syndrome, probably caused by an unidentified inborn error of metabolism (Carpenter et al, 1974). Gait impairment begins after age two. Affected children have curly, pale hair with decreased disulfide bonds and increased thiol groups.

Diagnosis. The EMG demonstrates fibrillations and fasciculations, but motor nerve conduction velocity is either normal or only mildly delayed. The protein content of the cerebrospinal fluid is normal. Axonal enlargement is observed by sural nerve biopsy in giant axonal neuropathy and in glue sniffing. The former is characterized by tightly packed neurofilaments and the latter by disrupted neurofilaments.

Treatment. Children with idiopathic axonal neuropathy usually have a slowly progressive weakness that does not respond to corticosteroids. It is only in acquired chronic demyelinating neuropathies that corticosteroids are indicated.

MYOPATHIES

Myotonic Dystrophy

Myotonic dystrophy is a multisystem disorder transmitted by autosomal dominant inheritance with variable penetrance. The onset of symptoms is usually during adolescence or later. A neonatal form, which occurs in children born to mothers with myotonic dystrophy, is described in Chapter 6.

Clinical Features. The major features are myotonia (a disturbance in muscle relaxation after contraction), weakness in the face and distal portion of the limbs, cataracts, frontal baldness, and multiple endocrinopathies. The pattern of muscle atrophy in the face is so stereotyped that all patients with the disease have a similar facies. The face is long and thin because of wasting of the temporal and masseter muscles, and the neck is thin because of atrophy of the sternocleidomastoid muscles. The eyelids and corners of the mouth droop, and the lower part of the face sags, producing the appearance of sadness.

Although patients rarely present to the physician before adolescence or adult life, myotonia is usually present in childhood and can be detected by the EMG, if not clinically. Myotonia is demonstrated by percussion of muscle, usually the thenar eminence, which dimples and remains dimpled at the site of percussion. In addition, the thumb abducts and remains in that position for several seconds. Myotonia can also be demonstrated by shaking hands with the patient. There is difficulty in letting go, and grip is released in part by forcing the flexors of the fingers open by flexion of the wrist.

Some patients have little or no evidence of muscle weakness, only cataracts, frontal baldness, or endocrine disturbances. However, when muscle weakness is present before age twenty, it is likely to be relentlessly progressive, causing severe distal weakness in the hands and feet by middle or adult life. Smooth and cardiac muscle involvement may be present and is characterized by disturbed gastrointestinal motility. Endocrine disturbances include testicular atrophy, infertility in women, hyperinsulinism, adrenal atrophy, and disturbances in growth hormone secretion.

Diagnosis. The diagnosis of myotonic dystrophy is usually based on clinical features and family history. EMG studies demonstrate myotonia (the appearance of motor unit potentials that wax and wane in amplitude and frequency), myopathic potentials, and involvement of peripheral large diameter motor and sensory fibers (Jamal et al, 1986).

Studies of muscle histology reveal a combination of internal nuclei and type I fiber atrophy. In addition, some fibers contain fibrils that are oriented in the wrong plane (ringbinden) and have undergone degeneration (sarcoplasmic masses). The serum concentration of creatine kinase is elevated.

Treatment. Myotonia frequently responds to drugs that stabilize membranes: quinidine, procainamide, phenytoin, and carbamazepine. However, it is weakness, for which there is no treatment, and not myotonia that disables the patient. Braces for footdrop are usually required as the disease progresses.

Hereditary Distal Myopathies

There are two different clinical forms of hereditary distal myopathy that run true within families. One occurs in infancy (Bautista et al, 1978) and the other in young adult life (Markesbery et al, 1974). Sporadic cases with early adult onset are reported as well. In one family, the father had late-onset oculopharyngeal dystrophy and his son had an infantile-onset distal myopathy (Fukuhara et al, 1982). It is not clear at the present time which of the hereditary distal myopathies are genetically distinct. All are transmitted by autosomal dominant inheritance.

Infant Onset

Clinical Features. Hereditary distal myopathy with onset in infancy begins anytime during the first two years. The first signs are footdrop and weakness in the hand extensors. There is little or no progression throughout the remainder of childhood. Occasionally, children demonstrate pseudohypertrophy of the calves, scoliosis, or pes cavus.

Diagnosis. Creatine kinase levels are usually normal, but the EMG demonstrates brief, small-amplitude polyphasic potentials; occasional fibrillations; and myotonia. Muscle biopsy reveals fiber type disproportion in which type I fibers are more numerous, but smaller in size, than type II fibers.

Treatment. Treatment is not available.

Adult Onset

Clinical Features. Adult-onset hereditary distal myopathy usually begins after age twenty and frequently not until middle life. The first symptoms are weakness of the hands and feet with very slow progression throughout adulthood.

Diagnosis. The serum concentration of creatine kinase is usually elevated, and the EMG reveals brief, small-amplitude polyphasic potentials. Muscle histology is variable and generally demonstrates fiber size variation, central nuclei, and vacuoles. Both fiber types are affected.

Treatment. Treatment is not available.

SCAPULO(HUMERAL)PERONEAL SYNDROMES

Progressive weakness and atrophy affecting the proximal muscles of the arms and the distal muscles of the legs may result from neuronopathy or myopathy, but most often the patients have features of both nerve and muscle disease.

Spinal Muscular Atrophy

Clinical Features. Scapuloperoneal neuronopathy is most often transmitted by autosomal dominant inheritance. The onset of symptoms is usually during adult life, but can be as early as the first decade. Weakness begins in the muscles around the shoulder, the anterior compartment of the legs, or both simultaneously. There is some spread to the proximal muscles of the legs, and the face may be involved as well. Tendon reflexes are lost early. The rate of progression is very slow.

Most cases of scapuloperoneal atrophy of early onset are either sporadic or believed to be transmitted by autosomal recessive inheritance (Mercelis et al, 1980). The initial symptoms are footdrop, followed later by weakness in the muscles of the shoulder girdle. The disease progresses relatively rapidly and may involve the forearms, hands, and occasionally the face. Although the disease is disabling, prolonged survivals are recorded.

Diagnosis. In both the autosomal dominant and the autosomal recessive forms, the concentration of serum creatine kinase is normal. The EMG may show mixed features of myopathy and neuropathy. Muscle biopsy is consistent either with a denervating process or with type I atrophy.

Treatment. Treatment is not available.

Emery-Dreifuss Muscular Dystrophy

This is an X-linked recessive muscle disease with onset between the ages of five and fifteen years (Merlini et al, 1986). A disorder identical to Emery-Dreifuss syndrome has also been described with transmission by autosomal dominant inheritance (Fenichel et al, 1982).

Clinical Features. The earliest feature of disease is the development of contractures in the flexors of the elbows, the Achilles tendon, and the extensors of the hand. This is followed by muscle weakness and wasting in the biceps and triceps and then the deltoid and other shoulder muscles. The peroneal muscles are severely affected in the legs. Calf hypertrophy does not occur. The progression of symptoms is very slow, and most patients stabilize by age twenty. In others, weakness progresses into adult life and ambulation is lost. In all patients, a cardio-myopathy develops with permanent atrial paralysis. Bradycardia and syncope may precede muscle weakness or be delayed until the third decade. The arrhythmia, if not treated by use of a permanent pacemaker, may be the cause of stroke and death.

Diagnosis. The EMG may demonstrate features of denervation and myopathy in the same patient or may be myopathic in one sibling and neuropathic in another. The most prominent feature on muscle biopsy is type I fiber atrophy. This histologic pattern is seen in many congenital myopathies in which it is uncertain whether the primary disease is in nerve or muscle (see Chapter 6). At the present time, there is reason to consider this disorder a dystrophy because of the early presence of muscle contractures and the absence of characteristic denervation patterns on biopsy.

Treatment. No treatment is available for the muscle weakness and wasting, but cardiac arrhythmia should be treated early by implantation of a permanent pacemaker.

Scapulohumeral Syndrome with Dementia

This disorder is transmitted by X-linked inheritance (Bergia et al, 1986).

Clinical Features. Affected children appear normal until age five and then develop mental deterioration, first recognized as a learning disability and then mental retardation. Weakness and atrophy of the scapular or humeral muscles and peroneal muscles follow shortly thereafter. Contractures do not develop in affected muscles, and pseudohypertrophy is not present. Symptomatic cardiomyopathy occurs during adolescence and proves fatal.

Diagnosis. This disorder is distinguished from Emery-Dreifuss dystrophy by the absence of contractures and the presence of mental deterioration. The EMG demonstrates a mixed myopathic-neuropathic pattern and muscle biopsy reveals excessive internal nuclei and fiber splitting. Serum CK concentration is elevated.

Treatment. Treatment is not available for the underlying disease. Fatalities may be prevented only by heart transplant.

■ Acute Generalized Weakness

The sudden onset or rapid evolution of generalized flaccid weakness, in the absence of symptoms of encephalopathy, is always due to disorders of the motor unit. Among the disorders listed in Table 7.5, acute polyradiculoneuropathy (the Guillain-Barré syndrome [GBS]) is by far the most common.

INFECTIOUS DISEASE

Enterovirus Infections

Poliovirus, coxsackievirus, and the echovirus group are small RNA viruses that inhabit the intestinal tract of humans. They are neurotropic and produce paralytic disease by destroying the motor neurons of the brainstem and spinal cord. Poliovirus causes the most severe and devastating disease in this group. Coxsackie and echoviruses are more likely to cause aseptic meningitis, but may also produce an acute paralytic syndrome similar to poliomyelitis.

Clinical Features. Enterovirus infections occur in epidemics during the spring and summer. The most common manifestation of poliovirus infection is a brief illness characterized by fever, malaise, and gastrointestinal symptoms. Aseptic meningitis occurs in more severe cases. The extreme situation is paralytic poliomyelitis. It begins with fever, sore throat, and malaise lasting one to two days. After a brief period of apparent well-being, fever recurs in association with headache, vomiting, and signs of meningeal irritation. Pain in the limbs or over the spine is an antecedent symptom of limb paralysis. Flaccid muscle weakness develops rapidly thereafter. The pattern of muscle weakness may vary from patient to patient, but it is generally asymmetric. One arm or leg is affected more than are other limbs.

Bulbar polio may occur with or without spinal cord disease and is life-threatening. Such children have prolonged episodes of apnea and require respiratory assistance. Several motor cranial nerves may be involved as well, but the extraocular muscles are spared.

The introduction of inactivated poliomyelitis vaccine in 1954, followed by the use of attenuated live poliomyelitis vaccine in 1960, has almost abolished the disease. Almost all presently reported cases are vaccine-related. Approximately one healthy child in 12 million immunized with trivalent oral polio vaccine will develop paralytic poliomyelitis. Most cases occur following the first immunization (Nkowane et al, 1987).

Diagnosis. The diagnosis can be suspected from clinical findings and confirmed by isolation and viral typing from stool and nasopharynx. The cerebrospinal fluid initially demonstrates a polymorphonuclear reaction with the cell count ranging from 50 to 200 per cu mm. After a week, lymphocytes predominate; after two to three weeks, the total cell count decreases. The protein content is elevated early and remains elevated for several months.

Treatment. Treatment, other than supportive care, is not available.

Acute Polyradiculoneuropathy
(Guillain-Barré Syndrome)

Guillain-Barré syndrome (GBS) is an acute, monophasic demyelinating neuropathy. It is generally accepted that the syndrome is immunologically mediated. More than 50 percent of patients describe an antecedent viral infection. Respiratory tract infections are most common, and the remainder are mainly gastrointestinal infections. There is some evidence that herpesviruses, especially Epstein-Barr virus and cytomegalovirus may cause a substantial number of cases (Dowling and Cook, 1981).

Clinical Features. Diagnostic criteria for GBS were developed in response to the increased incidence of cases following the swine flu vaccination program of 1976 (Asbury, 1981). In typical cases, the clinical features are so stereotyped that the diagnosis is established without laboratory confirmation. This is especially important, since the characteristic laboratory features of Guillain-Barré syndrome may not be present at the onset of clinical symptoms.

The two essential features of the Guillain-Barré syndrome are progressive motor weakness involving more than one limb and areflexia. Weakness is frequently preceded by insidious sensory symptoms that are usually ignored. These consist of fleeting dysesthesias and muscle tenderness in limbs that are soon to become paralytic. Weakness progresses rapidly, and approximately 50 percent of patients will reach a nadir by two weeks, 80 percent by three weeks, and the rest by four weeks. The weakness may be ascending or descending but is relatively symmetric qualitatively, if not quantitatively. Universal areflexia is the

rule and, if not present initially, is always present in weak muscles. Bilateral facial weakness occurs in half of cases. Autonomic dysfunction, characterized by arrhythmia, labile blood pressure, and gastrointestinal dysfunction, may be present as well.

Recovery of function usually begins two to four weeks after progression stops. In children, recovery is almost always complete. Prognosis is best when recovery begins early. The major concern in children with Guillain-Barré syndrome is that the muscular weakness will progress to respiratory paralysis and death. If the patient's respiratory function can be supported during the critical time of profound paralysis, complete recovery is to be expected.

Diagnosis. The concentration of protein in the cerebrospinal fluid is elevated after the first week of symptoms. During the first week, there are frequently ten or fewer mononuclear leukocytes per cu mm in the cerebrospinal fluid; however, these rapidly disappear and none are found in subsequent weeks. Approximately 90 percent of patients will have evidence of demyelinating lesions when electrodiagnostic studies are performed (McLeod, 1981). Since the proximal portion of the nerve is affected more than the distal portion, motor nerve conduction velocities and sensory latencies may be normal early in the course. The patchy demyelination can be demonstrated by abnormalities of the F wave response. The presence of abundant spontaneous fibrillations and other evidence of axonal degeneration is associated with a poor prognosis for complete recovery or at least a slower rate of recovery.

Treatment. In children who present with Guillain-Barré syndrome, respiratory function must be carefully monitored. If vital capacity falls rapidly to less than 50 percent of normal, an endotracheal tube should be placed. Most children who require respiratory support will need that support for several weeks, and many will require tracheostomy. Adequate control of respiration should completely prevent death from the disorder. Corticosteroids are not helpful in treatment, in that they may produce some initial improvement but tend to prolong the course. In severe cases, plasmapheresis has been shown to shorten the course in adults (The Guillain-Barré Syndrome Study Group, 1985). It is probably useful in children as well, but should be used selectively. The overall prognosis in children is excellent with only supportive care, and potentially dangerous procedures are rarely indicated.

ACUTE INFECTIOUS MYOSITIS

Acute myositis in children occurs most often secondary to influenza or other respiratory infections.

Clinical Features. Ordinarily, prodromal respiratory symptoms persist for one to seven days before the onset of severe symmetric muscle pain and weakness, which may lead to severe disability within twenty-four hours (McKinley and Mitchell, 1976). Proximal muscles are more severely affected than distal muscles, but generalized weakness may be present. The muscles are very tender to palpation. Tendon reflexes are present.

Diagnosis. The serum concentration of creatine kinase is elevated, usually more than ten times the upper limit of normal.

Treatment. Spontaneous resolution of the myositis occurs almost immediately. Bed rest is required for two to seven days until pain subsides, after which there is complete recovery.

NEUROMUSCULAR BLOCKADE

Tick Paralysis

The female of several species of North American ticks elaborates a salivary gland toxin that induces paralysis (Swift and Ignacio, 1975).

Clinical Features. The clinical syndrome is similar to the Guillain-Barré syndrome. There is rapid development of a severe generalized flaccid weakness, sometimes associated with bifacial palsy. Tendon reflexes are usually absent or greatly depressed. Dysesthesias may be present at the onset of weakness, but loss of sensation cannot be demonstrated on examination.

Diagnosis. The cerebrospinal fluid protein concentration is normal. Electrophysiologic studies demonstrate slowing of conduction velocities. The possibility of tick paralysis should be considered during the spring and summer in any child who presents with Guillain-Barré syndrome and has a normal protein content in the cerebrospinal fluid.

Treatment. Strength returns quickly once the tick is removed. However, the tick may be hard to find, frequently hidden in body hair.

Myasthenia Gravis

Myasthenia gravis is usually thought of as a slowly progressive disorder with fluctuations in strength in relation to exercise. It also occurs in a fulminating form in which generalized weakness progresses to respiratory distress within twelve to eighteen hours (Bastedo, 1950). Bulbar paralysis as well as limb paralysis is present. The rapid progression of limb weakness and respiratory insufficiency suggests the diagnosis of poliomyelitis.

Diagnosis. Cerebrospinal fluid is normal, as are most routine electrodiagnostic studies. Myasthenia should be at least suspected in every child with acute generalized weakness. The Tensilon test is critical to the diagnosis.

Treatment. The treatment of myasthenia is discussed in the section on limb-girdle myasthenia in this chapter and also in Chapters 5 and 15.

Botulism

Clostridium botulinum produces a toxin that interferes with the release of acetylcholine at the neuromuscular junction. An infantile form of botulism is described in Chapter 6, but most cases occur after infancy in individuals who ingest food, usually preserved at home, contaminated with the organism (Cherington, 1974).

Clinical Features. The first symptoms are blurred vision, diplopia, dizziness, dysarthria, and dysphagia, which have their onset twelve to thirty-six hours after the ingestion of toxin. Some patients have only bulbar signs; in others, flaccid paralysis develops in all limbs. Patients with generalized weakness always have ophthalmoplegia, but the pupillary response is usually spared. Tendon reflexes may be present or absent.

Diagnosis. Repetitive supermaximal nerve stimulation at a rate of 20 to 50/second produces an incremental response characteristic of a presynaptic defect. The electrical abnormality evolves with time and may not be demonstrable in all limbs on any given day.

Treatment. Botulism can be fatal because of respiratory depression. Treatment relies primarily on supportive care, which is similar to the management of patients with Guillain-Barré syndrome. Antitoxin does not influence the course of disease. Guanidine hydrochloride, a drug that enhances the release of acetylcholine from nerve terminals, may be of some benefit at an average dose of 250 mg every six hours in adults. In children and in adults, the dose should be titrated to the degree of weakness. Recovery is prolonged when paralysis has been severe, but all patients recover completely.

PERIODIC PARALYSES

The periodic paralyses are usually classified in relation to serum potassium: (1) hypokalemic, (2) hyperkalemic, and (3) normokalemic. In addition, periodic paralysis may be primary (genetically transmitted) or secondary. Secondary hypokalemic periodic paralysis is caused by urinary or gastrointestinal loss of potassium. Urinary loss accompanies primary hyperaldosteronism, licorice intoxication, amphotericin-B therapy, and several renal tubular defects. Gastrointestinal loss most often occurs with severe chronic diarrhea, prolonged gastrointestinal intubation and vomiting, and a draining gastrointestinal fistula. Hypokalemic periodic paralysis is also seen with thyrotoxicoses, especially in Orientals. Secondary hyperkalemic periodic paralysis is associated with renal or adrenal insufficiency.

Familial Hypokalemic Periodic Paralysis

This disorder is transmitted by autosomal dominant inheritance with decreased penetrance in women.

Clinical Features. The onset of symptoms occurs before sixteen years of age in 60 percent of cases and by twenty years of age in the remainder. Attacks of paralysis are at first infrequent, but then may occur several times a week. Factors that trigger an attack include rest after exercise (therefore, many attacks occur in the early hours of the morning); a large meal with high carbohydrate content; emotional or physical stress; alcohol ingestion; and exposure to cold. Preceding and during the attack there may be excessive thirst and oliguria. The weakness begins with a sensation of aching in the proximal muscles. Sometimes, only the proximal muscles are affected; at other times, there is complete paralysis so that the patient cannot even raise the head. Facial muscles are rarely affected, and extraocular muscles are never disturbed. Respiratory distress does not occur. When the weakness is most extreme, the muscles feel swollen and the tendon reflexes are absent. Most attacks last for six to twelve hours and some for the whole day. Strength recovers rapidly, but after several attacks residual weakness may be present.

Diagnosis. During the attack, serum potassium concentrations may fall to 1.5 mEq/L (1.5 mmol/L) and are associated with EKG changes: bradycardia, flattening of T waves, and prolon-

gation of the PR and QT intervals. The muscle is electrically silent and not excitable. Attacks can be provoked by the oral administration of glucose, 2 g/kg, with 10–20 units of crystalline insulin given subcutaneously. Serum potassium falls, and an attack of paralysis is initiated within two to three hours.

Treatment. Treatment of the acute attack in patients with good renal function is by repeated oral doses of potassium. In adolescents, 5 to 10 g is used. Smaller amounts should be considered for younger children. Daily use of acetazolamide is beneficial in many families to prevent attacks from occurring (Griggs et al, 1970).

Familial Hyperkalemic Periodic Paralysis

This disorder is transmitted by autosomal dominant inheritance and occurs with equal frequency in both sexes. Myotonia of the eyelids, face, and hands is sometimes associated, and such cases are described under the title *paramyotonia congenita.*

Clinical Features. The onset of weakness is in early childhood and sometimes in infancy. Like hypokalemic periodic paralysis, attacks may be provoked by rest shortly after exercise has ended. However, only moderate amounts of exercise are required. Weakness begins with a sensation of heaviness in the back and leg muscles. Sometimes the patient can delay the paralysis by walking or moving about. In infants and small children, the attacks are characterized by an episode of floppiness in which the child lies around and will not move. In older children and adults, both mild and severe attacks may occur. Mild attacks last for less than an hour and do not produce complete paralysis. More than one mild attack may occur in a day. Severe attacks are similar to the complete flaccid paralysis seen in hypokalemic periodic paralysis and may last for several hours. Residual weakness may persist after several severe attacks.

Diagnosis. Myotonia in patients with hyperkalemic periodic paralysis is mild and sometimes is demonstrated only on exposure to cold. To do this, a towel soaked in ice water is laid over the eyes for a few minutes. The patient is then asked to look upward briefly and then to look down quickly. When there is myotonia of the eyelids, the lids cannot come down quickly and a rim of sclera is exposed.

During attacks, the serum concentration of potassium increases but may not increase sufficiently to be abnormal. When potassium concentrations are very high, the EKG demonstrates changes consistent with hyperkalemia. The oral administration of potassium chloride given just after exercise in the fasting state provokes an attack. During the attack, the muscles are electrically silent.

Acute attacks seldom require treatment, since they are brief. Daily administration of acetazolamide is useful to prevent recurrence of attacks (Hoskins and Vroom, 1975). It is not clear why acetazolamide acts to prevent both hyperkalemic and hypokalemic periodic paralysis. The effect is apparently through stabilization of the muscle membrane.

Familial Normokalemic Periodic Paralysis

There are several families reported in the literature with an autosomal dominant inherited periodic paralysis in which no alteration in serum concentration of potassium can be detected. Some of these may represent cases of hyperkalemic period paralysis in which the flux of potassium into the serum was insufficient to be detected.

Acute Intermittent Porphyria

Acute intermittent porphyria is transmitted by autosomal dominant inheritance. It is characterized by at least 50 percent deficiency in the activity of porphobilinogen deaminase. Patients with similar degrees of enzyme deficiency may have considerable variation in phenotypic expression (Kappas et al, 1983).

Clinical Features. Approximately 90 percent of individuals with this disorder never have clinical symptoms. The minority who do become symptomatic have no difficulty before puberty. Symptoms and signs are periodic and occur at irregular intervals. The attacks are triggered by alterations in hormonal levels during a normal menstrual cycle or pregnancy and by exposure to certain drugs, of which barbiturates are especially notorious. Most attacks begin with abdominal pain, which is often followed by nausea and vomiting. Pain in the limbs is common, and many patients develop muscle weakness as well. The weakness is due to a motor neuropathy that causes greater weakness in proximal than distal muscles and in the arms more than the legs. Tendon reflexes are usually decreased and may be absent in weak muscles. Approximately half of patients have symptoms of cerebral dysfunction; mental changes are particularly com-

mon, and seizures can sometimes occur. Hypertension and tachycardia may accompany attacks. Chronic mental symptoms, such as depression and anxiety, sometimes continue even between attacks.

Diagnosis. Diagnosis is made by measuring porphobilinogen deaminase activity in red blood cells and urine.

Treatment. The most important aspect of managing patients with symptomatic disease is to prevent acute attacks. This is done in part by avoiding known precipitating factors. During an attack, patients frequently need to be hospitalized because of severe pain. Carbohydrates are believed to reduce porphyrin synthesis and should be administered intravenously daily at a dose of 300 to 500 grams as a 10 percent dextrose solution. More recently, intravenous infusions of hematin have been used and are said to be useful both in treating the acute attacks and as a preventive measure.

References

1. Angelini C, Engel AG: Comparative study of acid maltase deficiency. Biochemical differences between infantile, childhood, and adult types. Arch Neurol 26:344, 1972.
2. Asbury AK, Diagnostic considerations in Guillain-Barré syndrome. Ann Neurol 9:1, 1981.
3. Askansas V, Engel WK, Kwan HH, et al: Autosomal dominant syndrome of lipid neuromyopathy with normal carnitine: Successful treatment with long-chain fatty-acid-free diet. Neurology 35:66, 1985.
4. Bach JR, O'Brien J, Krotenberg R, et al: Management of end stage respiratory failure in Duchenne muscular dystrophy. Muscle Nerve 10:177, 1987.
5. Bailey RO, Marzulo DC, Hans MB: Infantile facioscapulohumeral muscular dystrophy: new observations. Acta Neurol Scand 74:51, 1986.
6. Bastedo DLA: Acute fulminating myasthenia gravis in children. Can Med Assoc J 63:388, 1950.
7. Bautista J, Rafel E, Castilla A, et al: Hereditary distal myopathy with onset in early infancy. J Neurol Sci 37:149, 1978.
8. Berciano J, Combarros O, Figols J, et al: Hereditary motor and sensory neuropathy Type II. Brain 109:897, 1986.
9. Bergia B, Sybers HD, Butler IJ: Familial lethal cardiomyopathy with mental retardation and scapuloperoneal muscular dystrophy. J Neurol Neurosurg Psychiatry 49:1423, 1986.
10. Bodensteiner JB, Schochet SS: Facioscapulohumeral muscular dystrophy: The choice of a biopsy site. Muscle Nerve 9:544, 1986.
11. Bowyer SL, Blane CE, Sullivan DB, et al: Childhood dermatomyositis: Factors predicting functional outcome and development of dystrophic calcification. J Pediatr 103:882, 1982.
12. Brooke MH, Fenichel GM, Griggs RC, et al: Clinical investigation in Duchenne dystrophy: 2. Determination

of the "power" of therapeutic trials based on the natural history. Muscle Nerve 6:91, 1983.

13. Brooke MH, Fenichel GM, Griggs RC, et al: Clinical investigation of Duchenne muscular dystrophy: Interesting results in a trial of prednisone. Arch Neurol 44: 812, 1987.

14. Bundey S, Lovelace RE: A clinical and genetic study of chronic proximal spinal muscular atrophy. Brain 98:455, 1975.

15. Carpenter S, Karpati G, Andermann F, et al: Giant axonal neuropathy. Arch Neurol 31:312, 1974.

16. Carroll JE, Brooke MH, Villadiego A, et al: "Dystrophic" lipid myopathy in two sisters. Arch Neurol 43:128, 1986.

17. Casey EB, Jellife AM, LeQuesne PM, et al: Vincristine neuropathy. Clinical and electrophysiological observations. Brain 96:69, 1973.

18. Cherington M: Botulism. Arch Neurol 30:432, 1974.

19. Cohen AS, Rubinow A: Amyloid neuropathy. In Dyck PJ, Thomas PK, Lambert EH, Bunge R, eds. Peripheral Neuropathy. WB Saunders Co, Philadelphia, 1984, p 1866.

20. Coleman WP III, Coleman WP, Derbes VJ, et al: Collagen disease in children. A review of 71 cases. JAMA 237:1095, 1977.

21. Dalakas MC, Engel WK: Chronic relapsing (dysimmune) polyneuropathy: pathogenesis and treatment. Ann Neurol 9:134, 1981.

22. DiMauro S, Bonilla E, Zeviani M, et al: Mitochondrial myopathies. Ann Neurol 17:521, 1985.

23. Dobkin BH, Verity MA: Familial neuromuscular disease with type I fiber hypoplasia, tubular aggregates, cardiomyopathy, and myasthenic features. Neurology 28:1135, 1978.

24. Dowling PC, Cook SD: Role of infection in Guillain-Barré syndrome: Laboratory confirmation of herpesviruses in 41 cases. Ann Neurol 9:44, 1981.

25. Dyck PJ: Inherited neuronal degeneration and atrophy affecting peripheral motor, sensory, and autonomic neurons. In Dyck PJ, Thomas PK, Lambert EH, Bunge R, eds. Peripheral Neuropathy. WB Saunders Co, Philadelphia, 1984, p 1600.

26. Dyck PJ, O'Brien PC, Oviatt KF, et al: Prednisone improves chronic inflammatory demyelinating polyradiculoneuropathy more than no treatment. Ann Neurol 11:136, 1982.

27. Dyck PJ, Oviatt KF, Lambert EH: Intensive evaluation of referred unclassified neuropathies yields improved diagnosis. Ann Neurol 10:222, 1981.

28. Evans OB: Polyneuropathy in childhood. Pediatrics 64:96, 1979.

29. Fenichel GM: Clinical syndromes of myasthenia gravis in infancy and childhood. Arch Neurol 35:97, 1978.

30. Fenichel GM, Sul YC, Kilroy AW, et al: An autosomal-dominant dystrophy with humeropelvic distribution and cardiomyopathy. Neurology 32:1399, 1982.

31. Fukuhara N, Kumamoto T, Tsubaki T, et al: Oculopharyngeal muscular dystrophy and distal myopathy. Intrafamilial difference in the onset and distribution of muscular involvement. Acta Neurol Scand 65:458, 1982.

32. Gibberd FB, Page NGR, Billimoria JD, et al: Heredopathia actactica polyneuritiformis (Refsum's disease) treated by diet and plasma-exchange. Lancet 1:575, 1979.

33. Griggs RC, Engel WK, Resnick JS: Acetazolamide treatment of hypokalemic periodic paralysis. Ann Int Med 73:39, 1970.

34. Griggs RC, Mendell JR, Brooke MH, et al: Clinical

investigation in Duchenne dystrophy: V. Use of creatine kinase and pyruvate kinase in carrier detection. Muscle Nerve 8:60, 1985.

35. Hagberg B, Lyon G: Pooled European series of hereditary peripheral neuropathies in infancy and childhood. Neuropediatria 12:9, 1981.

36. Harding AE, Thomas PK: Hereditary distal spinal muscular atrophy. A report on 34 cases and a review of the literature. J Neurol Sci 45:337, 1980.

37. Hausmanowa-Petrusewicz I, Zaremba J. Borkowska J: Chronic form of childhood spinal muscular atrophy. Are the problems of its genetics really solved? J Neurol Sci 43:317, 1979.

38. Henriksson K-G, Sandstedt P: Polymyositis—treatment and prognosis. Acta Neurol Scand 65:280, 1982.

39. Hoskins B, Vroom FQ: Hyperkalemic periodic paralysis: Effects of potassium, exercise, glucose and acetazolamide on blood chemistry. Arch Neurol 32:519, 1975.

40. Jamal GA, Weir AI, Hansen S, et al: Myotonic dystrophy. A reassessment by conventional and more recently introduced neurophysiological techniques. Brain 109:1279, 1986.

41. Johns TR, Campa J, Adelman L: Familial myasthenia with "tubular aggregates" treated with prednisone (abstract). Neurology 23:426, 1973.

42. Kappas A, Sassa S, Anderson KE: The prophyrias. In Stanbury JB, Wyngaarden JB, Fredrickson DS, et al, eds. The Metabolic Basis of Inherited Disease. 5th edition. McGraw-Hill, New York, 1983, p 1301.

43. Lander CM, Eadie MJ, Tyrer JH: Hereditary motor peripheral neuropathy predominantly affecting the arms. J Neurol Sci 28:389, 1976.

44. Loonen MCB, Busch HFM, Koster JF, et al: A family with different clinical forms of acid maltase deficiency (glycogenosis type II): Biochemical and genetic studies. Neurology 3l:1209, 1981.

45. Mantovani JF, Vidgoff J, Cass M: Brain dysfunction in an adolescent with the neuromuscular form of hexosaminidase deficiency. Dev Med Child Neurol 27:664, 1985.

46. Markesbery WR, Griggs RC, Leach RP, et al: Late onset hereditary distal myopathy. Neurology 24:127, 1974.

47. Martin J-J, Ceuterick C, Mercelis R, et al: Pathology of peripheral nerves in metachromatic leucodystrophy: a comparative study of ten cases. J Neurol Sci 53:95, 1982.

48. Martyn C, Jellinek EH, Webb JN: Lipid storage myopathy: successful treatment with propanolol. Br Med J 282:1997, 1981.

49. Mastaglia FL, Ojeda VJ: Inflammatory myopathies, parts 1 and 2. Ann Neurol 17:215, 1985; 18:317, 1985.

50. McGonigle RJS, Bewick M, Weston MJ, et al: Progressive, predominantly motor, uraemic neuropathy. Acta Neurol Scand 71:379, 1985.

51. McKinley IA, Mitchell A: Transient acute myositis in childhood. Arch Dis Child 51:135, 1976.

52. McLeod JG: Electrophysiological studies in the Guillain-Barré syndrome. Ann Neurol 9:20, 1981.

53. McLeod JG, Baker WC, Shorey CD, et al: Mitochondrial myopathy with multisystem abnormalities and normal ocular movements. J Neurol Sci 24:39, 1975

54. McQuillen M: Familial limb-girdle myasthenia. Brain 89:121, 1966.

55. Meadows JC, Marsden CD: A distal form of chronic spinal muscular atrophy. Neurology 19:53, 1969.

56. Mercelis R, Demeester J, Martin J-J: Neurogenic scapuloperoneal syndrome in childhood. J Neurol Neurosurg Psychiatry 10:888, 1980.

57. Merlini L, Granata C, Dominici P, et al: Emery-Dreifuss

muscular dystrophy: Report of five cases in a family and review of the literature. Muscle Nerve 9:481, 1986.

58. Miller RG, Gutmann L, Lewis RA, et al: Acquired versus familial demyelinative neuropathies in children. Muscle Nerve 8:205, 1985.

59. Moser H: Duchenne muscular dystrophy: Pathogenetic aspects and genetic prevention. Hum Genet 66:17, 1984.

60. Nkowane BH, Wassilak SGF, Orenstein WA: Vaccine associated paralytic poliomyelitis. United States: 1973 through 1984. JAMA 257:1335, 1987.

61. Ohnishi A, Mitsudome A, Murai Y: Primary segmental demyelination in the sural nerve in Cockayne's syndrome. Muscle Nerve 10:163, 1987.

62. Olson BJ, Fenichel GM: Progressive muscle disease in a young woman with family history of Duchenne's muscular dystrophy. Arch Neurol 39:378, 1982.

63. Ouvrier RA, McLeod JG, Conchin TE: The hypertrophic forms of hereditary motor and sensory neuropathy. A study of hypertrophic Charcot-Marie-Tooth disease (HMSN type I) and Déjérine-Sottas disease (HMSN type III) in childhood. Brain 110:121, 1987.

64. Ouvrier RA, McLeod JG, Morgan GJ, et al: Hereditary motor and sensory neuropathy of neuronal type with onset in early childhood. J Neurol Sci 51:181, 1981.

65. Parnes S, Karpati G, Carpenter S, et al: Hexosaminidase-A deficiency presenting as atypical juvenile-onset spinal muscular atrophy. Arch Neurol 42:1176, 1985.

66. Pearn JH: Incidence, prevalence, and gene-frequency studies of chronic childhood spinal muscular atrophy. J Med Genet 15:409, 1978a.

67. Pearn JH: Autosomal dominant spinal muscular atrophy. A clinical and genetic study. J Neurol Sci 38:263, 1978b.

68. Pearn JH, Bundey S, Carter CO, et al: A genetic study of subacute and chronic spinal muscular atrophy in childhood. A nosological analysis of 124 index patients. J Neurol Sci 227, 1978a.

69. Pearn JH, Hudgson P, Walton JN: A clinical and genetic study of adult-onset spinal muscular atrophy: The autosomal recessive form as a discrete entity. Brain 101:591, 1978b.

70. Petty RKH, Harding AE, Morgan-Hughes JA: The clinical features of mitochondrial myopathy. Brain 109:915, 1986.

71. Rebouche CJ, Engel AG: Carnitine metabolism and deficiency syndromes. Mayo Clin Proc 58:533, 1983.

72. Refsum S: Clinical and genetic aspects of Refsum disease. In Dyck PJ, Thomas PK, Lambert EH, Bunge R, eds. Peripheral Neuropathy. WB Saunders Co, Philadelphia, 1984, p 1680.

73. Riggs JE, Schochet SS, Gutmann L, et al: Lysosomal glycogen storage disease without acid maltase deficiency. Neurology 33:873, 1983.

74. Stumpf DA, Parker WD, Angelini C: Carnitine deficiency, organic acidemias, and Reye's syndrome. Neurology 35:1041, 1985.

75. Swift TR, Ignacio OJ: Tick paralysis: Electrophysiologic studies. Neurology 25:1130, 1975.

76. Taylor DA, Carroll JE, Smith ME, et al: Facioscapulohumeral dystrophy associated with hearing loss and Coats syndrome. Ann Neurol 12:395, 1982.L

77. The Guillain-Barré Study Group: Plasmapheresis and acute Guillain-Barré syndrome. Neurology 35:1096, 1985.

78. Vanasse M, Dubowitz V: Dominantly inherited peroneal muscular atrophy (hereditary motor and sensory neuropathy Type I) in infancy and childhood. Muscle Nerve 4:26, 1981.

79. Vignos PJ Jr: Physical models of rehabilitation in neuromuscular disease. Muscle Nerve 6:323, 1983.

80. Whitaker JN: Inflammatory myopathy: A review of etiologic and pathogenetic factors. Muscle Nerve 5:573, 1982.

81. Wulff JD, Lin JT, Kepes JJ: Inflammatory facioscapulohumeral muscular dystrophy and Coats syndrome. Ann Neurol 12:398, 1982.

82. Zeviani M, Wood DS, Bonilla E, et al: Gene product in Duchenne muscular dystrophy (DMD): Biochemical and morphological data indicate that nebulin is a candidate protein. Neurology 37(Suppl 1):116, 1987.

8 Cramps, Muscle Stiffness, and Exercise Intolerance

A cramp is an involuntary painful contraction of a muscle or part of a muscle. Cramps can occur in normal children during and after vigorous exercise and after excessive loss of fluid or electrolytes. Such cramps are characterized on electromyography (EMG) by the repetitive firing of normal motor unit potentials (Layzer, 1982). Stretching the muscle relieves the cramp, and it is generally believed, though without evidence, that muscle stretching prior to exercise may prevent cramps. Muscle that is partially denervated is particularly susceptible to cramping not only during exercise but also during sleep. Night cramps may awaken patients with neuronopathies, neuropathies, or root compression. Cramps during exercise occur also in patients with several different disorders of muscle energy metabolism. These cramps differ from other cramps in that they are electrically silent.

Muscle stiffness and spasms are sometimes called cramps by patients, but are actually prolonged contractions of several muscles that are able to impose postures. Such contractions may or may not be painful. When painful, they lack the explosive character of cramps (Layzer, 1985). Prolonged contractions occur when muscles fail to relax (myotonia) or when there is continuous motor unit activity (Table 8.1). Prolonged, painless muscle contractions occur also in dystonia and in other movement disorders (see Chapter 14).

Many normal children, especially preadolescent boys, complain of pain in their legs at night and sometimes during the day, especially after a period of increased activity. These pains are not true cramps. The muscle is not in spasm, the pain is diffuse and aching in quality, and the discomfort lasts for an hour or longer. Stretching the muscle does not relieve the pain. This is not a symptom of neuromuscular disease and, for want of better understanding, is usually referred to as *growing pains*. Symptoms are relieved by mild analgesics or heat.

Exercise intolerance is a relative term. Exercise becomes intolerable to everyone at some level. The term is used to include children who become fatigued or develop muscle cramps with only minimal effort. In general, children with weakness due to any neuromuscular disease have some degree of exercise intolerance. Most children with exercise intolerance, but no permanent weakness, have a defect in an enzyme needed to produce energy for muscular contraction (Table 8.2). Several such inborn errors of metabolism have been defined and others are yet to be defined. Even when the full spectrum of biochemical tests is available, there are still some children in whom cramps develop after exercise, and in whom there is clear-cut evidence of muscle disease, but for whom the metabolic defect cannot be identified.

Table 8.1 DISEASES WITH ABNORMAL MUSCLE ACTIVITY

Continuous Motor Unit Activity
1. Spinal (stiffman syndrome)
2. Neural (neuromyotonia)
3. Nerve terminal (Isaacs syndrome)
4. Schwartz-Jampel syndrome

Myotonia Congenita

Systemic Disorders
1. Uremia
2. Thyroid disease
3. Hypocalcemia (tetany)
4. Hypoadrenalism

Table 8.2 DISEASES WITH DECREASED MUSCLE ENERGY

Defects of carbohydrate utilization
  Myophosphorylase deficiency
  Phosphofructokinase deficiency
  Phosphoglycerate kinase deficiency
  Phosphoglycerate mutase deficiency
  Lactate dehydrogenase deficiency
Carnitine palmityltransferase deficiency
Mitochondrial (respiratory chain) myopathies
Myoadenylate deaminase deficiency

Myasthenia gravis is a disorder characterized by exercise intolerance, but it is not covered in this chapter because the usual initial symptoms are either isolated cranial nerve disturbances (see Chapter 15) or generalized weakness (see Chapters 6 and 7).

Conditions that produce some combination of cramps and exercise intolerance can be divided into three groups: (1) diseases with abnormal muscle activity, (2) diseases with decreased energy for muscle contraction, and (3) myopathies. As a rule, the first and third groups are symptomatic at all times, whereas the second group is symptomatic only with exercise.

■ Abnormal Muscle Activity

CONTINUOUS MOTOR UNIT ACTIVITY

The term continuous motor unit activity includes a heterogeneous group of disorders that have in common some combination of muscular pain, fasciculations, myokymia, contractures, and cramps (Table 8.3) (Valli et al, 1983). This group of disorders can be subdivided into those syndromes that are primarily due to dysfunction within the spinal cord (stiffman syndrome), within the peripheral nerve (neuromyotonia), and at the terminal nerve junction (Isaacs syndrome). The term *neuromyotonia* is also used to include Isaacs syndrome.

Table 8.3 ABNORMAL MUSCLE ACTIVITY

Fibrillation: Spontaneous contraction of a single muscle fiber. Not visible through the skin.
Fasciculations: Spontaneous, random twitching of a group of muscle fibers.
Myokymia: Repetitive fasciculations causing a quivering or undulating twitch.
Myotonic Discharges: Disturbance in muscle relaxation following voluntary contraction or percussion.
Neuromyotonia: The combination of generalized myokymia, muscle stiffness, and myotonia.

Disorders with continuous motor unit activity may be sporadic or familial in occurrence. When familial, they are usually transmitted by autosomal dominant inheritance. A major exception is the Schwartz-Jampel syndrome, which is transmitted by autosomal recessive inheritance.

An EMG should be the initial diagnostic test in patients with muscle stiffness that is not due to spasticity or rigidity. It will usually lead to the correct diagnosis (Table 8.4).

The Stiffman Syndrome

This is ordinarily a sporadic disease of adult life affecting both sexes equally. A genetic form, transmitted by autosomal dominant inheritance, has been recognized in children (Sander et al, 1980) and is also called hyperekplexia (Kurczynski, 1983). It is not clear if the genetic form is spinal or cerebral in origin.

Genetic Form

Clinical Features. Stiffness is present at birth and remains severe throughout the neonatal period. Apnea and an exaggerated startle response may be associated. Hypertonia in the newborn is unusual and has a limited differential diagnosis (Table 8.5). Rigidity diminishes, but is

Table 8.4 ELECTROMYOGRAPHY IN MUSCLE STIFFNESS

Normal Between Cramps (or may be myopathic)
1. Defects of carbohydrate metabolism
2. Defects of lipid metabolism
3. Mitochondrial myopathies
4. Myoadenylate deaminase deficiency
5. Brody disease
6. Tubular aggregates

Silent Cramps
1. Defects of carbohydrate metabolism
2. Brody disease
3. Tubular aggregates

Continuous Motor Activity
1. Stiffman syndrome
2. Neuromyotonia
3. Isaacs syndrome
4. Schwartz-Jampel syndrome

Myotonia
1. Myotonia congenita
2. Schwartz-Jampel syndrome

Myopathic
1. Rigid spine
2. Emery-Dreifuss syndrome
3. Trilaminar myopathy

Table 8.5 STIFFNESS (RIGIDITY) IN THE
NEWBORN

Tetany
Tetanus (bacterial)
Schwartz-Jampel syndrome
Stiffman syndrome
Isaacs syndrome
Hyperekplexia
Trilaminar myopathy

not absent, during sleep. Tendon reflexes are brisk and there is an increased spread of response.

The stiffness resolves spontaneously during infancy and by age three the children are normal. However, episodes of stiffness may recur during adolescence or early adult life in response to startle, cold exposure, or pregnancy. A prominent startle response and nocturnal myoclonus are present throughout adult life.

Diagnosis. A positive family history is usually the first clue to diagnosis. Because the trait is transmitted by autosomal dominant inheritance, several other family members will have a similar history. An EMG during the time of stiffness demonstrates continuous motor unit activity of normal configuration. General anesthesia or peripheral nerve block causes cessation of the continuous motor unit activity. The serum concentration of creatine kinase is normal.

Treatment. Diazepam relieves the stiffness in some but not all newborns. Failure of diazepam therapy may suggest a cerebral rather than a spinal origin of the motor unit activity. Indeed such children may have abnormal electroencephalograms (EEGs), but epilepsy and mental retardation are not associated.

Sporadic Form

Clinical Features. Following an initial period of aching and tightness in the truncal muscles, involuntary painful contractions occur, first in proximal muscles and then in distal muscles. Bulbar musculature may be involved, but the most severe contractions are in the trunk muscles. The patients become so rigid that they tend to walk or stand in a hyperextended fashion, unable to bend. They are described as "tin soldiers." Tightness in the abdominal muscles makes feeding difficult and respirations shallow. The spasms disappear during sleep, but are made worse by startle, fright, or emotional upset. Tendon reflexes are active or hyperactive. There is no evidence of muscle atrophy, and because

of the continued contraction, individual muscle bellies may stand out prominently.

Diagnosis. These cases are different from the neonatal genetic form in which the rigidity is not painful. Diagnosis relies upon an EMG, which demonstrates continuous motor unit activity of normal configuration. General anesthesia or peripheral nerve block causes immediate cessation of the continuous motor unit activity. The rigidity is also abolished by lidocaine, which produces selective blockade of the gamma system.

Treatment. Diazepam is the treatment of choice. The dose should be titrated according to the severity of symptoms and side effects. High doses are ordinarily required to relieve the spasms.

Neuromyotonia

The term neuromyotonia is used to describe a clinical syndrome in which the primary abnormality is in the nerve, but abnormal electrical activity apparently originates in both nerve and muscle. Adult onset cases are usually sporadic in occurrence. Childhood onset cases are transmitted by autosomal dominant inheritance (Ashizawa et al, 1983; Lazaro et al, 1980).

Clinical Features. The clinical triad includes involuntary muscle twitching (fasciculations or myokymia), muscle cramps or stiffness, and myotonia. Excessive sweating is frequently associated with the muscle stiffness.

The initial symptoms are muscle twitching and cramps brought on by exercise. Later, they occur also at rest, and even during sleep. In some families, the cramps affect only distal muscles, causing painful posturing of the hands and feet. In other families, pelvic girdle muscles are more severely affected. Legs are affected more severely than arms in all families. These disorders are not progressive and do not lead to permanent disability. Attacks of cramping become less frequent and less severe with age.

Muscle mass, muscle strength, and tendon reflexes are normal. Fasciculations are sporadic and are noted only after prolonged observation.

Diagnosis. An EMG demonstrates continuous motor unit activity of normal configuration, fasciculations, and sometimes myotonia. The continuous activity persists during general and spinal anesthesia, is progressively diminished by more distal nerve blocks, and is abolished by curare.

Treatment. Carbamazepine and phenytoin, at usual anticonvulsant doses, are both effective in reducing or abolishing symptoms.

Isaacs Syndrome

Isaacs syndrome is part of the spectrum of neuromyotonia and perhaps should not be discussed separately. The term refers to cases of continuous motor unit activity in which the abnormality is thought to occur at the very terminal portion of the nerve. Continuous motor unit activity is not diminished by nerve block, but is abolished by curare.

Clinical Features. Isaacs syndrome is only slightly different in its clinical form from disorders of the more proximal portion of the nerve (neuromyotonia). Cramps and fasciculations are not as prominent as stiffness, which causes abnormal limb posturing associated frequently with excessive sweating. The legs are more often affected than the arms and the presentation may suggest dystonia (see Chapter 14). Limb posturing may begin in one foot and may remain asymmetric for months. Most cases are sporadic in occurrence. The onset is anytime from birth (Black et al, 1972) to adult life. Some adult-onset cases are associated with malignancy, but this is never the case in children.

A hereditary form of Isaacs syndrome transmitted by autosomal dominant inheritance occurs in children (McGuire et al, 1984). Stiffness in the limbs produces flexion contractures. Stiffness of the chest muscles may be so severe as to restrict respiration. Increased muscle tone persists even during sleep. The tendon reflexes are normal or mildly diminished. Most patients have some evidence of myokymia as well as stiffness.

Diagnosis. The EMG demonstrates continuous firing of motor units of normal configuration. The serum concentration of creatine kinase may be normal or mildly elevated.

Treatment. Carbamazepine or phenytoin in ordinary anticonvulsant doses diminishes or completely abolishes symptoms. In some sporadic cases, symptoms may remit spontaneously, allowing cessation of drug therapy.

Schwartz-Jampel Syndrome

The Schwartz-Jampel syndrome (osteochondromuscular dystrophy) is a hereditary disorder transmitted by autosomal recessive inheritance. It is characterized by short stature, skeletal abnormalities, and persistent muscular contraction and hypertrophy.

Clinical Features. Progressive skeletal deformities are present in infancy, including hip dislocation, coxa vara or valga, pectus carina-tum, vertebral flattening, basilar impression, and dwarfism (Huttenlocher et al, 1969). The constellation of skeletal deformities suggests the diagnosis of the Morquio syndrome (osteochondrodystrophy). Continuous motor unit activity is most prominent in the face and produces a characteristic triad that includes narrowing of the palpebral fissures (blepharophimosis), pursing of the mouth, and puckering of the chin. Blepharospasm is provoked by striking or even blowing on the eyelids (see Chapter 14). Continuous motor unit activity in the limbs produces stiffness of gait and exercise intolerance. Motor development during the first year is slow, but intelligence is normal.

Diagnosis. The EMG demonstrates continuous discharge of motor units of normal configuration (Taylor et al, 1972). Initial reports suggested incorrectly that the abnormal activity seen on the EMG and expressed clinically was myotonia. Myotonia may be present, but continuous motor activity, generated in the nerve and abolished by curare, is responsible for the facial and limb symptoms. The serum concentration of creatine kinase can be mildly elevated. The muscle histologic appearance is usually normal, but may demonstrate variation in fiber size and an increased number of central nuclei.

Treatment. Muscle stiffness is diminished by phenytoin or carbamazepine. Early treatment with relief of muscle stiffness reduces the severity of subsequent muscle deformity.

MYOTONIA CONGENITA

Myotonia congenita is a genetic disorder characterized by muscle stiffness and hypertrophy. Dystrophy does not occur, although families are reported with features of both myotonic dystrophy and myotonia congenita. In 19 percent of families there is clear evidence of autosomal dominant inheritance. In the remainder, a smaller percentage is definitely transmitted by autosomal recessive inheritance, but most are sporadic and cannot be classified genetically (Kuhn et al, 1979). In general, the autosomal recessive form has a later age of onset and more severe myotonia than the dominant form. However, the overlap of clinical features is considerable, and the pattern of genetic transmission cannot be determined with certainty unless several family members are affected.

Clinical Features. Clinical features are stereotyped from patient to patient. After rest, muscles are stiff and difficult to move. With activity, the stiffness disappears and movement may be normal. One of our patients played Little League baseball and could not sit while he was waiting to bat for fear that he would be unable to get up from the bench. The autosomal dominant type is frequently present from birth or infancy, and the continuous muscle contraction produces generalized hypertrophy, which gives the infant a herculean appearance. The tongue, face, and jaw muscles are sometimes involved. Stiffness is painless and is exacerbated by exposure to cold. Percussion myotonia is present. Muscle mass, strength, and tendon reflexes are normal.

Diagnosis. Diagnosis is established by an EMG. Repetitive discharges are recorded when the needle is first inserted into the muscle and again on voluntary contraction. The amplitude and frequency of potentials wax and wane, producing a characteristic sound. No evidence of dystrophy is demonstrated. The serum concentration of creatine kinase is normal. Muscle biopsy specimens in patients with either the dominant or recessive form demonstrate the absence of type IIb fibers (Crews et al, 1976).

Treatment. Myotonia does not always require treatment but sometimes can be relieved by phenytoin or carbamazepine at ordinary anticonvulsant doses. Patients who do not respond to either of those drugs may be tried on quinine, quinidine, or procainamide, but the disease is unlikely to respond.

Acetazolamide has been found effective in relieving symptoms in one kindred with myotonia congenita transmitted by autosomal dominant inheritance (Trudell et al, 1987). It is not clear whether this is a unique kindred or whether acetazolamide will prove useful in other patients with myotonia.

SYSTEMIC DISORDERS

Uremia

Uremia is a known cause of polyneuropathy (see Chapter 7). However, 50 percent of patients complain of nocturnal leg cramps and flexion cramps of the hands even before clinical evidence of polyneuropathy is present (Nielsen, 1986). Excessive use of diuretics may be the triggering factor. Muscle cramps occur also in approximately one third of patients undergoing hemodialysis (Neal et al, 1981). Monitoring with an EMG during dialysis documents a build-up of spontaneous discharges, which after several

hours, usually toward the end of dialysis treatment, culminate in repetitive high-voltage discharges associated with clinical cramps. Because standard dialysis fluid is slightly hypotonic, many nephrologists have attempted to treat the cramps by the administration of hypertonic solutions. Either sodium chloride or glucose solutions are effective for treating most patients. The cramps are apparently secondary to either extracellular volume contraction or hypo-osmolarity. Similar cramps occur in children with severe diarrhea or vomiting.

Thyroid Disease

Muscle aches, cramps, and stiffness occur as an initial complaint in up to one half of patients with hypothyroidism. Stiffness is worse in the morning, especially on cold days, and is probably caused by slowing of both muscular contraction and relaxation. This is different from myotonia, in which only relaxation is affected. Indeed, the stiffness of hypothyroidism is made worse by activity and may be painful, whereas myotonia improves with activity and is painless. The slowing of muscular contraction and relaxation is sometimes demonstrated when tendon reflexes are tested. The response tends to "hang-up."

Percussion of a muscle produces a localized knot of contraction called *myoedema*. This localized contraction lasts for up to one minute before slowly returning to normal.

Myokymia, continuous motor unit activity of the face, tongue, and limbs, and muscle cramps develop in occasional patients with *thyrotoxicosis*.

All of the neuromuscular symptoms of hypothyroidism and hyperthyroidism can be reversed by restoring the euthyroid state.

Hypocalcemia (Tetany)

Tetany due to dietary deficiency of calcium is almost unheard of in modern times except in newborns fed cow's milk. Hypocalcemic tetany is more likely to occur secondary to hypothyroidism or to hyperventilation-induced alkalosis.

The initial symptom of tetany is tingling around the mouth, in the hands, and in the feet. With time, the tingling increases in intensity and becomes generalized. This is followed by spasms in the muscles of the face, hands, and feet. The hands assume a typical posture in which the fingers are extended, the wrist is flexed, and the thumb is adducted. Fasciculations may be present, and laryngeal spasm can occur as well. Percussion of the facial nerve, either just anterior to the ear or over the cheek, produces contraction of the muscles innervated by that branch of the nerve.

A similar syndrome is encountered with magnesium deficiency. In addition to the tetany, there is also encephalopathy.

The cramps associated with hypocalcemia and hypomagnesemia are reversed by restoring the proper concentration of serum electrolytes.

Hypoadrenalism

A small percentage of patients with Addison disease complain of cramps and pain in truncal muscles. At times, paroxysmal cramps occur in the lower torso and legs and cause the patient to double-up in pain. The symptoms are relieved by hormone replacement.

■ Decreased Muscle Energy

Glucose is the major substrate used to provide energy for muscular contraction. The glucose required to sustain a single powerful contraction can be provided by the breakdown of muscle glycogen (glycogenolysis) and the anaerobic metabolism of glucose to pyruvate (glycolysis) (Fig.

8.1). Anaerobic glycosis is not an efficient mechanism to produce energy. Therefore, muscle glycogenolysis and glycolysis are able to sustain muscle contraction for only a few seconds. Prolonged activity requires that glucose be delivered to working muscles via the bloodstream by glycogenolysis in the liver and that the pyruvate generated in muscle by glycolysis be metabolized aerobically in the mitochondria. Oxidative metabolism provides high levels of energy for every molecule of glucose (Fig. 8.2).

The central compound of oxidative metabolism in mitochondria is acetylcoenzyme A (acetyl-CoA). Acetyl-CoA is derived from pyruvate, from fatty acids, and from amino acids. When exercise is prolonged, glycogen stores are rapidly depleted. The energy for muscular contraction is then derived mainly from fatty acids. The changeover from glucose to fatty acid metabolism may provide, along with vascular dilation, the "second-wind" phenomenon experienced by distance runners. Acetyl-CoA is oxidized through the Krebs cycle and releases hydrogen ions that reduce nicotinamide-adenine dinucleotide (NAD). These reduced compounds then enter a sequence of oxidation-reduction steps in the respiratory chain that liberate energy. Energy is stored as adenosine triphosphate (ATP). This process of liberating and storing energy is called oxidation-phosphorylation coupling.

During anaerobic contraction, additional ATP

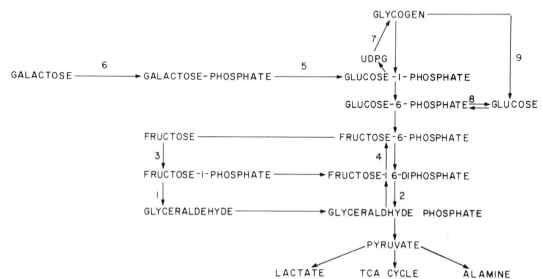

Figure 8.1 Carbohydrate metabolism. *1,* Fructose-1-phosphate aldolase. *2,* Fructose-1,6-diphosphate aldolase. *3,* Fructokinase. *4,* Fructose-1,6-diphosphatase. *5,* Galactose-1-phosphate uridyltransferase. *6,* Galactokinase. *7,* Glycogen synthase. *8,* Glucose-6-phosphatase. *9,* Acid maltase. (From Fenichel GM: Neonatal Neurology. Churchill Livingstone, New York, 1985.)

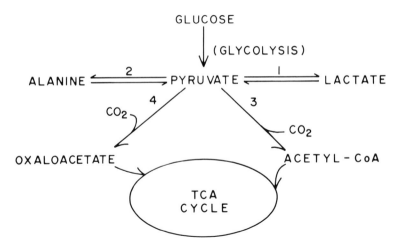

Figure 8.2 Pyruvate metabolism. *1,* Lactate dehydrogenase. *2,* Glutamic-pyruvate transaminase. *3,* Pyruvate dehydrogenase complex. *4,* Pyruvate carboxylase. (From Fenichel GM: Neonatal Neurology. Churchill Livingstone, New York, 1985.)

may be derived from adenosine diphosphate (ADP) via an alternate pathway using adenylate kinase and deaminase (Fig. 8.3).

The production of energy for muscular contraction is therefore impaired by disorders that prevent the delivery of glucose or fatty acids, the oxidation process in the mitochondria, or the creation of ATP.

THE ISCHEMIC EXERCISE TEST

The ischemic exercise test is the first step in the diagnosis of muscle energy disorders and should be performed by every patient who develops cramps on exercise (Fig. 8.4). Instructions for the procedure are outlined in Table 8.6.

In most normal individuals, serum lactate concentrations are raised more than 20 mg/dl (2 mmol/L) and serum ammonia concentrations are raised more than 100 μg/dl (60 μmol/L) over baseline (Coleman et al, 1986). If increased

concentrations of both lactate and ammonia fail to develop, it indicates that the subject did not exercise strenuously and the test should be repeated.

An abnormal increase in the concentration of serum creatine kinase, with or without failure to generate increased serum concentrations of lactate or ammonia, is an indication to proceed to muscle biopsy. It is likely to be diagnostic if histochemical and biochemical determinations can be applied. Patients with a normal lactate and ammonia response and a normal creatine kinase concentration are unlikely to have an abnormal muscle biopsy result, but an EMG should be done. Muscle biopsy is indicated if the EMG is abnormal or if there is a positive family history of cramps or muscle disease.

An elevated resting lactate concentration indicates a mitochondrial myopathy. Failure to raise the serum lactate concentration more than 5 mg/dl (0.5 mmol/L) above baseline, coupled with a normal rise in ammonia concentration is diagnostic of a glycogen storage disease. How-

Figure 8.3 Metabolic pathway utilizing myoadenylate deaminase (AMP deaminase). Ammonia (NH³) is formed when inosine monophosphate (IMP) is formed from adenosine monophosphate (AMP). S-AMP = Adenylosuccinate. (From Ashwal S, Peckham N: Pediatr Neurol 1:185, 1985.)

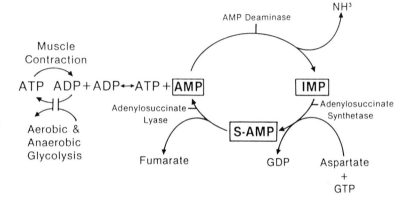

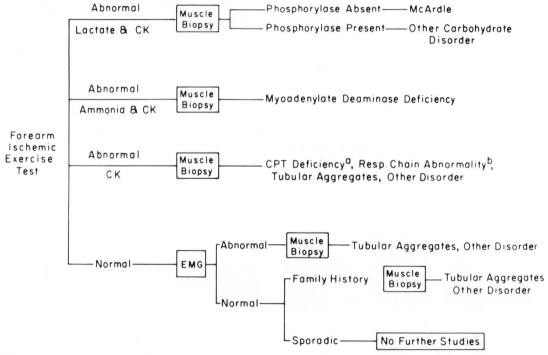

Figure 8.4 Approach to muscle cramps and exercise intolerance. a = Abnormal response to fasting; b = elevated serum lactate.

ever, patients who lack debrancher enzyme in liver and muscle may develop elevations between 5 and 10 mg/dl (0.5 to 1 mmol/L); those with only liver debrancher deficiency have a normal response.

Failure to increase ammonia concentrations more than 100 μg/dl (60 μmol/L) above baseline, coupled with a normal lactate response, suggests myoadenylate deaminase deficiency and is an indication for muscle biopsy (Sinkeler

Table 8.6 FOREARM ISCHEMIC EXERCISE TEST

1. Explain the procedure to the patient.
2. Patient should rest for at least 30 minutes before the test.
3. Place blood pressure cuff around arm.
4. Insert the indwelling catheter in the antecubital vein and obtain blood samples for lactate, ammonia and creatine kinase 10 minutes before exercise and immediately preceding it. Collect urine sample for myoglobin.
5. Inflate the cuff 20 mm Hg above systolic pressure and ask the patient to squeeze a hand dynamometer 40 times in 1 minute *or* two times/second for 1 minute.
6. Release the pressure in the cuff at the end of the exercise.
7. Collect blood samples at 1, 3, 5, 10, and 20 minutes following release of the cuff for lactate, ammonia, and creatine kinase determinations.
8. Collect a second urine sample for myoglobin at completion of blood collection.

et al, 1986). However, this aspect of the test produces many false-positive results.

DEFECTS OF CARBOHYDRATE UTILIZATION

Myophosphorylase Deficiency (McArdle Disease)

This disorder is ordinarily transmitted by autosomal recessive inheritance, but transmission by autosomal dominant inheritance occurs as well (Chui and Munsat, 1976). Phosphorylase activity is deficient only in muscle; the first step of glycogenolysis is prevented, and muscle glycogen is unavailable to produce glucose for energy. Liver phosphorylase concentrations are normal, and hypoglycemia does not occur.

Clinical Features. The severity of symptoms varies with the percentage of enzyme activity. Children with only mild deficiency states have little or no symptoms until adolescence. Aching becomes increasingly prominent and then, after an episode of vigorous exercise, severe cramps are noted in the exercised muscles. Myoglobinuria is sometimes associated. The pain can last for hours. Thereafter, on exercise repeated bouts of cramps are experienced that cause a decline in the overall level of activity. Pain begins soon after vigorous exercise is initiated and myoglobinuria is noted several hours later. Some patients exercise through the pain by slowing down just before the time of fatigue. Once they pass that point, exercise may continue unimpeded. This is probably due to (1) an increase in cardiac output, (2) the use of blood glucose and free fatty acids as a substrate for muscle metabolism, and (3) the recruitment of more motor units (Braakhekke et al, 1986).

Examination is generally unrevealing. Muscle mass and strength are normal and tendon reflexes are normoresponsive. Weakness is detected only in adult patients and even then the tendon reflexes are normal.

Myophosphorylase deficiency can also present as slowly progressive proximal weakness with onset during childhood or adult life (Abarbanel et al, 1987). Affected individuals may never complain of cramps on exercise or of myglobinuria. Tendon reflexes are preserved until late in the course of disease.

Diagnosis. The ischemic exercise test is the initial step to establish a defect in carbohydrate utilization. Patients with myophosphorylase deficiency develop cramps during the test and usually cannot complete the exercise, and the concentration of serum lactate increases less than 5 mg/dl (0.05 mmol/L) above baseline. Normal individuals have lactate concentrations between 15 and 25 mg/dl (0.15 to 0.25 mmol/L) within two to three minutes, which rapidly decline to normal levels after twenty minutes. Cramps are electrically silent by an EMG examination. The serum concentration of creatine kinase is elevated, and myoglobulin may appear in the urine coincidentally with the cramps.

Salient features on muscle biopsy specimens are histochemical evidence of subsarcolemmal blebs containing glycogen and the absence of phosphorylase. Muscle fiber degeneration and regeneration are present immediately after an episode of cramps and myoglobinuria. Definitive diagnosis requires the biochemical demonstration of decreased myophosphorylase activity.

Treatment. A high-protein diet consisting of 20 to 30 percent protein, 30 to 35 percent fat, and 40 to 45 percent carbohydrate was found to increase exercise tolerance in one patient (Slonim and Goans, 1985).

Other Disorders of Glucose Utilization

A syndrome identical to that of myophosphorylase deficiency—cramps on exercise and myoglobinuria—has also been described in four other enzyme deficiencies associated with the anaerobic glycolysis of carbohydrates (see Fig. 8.1). They are muscle phosphofructokinase deficiency (Layzer et al, 1967; Agamanolis et al, 1980), muscle phosphoglycerate kinase deficiency (DiMauro et al, 1981), muscle phosphoglycerate mutase deficiency (DiMauro et al, 1982), and lactate dehydrogenase deficiency (Kanno et al, 1980). Phosphofructokinase deficiency is the most common member of this group and has also been described as a cause of infantile hypotonia (see Chapter 6) and the scapuloperoneal syndrome (see Chapter 7).

These disorders are presumed to be transmitted by autosomal recessive inheritance. In some cases of phosphofructokinase deficiency, siblings are affected and there is consanguinity among parents. The other enzyme deficiencies have been sporadic in occurrence. Patients are suspected of having myophosphorylase deficiency because of the clinical presentation, evaluation of serum creatine kinase during attacks, and failure to produce a normal rise in venous lactate after ischemic exercise. Muscle biopsy results demonstrate subsarcolemmal collections of glycogen, but the histochemical reaction for phosphorylase is normal. It is only by biochemical analysis that these disorders are correctly identified. A high-protein diet should be tried in these patients.

DEFECTS OF LIPID UTILIZATION

Carnitine Palmityltransferase Deficiency

Long-chain fatty acids are the principal lipid oxidized to produce acetyl-CoA. Carnitine palmityltransferase is an essential enzyme that allows long-chain fatty acids to pass through the inner mitochondrial membrane to the inner portion of the mitochondria, where oxidation to acetyl-CoA occurs. A 50 to 75 percent deficiency in the activity of carnitine palmityltransferase produces a characteristic syndrome of exercise intolerance. The disorder is transmitted by autosomal recessive inheritance. However, the clinical expression of the deficiency will vary depending upon the percentage of enzyme activity and the organs involved (Angelini et al, 1981; DiDonato et al, 1981). Carnitine palmityltransferase deficiency may affect several tissues other than muscle: leukocytes, platelets, fibroblasts, and liver. During periods of prolonged fasting, patients with a liver deficiency of carnitine palmityltransferase are slow to make ketones and the concentration of long-chain fatty acids becomes elevated in the serum.

Clinical Features. The initial manifestations of muscle carnitine palmityltransferase deficiency usually begin during late childhood. No difficulty is experienced in performing even heavy exercise of short duration; energy for this activity is provided by glycogen. However, patients develop pain, tenderness, and swelling of muscles when sustained aerobic exercise is attempted. Severe muscle cramps, as in myophosphorylase deficiency, do not occur. Associated with the pain may be actual muscle injury characterized by increased concentrations of serum creatine kinase and the appearance of myoglobin in the urine. Muscle injury may also accompany periods of prolonged fasting, especially in patients on low-carbohydrate, high-fat diets. Prolonged exercise and prolonged fasting produce generalized muscle weakness that may lead to respiratory distress and death.

In the interval between attacks, results of muscle examination, serum concentration of creatine kinase, and EMG are usually normal but some children develop a permanent myopathy (Gieron and Korthals, 1987).

Diagnosis. The diagnosis is suspected by the demonstration of reduced or delayed production of ketone bodies in blood and urine during fasting. The fast should be ended by the administration of intravenous glucose at the first sign of clinical symptoms or the elevation of serum creatine kinase. Muscle biopsy can demonstrate an accumulation of lipid droplets within muscle fibers, but the results may also be normal. The definitive diagnosis requires measurement of carnitine palmityltransferase in platelets, fibroblasts, or muscle.

Treatment. Frequent carbohydrate feedings and the avoidance of prolonged aerobic activity minimize muscle destruction.

MITOCHONDRIAL (RESPIRATORY CHAIN) MYOPATHIES

The respiratory chain, located in the inner mitochondrial membrane, consists of four protein complexes: *complex I* (NADH–coenzyme Q reductase) carries hydrogen from NADH (the reduced form of NAD) to coenzyme Q; *complex II* (succinate–coenzyme Q reductase) carries hydrogen from succinate to coenzyme Q; *complex III* (reduced coenzyme Q–cytochrome-c-reduc-

tase) carries electrons from coenzyme Q to cytochrome-*c*, and contains cytochrome-*b*; and *complex IV* (cytochrome-c-oxidase) is composed of cytochrome-*a* and -a_3 (DiMauro et al, 1985) (Fig. 8.5).

Coenzyme Q is a shuttle between complexes I and II and complex III. A defect of coenzyme Q has been recorded in only one patient, who presented with neonatal seizures, abnormal ocular movements, and lactic acidosis (Fischer et al, 1986).

Three clinical syndromes have been associated with respiratory chain abnormalities: (1) a combination of progressive external ophthalmoplegia and limb weakness induced or increased by exertion, (2) exercise intolerance without progressive external ophthalmoplegia; and (3) an encephalomyopathy characterized by ataxia and some combination of dementia, deafness, involuntary movements, and seizures (Petty et al, 1986). Unfortunately, all three clinical syndromes occur with defects in each of the respiratory complexes; the phenotype does not predict the metabolic error.

Clinical Features. The age at onset ranges from birth to adult life, but is before age twenty in 61 percent of patients. Half of patients present with ptosis or ophthalmoplegia, a quarter with exertional complaints in the limbs, and a quarter with cerebral dysfunction. With time, there is considerable overlap among the three groups. Seventy-five percent eventually have ophthalmoplegia and 50 percent have exertional complaints. Pigmentary retinopathy occurs in 33 percent and neuropathy occurs in 25 percent (Yiannikas et al, 1986).

Exercise intolerance usually develops by age ten. With ordinary activity, active muscles become tight, weak, and painful, but cramps and myoglobinuria do not occur. Nausea, headache, and breathlessness are sometimes associated. During these episodes, the serum concentration of lactate and creatine kinase may be increased. Generalized weakness with ptosis and ophthalmoplegia may follow prolonged periods of activity or fasting. Such symptoms may last for several days, but recovery is usually complete.

Diagnosis. A mitochondrial myopathy should be considered in all children with exercise intolerance and ptosis or ophthalmoplegia. This combination of symptoms may also suggest myasthenia gravis, which can be differentiated with edrophonium chloride (Tensilon).

Some children with mitochondrial myopathies have increased concentrations of serum lactate at rest, but demonstrate lactic acidosis after

Figure 8.5 Respiratory complexes. Complex I (NADH–coenzyme Q reductase); complex II (succinate–coenzyme Q reductase); complex III (reduced coenzyme Q–cytochrome-c-reductase); complex IV (cytochrome-c-oxidase).

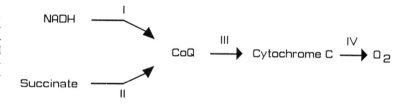

exercise. A simple screening test is the glucose-lactate tolerance test. An ordinary oral glucose tolerance test is administered, and lactate and glucose determinations are made at the same time. Children with mitochondrial disorders develop lactic acidoses and are slow to clear glucose.

Muscle biopsy reveals a clumping of the mitochondria, which are red when the Gomori trichrome stain is applied (see Fig. 7.6). These muscle cells are referred to as ragged, red fibers.

The demonstration of defects of specific respiratory complexes can be accomplished only in specialized laboratories.

Treatment. Attempts to treat selected patients with high doses of thiamine, menadione, or ubiquinone (coenzyme Q) have not been encouraging (Morgan-Hughes et al, 1984). At the present time, treatment is not available for any of these disorders.

MYOADENYLATE DEAMINASE DEFICIENCY

Deficiency of myoadenylate deaminase is clearly a familial trait, but the mode of inheritance has not been established (Keleman et al, 1982). This enzyme deficiency was discovered accidentally when a collection of muscle biopsy specimens taken from patients with several different clinical syndromes were surveyed for enzyme activity. The few biopsies that demonstrated myoadenylate deaminase deficiency were from patients with exercise intolerance. Myoadenylate deaminase deficiency has also been demonstrated in patients with infantile hypotonia, in patients with progressive myopathies beginning in childhood, and in asymptomatic individuals. While question remains whether permanent myopathy results from myoadenylate deaminase deficiency, there is considerable support for the notion that the deficiency may be responsible for familial syndromes of exercise intolerance.

Clinical Features. The typical history is one of intermittent muscle pain and weakness with exercise. A simple screening test is the glucose exercise (Ashwal and Peckham, 1985). The pain varies from a diffuse aching to a severe cramping type associated with muscle tenderness and swelling. Between attacks the children are normal. The duration of symptoms lasts from one to twenty years with the mean less than nine years.

Diagnosis. During attacks, the serum concentration of creatine kinase may be normal or markedly elevated. The EMG and muscle histologic studies are usually normal. The diagnosis is suggested by the ischemic exercise test (see Fig. 8.4). Patients with myoadenylate deaminase deficiency fail to generate ammonia but demonstrate normal elevations of lactate. However, ammonia levels may fail to rise even in normal individuals, and enzyme analysis of muscle is required for diagnosis.

Treatment. Treatment is not available.

■ Myopathic Stiffness and Cramps

This section comprises several different conditions that present as muscle stiffness or cramps, or both, in which the primary abnormality is thought to be in skeletal muscle.

Malignant Hyperthermia

This disorder is transmitted by autosomal dominant inheritance with variable penetrance. Attacks of muscular rigidity and necrosis in association with a rapid rise in body temperature is triggered by the administration of several inhalation anesthetics or by succinylcholine. Therefore, the syndrome is seen almost exclusively in the operating suite.

Clinical Features. The first symptoms are tachycardia, tachypnea, muscle fasciculations, and increasing muscle tone. Rise in body temperature is dramatic and may be as much as 2° C per hour. All muscles become rigid and there is a progressive and severe metabolic acidosis. Seizures and death may occur if the patient is not treated promptly.

Diagnosis. This is a clinical diagnosis based on the response to anesthesia or succinylcholine. Serum creatine kinase concentrations rise to ten times the upper limit of normal. A reliable test to identify susceptible individuals is not available.

Treatment. Treatment includes termination of anesthesia, body cooling, treatment of metabolic acidosis, and the intravenous injection of dantrolene, 1–2 mg/kg, which may be repeated every 5 to 10 minutes up to a total dose of 10 mg/kg (Gronert, 1980). All children in whom there is any suspicion of malignant hyperthermia should be pretreated with dantrolene prior to the use of anesthetics.

Neuroleptic Malignant Syndrome

Clinical Features. Several neuroleptics may induce an idiosyncratic response characterized by muscular rigidity, hyperthermia, altered states of consciousness, and autonomic dysfunction in susceptible individuals (Moore et al, 1986). Phenothiazines, butyrophenones, and thioxanthenes have all been implicated. All ages have been affected, but young males predominate. Symptoms develop over a period of one to three days. The first symptoms are rigidity and akinesia, followed by fever, excessive sweating, urinary incontinence, and hypertension. Consciousness fluctuates and there is a 20 percent mortality rate due to respiratory failure.

Diagnosis. The diagnosis is primarily clinical. The only helpful laboratory test results are an increased serum concentration of creatine kinase and a leukocytosis.

Treatment. The offending neuroleptic must be promptly withdrawn and general supportive care provided. Bromocriptine is effective in completely reversing the syndrome.

The Rigid Spine Syndrome

This term comprises a heterogeneous group of disorders, usually sporadic, with a male predominance (Van Munster et al, 1986). Emery-Dreifuss muscular dystrophy (see Chapter 7) has similar features, but is a distinct nosologic entity.

Clinical Features. Onset of symptoms is usually before age five. The first manifestation may be either stiffness or weakness. Stiffness is characterized by marked limitation of spinal flexion, especially in the cervical and dorsolumbar portions. Scoliosis is always associated and flexion contractures develop at the elbows, causing marked limitation of extension. The initial symptom of weakness is usually difficulty in climbing stairs or arising from the floor. Some children present with toe-walking and may be thought to have Duchenne dystrophy.

Examination reveals a pattern of scapuloperoneal or limb-girdle weakness in addition to spinal rigidity and scoliosis. Some patients have little subcutaneous fat. Tendon reflexes are always diminished in weak muscles and sometimes in strong muscles as well.

The subsequent course is variable. In some children, weakness and rigidity are only slowly progressive or remain stationary. In others, there is severe, progressive scoliosis that compromises respiratory effort. Contractures may form at the hip, knee, and ankle in addition to the elbow and spine. Some patients develop cardiomyopathy and should probably be classified as having Emery-Dreifuss muscular dystrophy.

Diagnosis. The serum concentration of creatine kinase is slightly elevated and the EMG is consistent with a myopathic process. Muscle biopsy usually reveals fibers undergoing degeneration with fatty replacement and fibrosis. Some patients have type I predominance and others have type II.

Treatment. Treatment for the myopathy is not available, but scoliosis should be treated surgically to prevent respiratory distress. Pacemakers are usually needed for patients with cardiomyopathy.

Trilaminar Myopathy

This is a single case report mentioned because it presents as rigidity in the newborn (Ringel et al, 1978).

Clinical Features. A term female newborn, the product of a normal pregnancy and delivery, had marked rigidity of the trunk and limbs immediately after birth that persisted during sleep. There was difficulty in sucking and swallowing with recurrent episodes of cyanosis and pneumonia. All skeletal muscles were firm to palpation and the limbs resisted efforts to move them. Tendon reflexes were normal.

Diagnosis. The EMG was normal. There was no evidence of continuous motor unit activity or fasciculations. Muscle biopsy results revealed fibers with three concentric zones: the innermost zone had densely packed myofibrils; the middle zone consisted of myofibrils; and the outer zone resembled a sarcoplasmic mass. The serum concentration of creatine kinase was elevated.

Treatment. Treatment is not available, but the child did improve spontaneously during infancy.

Cramps and Tubular Aggregates

Tubular aggregates are abnormal double-walled structures that originate from the sarcoplasmic reticulum and are located in a subsarcolemmal position (Fig. 8.6). They are found in muscle biopsy specimens with a variety of neuromuscular disorders, but are most often present in patients with cramps or myalgia (Niakan et al, 1985; Rosenberg et al, 1985). Indeed, cramps or myalgia may be the only symptom of neuromuscular disease.

Most cases of cramps and tubular aggregates are sporadic and have a male predominance (Lazaro et al, 1980). In addition, there is a genetic form transmitted by autosomal dominant inheritance (Pierobon-Bormioli et al, 1985).

Sporadic Cases

Clinical Features. Onset is usually in the second or third decade. Cramps may occur at rest or are exercise-induced. Thigh and calf muscles are usually affected and become swollen, stiff, and tender. Cramping occurs more often in cold weather and may also occur at night, interfering with sleep. Myalgia is present between cramps.

Episodic stiffness of the mouth and tongue occur and interfere with speech. Cramps are not associated with myoglobinuria. Muscle mass, strength, and tendon reflexes are normal.

Diagnosis. The serum concentration of creatine kinase is normal. The EMG is normal, except that in some patients the cramps are electrically silent. This suggests a disorder of carbohydrate metabolism. An ischemic tolerance test produces severe cramps, but there is normal generation of lactate with no elevation of the creatine kinase concentration.

Muscle biopsy results are diagnostic. Light and electron microscopic examination reveal tubular aggregates in type II fibers. There is no evidence of glycogen or lipid storage.

Treatment. The cramps are not responsive to medication.

Autosomal Dominant Cases

Clinical Features. Muscle aches, cramps, and proximal weakness begin in the second decade. The legs are usually more severely affected than the arms. Weakness is mild and progresses very slowly. Neck flexor and facial weakness occurs in occasional patients.

Diagnosis. The serum concentration of creatine kinase is moderately elevated. The EMG is consistent with a myopathic process. Muscle biopsy results reveal tubular aggregates in type I and type II fibers. Type I fiber predominance and type II hypotrophy are present in some patients.

Treatment. Treatment is not available for either the myopathy or the cramps.

Brody Disease

This myopathy is caused by a deficiency of calcium-activated ATP in sarcoplasmic reticulum (Karpati et al, 1986). The disorder is clearly familial, but occurs only in males, suggesting X-linked inheritance.

Clinical Features. The major clinical manifestation is difficulty in relaxation after contraction. Myotonia is suspected but not supported by the EMG. Symptoms of exercise-induced stiffness and cramping begin in the first decade and become progressively worse with age. Unlike myotonia, stiffness becomes worse rather than better with continued exercise. After a

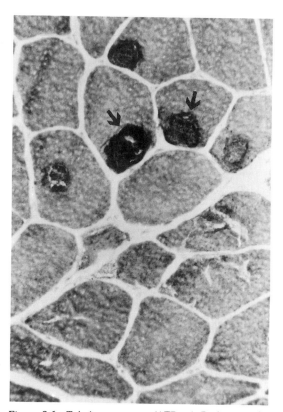

Figure 8.6 Tubular aggregates (ATPase). Dark material is present beneath the sarcolemma in type I and II fibers.

period of rest, exercise can be resumed. Muscle strength is normal, as are the tendon reflexes.

Diagnosis. Patients with Brody disease are thought to have myotonia, but the cramps are silent, suggesting myophosphorylase deficiency. The ischemic exercise test results are normal. Muscle biopsy results reveal type II atrophy. Definitive diagnosis requires the demonstration of the biochemical defect.

Treatment. Dantrolene and nifedipine have been tried without success.

References

1. Abarbanel JM, Potashnik R, Frisher S, et al: Myophosphorylase deficiency: The course of an unusual congenital myopathy. Neurology 37:316, 1987.
2. Agamanolis DP, Askari AD, DiMauro S, et al: Muscle phosphofructokinase deficiency: Two cases with unusual polysaccharide accumulation and immunologically active enzyme protein. Muscle Nerve 3:456, 1980.
3. Angelini C, Freddo L, Battistella P, et al: Carnitine palmityltransferase deficiency: Clinical variability, carrier detection, and autosomal-recessive inheritance. Neurology 31:883, 1981.
4. Ashizawa T, Butler IJ, Harati Y, et al: A dominantly inherited syndrome with continuous motor neuron discharges. Ann Neurol 13:285, 1983.
5. Ashwal S, Peckham N: Myoadenylate deaminase deficiency in children. Pediatr Neurol 1:185, 1985.
6. Black JT, Garcia-Mullin R, Good E, et al: Muscle rigidity in a newborn due to continuous peripheral nerve hyperactivity. Arch Neurol 27:413, 1972.
7. Braakhekke JP, de Bruin MI, Stegeman DF, et al: The second wind phenomenon in McArdle's disease. Brain 109:1087, 1986.
8. Chui LA, Munsat TL: Dominant inheritance of McArdle syndrome. Arch Neurol 33:636, 1976.
9. Coleman RA, Stajich JM, Pact VW, et al: The ischemic exercise test in normal adults and in patients with weakness and cramps. Muscle Nerve 9:216, 1986.
10. Crews J, Kaiser KK, Brooke MH: Muscle pathology of myotonic congenita. J Neurol Sci 28:449, 1976.
11. DiDonato S, Castiglione A, Rimoldi A, et al: Heterogeneity of carnitine-palmityltransferase deficiency. J Neurol Sci 50:207, 1981.
12. DiMauro S, Bonilla E, Zeviani M, et al: Mitochondrial myopathies. Ann Neurol 17:521, 1985.
13. DiMauro S, Dalakas M, Miranda AF: Phosphoglycerate kinase deficiency: A new cause of recurrent myoglobinuria (abstract). Ann Neurol 10:90, 1981.
14. DiMauro S, Miranda AF, Olarte M, et al: Muscle phosphoglycerate mutase deficiency. Neurology 32:584, 1982.
15. Fischer JC, Ruitenbeek W, Gabreels FJM, et al: A mitochondrial encephalomyopahy: the first case with an established defect at the level of coenzyme Q. Eur J Pediatr 144:441, 1986.
16. Gieron MA, Korthals JK: Carnitine palmityltransferase deficiency with permanent weakness. Pediatr Neurol 3:51, 1987.
17. Gronert GA: Malignant hyperthermia. Anesthesiology 53:395, 1980.
18. Huttenlocher PR, Landwirth J, Hanson V, et al: Osteochondro-muscular dystrophy. Pediatrics 44:945, 1969.
19. Kanno TK, Sudo I, Takeuchi, et al: Hereditary deficiency of lactate dehydrogenase M-subunit. Clin Chim Acta 108:267, 1980.
20. Karpati G, Charuk J, Jablecki C, et al: Myopathy caused by a deficiency of Ca^{2+}–adenosine triphosphatase in sarcoplasmic reticulum (Brody's disease). Ann Neurol 20:38, 1986.
21. Kelemen J, Rice DR, Bradley WG, et al: Familial myoadenylate deaminase deficiency and exertional myalgia. Neurology 32:857, 1982.
22. Kuhn E, Fiehn W, Seiler D, et al: The autosomal recessive (Becker) form of myotonia congenita. Muscle Nerve 2:109, 1979.
23. Kurcyznski TW: Hyperekplexia. Arch Neurol 40:246, 1983.
24. Layzer RB: Diagnostic implications of clinical fasciculation and cramps. In Rowland LP, ed. Human Motor Neuron Disease. Raven Press, New York, 1982, p 23.
25. Layzer RB: Neuromuscular Manifestations of Systemic Disease. FA Davis Company, Philadelphia, 1985, p 16.
26. Layzer RB, Rowland LP, Ranney HM: Muscle phosphofructokinase deficiency. Arch Neurol 17:512, 1967.
27. Lazaro RP, Fenichel GM, Kilroy AW, et al: Cramps, muscle pain, and tubular aggregates. Arch Neurol 37:715, 1980.
28. Lazaro RP, Rollinson RD, Fenichel GM: Familial cramps and muscle pain. Arch Neurol 38:22, 1981.
29. McGuire SA, Tomosovic JJ, Ackerman N: Hereditary continuous muscle fiber activity. Arch Neurol 41:395, 1984.
30. Moore A, O'Donohoe NV, Monagham H: Neuroleptic malignant syndrome. Arch Dis Child 61:793, 1986.
31. Morgan-Hughes JA, Hayes DJ, Clark JB, et al: Mitochondrial myopathies. Results of exploratory therapeutic trials. In Folkers K, Yamamura Y, eds. Biomedical and Clinical Aspects of Coenzyme Q. Elsevier Science Publishers, Amsterdam, 1984.
32. Neal CR, Resnikoff E, Unger Am: Treatment of dialysis-related muscle cramps with hypertonic dextrose. Arch Intern Med 141:171, 1981.
33. Niakan E, Harati Y, Danon MJ: Tubular aggregates: their association with myalgia. J Neurol Neurosurg Psychiatry 48:882, 1985.
34. Nielsen VK: The peripheral nerve function in chronic renal failure. I. Clinical symptoms and signs. Acta Med Scand 190:105, 1986.
35. Petty RKH, Harding AE, Morgan-Hughes JA: The clinical features of mitochondrial myopathy. Brain 109:915, 1986.
36. Pierobon-Bormioli S, Armani M, Ringel SP, et al: Familial neuromuscular disease with tubular aggregates. Muscle Nerve 8:291, 1985.
37. Ringel SP, Neville E, Duster MC, et al: A new congenital neuromuscular disease with trilaminar muscle fibers. Neurology 28:282, 1978.
38. Rosenberg NL, Neville HE, Ringel SP: Tubular aggregates: Their association with neuromuscular diseases, including the syndrome of myalgias/cramps. Arch Neurol 42:973, 1985.
39. Sander JE, Layzer RB, Goldsobel AB: Congenital stiffman syndrome. Ann Neurol 8:195, 1980.
40. Sinkeler SP, Wevers RA, Joosten EM, et al: Improvement of screening in exertional myalgia with a standardized ischemic forearm test. Muscle Nerve 9:731, 1986.

41. Slonim AE, Goans PJ: Myopathy in McArdle's syndrome. N Engl J Med 312:355, 1985.
42. Taylor RG, Layzer RB, Davis HS, et al: Continuous muscle fiber activity in the Schwartz-Jampel syndrome. EEG Clin Neurophysiol 33:497, 1972.
43. Trudell RG, Kaiser KK, Griggs RC: Acetazolamide-responsive myotonia congenita. Neurology 37:488, 1987.
44. Valli G, Barbieri S, Cappa S, et al: Syndromes of abnormal muscular activity: Overlap between continuous muscle fiber activity and the stiff man syndrome. J Neurol Neurosurg Psychiatry 46:241, 1983.
45. Van Munster ETL, Joosten EMG, Van Munster-Uijtdehaage MAM, et al: The rigid spine syndrome. J Neurol Neurosurg Psychiatry 49:1292, 1986.
46. Yiannikas C, McLeod JG, Pollard JD, et al: Peripheral neuropathy associated with mitochondrial myopathy. Ann Neurol 20:249, 1986.

9 Disturbances of Sensation

This chapter deals with disturbed or lost sensation in the limbs and trunk. Sensory disturbances of the face are considered in Chapter 17.

■ Sensory Symptoms

The important symptoms of disturbed sensation are pain, dysesthesias, and loss of sensibility. Peripheral neuropathy is the most common cause of disturbed sensation at any age. As a rule, discomfort is more likely than numbness to bring a patient to medical attention. Several different terms are used to describe sensory disturbances. Muscle aches, pains, and cramps are discussed in Chapters 7 and 8. Nerve root pain generally follows the course of a dermatome and is ordinarily described as deep and aching. The pain is more proximal than distal and may be constant or intermittent. When intermittent, the pain may radiate in a dermatomal distribution. The most common cause of root pain in adults is sciatica associated with lumbar disk disease. Disk disease also occurs in adolescents, usually due to trauma. In children, root pain is more likely due to radiculitis. Examples of radiculitis are the migratory aching of a limb preceding paralysis in the Guillain-Barré syndrome (see Chapter 7) and the radiating pain in a C5 distribution that heralds an idiopathic brachial neuritis (see Chapter 13).

Polyneuropathy involving small nerve fibers produces dysesthetic pain. This pain differs from previously experienced discomfort and is described as pins and needles, tingling, or burning. It is often compared with the abnormal sensation one feels when dental anesthesia is wearing off. The discomfort is superficial, distal, and usually symmetric.

The pattern of sensory loss as a guide to the anatomic site of abnormality is summarized in Table 9.1.

■ Hereditary Sensory and Autonomic Neuropathy

The classification of hereditary sensory and autonomic neuropathy provided in Table 9.2 is the one suggested by Dyck (1984). This classification attempts to synthesize information based on natural history, mode of inheritance, and electrophysiologic characteristics. It is likely that each of these disorders is heterogenous and that several different genetic errors may produce a similar phenotype.

Hereditary Sensory and Autonomic Neuropathy (HSAN I)

This disorder appears in the literature under several different names, most commonly as "hereditary sensory radiculoneuropathy" (Denny-Brown, 1951). The mode of transmission is by autosomal dominant inheritance. As with other dominantly inherited neuropathies, variable

Table 9.1 PATTERNS OF SENSORY LOSS

Pattern	Site
Glove and stocking	Peripheral nerve
One leg	Plexus or spinal cord
One arm	Plexus
Both legs	Spinal cord or peripheral nerve
Legs and trunk	Spinal cord
All limbs	Spinal cord or peripheral nerve
Unilateral arm and leg	Brain or spinal cord

214

Table 9.2 DISTURBANCES OF SENSATION

Hereditary Sensory and Autonomic Neuropathy (HSAN)
1. HSAN I: Autosomal dominant
2. HSAN II: Autosomal recessive
3. HSAN III: Familial dysautonomia
4. HSAN IV: With anhydrosis
5. HSAN: X-linked
6. HSAN: with spastic paraplegia
7. Familial amyloid neuropathy

Brachial Neuritis
1. Neuralgic amyotrophy
2. Recurrent familial brachial neuropathy
3. Sympathetic reflex dystrophy

Lumbar Disk Herniation

Syringomyelia

Foramen Magnum Tumors

Thalamic Syndromes

Congenital Insensitivity (Indifference) to Pain
1. Mental retardation
2. Lesch-Nyhan syndrome
3. With normal nervous system

expression is the rule. Therefore, history alone is unsatisfactory to determine if parents are affected; physical examination and electrophysiologic studies are required.

Clinical Features. The onset of symptoms is during the second decade or later. The major clinical features are lancinating pains in the legs and ulcerations of the feet. However, initial symptoms are usually insidious and it is often difficult to date the onset. A callus develops on the sole of the foot, usually in the skin overlying a weight-bearing bony prominence. The callus blackens, becomes necrotic, and breaks down into an ulcer that is difficult to heal. The ulcer had been preceded by sensory loss, but often it is the ulcer and not the sensory loss that first brings the patient to medical attention. Although plantar ulcers are an important feature, they are not essential for diagnosis. Most patients with HSAN I do not have ulcers. When a kindred is studied in which the proband has typical features of plantar ulcers and lancinating pain, other family members may have sensory loss in the feet, mild pes cavus or peroneal atrophy, and loss of the Achilles tendon reflex.

Sensory loss in the feet is a constant feature, whereas sensory loss in the hands is variable. The hands are never affected as severely as are the feet, and finger ulcers do not occur. The sensations of pain and temperature are lost before the sensations of touch and pressure. In some patients, the dissociation of sensory loss is constant, whereas in others, the dissociation is

only a first stage before the development of global sensory loss. The Achilles tendon reflex is always absent, and the quadriceps tendon reflex may be absent as well. Tendon reflexes in the arms are preserved.

Foot ulcers are caused by trauma to the insensitive skin of the feet. They occur more often and are more difficult to heal in boys than in girls, in individuals who wear ill-fitting shoes, and in individuals who are on their feet much of the day. Lancinating pains are a late occurrence. They come as recurring attacks usually affecting a single arm or leg. Other limbs may be affected on subsequent days. The intensity of pain is variable.

Diagnosis. Autosomal dominant inheritance and sensory loss in the feet is essential for the diagnosis. The presence of plantar ulcers and lancinating pain add substantially to, but are not critical, for the diagnosis. HSAN I can be differentiated from familial amyloid polyneuropathy on clinical grounds. Urinary incontinence, impotence, and postural hypotension are frequent features of amyloidosis but do not occur in HSAN I.

Electrophysiologic studies demonstrate slowing of sensory nerve conduction velocity and reduced amplitude of sensory action potentials. Sural nerve biopsy reveals a marked decrease or absence of myelinated fibers and a mild to moderate reduction of small myelinated fibers.

Treatment. Treatment is not available for the neuropathy, but plantar ulcers can be prevented by good foot care. Tight shoes and activities that produce trauma to the feet should be avoided. Weight bearing must be discontinued at the first sign of a plantar ulcer. Much of the foot mutilation reported in previous years was due to secondary infection of the ulcers. This should be avoided by warm soaks, elevation, and antibiotics.

Hereditary Sensory and Autonomic Neuropathy II (HSAN II)

The term HSAN II probably includes several different disorders transmitted by autosomal recessive inheritance. Many of the cases are sporadic, there are instances of parental consanguinity, and kindred exist in which siblings are affected.

Clinical Features. The onset of symptoms is probably during infancy and possibly at the time of birth. Unlike HSAN I, which affects primarily the feet, HSAN II involves the arms and legs equally, and also affects the trunk and the forehead. The result is a diffuse loss of all sensation; touch and pressure are probably affected earlier and to a greater extent than are temperature and pain. Affected infants and children are constantly hurting themselves without a painful response and are sometimes believed to have "congenital absence of pain" (Winkelmann et al, 1962). The absence of pain as a protective measure against injury results in ulcerations and infections of the fingers and toes, stress fractures, and injuries to long bones. Loss of deep sensibility causes injury and swelling of joints, and loss of touch makes simple tasks, such as tying shoes, manipulating small objects, and buttoning buttons, difficult, if not impossible. Tendon reflexes are absent throughout. Sweating is diminished in all areas of decreased sensibility, but there are no other symptoms or signs of autonomic dysfunction. Some children have been described with features of HSAN II and retinitis pigmentosa (Landwirth, 1964), and there is one family with features of HSAN II and the early onset of cataracts (Donaghy et al, 1987). It is not clear if such children represent separate genetic disorders or are part of the phenotypic spectrum of a single genetic disorder. Anhydrosis is prominent also in HSAN IV (discussed subsequently) and the boundary between HSAN II and HSAN IV is difficult to delineate.

Diagnosis. The diagnosis relies primarily on the history and examination. Absence of sensory potentials confirms that the congenital absence of pain is due to peripheral neuropathy and not to a cerebral abnormality (Johnson and Spalding, 1964). Motor nerve conduction velocities are normal as are the morphologic characteristics of motor unit potentials. Fibrillations are sometimes present. Sural nerve biopsy reveals an almost complete absence of myelinated fibers (Nukada et al, 1982).

Treatment. No treatment is available for the neuropathy. However, there must be constant vigilance for painless injuries. Discoloration of the skin and swelling of joints or limbs should raise the possibility of fracture. Children must be taught to avoid activities that might cause injury and to examine themselves for signs of superficial infection.

Hereditary Sensory and Autonomic Neuropathy III (HSAN III)

HSAN III is ordinarily referred to as familial dysautonomia or the Riley-Day syndrome. This disorder is present at birth. Hypotonia is a cardinal feature, as are feeding difficulties and poor control of autonomic function. Because neonatal hypotonia is prominent, the disorder is discussed in Chapter 6.

Hereditary Sensory Autonomic Neuropathy IV (HSAN IV)

This is probably a heterogeneous group of disorders transmitted by autosomal recessive inheritance. The major features are congenital insensitivity to pain, anhydrosis, and mental retardation (Vardy et al, 1979). There is some support for the notion that the disorder is caused by a defect in the development of the neural crest (Brown and Podosin, 1966). Table 9.3 summarizes the tissues derived from the neural crest and the clinical abnormalities that would correlate with their deficiency. All of the clinical abnormalities are present at birth, and although complications of the pain-free state are a continuous problem, the underlying disease may not be progressive.

Clinical Features. The initial symptoms may be due to anhydrosis or to insensitivity to pain. Many affected children present during infancy with repeated episodes of fever, sometimes associated with convulsions. These episodes are most likely to occur during the summer and are caused by the inability to sweat in response to exogenous heat. Sweat glands are present in the skin, but sympathetic innervation of the sweat glands is lacking. Most infants are hypotonic and areflexic. Developmental milestones are attained slowly, and by two or three years of age it is apparent that the child has had several self-inflicted injuries due to pain insensitivity. The injuries include ulcers of the fingers and toes, stress fractures, self-mutilation of the tongue, and Charcot joints. Sensory examination reveals widespread absence of pain and temperature sensation. Touch, vibration, and stereognosis are intact in some patients, but not in others. Mild to moderate retardation is present in almost every case.

Table 9.3 NEURAL CREST SYNDROME*

Tissue	Clinical Symptoms
Spinal ganglia	Absence of pain
Sympathetic ganglia	Anhydrosis
Pia-arachnoid	Dural thickening
Induction of enamel	Enamel aplasia
Skin pigment	Blond hair, fair skin
Forebrain cells	Mental retardation

*Modified from Brown JW, Podosin R: Arch Neurol 15:294, 1966.

Other features, present in some but not all patients, are blond hair and fair skin, Horner syndrome, and aplasia of dental enamel.

Diagnosis. Familial dysautonomia (HSAN III) and HSAN IV have many features in common and are easily confused. However, insensitivity to pain is not prominent in HSAN III and fungiform papillae of the tongue are present in HSAN IV. Anhydrotic ectodermal dysplasia is another hereditary disorder that shares many features with HSAN IV. Affected children also present with unexplained fevers and abnormalities of tooth formation. However, children with ectodermal dysplasia are anhydrotic because sweat glands are present. The nervous system is intact, and sensation to pain is present. Diagnosis of HSAN IV depends primarily on the clinical features but can be confirmed by demonstrating the absence of sensory evoked potentials, the absence of an axon reflex when histamine is injected into the skin, and the presence of sweat glands on skin biopsy specimens.

Treatment. Treatment is not available for the underlying disease. However, constant vigilance is required to prevent injuries to the skin and bones with secondary infection.

X-linked Hereditary Sensory Neuropathy

This disorder was described in five members of one family (Jestico et al, 1985).

Clinical Features. Painless deformities of the feet characterized by calcaneovalgus and loss of arch are noted between the ages of three and thirteen. Family members who experience repeated trauma to the feet develop painless ulcerations as well. Pain and touch sensation in the feet is reduced but not absent. The ankle tendon reflex is difficult to elicit but may be obtained with reinforcement. Other tendon reflexes are present. Autonomic function is preserved.

The rate of progression is variable. Ulcers tend to enlarge and lead to osteomyelitis. Amputation may be required. The neuropathy remains limited to the feet.

Diagnosis. The only abnormality on electromyogram (EMG) is reduction or absence of the sural nerve potential. Motor conduction velocities are normal, as are motor unit potentials. Sural nerve biopsy results demonstrate selective loss of the small-diameter myelinated fibers.

Treatment. Treatment is not available, but management requires the same concern for foot care as outlined for HSAN I.

Hereditary Sensory Autonomic Neuropathy with Spastic Paraplegia

This syndrome may be caused by more than one genetic error. Some of the cases are sporadic, and others have occurred in siblings (Cavanagh et al, 1979). Autosomal recessive inheritance is suspected, but other modes of transmission cannot be excluded. Some patients with HSAN I and HSAN II have demonstrated mild signs of corticospinal tract dysfunction such as brisk reflexes and extensor plantar responses. Possibly, cases with spastic paraplegia are variant phenotypes of either HSAN I or HSAN II. However, it is reasonable to consider these cases separately at the present time.

Clinical Features. Progressive spastic paraplegia and sensory neuropathy are the major clinical features. The spasticity occurs first, or at least simultaneously with, the sensory symptoms (see Chapter 12). A stiff-legged gait is noted during infancy or early childhood. Developmental motor milestones may be delayed. Tendon reflexes in the legs are increased, plantar responses are extensor, and sphincter control may not be attained. Either coinciding with the development of paraplegia, or following it by several years, a relative insensitivity to pain is appreciated by parents. This is characterized by repeated episodes of injury, ulcerations of the fingers and toes, and fractures. Pain and temperature sensations are much more severely affected than are the sensations of touch and vibration.

Intelligence is normal, and cranial nerves are unaffected. As the neuropathy becomes more profound, tendon reflexes, which initially were brisk, become depressed and are lost.

When disease onset is during infancy and early childhood, the course is relentlessly progressive and may lead to early death. Patients with onset in the second decade show a slower progression.

Diagnosis. A diagnosis cannot be established during early stages of the disease when spastic paraplegia is present but neuropathy is not. The development of insensitivity to pain and ulcers of the feet and fingers is essential for the diagnosis. Nerve conduction studies demonstrate prolonged sensory latencies and a reduced amplitude of action potentials. Motor conduction velocity may be normal. Sural nerve biopsy results demonstrate a profound loss of myelinated and unmyelinated fibers.

Treatment. Treatment for the underlying disease is not available, but symptomatic care is needed to prevent injury to the hands and feet.

Familial Amyloid Neuropathy

This is a heterogeneous group of disorders, all transmitted by autosomal dominant inheritance, in which amyloid is deposited in the peripheral somatic and autonomic nervous systems. Other organs may be affected as well. The disorder has been described in several different ethnic groups (Andersson, 1970; Olofsson et al, 1980; Van Allen et al, 1969). It is not clear whether the genetic defect responsible for familial amyloid polyneuropathy is common among the different nationalities.

Clinical Features. The onset of symptoms is usually between the second and seventh decades, most often between the ages of twenty-five and thirty-five. Dysesthesias are an early feature. Pain and temperature sensations are lost first, followed by touch, pressure, and vibration sensations. Lancinating pains and foot ulcers may be present, suggesting the diagnosis of HSAN I. However, autonomic dysfunction is much more profound and occurs earlier in the course of amyloid neuropathy than in HSAN I. Symptoms of autonomic dysfunction include impotence, constipation, diarrhea, fecal or urinary incontinence, and anhydrosis. Cardiac involvement is relatively common as evidenced by bundle branch block, left ventricular hypertrophy, and atrioventricular dissociation. Postural hypotension occurs in approximately 10 percent of patients.

Motor involvement is a late feature; weakness and atrophy occur both in the hands and feet. Tendon reflexes are depressed or absent in all limbs. Symptoms of other organ involvement tend to be mild. Vitreous opacities and perivascular amyloid deposition in retinal vessels are common. Some patients have proteinuria, but few develop renal insufficiency.

The course of disease is one of steady progression, leading to cachexia and death within fifteen years. Postmortem studies demonstrate amyloid deposition predominantly in peripheral nerves and blood vessels, and to a lesser degree in cardiac muscle, smooth muscle, spleen, and kidneys.

Diagnosis. The clinical presentation of a hereditary mixed motor sensory neuropathy with prominent autonomic dysfunction should suggest the diagnosis of familial amyloid polyneuropathy. Electrophysiologic studies are consistent with a mixed motor sensory neuropathy of the axonal type. Examination of the sural nerve reveals amyloid deposition around the nerve causing compression within the endoneurium and in the walls of the vasa nervorum.

Treatment. Treatment is not available for the underlying disease. However, cardiac arrhythmias may require a permanent cardiac pacemaker. Other manifestations of autonomic dysfunction are managed symptomatically.

■ Brachial Neuritis

There are three painful arm syndromes: acute idiopathic brachial neuritis (neuralgic amyotrophy), familial recurrent brachial neuritis, and sympathetic reflex dystrophy. The first two are characterized by some initial pain in the shoulder or arm, which then subsides and is followed by muscle atrophy. Weakness is the prominent feature and these two syndromes are therefore discussed in Chapter 13. Although muscle atrophy also occurs in sympathetic reflex dystrophy, pain is the prominent feature and this syndrome is discussed next.

Reflex Sympathetic Dystrophy

This syndrome has several different names in the medical literature, including causalgia, algodystrophy, neurovascular reflex dystrophy, posttraumatic sympathetic dystrophy, and Sudeck atrophy. The essential features are sustained burning pain in a limb, combined with vasomotor and pseudomotor dysfunction, leading to atrophic changes in skin, muscle, and bone following trauma. The inciting trauma, which may be accidental or surgical, injures the nerves in a limb or the cervical spinal cord. The mechanism of reflex sympathetic dystrophy remains a debated issue, but it is likely that abnormal sensory input and processing are present in both peripheral and central pathways.

Clinical Features. Reflex sympathetic dystrophy in children most often occurs following trauma to one arm (or leg) with or without fracture. The trauma may be relatively minor and the clinical syndrome is so unusual that many affected individuals are first labeled "hysterical" or "malingering." Time of onset after injury is usually within one or two months, but may be longer. The first symptom is pain in the shoulder, followed by generalized swelling and stiffness of the hand and fingers. Pain is intense, is described as burning or aching, and is out of proportion to the injury. It may be maximally severe at onset or may become progressively worse for three to six months. Pain is exacerbated by movement or dependency, causing the arm to be held in a position of abduction and internal rotation, as if it were swaddled to the body. The hand becomes swollen and hyperesthetic and feels warmer.

In most patients, the pain and swelling resolve in three to six months. However, some continue to experience pain for as long as seven years (Horowitz, 1984). The edematous part becomes indurated, and the skin is cool and hyperhidrotic. During this time, the nails become brittle, osteoporosis develops in the bones of the hand and shoulder, and flexion contractures occur in the fingers on the ulnar side of the hand (Marsden et al, 1984).

Reflex sympathetic dystrophy can spread to other limbs without new injury (Schwartzman and McLellan, 1987).

Diagnosis. This is a clinical diagnosis and cannot be confirmed by laboratory tests during the early stages. Because the syndrome follows either accidental or surgical trauma, litigation is commonplace, and careful documentation of the examination is needed. One simple test is to immerse the affected hand in warm water. Wrinkling of the fingers requires an intact sympathetic innervation. The absence of wrinkling is evidence of a lesion in either the central or peripheral sympathetic pathway (Braham et al, 1979).

Relief of pain by selective blockade of the stellate ganglion is considered the best diagnostic test. Radiographs of the affected limb eventually demonstrate osteoporosis of bone in every case.

Treatment. The oral administration of guanethidine, at a dose of 20 to 30 mg/day, is used in adults. The major side effect is orthostatic hypotension. Both pain and edema are said to resolve within days or weeks (Tabira et al, 1983). Prednisone, with or without stellate ganglion blockade, is also reported to be effective in some cases (Kozin et al, 1981). High doses are started and tapered over a period of four weeks. Patients who are unresponsive to medical therapy may respond only to sympathectomy. Physical therapy should be initiated as early as is tolerable in order to prevent permanent disability from disuse.

■ **Lumbar Disk Herniation**

Lumbar disk herniation in children is usually traumatic. Almost all cases occur after the age of ten; they are more common in boys than in girls and are frequently sports-related (Epstein et al, 1984; Kurihara and Kataoka, 1980). Because the index of suspicion for lumbar disk herniation in children is low, diagnosis may be delayed for months to years.

Clinical Features. Sciatica or back pain, or both, are the initial manifestations. Twenty percent of patients never experience back pain, but all develop sciatica at some time in the course. Bilateral sciatica is reported by almost half of patients.

Physical findings may include diminished lumbar lordosis, vertebral muscle spasm, and scoliosis. Some effort is made to hold the lumbar spine rigid in almost every patient. Point tenderness may be present over the involved disk space. Straight-leg raising routinely provokes sciatica. Sensation to pinprick may be diminished in the distribution of the L–5 and S-1 dermatome, and the ankle tendon reflex is diminished or absent in more than half of patients.

Diagnosis. Radiographs of the lumbosacral spine reveal minor congenital anomalies (hemivertebrae, sacralization of the lumbar spine) in an unusually large number of cases. The diagnosis is confirmed by computerized tomography (CT) of the spine or by myelography.

Treatment. Conservative treatment (bed rest and traction) provides immediate relief in the majority of patients, but surgery is usually required for permanent relief of symptoms.

■ **Syringomyelia**

Syringomyelia is a generic term for disorders in which there is cavitation within the spinal cord. The length of the cavity is variable and may extend into the brainstem. Such a cephalic extension is termed *syringobulbia*. The cavity, or syrinx, is centrally placed in the gray matter and may enlarge in all directions. The cervicothoracic region is a favorite site, but thoracolumbar syrinx occurs as well, and occasionally a syrinx may extend from the brainstem to the conus medullaris (Epstein and Epstein, 1981).

The mechanism of syrinx formation is much debated (Newman et al, 1981). It is clear that cavitation of the spinal cord may follow trauma and infarction, but these are not important mechanisms of syringomyelia in children. In childhood, primary syringomyelia is generally regarded to be either a congenital malformation or a cystic astrocytoma. In the past, the distinction between congenital cysts and astrocytoma could be achieved only by postmortem examination. Astrocytomas of the spinal cord, like those of the cerebellum, may have very large cysts with only a nubbin of solid tumor. The development of magnetic resonance imaging has greatly enhanced antemortem diagnosis of cystic astrocytoma by demonstrating small areas of increased signal intensity in one or more portions of the cyst. As a rule, cystic astrocytoma is more likely to produce symptoms during the first decade (Epstein and Epstein, 1982), whereas congenital syringomyelia presents in the second decade or later and is usually associated with the Chiari anomaly (Newman et al, 1981). Cystic astrocytoma of the spinal cord is considered further in Chapters 12 and 13; this section deals primarily with congenital syringomyelia.

Clinical Features. The initial symptoms of syringomyelia depend upon the location of the cyst. Because the cavity is located near the central canal, crossing fibers subserving pain and temperature are often affected first. When the syrinx is in the cervical area, pain and temperature are typically lost in a "cape" or "vest" distribution. However, early involvement is often unilateral or at least asymmetric and sometimes involves the fingers before the shoulders. Touch and pressure are ordinarily preserved until the cyst enlarges into the posterior columns or the dorsal root entry zone. Loss of pain sensibility in the hands often leads to injury, ulceration, and infection as seen in hereditary sensory and autonomic neuropathies. Pain is not ordinarily a feature of syringomyelia, but lancinating limb pain is occasionally reported.

Scoliosis is commonplace, and torticollis may be an initial sign in children with cervical cavities (Kiwak et al, 1983). As the cavity enlarges into the ventral horn, weakness and atrophy develop in the hands and may be associated with fasciculations; pressure on the lateral columns causes hyperreflexia and spasticity in the legs. Very long cavities may produce lower motor neuron signs in all four limbs. Sphincter control is sometimes impaired. The posterior columns are generally the last to be affected so that vibration sense and touch is preserved until relatively late in the course. It is important to emphasize that the progress of symptoms is extremely slow and insidious. The spinal cord accommodates well to the slowly developing pressure within. Thus, at the time of presentation a long history of minor neurologic handicap such as clumsiness or difficulty running may be elicited.

Bulbar signs are relatively uncommon and usually asymmetric. They include hemiatrophy of the tongue with deviation on protrusion, facial weakness, dysphasia, and dysarthria. The descending pathway of the trigeminal nerve is frequently affected, causing loss of pain and temperature sensations on the same side of the face as the facial weakness and tongue hemiatrophy.

Diagnosis. The primary diagnostic procedure in previous years has been myelography. The usual finding is an elongated fusiform widening of the spinal cord. Diagnostic accuracy can be improved by the combination of metrizamide myelography and CT scans. Magnetic resonance imaging (MRI) is now the diagnostic modality of choice. This noninvasive test not only allows visualization of the cavity (Fig. 9.1) and the Chiari malformation but also detects the presence of small foci of glioma.

Treatment. Several different surgical approaches have been used in treating syringomyelia. Syringoperitoneal shunting has provided the most favorable results (Barbaro et al, 1984). Some degree of stabilization is achieved in the majority of patients. Children with syringomyelia secondary to spinal cord astrocytoma should have direct removal of the tumor through the use of an ultrasonic surgical aspirator (Epstein and Epstein, 1982).

■ Foramen Magnum Tumors

Extramedullary tumors in and around the foramen magnum are known for false localizing

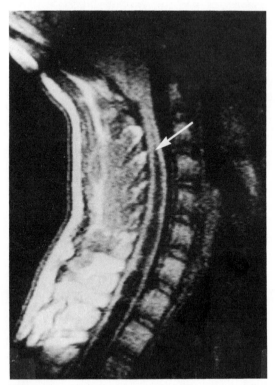

Figure 9.1 Cervical syringomyelia. Magnetic resonance image demonstrates a long cavity, beginning (arrow) just below the foramen magnum.

signs and for mimicking other disorders, especially syringomyelia and multiple sclerosis. In children, neurofibroma secondary to neurofibromatosis is the only tumor found in this location (Yasuoka et al, 1978).

Clinical Features. The most frequent initial symptom is unilateral or bilateral dysesthesias of the fingers. Suboccipital or neck pain is present in half of patients. These two symptoms are often ignored early in the course. Numbness and tingling usually begin in one hand and then migrate to the other. Dysesthesias in the feet are a late occurrence. Gait disturbances, incoordination of the hands, and bladder disturbances generally follow the onset of sensory symptoms and are so alarming that they prompt medical consultation.

Many patients will have café-au-lait spots, but few have evidence of subcutaneous neuromas. Weakness may be confined to one arm, one side, or both legs; 25 percent of patients have weakness in all limbs. Atrophy of the hands is uncommon. Sensory loss may involve only one segment or may have a "cape" distribution. Pain and temperature are usually diminished, and disturbances of other modalities may be associated or dissociated. Tendon reflexes are brisk in the arms and legs.

Patients with neurofibromatosis may have multiple neurofibromas causing segmental abnormalities in several levels of the spinal cord.

Diagnosis. Magnetic resonance imaging is the best method for demonstrating abnormalities at the foramen magnum.

Treatment. Neurofibroma of the C2 root can be surgically excised with complete relief of symptoms.

■ Thalamic Pain

The thalamic pain syndrome of Déjérine and Roussy occurs almost exclusively in adults following infarction of the thalamus or of the white matter of the parietal lobe. Similar symptoms sometimes occur in patients with thalamic glioma. Such tumors more often produce hemiparesis than thalamic pain.

Clinical Features. Touching the affected limb or part of the body produces intense discomfort described as "sharp," "crushing," or "burning." Suffering is considerable, and the quality of pain is unfamiliar to the patient. Several different modes of stimulation, such as changes in ambient temperature, auditory stimulation, and even changes in emotional state can accentuate the pain. Despite the severity of these dysesthesias, the affected limb is otherwise anesthetic to ordinary sensory testing.

Diagnosis. The presence of thalamic pain should prompt imaging studies to determine the presence of tumor, infarction, or demyelinating disease.

Treatment. The combination of levodopa and a peripheral decarboxylase inhibitor may be helpful for relieving pain (Plasencia et al, 1987). If this does not prove satisfactory, some combination of analgesic and tranquilizing medication should be administered.

■ Congenital Insensitivity (Indifference) to Pain

Most children with congenital insensitivity to pain have a hereditary sensory neuropathy. In many early reports of this entity, specific tests for sensory neuropathy and complete postmortem examinations were not performed. However, there are children and families with congenital universal insensitivity to pain in whom sensory neuropathy has been excluded. Many such children are mentally retarded as well, and testing pain sensation is difficult. The Lesch-Nyhan syndrome is a specific disorder characterized by self-mutilation and mental retardation without any evidence of sensory neuropathy (see Chapter 5).

Clinical Features. An occasional child is reported with congenital insensitivity to pain in whom a structural disturbance of the central or peripheral nervous system cannot be demonstrated after extensive antemortem and postmortem evaluation (Baxter and Olszewski, 1960). Such children do not come to medical attention until the end of their first year when they begin to move around the environment independently. It is then noted that injuries do not produce crying and there is a failure to learn the potential of injury from experience. The result is repeated bruising, fractures, ulcerations of the fingers and toes, and mutilation of the tongue. Sunburn and frostbite are frequent occurrences.

Examination reveals absence of the corneal reflex and insensitivity to pain and temperature, but relative preservation of touch and vibration sensations. Tendon reflexes are present.

Diagnosis. Intelligence tests, electroencephalograms, and examination of the cerebrospinal fluid provide normal results.

Treatment. Treatment is not available for the underlying insensitivity, but supportive care is needed for the repeated injuries. Life is shortened by repeated injuries and recurrent infections.

References

1. Andersson R: Familial amyloidosis with polyneuropathy. Acta Med Scand 188:85, 1970.
2. Barbaro NM, Wilson CB, Gutin PH et al: Surgical treatment of syringomyelia. Favorable results with syringoperitoneal shunting. J Neurosurg 61:531, 1984.
3. Baxter DW, Olszewski J: Congenital universal insensitivity to pain. Brain 83:381, 1960.
4. Braham J, Sadeh M, Sarova-Pinhas I: Skin wrinkling on immersion of hands. A test of sympathetic function. Arch Neurol 36:113, 1979.
5. Brown JW, Podosin R: A syndrome of the neural crest. Arch Neurol 15:294, 1966.
6. Cavanagh NPC, Eames RA, Galvin RJ, et al: Hereditary sensory neuropathy with spastic paraplegia. Brain 102:79, 1979.
7. Denny-Brown D: Hereditary sensory radicular neuropathy. J Neurol Neurosurg Psychiatry 14:237, 1951.
8. Donaghy M, Hakin RN, Bamford JM, et al: Hereditary sensory neuropathy with neurotrophic keratitis. Description of an autosomal recessive disorder with a selective reduction of small myelinated nerve fibres and a discussion of the classification of the hereditary sensory neuropathies. Brain 110:563, 1987.
9. Dyck PJ: Neuronal atrophy and degeneration predominantly affecting peripheral sensory and autonomic neurons. In Dyck PJ, Thomas PK, Lambert EH, Bunge R, eds. Peripheral Neuropathy. WB Saunders Co, Philadelphia, 1984, p 1557.
10. Epstein F, Epstein N: Surgical management of holocord intramedullary spinal cord astrocytomas in children. Report of three cases. J Neurosurg 54:829, 1981.
11. Epstein F, Epstein N: Surgical treatment of spinal cord astrocytomas of childhood. A series of 19 patients. J Neurosurg 57:685, 1982.
12. Epstein JA, Epstein NE, Marc J, et al: Lumbar intervertebral disk herniation in teenage children: Recognition and management of associated anomalies. Spine 9:427, 1984.
13. Horowitz SH: Iatrogenic causalgia. Classification, clinical findings, and legal ramifications. Arch Neurol 41:821, 1984.
14. Jestico JV, Urry PA, Efphimiou J: An hereditary sensory and autonomic neuropathy transmitted as an X-linked recessive trait. J Neurol Neurosurg Psychiatry 48:1259, 1985.
15. Johnson RH, Spalding JMK: Progressive sensory neuropathy in children. J Neurol Neurosurg Psychiatry 27:125, 1964.
16. Kiwak KJ, Deray MJ, Shields WD: Torticollis in three children with syringomyelia and spinal cord tumor. Neurology 33:946, 1983.
17. Kozin F, Ryan LM, Carerra GF, et al: The reflex sympathetic dystrophy syndrome (RSDS). III. Scintigraphic studies, further evidence for the therapeutic efficacy of systemic corticosteroids, and proposed diagnostic criteria. Am J Med 70:23, 1981.
18. Kurihara A, Kataoka O: Lumbar disc herniation in children and adolescents. A review of 70 operated cases and their minimum 5-year follow-up studies. Spine 5:443, 1980.
19. Landwirth J: Sensory radicular neuropathy and retinitis pigmentosa. Pediatrics 34:519, 1964.
20. Marsden CD, Obeso JA, Traub MM, et al: Muscle spasms associated with Sudeck's atrophy after injury. Br Med J 288:173, 1984.
21. Newman PK, Terenty TR, Foster JB: Some observations on the pathogenesis of syringomyelia. J Neurol Neurosurg Psychiatry 44:964, 1981.
22. Nukada H, Pollock M, Haas LF: The clinical spectrum and morphology of type II hereditary sensory neuropathy. Brain 105:647, 1982.
23. Olofsson BO, Andersson R, Furgerg B: Atrioventricular and intraventricular conduction in familial amyloidosis with polyneuropathy. Acta Med Scand 208:77, 1980.
24. Plasencia RJ, Gilroy J, Cullis P: Treatment of thalamic pain syndrome with levodopa. Neurology 34:137, 1984.
25. Schwartzman RJ, McLellan TL: Reflex sympathetic dystrophy. Arch Neurol 44:555, 1987.
26. Tabira T, Shibasaki H, Kuroiwa Y: Reflex sympathetic dystrophy (causalgia) treatment with guanethidine. Arch Neurol 40:430, 1983.
27. Van Allen MW, Frolich JA, Davis JR: Inherited predisposition to generalized amyloidosis. Neurology 19:10, 1969.
28. Vardy PA, Greenberg LW, Kachel C, et al: Congenital insensitivity to pain with anhydrosis. Am J Dis Child 133:1153, 1979.
29. Winkelmann RK, Lambert EH, Hayles AB: Congenital absence of pain. Arch Dermatol 85:325, 1962.
30. Yasuoka S, Okazaki H, Daube JR, et al: Foramen magnum tumors. J Neurosurg 49:828, 1978.

10 Ataxia

The term ataxia can be used generically for any disturbance in gait, but is used here in a more restricted sense to denote disturbances of coordination rather than strength. Disturbances of coordination are typically caused by dysfunction of the cerebellum or its major input systems from the frontal lobes or the posterior columns of the spinal cord. An ataxic gait is wide-based, lurching and staggering, and it provokes disquiet in the observer for fear that the patient is in imminent danger of falling. The same gait is seen in people attempting to walk in a vehicle that has several directions of movement at once, such as a train. When there is abnormality in the vermis of the cerebellum, the child cannot sit still, and there is constant to-and-fro movement of the body and bobbing of the head (titubation). In contrast, disturbances of the cerebellar hemispheres cause a tendency to veer in the direction of the affected hemisphere, with dysmetria and hypotonia in the ipsilateral limbs. Bifrontal lobe disease may produce symptoms and signs that are indistinguishable from cerebellar disease.

Loss of sensory input to the cerebellum, because of peripheral nerve or posterior column disease, requires constant looking at the feet in order to know their location in space. The gait is also wide-based, but is not so much lurching as it is careful. The foot is raised high with each step and then slaps down too heavily on the ground (steppage gait). Station and gait are considerably worse with the eyes closed and the patient may actually fall to the floor (positive Romberg sign).

The differential diagnosis of a child with acute ataxia or recurrent attacks of ataxia (Table 10.1) is quite different from that of a child with chronic static or progressive ataxia (Table 10.2). There-

fore, these two presentations are dealt with separately in the text. However, it must be kept in mind that a slowly progressive ataxia may be noticed "acutely," and children with recurrent ataxia may never return to baseline after each attack and may have a progressive ataxia superimposed upon the acute attacks.

Table 10.1 ACUTE OR RECURRENT ATAXIA

Drug Ingestion

Postinfectious/Immune
1. Acute postinfectious cerebellitis
2. Miller-Fisher syndrome
3. Myoclonic encephalopathy
4. Neuroblastoma
5. Multiple sclerosis

Encephalitis—Brainstem

Traumatic
1. Postconcussion
2. Hematoma
3. Vertebrobasilar occlusion

Migraine
1. Basilar
2. Benign paroxysmal vertigo

Genetic Disorders
1. Dominant recurrent ataxia
2. Pyruvate decarboxylase deficiency
3. Carnitine acetyltransferase deficiency
4. Maple syrup urine disease
5. Hartnup disease

Vascular Disorders
1. Cerebellar hemorrhage
2. Lupus erythematosus
3. Kawasaki disease

Pseudoataxia (Epileptic)

Brain Tumor

Conversion Reaction

Table 10.2 CHRONIC OR PROGRESSIVE
ATAXIA

Primary Brain Tumors
1. Cerebellar astrocytoma
2. Medulloblastoma
3. Ependymoma
4. Cerebellar hemangioblastoma (von Hippel–Lindau disease)
5. Supratentorial tumors (see Chapter 4)

Congenital Ataxias
1. Cerebellar aplasia
2. Vermal aplasia
   a. Dandy-Walker malformation
   b. Joubert syndrome
3. Chiari malformation
4. Basilar impression

Hereditary Ataxias
1. Autosomal dominant inheritance
   a. Machado-Joseph syndrome
   b. Olivopontocerebellar degeneration
   c. Ramsay Hunt syndrome
      (1) With pallidoluysian atrophy
      (2) With mitochondrial myopathy
2. Autosomal recessive inheritance
   a. Friedreich ataxia
   b. Ramsay Hunt syndrome
   c. Ataxia-telangiectasia
   d. Marinesco-Sjögren syndrome
   e. Abetalipoproteinemia
   f. Hypobetalipoproteinemia
   g. Juvenile sulfatide lipidoses
   h. Juvenile GM$_2$ gangliosidosis
   i. Sea-blue histiocytosis
   j. Refsum disease (HSMN-IV) (see Chapter 7)
   k. Disorders of pyruvate metabolism (see Chapters 5, 7, 8)
   l. Respiratory chain disorders (see Chapter 8)
   m. Hartnup disease
   n. Maple syrup urine disease
3. X-linked inheritance
   a. Adrenoleukodystrophy (see Chapter 5)
   b. Leber optic neuropathy (see Chapter 16)
   c. With adult-onset dementia

■ Acute or Recurrent Ataxia

The two most common causes of ataxia among children who were previously healthy and then in one day developed an ataxic gait are drug ingestion and acute postinfectious cerebellitis (Fig. 10.1). Migraine, brainstem encephalitis, and an underlying neuroblastoma are the next considerations. In preadolescent and adolescent girls, the possibility of a conversion reaction is always a consideration. Recurrent ataxia is uncommon and is usually caused by hereditary disorders. Migraine is the most common cause and disorders of pyruvate metabolism are second.

DRUG INGESTION

The incidence of accidental drug ingestion is highest among children between one and four years of age.

Clinical Features. Most psychoactive drugs can produce ataxia when an overdose is taken. The ataxia is usually associated with some change in personality or sensorium. Toxic doses of anticonvulsant drugs, especially phenytoin, may produce marked ataxia without an alteration in sensorium. Nystagmus usually is present as well. Excessive use of antihistamines in the treatment of an infant or young child with allergy or an upper respiratory infection may produce ataxia. This is especially true in children with otitis media who may have underlying unsteadiness due to middle ear infection.

Diagnosis. The parents or care providers of every child with acute ataxia should be carefully questioned concerning drugs intentionally administered to the child and others accessible in the home. It is worthwhile to specifically inquire if anyone in the family is using anticonvulsants or psychoactive drugs. Urine should be screened for drug metabolites, and blood should be sent for analysis when a specific drug is suspected.

Treatment. Treatment must be individualized depending upon the specific drug ingested and its blood concentration. In most cases of ataxia due to drug ingestion, the drug can be safely eliminated spontaneously if vital function is not compromised, if acid-base balance is not disturbed, and if liver and kidney function are normal. In life-threatening situations, dialysis may be necessary while vital function is supported in an intensive care unit.

POSTINFECTIOUS/IMMUNE DISORDERS

In all of the conditions discussed in the following sections, an altered immune state is blamed for cerebellar dysfunction and sometimes for other neurologic deficits. Preceding viral infections are usually incriminated, but are documented in only half of cases. When one considers that children have an average of four to six viral infections a year, it is not surprising to obtain a positive history of a viral illness during the preceding thirty days in 50 percent of any group of children. There is no evidence that acute cerebellar ataxia is caused by immunization.

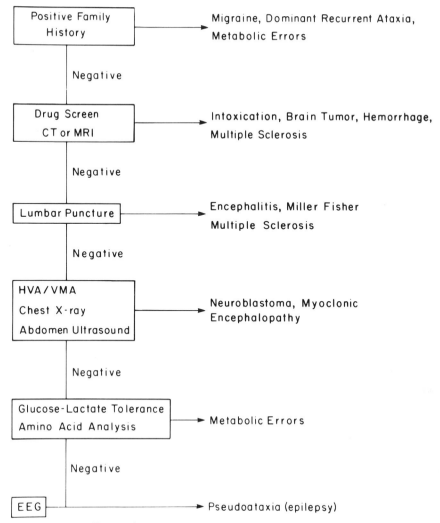

Figure 10.1 Diagnostic studies in acute cerebellar ataxia.

Acute Postinfectious Cerebellitis

Acute postinfectious cerebellitis affects children between ages one and five, but it may occur as late as fourteen years of age (Weiss and Carter, 1959). Males and females are affected equally, and there have been no reports of an increased incidence among family members.

Clinical Features. The onset is explosive. A previously healthy infant awakens from a nap and cannot stand. Ataxia is almost maximal from onset. Some worsening may occur during the first day, but a longer progression, or a waxing and waning course, makes the diagnosis unlikely. Ataxia varies from mild unsteadiness while walking to complete inability to stand or walk. Even when ataxia is severe, sensorium is clear

and the child is otherwise normal. Tendon reflexes may be present or absent; when absent, Miller Fisher syndrome should be considered. Nystagmus, when present, is usually mild. Chaotic movements of the eyes (opsoclonus) should suggest either myoclonic encephalopathy or an occult neuroblastoma.

Symptoms may begin to remit after only a few days, but complete recovery takes three weeks to five months. Those with pure ataxia of the trunk or limbs and only mild nystagmus are likely to recover completely. Marked nystagmus or opsoclonus (myoclonic encephalopathy), tremors of the head and trunk, or moderate irritability is likely to be followed by persistent neurologic sequelae.

Diagnosis. The diagnosis of acute postinfectious cerebellitis is a diagnosis of exclusion.

Every child should undergo a drug screen and computerized tomography (CT) of the head. One possible exception is a child in whom ataxia develops during varicella infection. The association between the two is well established, and further diagnostic tests may not be needed. If the CT scan is normal, lumbar puncture is indicated to exclude encephalitis (Fig. 10.1). All children with severe nystagmus or opsoclonus must be screened for neuroblastoma. Further evaluation depends upon associated features of the history or physical examination.

Treatment. Acute postinfectious cerebellitis is a self-limited disease. Treatment is not required.

Miller Fisher Syndrome

The Miller Fisher syndrome is characterized by ataxia, ophthalmoplegia, and areflexia (see Chapter 15). It is generally regarded as a disorder of peripheral myelin (Ropper, 1983) and is classified as a variant of the Guillain-Barré syndrome (Asbury, 1981). Others believe that it may represent a brainstem encephalitis (Al-Din et al, 1982). All agree that the disorder is harmless and recovery is expected.

Clinical Features. A viral illness precedes the neurologic symptoms by five to ten days in 50 percent of cases. Either ophthalmoparesis or ataxia may be the presenting feature. Both are present early in the course. The most common ocular motor disturbance is paralysis of vertical gaze; upward gaze is more severely affected than downward gaze. The Bell phenomenon may be preserved despite paralysis of voluntary upward gaze, suggesting the possibility of a supranuclear palsy (Meienberg and Ryffel, 1983). Horizontal gaze is generally preserved but dissociated nystagmus, most marked in the abducting eye, may be present. Ptosis occurs but is less severe than the vertical gaze palsy.

Ataxia is more prominent in the limbs than in the trunk and, like the areflexia, is probably caused by decreased peripheral sensory input. Weakness of the limbs may be noted as well. Unilateral or bilateral facial weakness occurs in a significant minority of children. The course is similar to that of the Guillain-Barré syndrome. Recovery generally begins within two to four weeks after symptoms become maximal and is complete within six months.

Diagnosis. The clinical distinction between the Miller Fisher syndrome and brainstem encephalitis can be difficult. Disturbances of sensorium, multiple cranial nerve palsies, an abnormal electroencephalogram (EEG), or pro-

longation of the interpeak latencies of the brainstem auditory evoked response should suggest a brainstem encephalitis. The cerebrospinal fluid profile in the Miller Fisher syndrome parallels that of the Guillain Barré syndrome. A cellular response is noted early in the course, and protein elevation occurs later.

Treatment. There is no evidence that corticosteroids, adrenocorticotropic hormone (ACTH), or plasmapheresis is beneficial in treating the Miller Fisher syndrome. The outcome in untreated children is excellent.

Myoclonic Encephalopathy

Myoclonic encephalopathy is a syndrome characterized by chaotic eye movements (dancing eyes, opsoclonus), myoclonic ataxia, and encephalopathy. It may occur either as a postviral syndrome or secondary to an occult neuroblastoma. The common pathophysiologic mechanism is an altered immune state. The clinical presentation and the neurologic outcome are the same whether or not a tumor is present (Bolthauser et al, 1979).

Clinical Features. The mean age at onset is nineteen months with a range from six months to six years. Unlike acute postinfectious cerebellitis and the Miller Fisher syndrome, in which neurologic symptoms are fully expressed within one to two days, the evolution of symptoms in myoclonic encephalopathy may take a week or longer.

Either ataxia or chaotic eye movements may bring the child to medical attention. Almost half of these children demonstrate personality change or irritability, suggesting the presence of a more diffuse encephalopathy. Some children are described as having a cerebellar ataxia, whereas others are said to be incoordinated because of myoclonus, constant rapid muscular contractions that are irregular in occurrence and widespread in distribution (see Chapter 14). Opsoclonus probably represents a disorder of ocular muscles similar to myoclonus. It is characterized by spontaneous, conjugate, irregular jerking of the eyes in all directions (Dyken and Kolar, 1968). The movements are most prominent with attempts to change fixation and are then associated with blinking or eyelid flutter. Opsoclonus persists even in sleep and becomes more severe with agitation.

Diagnosis. The myoclonic encephalopathy syndrome can be diagnosed on clinical grounds, but laboratory investigation is required to determine the underlying cause (Fig. 10.1). The presence of an occult neuroblastoma should be suspected in all children with acute ataxia, recurrent ataxia, or the myoclonic encephalopathy syndrome. An acute ataxia that progresses over several days or waxes and wanes in severity is more likely to be caused by neuroblastoma than by a preceding viral infection.

In children with myoclonic encephalopathy due to occult neuroblastoma, there is an equal chance that the tumor is in the chest or the abdomen. In contrast, only 10 to 15 percent of neuroblastomas are in the chest when myoclonic encephalopathy is not present. The evaluation for neuroblastoma should include radiographs of chest and abdomen, careful palpation and ultrasonography of the abdomen, and measurement of the urinary excretion of homovanillic acid (HVA) and vanillylmandelic acid (VMA) and of serum metanephrine (Tuchman et al, 1985).

The other important diagnostic consideration in children with myoclonic encephalopathy syndrome is brainstem encephalitis.

Treatment. Partial or complete spontaneous remission of the neurologic syndrome occurs occasionally whether or not neuroblastoma is present. In most patients, the course is prolonged with some waxing and waning in the severity of neurologic dysfunction. Either ACTH or oral corticosteroids provide partial or complete relief of symptoms in 80 percent of patients, including those with neuroblastoma. Oral corticosteroids are the treatment of choice because of ease of administration. Marked improvement usually occurs one to four weeks after initiating therapy. Relapses occur when therapy is discontinued, but may occur also while treatment is in progress.

Neuroblastoma, when present, must be removed. However, the long-term neurologic outcome is the same whether or not neuroblastoma is present or corticosteroids are used. Approximately half of these children will have an impairment of motor ability and one third will have some disturbance in intellectual function (Bolthauser et al, 1979).

Multiple Sclerosis

Multiple sclerosis is usually a disease of young adults. Epidemiologic evidence suggests that the cause is infectious, acquisition occurs after age eleven, and there is at least a two-year delay from acquisition to development of symptoms (Kurtzke and Hyllested, 1986). If this suggestion proves to be correct, symptomatic multiple

sclerosis should not occur in prepubertal children. Yet children are reported who fulfill the criteria for multiple sclerosis with first episodes as early as twenty-four months (Bejar and Ziegler, 1984). Whether the childhood forms of multiple sclerosis are etiologically distinct from adult counterparts cannot be determined at this time.

Clinical Features. The female to male ratio varies from 2:1 to 4:1 (Bye et al, 1985). Ataxia and blindness, alone or in combination, are the most common initial features. The first episode is usually concurrent with a febrile episode. Alternate initial manifestations are encephalopathy, hemiparesis, or seizures. One third of patients develop an intranuclear ophthalmoplegia that may be unilateral or bilateral (see Chapter 15).

Clinical features are sufficiently protean that a single prototype cannot be provided. The essential feature is repeated episodes of demyelination in noncontiguous areas of the central nervous system. Each episode is characterized by the rapid development of focal neurologic deficits that persist for weeks and months; afterward there is partial or complete recovery. Recurrences are separated by months or years and are frequently associated with febrile illnesses. Lethargy, nausea, and vomiting sometimes accompany the attacks in children, but rarely in adults.

The child is usually irritable and demonstrates truncal and limb ataxia. Tendon reflexes are generally brisk throughout. Long-term outcome is unpredictable.

Diagnosis. Multiple sclerosis can be suspected at the time of the first attack, but definitive diagnosis requires recurrence to establish a polyphasic course. The EEG is frequently abnormal but nonspecific, characterized by focal or diffuse slowing. Examination of the cerebrospinal fluid at the time of exacerbation reveals less than twenty-five lymphocytes, a normal or mildly elevated protein content, and sometimes the presence of oligoclonal bands.

Low-density lesions in the white matter can often be seen on a contrasted CT scan, but magnetic resonance imaging (MRI) is a considerably more powerful technique to image areas of demyelination (Fig. 10.2). Visual evoked responses are useful to document prior or concurrent optic neuritis, and peroneal somatosensory evoked responses can be used to document myelitis.

Treatment. A course of ACTH or corticosteroids is recommended at the time of acute ex-

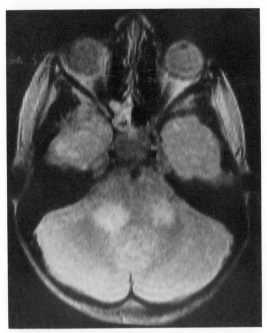

Figure 10.2 Magnetic resonance image in multiple sclerosis. Two areas of increased signal intensity are present in the cerebellum.

acerbations. Prednisone is generally administered orally at a dose of 2 mg/kg/day for one week and is then rapidly tapered and discontinued at the end of a month. Many authorities believe that ACTH is superior to corticosteroids in adults with multiple sclerosis. Aqueous ACTH, 80 units, is given intravenously over eight hours in 5 percent dextrose and water each day for three days. Forty units of ACTH gel is then given intramuscularly every twelve hours for seven days. Each injection is reduced by 5 units every three days. Improvement, when it occurs, is expected during the first two weeks.

BRAINSTEM ENCEPHALITIS

Ataxia may be a presenting feature of viral encephalitis affecting primarily the structures of the posterior fossa. Echoviruses, coxsackie viruses, and adenoviruses have been implicated as etiologic agents.

Clinical Features. Cranial nerve dysfunction is often associated with the ataxia. A more diffuse encephalitis characterized by states of decreased consciousness and seizures may develop later. Meningismus is sometimes present. The course is variable, and though most children recover completely, some may be left with considerable neurologic impairment. Those who

have only ataxia and cranial nerve palsies, with no disturbance of neocortical function, tend to recover best. Such cases cannot be distinguished from the Miller Fisher syndrome on clinical grounds alone.

Diagnosis. Diagnosis requires the demonstration of a cellular response, primarily mononuclear leukocytes, in the cerebrospinal fluid, with or without some elevation of the protein content. Prolonged interpeak latencies of the brainstem auditory evoked response are supporting evidence of an abnormality within the brainstem parenchyma and not the peripheral sensory input system. The EEG is usually normal in children with brainstem encephalitis who have a normal sensorium. A mild increase in *theta* activity may be recorded as well.

Treatment. Specific treatment is not available for the viral infection.

TRAUMA

Mild head injuries are common in childhood and almost constant in toddlers. Recovery is almost always complete despite considerable parental concern. More serious head injuries, associated with loss of consciousness, seizures, and cerebral contusion, are fortunately less common, but still account for several thousand deaths in children annually. Ataxia may follow head injuries, sometimes even mild head injuries. In most of these cases the ataxia is part of the so-called post-concussion syndrome, in which no structural derangement of the nervous system can be demonstrated. In others, a cerebellar contusion or posterior fossa hematoma may be present (see Chapter 2).

Ataxia may also follow cervical injuries. These are frequently sports-related and due to occlusive disease of the vertebrobasilar artery.

Postconcussion Syndrome

Clinical Features. Many adults complain of headache, dizziness, and mental changes following even a mild head injury. The frequency of such complaints is greater and the symptoms more severe and long-lasting when litigation is pending. Some of these symptoms also occur after head injury in children and probably represent a transitory derangement of cerebral function caused by the trauma. Even mild head trauma can at times produce structural disturbances in the brain, and this may explain the persistence of symptoms.

In infants and small children, the most prominent postconcussive symptom is ataxia. This is not necessarily a typical cerebellar ataxia but may be only an unsteadiness of gait. Limb dysmetria is not present, and the remainder of the neurologic examination is normal.

In older children, postconcussive symptoms include an equal frequency of headache and dizziness ataxia. The headache is usually described as low grade and constant, sometimes made worse by movements of the head. Gait is less disturbed, possibly because the older child is better able to compensate for dizziness, but the sensation of unsteadiness is still described.

Diagnosis. A CT scan should be performed in all children with postconcussive symptoms to exclude the possibility of posterior fossa hematoma.

Treatment. Ataxia usually clears completely within one month and always within six months. Decreased activity during this time is recommended. Further treatment is usually not required.

Vertebrobasilar Occlusion

Traumatic injuries to the vertebrobasilar arteries are reported with chiropractic manipulation and from sports injuries (Zimmerman et al, 1978). The vertebral arteries are encased within bony canals from C2 to the foramen magnum. Sudden stretching of the arteries by hyperextension or hyperflexion of the neck causes endothelial injury and thrombosis.

Clinical Features. Symptoms are noted within minutes or hours of injury. Vertigo, nausea, and vomiting are the initial manifestations of brainstem ischemia. Occipital headache may be present as well. Ataxia is due to incoordination of the limbs on one side. It may be maximal at onset or progress over several days.

Examination demonstrates some combination of unilateral brainstem disturbances (diplopia, facial weakness) and ipsilateral cerebellar dysfunction.

Diagnosis. A CT scan or MRI demonstrates a unilateral infarction in the cerebellar hemisphere and may reveal an infarction of the lateral medulla as well. The location of arterial thrombosis is visualized by arteriography.

Treatment. Many children recover completely in the months that follow injury. The value of anticoagulation has not been established.

MIGRAINE

Basilar Migraine

The term basilar (artery) migraine is used to characterize recurrent attacks of brainstem or cerebellar dysfunction that occur as a manifestation of migraine. Girls are affected more often than boys. The peak incidence is during adolescence, but attacks may occur at any age (Lapkin and Golden, 1978). Infant onset cases are more likely to present as benign paroxysmal vertigo.

Clinical Features. Gait ataxia occurs in approximately 50 percent of patients. Other symptoms include visual loss, vertigo, tinnitus, alternating hemiparesis, and paresthesias of the fingers, toes, and corners of the mouth. An abrupt loss of consciousness, usually lasting for only a few minutes, may be reported. Rare life-threatening complications are cardiac arrhythmia and brainstem stroke. Neurologic disturbances are usually followed by a severe, throbbing, occipital headache. Nausea and vomiting occur in less than one third of cases.

Several authors have stressed the association of seizures and occipital lobe spike discharges with attacks of basilar migraine. The migraine attack appears to serve as a trigger for the seizure. In one patient, routine photic stimulation provoked repetitive slow spike discharges from the occipital lobe that was concurrent with a loss of consciousness (Swanson and Vick, 1978). Upon regaining consciousness, the patient experienced ataxia, was nauseated, and had a generalized throbbing headache. It is likely that such cases are actually benign occipital epilepsy and not migraine (see Chapter 1).

Children may have repeated basilar migraine attacks, but with time the episodes evolve into a pattern of classic migraine. Even during attacks of classic migraine, the patient may continue to complain of vertigo and even ataxia.

Diagnosis. The diagnosis of basilar migraine, as in other forms of migraine, relies heavily upon a positive family history. The trait is transmitted by autosomal dominant inheritance. The parents, and the grandparents when possible, should be questioned concerning migraine symptomatology. A casual inquiry of "Is there migraine in the family?" is not sufficient. Many people do not realize that their headaches are migrainous in nature. Further, many parents are unaware that they suffered from migraine, even basilar migraine, in childhood and have had no attacks in adult life.

An EEG is the only informative laboratory test. The most common EEG abnormality in children with basilar migraine is occipital intermittent rhythmic *delta* activity (Fig. 10.3). It is present only during and just after an attack and suggests ischemia in the territory supplied by the posterior cerebral artery. Posterior circulation ischemia is further confirmed by caloric testing, which may be abnormal even between attacks.

Treatment. Many authors have recommended the use of anticonvulsant drugs for the treatment of basilar migraine. This is probably a result of confusing benign occipital epilepsy with basilar migraine. Anticonvulsant drugs are clearly indicated in children with epilepsy, whether or not they are triggered by migraine (see Chapter 1), but cannot be recommended for the prevention of migraine.

Basilar migraine is a potentially lethal form of migraine because of the potential for loss of consciousness, cardiac arrhythmia, and brainstem stroke. Therefore, prophylactic antimigraine therapy is indicated. The most effective agent for this purpose is propranolol, 1 to 2 mg/kg/day, which can be given once a day in the long-acting preparation. Despite the potential for hypotension, pulse rate reduction, and the provocation of asthma, propranolol is a remarkably safe drug in healthy children. Patients do not develop tolerance, but rebound headaches of increased frequency and intensity may occur when the drug is stopped abruptly (Diamond et al, 1982).

Benign Paroxysmal Vertigo

Benign paroxysmal vertigo is primarily a disorder of infants and preschool children but may occur in older children as well.

Clinical Features. Episodes are characterized by the sudden onset of vertigo. True cerebellar ataxia is not present, but vertigo is so profound that posture cannot be maintained. The child either lies motionless on the floor or indicates the need to be held by a parent. Consciousness is not altered and headache is not reported. Instead, the predominant symptoms are pallor, nystagmus, and fright. Episodes last only minutes and may recur at irregular intervals. With time, attacks of paroxysmal vertigo are replaced

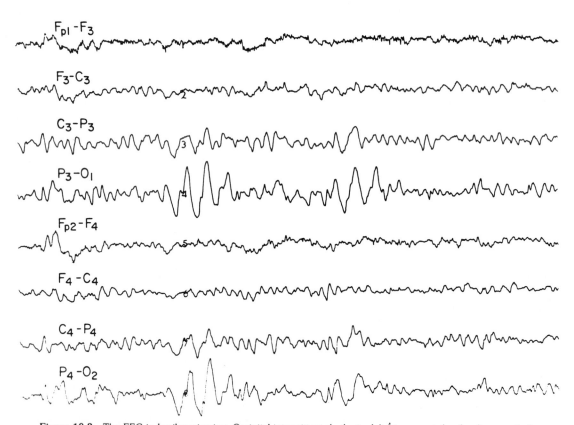

Figure 10.3 The EEG in basilar migraine. Occipital intermittent rhythmic delta is present shortly after an attack.

by episodes of headache and vomiting, which are more readily recognized as migraine (Fenichel, 1967).

Diagnosis. This is primarily a clinical diagnosis, and laboratory tests are useful only to exclude other possibilities. A positive history of migraine, though not necessarily paroxysmal vertigo, should be obtained in almost every case. Only in rare cases is there a history of benign paroxysmal vertigo in a parent.

Treatment. The attacks are so brief and harmless that treatment is usually not indicated. Standard migraine therapy can be employed when the child grows older and vertiginous episodes are replaced by headache and vomiting.

GENETIC DISORDERS

Dominant Recurrent Ataxia

More than twenty families have been reported in which episodic ataxia is transmitted by autosomal dominant inheritance (Zasorin et al, 1983). The underlying metabolic defect has not been identified and may not be the same in all families. However, the clinical findings are sufficiently similar from family to family to suggest a uniform cause.

Clinical Features. The onset of symptoms is usually in childhood, often during the first three years, but may be delayed until adult life (Farmer and Mustian, 1963; Farris et al, 1986). The child first becomes unsteady, then is totally unable to maintain posture because of vertigo and ataxia. Vomiting is frequent and severe. Jerk nystagmus, sometimes with a rotary component, is observed during attacks. In young children, the frequency of attacks is one to three per month with symptoms lasting from one hour to one day. Attacks become less frequent and less severe with age. In some patients, ataxia is the only symptom (Griggs et al, 1978); others have only vertigo (Donat and Auger, 1979), and some have only nystagmus (Farris et al, 1986; Sogg and Hoyt, 1962).

Most affected individuals are normal between attacks, but some demonstrate nystagmus and clumsiness (Farris et al, 1986).

Diagnosis. Diagnosis relies upon the clinical features and a positive family history. Basilar artery migraine and benign paroxysmal vertigo must be distinguished. In these conditions, older family members have migraine but do not have recurrent ataxia. In addition, attacks of benign paroxysmal vertigo are brief, never lasting more than a few minutes.

None of the hereditary recurrent ataxias, other than migraine, are transmitted by autosomal dominant inheritance. Nevertheless, disorders of pyruvate metabolism, many of which produce intermittent ataxia, must be excluded.

Treatment. Daily oral acetazolamide prevents recurrence of attacks in almost every case. Its mechanism of action is unknown. In young children, the dose is generally 125 mg twice a day and in older children, 250 mg twice a day. Anticonvulsant and antimigraine medications are without value.

Pyruvate Decarboxylase Deficiency

Pyruvate decarboxylase comprises the first enzyme system in the pyruvate dehydrogenase complex. This complex is responsible for the oxidative decarboxylation of pyruvate to carbon dioxide and acetylcoenzyme A (acetyl-CoA). Disorders of this complex are associated with several neurologic conditions, including subacute necrotizing encephalomyelopathy (Leigh syndrome), mitochondrial myopathies, and lactic acidosis.

An X-linked form of pyruvate decarboxylase deficiency is characterized by episodes of intermittent ataxia and lactic acidosis (Evans, 1984; Evans et al, 1978; Livingstone et al, 1984).

Clinical Features. Most patients demonstrate mild developmental delay during early childhood. Episodes of ataxia, dysarthria, and sometimes lethargy usually begin after age three. In more severely affected cases, episodes may begin during infancy and are associated with generalized weakness and states of decreased consciousness. Some attacks are spontaneous, but others are provoked by intercurrent infection, stress, or a high-carbohydrate meal. Attacks recur at irregular intervals and may last from one day to several weeks.

The severity of neurologic dysfunction in any individual probably reflects the level of residual enzyme activity. Those with generalized weakness are also areflexic and have nystagmus or other disturbances in ocular motility. Ataxia is the predominant symptom. Intention tremor and dysarthria may be present as well. Hyperventilation is frequent and may be secondary to metabolic acidosis.

Patients with almost complete decarboxylase deficiency die during infancy of lactic acidosis and central hypoventilation.

Diagnosis. Many patients have mild elevation in the concentration of blood lactate between attacks; all demonstrate elevated concentrations of blood lactate and pyruvate during attacks. Some have hyperalaninemia as well. The diagnosis of a pyruvate dysmetabolism state is further verified by an oral glucose tolerance test. When oral glucose is administered, hyperglycemia is prolonged and blood concentrations of lactate are elevated. The test may provoke clinical symptoms. Definitive diagnosis requires analysis of enzyme activity in cultured fibroblasts, leukocytes, or muscle.

Treatment. In patients with disorders of pyruvate metabolism, a high-fat (ketogenic) diet is useful to provide substrate that bypasses carbohydrate metabolism. In addition, daily oral acetazolamide, 125 mg twice a day in small children and 250 mg twice a day in older children, may significantly abort the attacks. Biotin and thiamine supplements have been employed in several patients, but the value of vitamin supplementation has not been established.

Carnitine Acetyltransferase Deficiency

Carnitine acetyltransferase is a putative enzyme in the control of acetyl-CoA flux in mitochondria. Enzyme deficiency has been described in a single patient (DiDonato et al, 1979).

Clinical Features. A previously healthy girl had recurrent episodes of confusion, ataxia, and decreased states of consciousness beginning at age two. Hypotonia with reduced tendon reflexes and ophthalmoparesis accompanied episodes. She recovered most functions within three days, but mild ataxia and dysmetria persisted after several episodes. Episodes became progressively more severe between ages three and six. They were characterized by vomiting, delirium, ptosis, large or small pupils, and ataxia. The clinical syndrome suggests a disturbance in the pyruvate dehydrogenase complex, except that the liver is enlarged. Death occurred during one of the episodes.

Diagnosis. The EEG is normal between episodes and diffusely slow during an episode. Serum transaminase concentrations are first normal and then become progressively elevated. Serum concentrations of lactate and pyruvate are normal. Definitive diagnosis requires demonstration of enzyme deficiency in liver or cultured fibroblasts.

Treatment. Treatment is not available.

Maple Syrup Urine Disease (Intermittent)

Maple syrup urine disease is a disorder of branched-chain amino acid metabolism caused by deficiency of the enzyme branched-chain ketoacid dehydrogenase. It is transmitted by autosomal recessive inheritance. Three different phenotypes are associated with this enzyme deficiency. The *classic* form presents as seizures in the newborn (see Chapter 1), the *mild* form produces progressive mental retardation (see Chapter 5), and the *intermittent* form produces recurrent attacks of ataxia and encephalopathy (Dancis et al, 1967; Zaleski et al, 1973).

Clinical Features. Affected individuals are normal during the first year. During the second year, episodes of ataxia, irritability, and progressive lethargy are provoked by minor infections, vaccination, surgery, or a diet rich in protein. The length of an attack is variable; most children recover spontaneously, but some develop severe metabolic acidosis and die. Psychomotor development remains normal in survivors.

Diagnosis. The urine has a maple syrup odor during the attack, and the blood and urine have an elevated concentration of branched-chain amino acids and ketoacids. Preliminary screening is accomplished by demonstrating a yellow precipitate when 0.2 ml of a 0.5 percent solution of 2,4-dinitrophenylhydrazine in 2N hydrochloride is added to 1 ml of urine, or a navy blue color when five to ten drops of 5 to 10 percent solution of ferric chloride are added to 1 ml of urine. Between attacks, the concentration of branched-chain amino acids and ketoacids is normal in both blood and urine. Definitive diagnosis requires the demonstration of enzyme deficiency in cultured fibroblasts.

Treatment. Children with intermittent maple syrup urine disease should be put on a protein-restricted diet. In addition, the enzyme defect in some children is thiamine-responsive and doses up to 1 g a day should be tried for the acute attack (Pueschel et al, 1979). If this is successful, a maintenance dose of 100 mg/day is recommended. The major objective during an acute attack is to reverse ketoacidosis. Protein should not be given. Peritoneal dialysis may be helpful in life-threatening situations.

Hartnup Disease

Hartnup disease is a rare disorder transmitted by autosomal recessive inheritance (Pomeroy et al, 1968). The basic error is a defect of amino acid transport in cells of the proximal renal tubules and small intestine. The result is massive aminoaciduria and the retention of amino acids in the small intestine, where they are converted by bacteria into useless or toxic products that may be absorbed. Tryptophan is converted to nonessential indole products instead of nicotinamide.

Clinical Features. Affected children are normal at birth, but may be slow in attaining developmental milestones. Most will achieve only borderline intelligence; others are normal. Affected individuals are photosensitive and develop a severe pellagra-like skin rash after exposure to sunlight. The rash is attributed to nicotinamide deficiency. Many patients have episodes of limb ataxia, sometimes associated with nystagmus (Baron et al, 1956). Mental changes, ranging from emotional instability to delirium, or states of decreased consciousness may occur. Tone is decreased and the tendon reflexes are normal or exaggerated. The neurologic disturbances are triggered by stress or intercurrent infection and may be due to the intestinal absorption of toxic amino acid breakdown products.

Most patients have both rash and neurologic disturbances, but each can occur without the other. Neurologic symptoms progress over several days and last from a week to a month before recovery occurs.

Diagnosis. The constant feature of Hartnup disease is massive aminoaciduria involving neutral monoaminomonocarboxylic amino acids. These include alanine, serine, theonine, asparagine, glutamine, valine, leucine, isoleucine, phenylalanine, tyrosine, tryptophan, histidine, and citrulline.

Treatment. The rash can be prevented by continuous oral administration of nicotinamide. It is not clear whether nicotinamide has a beneficial effect on the neurologic symptoms.

VASCULAR DISORDERS

Cerebellar Hemorrhage

Spontaneous cerebellar hemorrhage in children, in the absence of a coagulopathy, is due to arteriovenous malformation.

Clinical Features. Hemorrhage is the presenting feature in half of arteriovenous malformations (Kelly et al, 1978) and though bleeding may occur at any age, it is less common before ten years (Graf et al, 1983). After the initial hemorrhage, the risk of recurrence is 2 percent per year.

Less than 10 percent of all intracranial arteriovenous malformations in children are in the cerebellum. The two major features of cerebellar hemorrhage are ataxia and headache. Obtundation also occurs but may be mild.

Diagnosis. Cerebellar hemorrhage is easily identified on a CT scan. Blood in the posterior fossa should lead to arteriography in order to further define the source of bleeding.

Treatment. A posterior fossa hematoma producing hydrocephalus or brainstem compression must be removed, but the decision concerning surgical removal of the malformation can be individualized. Critical factors include the size of the malformation, the number of feeding vessels, and the potential damage to posterior fossa structures.

Lupus Erythematosus

Cerebellar disturbances occur in systemic lupus erythematosus (Sergent et al, 1975) and in other systemic vasculitides (Moore and Fauci, 1981). The peak incidence of lupus erythematosus is in girls near the time of puberty. In general, children with systemic lupus are much sicker than are adults with the disease (Coleman et al, 1977).

Clinical Features. The major clinical features are fever, rash, arthritis or arthralgia, and cardiac abnormalities, including cardiomegaly, pericarditis, myocarditis, and congestive heart failure. Gastrointestinal bleeding, abnormal renal function, and cardiac disturbances indicate a poor prognosis for survival. Neurologic complications of lupus erythematosus ordinarily occur late in the course of disease, after the diagnosis is already established. The most common neurologic manifestations are seizures, personality changes, and chorea. However, cerebellar ataxia is sometimes noted as an isolated finding or in association with other neurologic manifestations. The pathophysiology of cerebral dysfunction in lupus erythematosus has not been established, but probably the dysfunction is not from ischemia. Immune complex deposition within the brain is a more likely mechanism.

Diagnosis. Systemic lupus erythematosus is an unlikely diagnosis in a previously healthy child with acute ataxia. When clinical symptoms and signs are compatible with the diagnosis, the demonstration of high concentrations of antinuclear antibody is confirmatory.

Treatment. Corticosteroids alone or in combination with cytotoxic agents are used to treat the underlying disease and its neurologic complications. Every-day high-dose corticosteroids are recommended, even though their benefit has not been established.

Kawasaki Disease

Kawasaki disease is a systemic vasculitis that occurs predominantly in infants and children.

Clinical Features. Five of the following six criteria are required for diagnosis: (1) fever, (2) conjunctival congestion, (3) reddening of the oropharynx and lips, (4) indurative edema of the limbs, (5) polymorphic exanthems, and (6) lymphadenopathy. Arthralgia, carditis, and aseptic meningitis may be associated. The disease is thought to be identical to childhood polyarteritis nodosa.

Multiple infarcts may occur in the brain. Acute ataxia, facial palsy, ocular motor palsies, and hemiplegia have been reported (Scully et al, 1986). Prognosis is guarded, not only because of neurologic complications but also mainly because of coronary artery disease.

Diagnosis. Clinical features of multisystem disease are essential for diagnosis. Abnormal laboratory findings include an increased sedimentation rate, a positive test for C-reactive protein, and increased serum complement and globulin levels. Typical changes of arteritis are demonstrated by skin biopsy.

Treatment. An effective method of treatment has not been established. Aspirin is usually recommended. Corticosteroids are thought to increase coronary artery disease. Recent studies suggest that intravenous high-dose gamma globulin may be useful.

PSEUDOATAXIA (Epileptic)

Clinical Features. Ataxia and other gait disturbances can be the only manifestation of epileptiform activity (Bennett et al, 1982). The child may not have been identified as being epileptic prior to the onset of ataxia. If the child is already on anticonvulsant medication, the gait disturbance may be blamed on overdose. However, the absence of nystagmus should raise suspicion that ataxia is a seizure manifestation and is not due to anticonvulsant drug toxicity.

Both gait and limb ataxia may be present. Dysmetria can interfere with voluntary movement. Concurrent with the ataxia are prolonged generalized 2 to 3 Hz spike-wave complexes that have a frontal predominance. This is the typical EEG finding in the Lennox-Gastaut syndrome (see Chapter 1). Such discharges are ordinarily associated with either myoclonic jerks or akinetic seizures. Either one occurring momentarily, but repeatedly, could interrupt smooth movement and produce ataxia (Brett, 1966). During the ataxic episode, the child may also appear to be inattentive or confused. As with other seizure manifestations, ataxia is sudden in onset and episodic.

Diagnosis. The demonstration of epileptiform activity concurrent with ataxia is essential to diagnosis.

Treatment. Pseudoataxia usually responds to anticonvulsant drugs. Clonazepam and valproic acid are the ones used most widely for slow spike-wave discharges (see Chapter 1).

BRAIN TUMOR

Primary brain tumors ordinarily produce chronic progressive ataxia and are discussed in the section that follows. However, tumors may also present as acute ataxia because of bleeding, sudden shifts in position that cause hydrocephalus, or growth. In addition, early clumsiness may be overlooked until it "suddenly" becomes sufficiently severe to cause an obvious gait disturbance. For this reason, brain imaging is recommended in all children with acute cerebellar ataxia (see Fig. 10.1).

CONVERSION REACTION

Clinical Features. Hysterical gait disturbances are common in children, especially in girls between the ages of ten and fifteen. The disturbance is involuntary, usually provides some secondary gain, and should be distinguished from malingering, which is a voluntary act. Hysterical gait disturbances are often outrageous and are termed *astasia-abasia*. The child appears to sit without difficulty, but when brought to standing immediately begins to sway from the waist. A wide-based stance is not assumed to increase stability. Instead, the child lurches, staggers, and otherwise propels across the room from object to object. The lurching maneuvers are often quite complex and require extraordinary balance. Strength, tone, sensation, and tendon reflexes are normal.

Diagnosis. Hysterical ataxia is usually diagnosed by observation; laboratory tests are not ordinarily required to exclude other possibilities.

Treatment. It is important to determine the precipitating stress. Conversion may represent a true call for help in a desperate situation such as child abuse. Such cases require referral to a multispecialty team able to deal with the whole family.

Most children with hysterical ataxia are responding to a more immediate and less serious difficulty. Symptoms disappear promptly when the life-stress is relieved or with time. In such circumstances, psychiatric referral is necessary only when conversion is used repeatedly to handle stress.

■ Chronic or Progressive Ataxia

Brain tumor is always an initial consideration in children who were previously normal and then develop progressive ataxia, especially if headache is present as well (see Table 10.2). Congenital abnormalities that cause ataxia are frequently associated with some degree of mental deficiency. The onset of symptoms may occur during infancy or may be delayed until adult life. With the exception of Friedreich ataxia, hereditary causes of chronic ataxia are rare. However, most are easily diagnosed and many are treatable. Failure to diagnose can have unfortunate consequences for the child.

PRIMARY BRAIN TUMORS

Neuroectodermal tumors are the second most common malignancy of childhood. In most childhood brain tumor series, posterior fossa tumors account for approximately 50 percent of the total number (Schulte, 1984; Yates et al, 1979). The four major tumors of the posterior fossa are cerebellar astrocytoma, medulloblastoma, ependymoma, and brainstem glioma. Ataxia is a late manifestation of brainstem glioma; the initial features are disturbances of cranial nerve function (see Chapter 15). Although this section is limited to tumors of the posterior fossa, it is important to remember that supratentorial brain tumors may produce ataxia as well. Twenty-two percent of children with supratentorial brain tumors complain of gait disturbances at the time of their first hospitalization and 17 percent have "cerebellar signs" (Gjerris, 1978). Gait disturbances occur with equal frequency whether supratentorial tumors are located in the midline or in the hemispheres, whereas cerebellar signs are more common with midline tumors.

Cerebellar Astrocytoma

Cerebellar astrocytoma comprises 16 to 20 percent of all brain tumors in children. Less than 20 percent are malignant. The tumor may be located in the hemisphere or the vermis, in both the hemisphere and vermis, or may occupy the fourth ventricle (Tomita, 1983).

Clinical Features. Girls and boys are affected equally. The onset of symptoms is usually after age three, but may be as early as infancy. Headache is the most common initial complaint in school-aged children, whereas unsteadiness of gait and vomiting are the initial symptoms in preschool children. Headache can be insidious and intermittent; only rarely is there typical morning headache and vomiting. The first complaints of headache and nausea are usually attributed to a flu-like illness. It is only when symptoms persist that the possibility of increased intracranial pressure is considered. In infants and small children, symptoms of increased intracranial pressure are often relieved by the separation of cranial sutures. For this reason, gait disturbances without headache or vomiting are the common presentation of cerebellar astrocytoma in infants.

Papilledema is present in almost 83 percent of children at the time of initial examination, but is often absent in infants with separation of cranial sutures. Ataxia is present in 72 percent, dysmetria in 50 percent, and nystagmus in only 22 percent of these children.

Ataxia varies in severity from a wide-based lurching gait to a subtle alteration of gait observed only with tandem walking or quick turning. It is caused in part by the cerebellar location of the tumor and in part by hydrocephalus. When tumor is located in the cerebellar hemisphere, ipsilateral or bilateral dysmetria may be present. Other neurologic signs sometimes present in children with cerebellar astrocytoma include abducens palsy, multiple cranial nerve palsies, stiff neck, and head tilt.

Diagnosis. A CT scan and MRI are excellent noninvasive tests for diagnosis.

Treatment. Children with life-threatening hydrocephalus should undergo a shunting procedure as the first step in treatment. Many of the symptoms and signs, including ataxia, are relieved by the shunt (Hendrick, 1983).

Corticosteroids are sufficient to relieve pressure in many children with less severe hydrocephalus. Complete surgical extirpation of the tumor is possible when the astrocytoma is located in the cerebellar hemisphere. Such tumors are usually cystic, and removal of the mural nodule is curative. Deeper tumors that involve the floor of the fourth ventricle are rarely removed in toto. Local recurrence is common after partial resection. Repeat surgery may be curative in some cases, but postoperative radiotherapy appears to offer a better prognosis following partial resection. In one series (Leibel, 1975), partial resection and radiotherapy resulted in a 93 percent five-year survival rate, a 70 percent ten-year survival rate, and a 40 percent twenty-year survival rate. Chemotherapy is not currently recommended for low-grade cerebellar astrocytomas regardless of the degree of surgical resection.

In rare cases, high-grade cerebellar astrocytoma (glioblastoma) has been reported in children. More than 30 percent of such patients have dissemination of tumor through the neuraxis (spinal cord drop metastases). Examination of cerebrospinal fluid for cytologic features and complete myelography are recommended following surgical resection in all patients with glioblastoma. If either result is abnormal, whole-axis radiation is indicated.

Medulloblastoma

Medulloblastoma is a primitive neuroectodermal tumor with the capacity to differentiate into neuronal and glial tissue. Most tumors are located in the vermis or fourth ventricle with or without extension into the cerebellar hemispheres. Approximately 10 percent are in the hemisphere alone (Tomita, 1983).

Clinical Features. Most series indicate a male to female ratio of 3:2. Ninety percent of cases have their onset during the first decade and the remainder during the second decade. Medulloblastoma is the most common primary brain tumor with onset of symptoms during infancy.

The tumor grows rapidly and the interval between onset of symptoms and medical consultation is generally brief; 25 percent of cases within two weeks and 50 percent in less than a month. Vomiting is the initial symptom in 58 percent of children, headache in 40 percent, and an unsteady gait in 20 percent. Ten percent

of children present with torticollis or stiff neck. The predominance of vomiting as a presenting symptom, with or without headache, is probably caused by the position of the tumor irritating the floor of the fourth ventricle. Gait disturbances are more common in young children and are characterized by refusal to stand or walk rather than by ataxia.

Two thirds of children have papilledema at the time of initial examination. Truncal ataxia or limb ataxia, or both, are equally common. Nystagmus is present in only 22 percent of children. Tendon reflexes are hyperactive when hydrocephalus is present and hypoactive when tumor is primarily causing cerebellar dysfunction.

Diagnosis. Medulloblastoma is readily diagnosed by CT scan or magnetic resonance imaging (Fig. 10.4). The tumors are highly vascular and become enhanced when contrast medium is used.

Treatment. The prognosis for children with medulloblastoma is markedly improved by the combined use of surgical extirpation, radiation therapy, and chemotherapy. The role of surgery is to provide histologic identification, debulk the tumor, and relieve obstruction of the fourth ventricle.

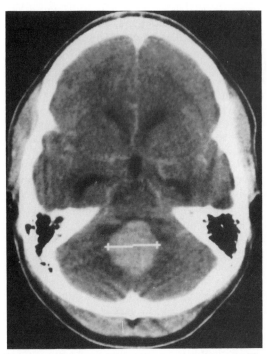

Figure 10.4 Image (CT scan) of medulloblastoma. The tumor is demonstrated as an enhancing mass in the vermis of the cerebellum.

Children with medulloblastoma are divided into high-risk and low-risk groups for the purpose of designing therapy. The high-risk or poor-prognosis group includes those with any evidence of tumor dissemination, residual tumor more than 1.5 cm^2 following initial surgery, tumors invading two structures or completely filling the fourth ventricle, or tumor filling the fourth ventricle and extending to the third ventricle or the cervical cord. Radiation therapy is necessary for children in both the high-risk and low-risk groups. Medulloblastoma is more radiosensitive than is glioma, and a lower total dose of radiation can be used (Tomita and McLone, 1986). Before radiation is begun, a complete myelogram must be performed to determine if drop metastases are present. Areas with visible metastatic disease receive a "boosted" radiation dose.

Children in the high-risk group are treated with chemotherapy as well. The currently recommended regimen includes vincristine, CCNU, and prednisone. This combination has improved five-year survival rates by more than 10 percent. Other experimental protocols are being tested at present and children with medulloblastoma should be referred to specialized centers for chemotherapy.

Using the combined approaches of surgery, radiation, and chemotherapy, the five-year survival rate is 50 to 70 percent.

Ependymoma

Posterior fossa ependymoma is derived from the cells that line the roof and floor of the fourth ventricle. The tumor can extend into both lateral recesses and grow out to the cerebellopontine angle. They account for 10 percent of all primary brain tumors in children.

Clinical Features. Ependymoma is primarily a tumor of young children; 50 percent become symptomatic before the age of three (Choux, 1983). Both sexes are affected equally.

Symptoms evolve more slowly in children with ependymoma than in those with medulloblastoma. It is common for symptoms to be present for several months before medical consultation is sought. Symptoms of increased intracranial pressure are the first manifestation in 90 percent of patients. Disturbances of gait and coordination, neck pain, and cranial nerve dysfunction account for the remainder. Fifty percent have ataxia, usually of the vermal type, and 33 percent have nystagmus. Head tilt or neck stiffness is present in one third of children and

indicates extension of tumor into the cervical canal.

Although steady, progressive deterioration is expected in most children, some have an intermittent course. Transient episodes of headache and vomiting, ataxia, and even nuchal rigidity lasting for days or weeks are followed by periods of well-being. These intermittent symptoms are caused by transitory obstruction of the fourth ventricle or aqueduct by the tumor acting in a ball-valve fashion.

Diagnosis. CT and MRI are equally effective diagnostic procedures. Marked dilation of the ventricular system is almost always present. MRI has the advantage over CT in better demonstrating the location of the tumor within the fourth ventricle and its extraventricular extensions.

Treatment. The goals of surgical therapy are to relieve the hydrocephalus and to remove as much tumor as possible without causing damage to the fourth ventricle. Postoperative irradiation to the posterior fossa, but not the neuraxis, is usually indicated. A postoperative mortality rate of approximately 30 percent is noted in several series. Five-year survival rates vary from 33 to 70 percent.

High-grade ependymomas and ependymoblastomas are likely to seed the spinal subarachnoid space and require whole neuraxis radiation. In addition, chemotherapeutic agents, similar to those used for medulloblastoma, should be administered.

Cerebellar Hemangioblastoma
(Von Hippel–Lindau Disease)

Von Hippel–Lindau disease is a multisystem disorder transmitted by autosomal dominant inheritance. The most prominent features are hemangioblastomas of the cerebellum and retina (Huson et al, 1986). All children presenting with cerebellar hemangioblastoma have von Hippel–Lindau disease. Among adults, 60 percent have isolated tumors and do not have the genetic defect. The expression of von Hippel–Lindau disease is variable even within the same kindred. Postmortem examination reveals the following incidence of major manifestations: cerebellar hemangioblastoma, 83 percent; retinal hemangioblastoma, 46 percent; other cerebral hemangioblastoma, 20 percent; renal carcinoma, 51 percent; renal cysts, 49 percent; pancreatic cysts, 69 percent; and pheochromocytoma, 17 percent.

Clinical Features. Mean age at onset of cerebellar hemangioblastoma in von Hippel–Lindau disease is thirty-two years; presentation before fifteen is unusual. The initial features are headache and ataxia. Retinal hemangioblastomas occur at a younger age and may cause visual impairment resulting from hemorrhage as early as the first decade. They may be multiple and bilateral and appear on ophthalmoscopic examination as a dilated artery leading from the disk to a peripheral tumor with an engorged vein.

Diagnosis. The diagnosis of von Hippel–Lindau disease is made by any of the following criteria: (1) more than one hemangioblastoma of the central nervous system, (2) an isolated hemangioblastoma associated with a visceral cyst or renal carcinoma, (3) any known manifestation with a positive family history.

A contrasted head CT scan is usually successful in demonstrating cerebellar hemangioblastoma. Arteriography is required to fully visualize the blood supply. Visceral manifestations can be identified by abdominal CT scan and ultrasound.

Treatment. Children at risk for von Hippel–Lindau disease should be screened for retinal hemangioblastomas by indirect ophthalmoscopy every five years. Cryotherapy or photocoagulation of smaller lesions can lead to complete tumor regression without visual loss.

CT scans should be performed in any child who develops ataxia, and at five-year intervals after the age of fifteen in children with genetic risk factors. Cerebellar hemangioblastoma should be treated surgically and can often be totally extirpated.

Visceral manifestations are uncommon in childhood, but must be screened with abdominal CT scans in adults.

CONGENITAL MALFORMATIONS

Cerebellar Hypoplasia

Congenital hypoplasia of the cerebellum occurs in humans as an autosomal recessive disease and can be experimentally induced in immature animals by cytotoxic drugs, irradiation, or viral infection. The common histologic feature is the absence of granular cells with a relative preservation of Purkinje cells. In the human hereditary form, granular cell degeneration may continue postnatally and cause progressive cerebellar dysfunction during infancy. Most cases of human cerebellar hypoplasia are sporadic, and though the causes are probably diverse, the clinical features are relatively constant (Sarnat and Alcala, 1980).

Clinical Features. Developmental delay and hypotonia are the first features suggesting a cerebral abnormality in the infant. Titubation of the head is constant, and some combination of ataxia, dysmetria, and intention tremor is noted as well. A jerky coarse nystagmus is usually present. Tendon reflexes may be increased or diminished. Those with hyperactive reflexes probably have congenital abnormalities of the corticospinal tract in addition to cerebellar hypoplasia. Seizures occur in some hereditary and some sporadic cases. Other neurologic signs and symptoms may be present, depending upon associated malformations. Mental retardation is a constant feature, but varies from mild to severe.

Diagnosis. Cerebellar hypoplasia can be demonstrated by CT or MRI. The folial pattern of the cerebellum is prominent and there is compensatory enlargement of the fourth ventricle, cisterna magna, and vallecula.

Treatment. Treatment is not available.

Vermal Aplasia

Aplasia of the vermis is relatively common and often associated with other cerebral malformations. The vermis may be missing in part or in whole, and when incomplete the caudal portion is usually lacking.

Clinical Features. Partial agenesis of the cerebellar vermis may be asymptomatic. A family with dominantly inherited aplasia of the anterior vermis demonstrated only mild gait ataxia and upbeating nystagmus (Furman et al, 1985). Complete agenesis causes titubation of the head and truncal ataxia. Vermal agenesis is frequently associated with other cerebral malformations, producing a constellation of symptoms and signs referable to neurologic dysfunction. Two such examples are the Dandy-Walker malformation (see Chapter 18) and the Joubert syndrome (Joubert et al, 1969).

Cerebellar vermal agenesis is a constant feature of the Joubert syndrome, but several other cerebral malformations are usually present as well. More than one sibling in a family may be involved, but the parents are normal. The typical clinical manifestation in newborns and infants is periods of hyperpnea, usually around 120 breaths/minute and lasting for up to 16 seconds, alternating with episodes of apnea lasting up to 12 seconds. Abnormal, conjugate jerking eye movements are observed in half of infants. Most are hypotonic. Tendon reflexes may be normal or exaggerated. All are mentally retarded and some are microcephalic. Several affected children have died unexpectedly, possibly from respiratory failure.

Diagnosis. CT demonstrates agenesis of the vermis of the cerebellum with enlargement of the cisterna magna (Curatolo et al, 1980). Other cerebral malformations, such as agenesis of the corpus callosum, may be observed as well.

Treatment. Treatment is not available.

The Chiari Malformation

The Chiari malformation is a displacement of the cerebellar tonsils into the upper cervical canal, sometimes accompanied by caudal dislocation of the hindbrain. Children with the Chiari malformation usually have myelomeningocele as well, and the combination is referred to as the Arnold-Chiari malformation (see Chapter 12). When the Chiari malformation is present without meningocele, the onset of symptoms is frequently delayed until adolescence or adult life.

Clinical Features. Major clinical features are headache, pain in the neck and shoulders, ataxia, and lower cranial nerve dysfunction (Levy et al, 1983). Physical signs are variable from patient to patient. The following features are found in approximately half of cases: weakness of the arms, hyperactive tendon reflexes in the legs, nystagmus, and ataxia.

Diagnosis. Magnetic resonance imaging provides the best visualization of posterior fossa structures. The distortion of the cerebellum and the hindbrain are precisely identified (Fig. 10.5).

Treatment. Surgical decompression of the foramen magnum to at least the C3 vertebrae is recommended (Park et al, 1983). More than half of patients will be significantly improved by surgery.

Basilar Impression

Basilar impression is a disorder of the craniovertebral junction in which the odontoid process is displaced posteriorly and compresses the spinal cord or brainstem.

Clinical Features. The first symptoms are often head tilt, neck stiffness, and headache. The onset of symptoms is frequently precipitated by minor trauma to the head or neck. Examination reveals ataxia, nystagmus, and hyperreflexia (Teodori and Painter, 1984).

Diagnosis. On a lateral skull radiograph, a line is drawn from the posterior edge of the hard palate to the inferior aspect of the occiput

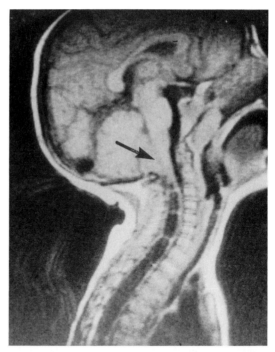

Figure 10.5 Chiari malformation. Magnetic resonance image demonstrates displacement of the cerebellar tonsils (arrow) into the foramen magnum. (Courtesy of Drs. Partain, Heller, and Kessler, Department of Radiology and Radiological Sciences, Vanderbilt University, Nashville.)

(McGregor's line). The tip of the odontoid should not be more than 7 mm above this line. CT demonstrates invagination of the odontoid process into the foramen magnum. Magnetic resonance imaging may be useful to delineate an associated Chiari malformation or syringobulbia (Fig. 10.5).

Treatment. Surgical decompression of the foramen magnum is usually successful in relieving symptoms.

HEREDITARY ATAXIA

Dominant Hereditary Ataxia

There are probably several different ataxic disorders transmitted by autosomal dominant inheritance. Unfortunately, they are difficult to separate on clinical grounds, because there is considerable phenotypic variability even within a single kindred. Two terms are used in the literature to describe families with progressive dominantly inherited ataxia: *olivopontocerebellar degeneration* and *Machado-Joseph* disease.

Olivopontocerebellar Degeneration

The olivopontocerebellar degenerations have their onset between the ages of fifteen and thirty-five. They may be broadly divided into two subgroups: one in which the genetic defect is linked to the HLA-locus on chromosome 6 and the other in which this linkage is not present (Nino et al, 1980). When the linkage is present, the risk of having the defective gene can be calculated in an asymptomatic child to provide genetic counseling (Jackson and Currier, 1983).

Clinical Features. Cerebellar ataxia is invariably present and is frequently the initial manifestation. There is gait ataxia, dysmetria, dysdiadochokinesia, finger-nose ataxia, and decomposition of movement. Tendon reflexes are exaggerated and the plantar response is usually extensor. Optic nerve atrophy is a constant finding in some families, but not in others (Landis et al, 1974). Other variable features include nystagmus, dysarthria, decreased pupillary response, ptosis, and impaired position sense.

Diagnosis. Diagnosis depends upon the clinical features and a positive family history.

Treatment. Treatment is not available.

Machado-Joseph Disease

In contrast to the olivopontocerebellar degenerations, Machado-Joseph disease is genetically homogeneous. It originated in Portuguese-Azorean populations and was transmitted worldwide by Portuguese sailors during the age of exploration. The age of onset appears to be earlier with each generation (*anticipation*), and presentation during adolescence is relatively common.

Clinical Features. The disorder is characterized by a degeneration of all motor systems: cerebellar, extrapyramidal, pyramidal, and motor unit. However, ataxia is almost always the first symptom. There is unsteadiness of gait first and then dysmetria of the hands. Nystagmus is often present and tendon reflexes may be diminished or brisk if corticospinal tract involvement is present.

Within the same family, some members have predominantly a dystonic disorder, others have ataxia and pyramidal signs, and still others demonstrate amyotrophy (Fowler, 1984; Lima and Coutinho, 1980). Dystonia is somewhat more common than ataxia as a presenting sign in children. Bulging eyes are a characteristic, but not constant, early feature of the disorder. All affected individuals eventually develop multi-motor system degeneration, with death occurring in middle to late adult life.

Diagnosis. Diagnosis depends upon the clinical features and a positive family history. Neurodiagnostic studies do not add to the physical examination. In families with several affected members, individuals recognize the disease in themselves and may not seek medical attention.

Treatment. Treatment is not available for the underlying genetic defect, but Parkinson-like symptoms may be reversed by L-dopa and dystonia may respond to trihexyphenidyl hydrochloride.

Ramsay Hunt Variants

The Ramsay Hunt syndrome is discussed with genetic ataxias transmitted by autosomal recessive inheritance (see later discussion). However, the same complex of symptoms also occurs in two dominantly inherited disorders in which dentatorubral degeneration is associated with (1) progressive atrophy of the globus pallidus and subthalamic nucleus (Naito and Oyanagi, 1982; Suzuki et al, 1985), or (2) a mitochondrial myopathy (Feit et al, 1983; Fitzsimons et al, 1981).

Clinical Features. In families with combined dentatorubral-pallidoluysian degeneration, the onset of symptoms may be in childhood or adult life. Those with a childhood onset have epilepsy and early dementia, whereas those with an adult onset present with ataxia. Dementia, dysarthria, and ataxia of gait and limbs occurs in all cases; myoclonus occurs in 90 percent; convulsions occur in 70 percent; and choreoathetosis occurs in 50 percent of patients.

Patients with widespread mitochondrial disease have mental retardation and proximal weakness in addition to the cerebellar ataxia and myoclonus.

Diagnosis. Ramsay Hunt variants transmitted by autosomal dominant inheritance are easy to separate from sporadic cases by family history. A glucose-lactate tolerance test should be performed in every patient to screen for a mitochondrial disorder (see Chapters 7 and 8).

Treatment. Myoclonus and seizures are best treated with valproic acid. One patient with a mitochondrial disorder responded to oral doses of L-5 hydroxytryptophan and carbidopa.

Autosomal Recessive Inheritance

Friedreich Ataxia

The term *Friedreich ataxia* has been used in a generic sense as a prototype for all spinocerebellar degenerations. This usage is not helpful. When strict clinical criteria are applied, there emerges a more homogeneous group of patients who have a predictable course (Harding, 1981; Stumpf, 1985). These criteria include autosomal recessive inheritance, onset of ataxia or scoliosis before age twenty, rapid early progression, and the absence of ophthalmoplegia and dementia. Several lines of investigation have suggested a defect in pyruvate metabolism as a cause of Friedreich ataxia, but there is currently no evidence to support this notion.

Clinical Features. It is well recognized that clinical features are similar in members of the same family. Several large kindreds of French-Canadians with Friedreich ataxia have all descended from a single couple (Bouchard et al, 1979). These families have many clinical features that are not ordinarily seen in other families with the disease. The French-Canadian families are probably genetically distinct and will not be discussed here.

Heterozygotes have no manifestations of disease, and the presence of abnormal signs, such as pes cavus or scoliosis, in parents should suggest a dominantly inherited ataxia or Charcot-Marie-Tooth disease (Harding, 1981).

Age of onset in the majority of cases is between two and sixteen years, but occasional patients present after twenty and some present during infancy. The initial manifestation in 95 percent of cases is ataxia or clumsiness of gait; the remaining 5 percent present with scoliosis. The course is one of steady deterioration; most patient are confined to a wheelchair within twenty years of onset. All patients develop dysarthria. Disturbances of ocular motility occur in 32 percent and deafness occurs in 8 percent of patients. Titubation of the head occurs in only 4 percent of cases. Symptoms of cerebellar dysfunction are more severe and more common in the arms than in the legs. Almost every patient will develop finger-nose ataxia and difficulty in performing rapid alternating movements. Only 28 percent of patients demonstrate the same symptoms in the legs, but spastic weakness is often present and may hide the cerebellar signs. All tendon reflexes are absent in 75 percent of patients. In the other 25 percent, reflexes are obtained only at the biceps. Extensor plantar responses are present in 89 percent. Joint position sense is absent in the feet in 90 percent and in the hands in 27 percent of cases. Vibration sense is equally impaired, but disturbances of light touch and pain occur in less than 10 percent of patients.

Scoliosis develops in 79 percent of patients, and pes cavus develops in 55 percent. The severity of the skeletal deformities varies and is usually mild. A cardiomyopathy, characterized by dyspnea on exertion, palpitations, and angina, develops in 40 percent of patients. Systolic ejection murmurs, heard best over the apex or left sternal edge, are relatively common.

Diabetes is present in 10 percent of patients and has its onset during the third decade. The diabetes tends to be severe, may be difficult to control with insulin, and can significantly contribute to death from the disease.

Diagnosis. The diagnosis relies primarily upon the clinical features. Motor nerve conduction velocities in the arms and legs are slightly slower than normal. In contrast, sensory action potentials are either absent or markedly reduced in amplitude. Spinal somatosensory evoked responses are usually absent as well.

The common electrocardiogram (EKG) changes are a reduced amplitude of T waves and left or right ventricular hypertrophy. Arrhythmias and conduction defects are uncommon.

Treatment. The underlying disturbance is not curable, but symptomatic treatment is available. Severe scoliosis should be prevented by orthopedic intervention. The development of cardiomyopathy must be monitored by regular EKG and chest radiographs to determine heart size. Chest pain on exertion responds to propranolol and congestive heart failure responds to digitalis. Patients should be checked for diabetes, and insulin should be administered when necessary.

Ramsay Hunt Syndrome

This syndrome, also termed *dyssynergia cerebellaris myoclonica*, is a progressive degeneration of the dentate nucleus and superior cerebellar peduncle characterized by myoclonus, cerebellar ataxia, and seizures (see Chapter 1). Many cases are sporadic and autosomal recessive inheritance is only presumed.

Clinical Features. Sporadic cases are not homogeneous, but a general clinical picture can be delineated. The initial symptom is clumsiness, usually noted during the first decade, which evolves into progressive ataxia. Intention tremor and dysarthria may follow. Myoclonus usually begins in the second decade. It is present at rest, but is made worse by attempted movement. Myoclonus may be so severe as to throw the patient to the floor. The combination of ataxia

and myoclonus is severely disabling. Generalized tonic-clonic convulsions are not a constant
feature and develop late in the course. Tendon
reflexes are depressed and scoliosis may be
present.

Diagnosis. The Ramsay Hunt syndrome is
diagnosed by the combination of cerebellar
ataxia and myoclonus. However, diagnosing the
syndrome does not diagnose a disease. Variants
with autosomal dominant inheritance as well as
other syndromes causing myoclonic epilepsy
must be considered (see Chapter 1). CT or MRI
may reveal atrophy of the pons, cerebellar pe-
duncles, and cerebellum. EEG frequently demonstrates epileptiform activity of the slow spike-
wave type.

Treatment. Seizures usually respond to ordinary anticonvulsant drugs. Valproic acid has
been found specifically useful in reducing the
amplitude and frequency of myoclonus (Somerville and Olanow, 1982).

Ataxia Telangiectasia

This is a disorder affecting both the nervous
and immune systems. It is transmitted by autosomal recessive inheritance. The disease is
worldwide in distribution, occurs in all races, and
may be more frequent than Friedreich ataxia.

Clinical Features. The principal feature is a
progressive ataxia that has its onset during the
first year. Some infants develop choreoathetosis
instead of, or in addition to, ataxia. The ataxia,
which begins as clumsiness, progresses so slowly
that many affected infants are diagnosed as
having cerebral palsy. Oculomotor apraxia is
present in 90 percent of patients, but may be
mild and overlooked (see Chapter 15). It is a
disturbance of voluntary gaze with intact following responses. Consequently, the head turns
first and the eyes follow after. Many children are
said to have a dull or expressionless face. Intellectual development is normal at first, but tends
to slow with time. One third of children will
ultimately function in the mildly retarded range.

Telangiectasias usually develop after age two
and sometimes as late as age ten. They are first
noted on the bulbar conjunctivae, giving the
eyes a bloodshot appearance. Similar telangiectasias also appear on the upper half of the ears,
the flexor surfaces of the limbs, and the butterfly
area of the face. Telangiectasia may be exacerbated by exposure to sun or by irritation or
friction (Hosking, 1982).

Recurrent sinopulmonary infection is one of
the more serious features of the disease and

reflects an underlying immunodeficiency. The
synthesis of antibodies and certain immunoglobulin subclasses is disturbed as a result of disorders of B-cell and helper T-cell function. Serum
and salivary IgA are absent in 70 to 80 percent
and IgE is absent or diminished in 80 to 90
percent of children. IgM may be elevated in
compensation for the IgA deficiency. The thymus has an embryonic appearance, and alpha-
fetoprotein concentrations are elevated in the
majority of patients (Waldmann et al, 1983).

Taken together, the many features of this
disease suggest a generalized disorder of tissue
differentiation and cellular repair. The result is
an increased incidence of neoplasia, especially
lymphoma and lymphocytic leukemia. Two
thirds of patients are dead by age twenty. After
infection, neoplastic disease is the most common
cause of death.

Diagnosis. The diagnosis should be suspected in infancy by the combination of ataxia,
chronic sinopulmonary infections, and oculomotor apraxia. As the child gets older, the
addition of telangiectasia to the other clinical
features makes the diagnosis a certainty. Complete studies of immunocompetence should be
performed. Elevated concentrations of alpha-
fetoprotein provide further confirmation.

Treatment. All infections must be treated
vigorously. Intravenous antibiotics are sometimes required for what would otherwise be a
trivial sinusitis in a normal child. Patients with
ataxia telangiectasia are exquisitely sensitive to
radiation, which produces cellular and chromosomal damage. This may be a precipitating
cause in the development of neoplasia. Therefore, despite the frequency of sinopulmonary
infections, radiologic exposure must be mini-
mized.

Marinesco-Sjögren Syndrome

The Marinesco-Sjögren syndrome, characterized by cerebellar ataxia, congenital cataracts,
and mental retardation, is transmitted by autosomal recessive inheritance. It is a rare disorder
and by 1985, slightly more than sixty patients
had been reported. The inherited abnormality is
unknown, but electron microscopic studies suggest the possibility of a lysosomal storage disorder (Walker et al, 1985).

Clinical Features. Cataracts are a constant
feature; they may be congenital or develop
during infancy. The type of cataract is variable
and not specific. Cerebellar dysfunction during
infancy is characterized by dysarthria, nystag-

mus, and ataxia of trunk and limbs. Strabismus and hypotonia are frequently associated in childhood. Developmental delay is a constant feature, but varies from mild to severe. Other features include short stature, delayed sexual development, pes valgus, and scoliosis.

Although the onset of symptoms is in infancy, the progress is very slow or stationary. Ataxia leads to a wheelchair existence by the third or fourth decade and the life span is significantly shortened.

Diagnosis. Diagnosis of the Marinesco-Sjögren syndrome relies primarily on the triad of bilateral cataracts, progressive cerebellar ataxia, and mental retardation. The underlying biochemical defect is unknown and laboratory tests are not helpful.

Treatment. Treatment is not available.

Abetalipoproteinemia

This is a disorder of lipid metabolism transmitted by autosomal recessive inheritance. Other terms for the disorder are *acanthocytosis* and the *Bassen-Kornzweig syndrome*. Apolipoprotein-B, which is essential for the synthesis and structural integrity of chylomicrons, very low-density lipoproteins, and low-density lipoproteins, is missing from the serum. The result is fat malabsorption and a progressive deficiency of vitamins A, E, and K.

Clinical Features. Fat malabsorption is present from birth, and most newborns come to medical attention because of failure to thrive, vomiting, and large volumes of loose stools. The correct diagnosis may be made at that time.

Psychomotor development during infancy is delayed. A cerebellar ataxia develops in one third of children during the first decade and in almost every child by the end of the second decade. The progression of symptoms may suggest Friedreich ataxia. Tendon reflexes are usually lost by age five. Progressive limb ataxia is characterized by disturbances of gait, dysmetria, and difficulty with performing rapid, alternating movements. Ataxia progresses until the third decade and then becomes stationary. Proprioceptive sensation is lost in the hands and feet, and mild reduction of pinprick and temperature sensations may be present as well. Sensory loss results from demyelination in the posterior columns of the spinal cord and the peripheral nerves (Wichman et al, 1985).

Retinitis pigmentosa is an almost constant feature of abetalipoproteinemia. The age of onset is variable, but is usually during the first decade. The initial symptom is night blindness. Nystagmus is common and may be caused either by the cerebellar disturbance or by loss of central vision.

Diagnosis. The acanthocyte is the hallmark of abetalipoproteinemia and other lipoprotein deficiencies. It is an abnormal erythrocyte characterized by thorny projections from the cell surface which prevent normal rouleau formation and cause a very low erythrocyte sedimentation rate. Fifty to 70 percent of peripheral erythrocytes undergo transformation to acanthocytes. Severe anemia, with hemoglobulin levels below 8 g/dl (5 mmol/L), is common in young children, but not in adults. The anemia may be secondary to malabsorption and can be corrected with parenteral supplementation of iron or folate. Plasma cholesterol levels are less than 100 mg/dl (2.5 mmol/L) and triglyceride levels are less than 30 mg/dl (0.3 mmol/L). The diagnosis is confirmed by the absence of apolipoprotein-B in plasma. Parents should be screened for apolipoprotein-B as well. In abetalipoproteinemia, the heterozygote is normal; if partial deficiency is present, the diagnosis of familial hypobetalipoproteinemia is more likely.

Treatment. It is not clear how much of the neurologic abnormality is a direct effect of lipoprotein deficiency and how much is secondary to fat-soluble vitamin deficiency. Steatorrhea in the newborn responds to a restricted intake of triglycerides containing long-chain fatty acids. In addition to the low-fat diet, patients should be maintained for life on 200 to 300 IU/kg/day of vitamin E and 200 to 400 IU/kg/day of vitamin A (Illingworth et al, 1980). There is evidence that vitamin supplementation not only prevents or retards the development of neurologic sequelae, but also may reverse a neuropathy or myopathy already present (Hegele and Angel, 1985).

Hypobetalipoproteinemia

Clinical Features. Several different disorders are described in which serum lipid profiles reveal hypocholesterolemia and reduced, but not absent, concentrations of apolipoprotein-B and apolipoprotein-A. Some individuals have no neurologic symptoms. Others have severe ataxia beginning in infancy (Agamanolis et al, 1986). Malabsorption does not occur, but there is failure to thrive and progressive fatty cirrhosis of the liver. Severe hypotonia and absent tendon reflexes are noted in the first months. The course is characterized by inanition, slow development, and recurrent infection. Death occurs in the second year.

Diagnosis. Total serum lipid content is normal and the concentration of triglycerides is increased. Total high-density lipoprotein (HDL) and low-density lipoprotein (LDL) cholesterol concentrations are reduced, as are apolipoprotein-B and apoprotein-A-1.

Treatment. Treatment is not available.

Juvenile Sulfatide Lipidosis

Sulfatide lipidosis (metachromatic leukodystrophy) is a disorder of central and peripheral myelin metabolism due to deficient activity of the enzyme arylsulfatase-A (ASA). It is transmitted by autosomal recessive inheritance. The late infantile form is discussed in Chapters 5 and 7. The juvenile form is genetically distinct and affects central myelin more than peripheral myelin.

Clinical Features. The age at onset is usually after age five, but may be as early as infancy or as late as adult life. When onset is in infancy, the initial symptoms are developmental delay and clumsiness. In school-aged children, the disease presents with spasticity and progressive ataxia of the trunk and limbs and generalized tonic-clonic convulsions (Haltia et al, 1980; MacFaul et al, 1982). Mental deterioration follows. Peripheral neuropathy is not a prominent clinical feature, but motor conduction velocities are usually prolonged late in the course. Protein concentration in the cerebrospinal fluid may be normal or only slightly elevated.

Once symptoms start, progression is relatively rapid. Most children deteriorate into a vegetative state and die within ten years. The duration from onset to death ranges from three to seventeen years and cannot be predicted by age at onset.

Diagnosis. Among the many causes of progressive ataxia, this one demonstrates rapid and severe degeneration of multiple neurologic systems. It should be especially considered when there is a family history of a similar illness. Nevertheless, many such families have gone for years without diagnosis. Physicians are frequently misled by normal motor conduction velocities early in the course. CT and MRI demonstrate widespread demyelination of the cerebral hemispheres. Patients with late-onset disease are often thought to have multiple sclerosis. Diagnosis requires the demonstration of markedly reduced or absent ASA in peripheral leukocytes.

Treatment. Treatment is not available.

Juvenile GM₂ Gangliosidosis

There are several juvenile forms of both *alpha* and *beta* hexosaminidase-A deficiency (Johnson, 1981). All are transmitted by autosomal recessive inheritance. Some, like Tay-Sachs disease, are restricted in occurrence to Ashkenazi Jews, whereas others occur in individuals of non-Jewish descent (see Chapter 5). In all of these conditions, there is storage of GM₂ gangliosides within the central nervous system.

Clinical Features. Several different syndromes have been described; some resemble the Ramsey Hunt syndrome, and others mimic Friedreich ataxia or other spinocerebellar degenerations (Willner et al, 1981). Clumsiness of gait and ataxia are the usual presenting features. Onset is usually after age two, but can be as late as adult life. Intention tremor is frequently associated. Affected children may be considered clumsy for several years before neurologic deterioration is evident. Although ataxia is a constant feature, the variety of other neurologic findings and the rate of progression varies from family to family, but is relatively constant within a kindred. Associated neurologic disturbances may include spasticity, dysarthria, optic atrophy, athetoid posturing of the hands, and dementia. Many patients progress to a vegetative state.

Other findings in some families include pes cavus, scoliosis, and visceromegaly.

Diagnosis. Any child with an apparent "spinocerebellar degeneration" should be evaluated for GM₂ gangliosidosis by measuring alpha- and beta-hexosaminidase activity in fibroblasts. Ganglioside storage in neurons is demonstrated by rectal biopsy.

Treatment. Treatment is not available.

Sea-Blue Histiocytoses

This is a group of neurovisceral storage diseases, similar to Niemann-Pick disease, for which the enzymatic error has not been established. Sea-blue histiocytes are large macrophages 20 to 60 μ in diameter with a single eccentric nucleus and a prominent nucleolus. Wright-Giemsa staining reveals blue or blue-green granules in the cytoplasm that contain ceroid, lipofuscin, and sphingomyelin. The histiocytes are present in the bone marrow, liver, and lymph glands.

Clinical Features. Several different clinical presentations have been described (Ashwal et al, 1984; Gartner et al, 1986). Hepatosplenomegaly is usually the first manifestation, but neurologic deterioration may precede the visceral dysfunction. Onset of symptoms can be as early as two months, but more frequently occurs after one year and sometimes after age ten. Ataxia and spasticity are prominent features. The initial progress of neurologic dysfunction is sufficiently slow that the child is thought to have cerebral palsy. Involuntary movements and tremor may be present as well.

Neurologic deterioration accelerates as the child gets older. Further symptoms include dementia, seizures, speech disturbances, and supranuclear ophthalmoplegia. Severe bulbar palsy leads to aspiration and death.

Diagnosis. Sea-blue histiocytes are present in the bone marrow or liver, and lysosomal enzyme activity is normal.

Treatment. Treatment is not available. Liver transplantation was tried in one patient without success.

Ataxia with Episodic Dystonia

Families are described with the combination of ataxia, brisk tendon reflexes, and episodic dystonia, in which transmission of the trait is by autosomal recessive inheritance (Graff-Radford, 1986). An underlying metabolic disturbance has not been identified. Onset is always in the first decade. The child first develops progressive ataxia and then episodes of dystonia, which may be unilateral. The dystonia responds to anticonvulsant drugs. This syndrome shares many features with the syndrome of familial paroxysmal choreoathetosis, except for the pattern of inheritance and the progressive nature of the ataxia (see Chapter 1).

Other Metabolic Disorders

Hartnup disease and maple syrup urine disease were both described in the section on Acute or Recurrent Ataxia. After an acute attack, some patients never return to baseline and present with chronic progressive ataxia. Such patients should be screened for metabolic disorders (Table 10.3). Refsum disease is an inborn error of phytanic acid metabolism and is transmitted by autosomal recessive inheritance. The cardinal features are retinitis pigmentosa, chronic or recurrent polyneuropathy, and cerebellar ataxia. Affected individuals usually present with either night blindness or neuropathy (see Chapter 7).

Disorders of pyruvate metabolism and the respiratory chain enzymes produce widespread disturbances in the nervous system and are

Table 10.3 METABOLIC SCREENING IN PROGRESSIVE ATAXIAS

Disease	Abnormality
Blood	
Adrenoleukodystrophy	Very-long-chain fatty acids
Ataxia-telangiectasia	IgA, IgE, alpha-fetoprotein
Abetalipoproteinemia	Lipoproteins, cholesterol
Hypobetalipoproteinemia	Lipoproteins, cholesterol
Mitochondrial disorders	Lactate, glucose-lactate tolerance
Sulfatide lipidoses	Arylsulfatase-A
Urine	
Hartnup disease	Amino acids
Maple syrup urine disease	Amino acids
Fibroblasts	
GM$_2$ gangliosidosis	Hexosaminidase
Refsum disease	Phytanic acid
Carnitine acetyltransferase deficiency	Carnitine acetyltransferase
Bone Marrow	
Neurovisceral storage	Sea-blue histiocytes

described in Chapters 5, 7, and 8. The common features among the several disorders of mitochondrial metabolism include lactic acidosis, ataxia, hypotonia, ophthalmoplegia, mental retardation, and peripheral neuropathy. These disorders are suggested by a raised concentration of blood lactate or the production of lactic acidosis by administration of a standard glucose tolerance test. A deficiency of pyruvate decarboxylase may produce acute, recurrent, or chronic ataxias and is discussed in the section on Acute or Recurrent Ataxia. Respiratory chain disorders produce a combination of ataxia, dementia, myoclonus, and seizures.

X-Linked Inheritance

The infantile form of adrenoleukodystrophy and Leber optic neuropathy may present with ataxia. Both are discussed elsewhere in the text. Leber optic atrophy is readily distinguished from other cerebellar degenerations because other family members have characteristic ophthalmologic features. Adrenoleuokodystrophy may mimic a spinocerebellar degeneration more closely and should be considered in any family with only males affected (Kobayashi et al, 1986).

Ataxia with Dementia

Clinical Features. Age at onset is two to three years. The initial features are delayed milestones, clumsiness, and intention tremor. Early school performance is acceptable. During the second decade, affected males develop progressive ataxia and spasticity. Incoordination becomes progressively severe, leading to loss of ambulation. Progressive dementia begins in the third and fourth decades. Death usually occurs in the seventh decade (Farlow et al, 1987).

Examination reveals disturbances of cerebellar, corticospinal, and intellectual function. Other neurologic systems are intact.

Diagnosis. CT or MRI reveals cerebellar atrophy. No biochemical defect has been identified. Adrenoleukodystrophy is a major consideration, and plasma concentrations of very-long-chain fatty acids should be determined.

Treatment. Treatment is not available.

References

1. Agamanolis DP, Potter JL, Naito HK, et al: Lipoprotein disorder, cirrhosis and olivopontocerebellar degeneration in two siblings. Neurology 36:674, 1986.
2. Al-Din AN, Anderson M, Bickerstaff ER et al: Brainstem encephalitis and the syndrome of Miller Fisher. A clinical study. Brain 105:481, 1982.
3. Asbury AK: Diagnostic considerations in Guillain-Barré syndrome. Ann Neurol 9:1, 1981.
4. Ashwal S, Thrasher TV, Rice DR, et al: A new form of sea-blue histiocytosis associated with progressive anterior horn cell and axonal degeneration. Ann Neurol 16:184, 1984.
5. Baron DN, Dent CE, Harris H, et al: Hereditary pellagra-like skin rash with temporary cerebellar ataxia. Constant renal amino-aciduria and other bizarre biochemical features. Lancet 2:6940, 1956.
6. Bejar JM, Ziegler DK: Onset of multiple sclerosis in a 24-month-old child. Arch Neurol 41:881, 1984.
7. Bennett HS, Selman JE, Rapin I, et al: Nonconvulsive epileptiform activity appearing as ataxia. Am J Dis Child 136:30, 1982.
8. Bolthauser E, Deonna A, Hirt HR: Myoclonic encephalopathy of infants or "dancing eyes syndrome." Helv Paediat Acta 34:119, 1979.
9. Bouchard JP, Barbeau A, Bouchard R, et al: A cluster of Friedreich's ataxia in Rimouski, Quebec. Can J Neurol Sci 6:205, 1979.
10. Brett EM: Minor epileptic status. J Neurol Sci 3:52, 1966.
11. Bye AME, Kendall B, Wilson J: Multiple sclerosis in childhood: A new look. Dev Med Child Neurol 27:215, 1985.
12. Choux M: Ependymomas in the posterior fossa of children. In Amador LV, ed. Brain Tumors in the Young. Charles C Thomas, Springfield, Ill, 1983, p 526.
13. Coleman WP III, Coleman WP, Derbes VJ, et al: Collagen disease in children. A review of 71 cases. JAMA 237:1095, 1977.
14. Curatolo P, Mercuri S, Cotroneo E: Joubert syndrome: a case confirmed by computerized tomography. Dev Med Child Neurol 22:362, 1980.
15. Dancis J, Hutzler J, Rokkones T: Intermittent branched-chain ketonuria. Variant of maple-syrup-urine disease. N Engl J Med 276:84, 1967.
16. Diamond S, Kudrow L, Stevens J, et al: Long-term

17. DiDonato S, Rimoldi M, Moise A, et al: Fatal ataxic encephalopathy and carnitine acetyltransferase deficiency: A functional defect of pyruvate oxidation? Neurology 29:1578, 1979.
18. Donat JR, Auger R: Familial periodic ataxia. Arch Neurol 36:568, 1979.
19. Dyken P, Kolar O: Dancing eyes, dancing feet: Infantile polymyoclonia. Brain 91:305, 1968.
20. Evans OB: Episodic weakness in pyruvate decarboxylase deficiency. J Pediatr 105:961, 1984.
21. Evans OB, Kilroy AW, Fenichel GM: Acetazolamide in the treatment of pyruvate dysmetabolism syndromes. Arch Neurol 35:502, 1978.
22. Farlow MR, DeMyer W, Dlouhy SR, et al: X-linked recessive inheritance of ataxia and adult-onset dementia: Clinical features and preliminary linkage analysis. Neurology 37:602, 1987.
23. Farmer TW, Mustian VM: Vestibulocerebellar ataxia: A newly defined hereditary syndrome with periodic manifestations. Arch Neurol 88:471, 1963.
24. Farris BK, Smith JL, Ayyar R: Neuro-ophthalmologic findings in vestibulocerebellar ataxia. Arch Neurol 43:1050, 1986.
25. Feit H, Kirkpatrick J, Van Woert MH, et al: Myoclonus, ataxia, and hypoventilation: Response to L-5-hydroxytryptophan. Neurology 33:109, 1983.
26. Fenichel GM: Migraine as a cause of benign paroxysmal vertigo in childhood. J Pediatr 71:114, 1967.
27. Fitzsimons RB, Clifton-Bligh P, Wolfenden WH: Mitochondrial myopathy and lactic acidemia with myoclonic epilepsy, ataxia and hypothalamic infertility: A variant of Ramsay-Hunt syndrome? J Neurol Neurosurg Psychiatry 44:79, 1981.
28. Fowler HL: Machado-Joseph-Azorean disease: A ten-year study. Arch Neurol 41:921, 1984.
29. Furman JM, Baloh RW, Chugani H, et al: Infantile cerebellar atrophy. Ann Neurol 17:399, 1985.
30. Gartner JC, Bergman I, Malatack J, et al: Progression of neurovisceral storage disease with supranuclear ophthalmoplegia following orthotropic liver transplantation. Pediatrics 77:104, 1986.
31. Gjerris F: Clinical aspects and long-term prognosis in supratentorial tumors of infancy and childhood. Acta Neurol Scand 57:445,1978.
32. Graf CJ, Perret GE, Torner JC: Bleeding from cerebral arteriovenous malformations as part of their natural history. J Neurosurg 58:331, 1983.
33. Graff-Radford NR: A recessively inherited ataxia with episodes of dystonia. J Neurol Neurosurg Psychiatry 49:591, 1986.
34. Griggs RC, Moxley RT, Lafrance RA, et al: Hereditary paroxysmal ataxia: Response to acetazolamide. Neurology 28:1259, 1978.
35. Haltia T, Palo J, Haltia M, et al: Juvenile metachromatic leukodystrophy. Clinical, biochemical, and neuropathologic studies in nine new cases. Arch Neurol 37:42, 1980.
36. Harding AE: Friedreich's ataxia: A clinical and genetic study of 90 families with an analysis of early diagnostic criteria and intrafamilial clustering of clinical features. Brain 104:589, 1981.
37. Hegele RA, Angel A: Arrest of neuropathy and myopathy in abetalipoproteinemia with high-dose vitamin E therapy. Can Med Assoc J 132:41, 1985.
38. Hendrick EB: Medulloblastomas, astrocytomas, and sarcomas of the posterior fossa. In Amador LV, ed. Brain

Tumors in the Young. Charles C. Thomas, Springfield, Ill, 1983, p 498.

39. Hosking GM: Ataxia telangiectasia. Dev Med Child Neurol 24:77, 1982.

40. Huson SM, Harper PS, Hourihan MD, et al: Cerebellar haemangioblastoma and Von Hippel-Landau disease. Brain 109:1297, 1986.

41. Illingworth DR, Connor WE, Miller RG: Abetalipoproteinemia. Report of two cases and review of therapy. Arch Neurol 37:659, 1980.

42. Jackson JF, Currier RD: Dominant spinocerebellar ataxia: Genetic counseling. J Neurogenet 1:87, 1983.

43. Johnson WG: The clinical spectrum of hexosaminidase deficiency diseases. Neurology 31:1453, 1981.

44. Joubert M, Eisenring JJ, Robb JP, et al: Familial agenesis of the cerebellar vermis. Neurology 19:813, 1969.

45. Kelly JJ Jr, Mellinger JF, Sundt TM Jr: Intracranial arteriovenous malformations in childhood. Ann Neurol 3:338, 1978.

46. Kobayashi T, Noda S, Umezaki H, et al: Familial spinocerebellar degeneration as an expression of adrenoleukodystrophy. J Neurol Neurosurg Psychiatry 49:1438, 1986.

47. Kurtzke JF, Hyllested K: Multiple sclerosis in the Faroe Islands. II. Clinical update, transmission, and the nature of MS. Neurology 36:307, 1986.

48. Landis DMD, Rosenberg RN, Landis SC, et al: Olivopontocerebellar degeneration. Clinical and ultrastructural abnormalities. Arch Neurol 31:295, 1974.

49. Lapkin ML, Golden GS: Basilar artery migraine. Am J Dis Child 132:278, 1978.

50. Leibel SA, Sheline GE, Wara WM, et al: The role of radiation therapy in the treatment of astrocytomas. Cancer 35:1551, 1975.

51. Levy WJ, Mason L, Hahn JF: Chiari malformation presenting in adults: A surgical experience in 127 cases. Neurosurgery 12:377, 1983.

52. Lima L, Coutinho P: Clinical criteria for diagnosis of Machado-Joseph disease: Report of a non-Azorean Portuguese family. Neurology 30:319, 1980.

53. Livingstone IR, Gardner-Medwin D, Pennington RJT: Familial intermittent ataxia with possible X-linked recessive inheritance. J Neurol Sci 64:89, 1984.

54. MacFaul R, Cavanagh N, Lake BD, et al: Metachromatic leucodystrophy: Review of 38 cases. Arch Dis Child 3:168, 1982.

55. Meienberg O, Ryffel R: Supranuclear eye movement disorders in Fisher's syndrome of ophthalmoplegia, ataxia, and areflexia. Report of a case and literature review. Arch Neurol 40:402, 1983.

56. Moore PM, Fauci AS: Neurologic manifestations of systemic vasculitis. A retrospective and prospective study of the clinicopathologic features and responses to therapy in 25 patients. Am J Med 71:517, 1981.

57. Naito H, Oyanagi S: Familial myoclonus epilepsy and choreoathetosis: Hereditary dentatorubral-pallidoluysian atrophy. Neurology 32:798, 1982.

58. Nino HE, Noreen HJ, Dubey DP, et al: A family with hereditary ataxia: HLA typing. Neurology 30:12, 1980.

59. Park TS, Hoffman HJ, Hendrick EB, et al: Experience with surgical decompression of the Arnold-Chiari malformation in young infants with myelomeningocele. Neurosurgery 13:147, 1983.

60. Pomeroy J, Efron ML, Dayman J, et al: Hartnup disorder in New England family. N Engl J Med 278:1214, 1968.

61. Pueschel SM, Bresnan MJ, Shih VE, et al: Thiamine-responsive intermittent branched chain ketoaciduria. J Pediatr 94:629, 1979.

62. Ropper AH: The CNS in Guillain Barré syndrome. Arch Neurol 40:397, 1983.

63. Sarnat HB, Alcala H: Human cerebellar hypoplasia. A syndrome of diverse causes. Arch Neurol 37:300, 1980.

64. Schulte FJ: Intracranial tumors in childhood - Concepts of treatment and prognosis. Neuropediatrie 15:3, 1984.

65. Scully RE, Mark EJ, McNeely BU: Case records of the Massachusetts General Hospital. N Engl J Med 315:1143, 1986.

66. Sergent JS, Lockshin MD, Klempner MS, et al: Central nervous system disease in systemic lupus erythematosus. Am J Med 58:644, 1975.

67. Sogg RL, Hoyt WF: Intermittent vertical nystagmus in father and son. Arch Ophthalmol 68:515, 1962.

68. Somerville ER, Olanow CW: Valproic acid. Treatment of myoclonus in dyssynergia cerebellaris myoclonica. Arch Neurol 39:527, 1982.

69. Stumpf DA: The inherited ataxias. Pediatr Neurol 1:129, 1985.

70. Suzuki S, Kamoshita S, Ninomura S: Ramsay Hunt syndrome in dentatorubralpallidoluysian atrophy. Pediatr Neurol 1:298, 1985.

71. Swanson JW, Vick NA: Basilar artery migraine. 12 patients, with an attack recorded electroencephalographically. Neurology 28:782, 1978.

72. Teodori JB, Painter MJ: Basilar impression in children. Pediatrics 74:1097, 1984.

73. Tomita T: Statistical analysis of symptoms and signs in cerebellar astrocytoma and medulloblastoma. In Amador LV, ed. Brain Tumors in the Young, Charles C. Thomas, Springfield, Ill, 1983, p 514.

74. Tomita T, McLone DG: Medulloblastoma in childhood: results of radical resection and low-dose neuraxis radiation therapy. J Neurosurg 64:238, 1986.

75. Tuchman M, Morris CL, Ramnaraine ML, et al: Value of random urinary homovanillic acid and vanillylmandelic acid levels in diagnosis and management of patients with neuroblastoma. Pediatrics 75:324, 1985.

76. Waldmann TA, Misiti J, Nelson DL, et al: Ataxia-telangiectasia: A multisystem hereditary disease with immunodeficiency, impaired organ maturation, X-ray hypersensitivity, and a high incidence of neoplasia. Ann Intern Med 99:367, 1983.

77. Walker PD, Blitzer MG, Shapira E: Marinesco-Sjogren syndrome: Evidence for a lysosomal storage disorder. Neurology 35:415, 1985.

78. Weiss S, Carter S: Course and prognosis of acute cerebellar ataxia in children. Neurology 9:711, 1959.

79. Wichman A, Buchthal F, Pezeshkpour GH, et al: Peripheral neuropathy in abetalipoproteinemia. Neurology 35:1279, 1985.

80. Willner JP, Grabowski GA, Gordon RE, et al: Chronic GM$_2$ gangliosidosis masquerading as atypical Friedreich ataxia: Clinical, morphologic, and biochemical studies of nine cases. Neurology 31:787, 1981.

81. Yates AJ, Becker LE, Sachs LA: Brain tumors in childhood. Child Brain 5:31, 1979.

82. Zaleski LA, Dancis J, Cox RP, et al: Variant maple syrup urine disease in mother and daughter. Can Med Assoc J 109:299, 1973.

83. Zasorin NL, Baloh RW, Myers LB: Acetazolamide-responsive episodic ataxia syndrome. Neurology 33:1212, 1983.

84. Zimmerman AW, Kumar AJ, Gadoth N, et al: Traumatic vertebrobasilar occlusive disease in childhood. Neurology 28:185, 1978.

Hemiplegia

In the approach to children with hemiplegia, it is important to distinguish acute hemiplegia, in which weakness is maximal within a few hours, from chronic progressive hemiplegia, in which weakness evolves over a period of days, weeks, or months. The distinction between an acute and an insidious onset should be easy, but sometimes poses a problem. In children with a slowly evolving hemiplegia, early weakness may be missed completely until an obvious level of functional disability is attained; then the hemiplegia seems a new and acute problem.

■ Acute Hemiplegia

The sudden onset of an acute, focal neurologic deficit suggests either a vascular or an epileptic mechanism (Table 11.1). Infants and children who present with acute hemiplegia can be divided almost equally into two groups according to whether or not the hemiplegia was preceded by epilepsia partialis continua (Gastaut et al, 1979). Both groups may have seizures on the paretic side after hemiplegia is established. Cerebral infarction, usually in the distribution of the middle cerebral artery, accounts for 23 percent of cases in which seizures precede the hemiplegia and 57 percent of cases in which hemiplegia is the first manifestation. Whatever the cause, the probability of a permanent motor deficit is almost 100 percent when the initial manifestation is epilepsia partialis continua and about 50 percent when it is not (Solomon et al, 1970).

CEREBROVASCULAR DISEASE

The annual incidence of stroke in children is 2.5/100,000, which is about half the incidence

of brain tumors (Schoenberg et al, 1976). Some children with acute hemiplegia from stroke have a known predisposing condition, such as congenital heart disease or sickle cell anemia. In such children, the index of suspicion for stroke is very high whenever an acute neurologic disturbance occurs. Stroke may also occur in the absence of known risk factors (Table 11.2). In a previously healthy child, stroke is usually considered because of the sudden onset of a focal neurologic disturbance and is then confirmed by computerized tomography (CT). Infarction is identified as an area of increased lucency that becomes enhanced with contrast (Fig. 11.1). As a rule, the lucency cannot be visualized in the first twenty-four hours after stroke. Cerebral infarction is often superficial, affecting both gray and white matter, and is in the distribution of a single artery. Multiple infarcts suggest either embolism or vasculitis. Small, deep lesions of the internal capsule are rare, but can occur in infants.

The evaluation of a child with cerebral infarction is summarized in Table 11.3. The usual line of investigation includes tests for blood dyscrasias, a search for cardiac sources of emboli, and cerebral arteriography to identify the site of vascular occlusion.

Children of all ages, who are otherwise healthy, may experience a single episode of cerebral infarction. Despite the most extensive evaluation, an underlying cause cannot be

Table 11.1 DIFFERENTIAL DIAGNOSIS OF ACUTE HEMIPLEGIA

Cerebrovascular disease
Epilepsy
Migraine
Diabetes mellitus
Infection
Trauma

248

Table 11.2 CAUSES OF STROKE

Idiopathic Infarction

Moyamoya Disease

Carotid Disorders
1. Trauma
2. Infection
3. Fibromuscular dysplasia

Heart Disease
1. Congenital
2. Rheumatic
3. Mitral valve prolapse

Sickle Cell Anemia

Vasculopathies
1. Systemic lupus erythematosus
2. Takayasu arteritis
3. Hypersensitivity vasculitis
4. Kawasaki disease (see Chapter 10)

MELAS

Lipoprotein Disorders

Cancer
1. Disseminated intravascular coagulation
2. L-Asparginase-induced thrombosis
3. Methotrexate-induced infarction
4. Metastatic neuroblastoma

Venous Thrombosis

Intracerebral Hemorrhage
1. Neonatal
2. Arteriovenous malformations

Homocystinuria (see Chapter 5)

Table 11.3 EVALUATION OF CEREBRAL INFARCTION

	Evaluation	Condition
Blood	CBC, ESR, culture anti-DNA, lipid profile lactic acid	Bacterial endocarditis Hyperlipidemia Leukemia Lupus erythematosus MELAS Polycythemia Sickle cell anemia
Urine	Nitroprusside reaction Urinalysis	Homocystinuria Nephritis Nephrosis
Heart	EKG Echocardiogram	Bacterial endocarditis Congenital heart disease Mitral valve prolapse Rheumatic heart disease
Brain	Arteriography	Arterial dissection Arterial thrombosis Arteriovenous malformation Fibromuscular hypoplasia Moyamoya disease, vasculitis

Cerebral hemorrhage is readily identified as an area of increased density on an uncontrasted CT scan (Fig. 11.2). It is frequently surrounded by edema and may produce a mass effect with shift of midline structures. The differential diagnosis of intracerebral hemorrhage is summarized in Table 11.4.

Neonatal Infarction

Cerebral infarction from arterial occlusion occurs more often in term newborns than in premature newborns and may result from (1) disseminated intravascular coagulation, (2) polycythemia, or (3) injury to the carotid or middle

found. Clinical features vary with age and site of infarction. Hemiplegia, either immediately or as a late sequela, is one of the more constant features.

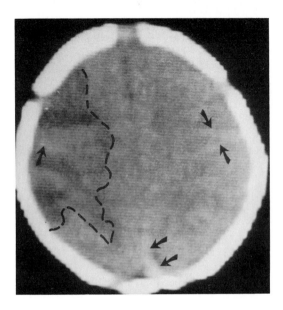

Figure 11.1 Cerebral infarction. An area is outlined that represents early changes resulting from infarction in the middle cerebral artery distribution. Arrows indicate hemorrhage.

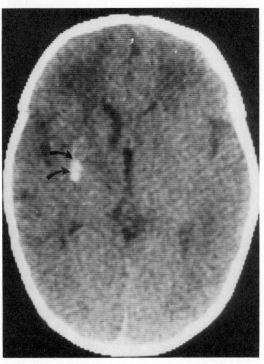

Figure 11.2 Cerebral hemorrhage. A small hemorrhage is indicated by arrows.

cerebral arteries during delivery (Barmada et al, 1979; Roessmann and Miller, 1980).

Clinical Features. Small unilateral infarcts, usually frontal or parietal in location, occur in newborns without systemic disease or obvious risk factors (Fenichel et al, 1984). Subarachnoid hemorrhage is frequently associated. Such newborns appear normal at birth, then develop repetitive, focal, or generalized seizures during the first four days post partum (Clancy et al, 1976; Levy et al, 1985). Some recover fully, whereas others are left with hemiparesis.

Table 11.4 DIFFERENTIAL DIAGNOSIS OF INTRACEREBRAL HEMORRHAGE

Arteriovenous Malformations

Blood Dyscrasias
1. Disseminated intravascular coagulation
2. Idiopathic thrombocytopenic purpura
3. Leukemia

Brain Tumors

Hemorrhagic Infarction
1. Cerebral emboli
2. Sagittal sinus thrombosis
3. Sickle cell anemia
4. Systemic lupus erythematosus

Hypersensitivity Vasculitis

Diagnosis. A CT scan is required to demonstrate small infarcts, but large infarcts in the complete distribution of the middle cerebral artery can be detected by ultrasound. A follow-up CT scan demonstrates two different patterns of abnormality (Kotlarek et al, 1981). Approximately half of these children develop unilateral enlargement of the lateral ventricle contralateral to the hemiparesis (Fig. 11.3). In these cases, venous hemorrhage is considered the mechanism of brain injury and a history of an abnormal pregnancy or of prematurity is common. The other half of patients develop porencephaly in the distribution of the middle cerebral artery contralateral to the hemiparesis. Hemiplegia associated with porencephaly is usually more severe and more often associated with epilepsy and mental retardation than is hemiplegia associated with ventricular enlargement.

Treatment. Anticonvulsant drugs are usually effective for seizure control (see Chapter 1). Hemispherectomy or commissurotomy should be considered in children with intractable focal seizures (Goodman, 1986).

Idiopathic Capsular Stroke

Small, deep infarcts involving the internal capsule are usually seen in adults with hyperten-

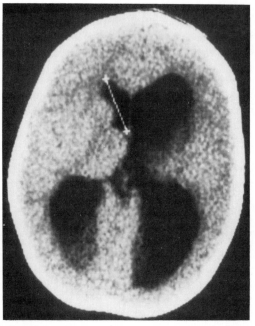

Figure 11.3 Cerebral hemiatrophy with ventricular enlargement. The lateral ventricle on the right side is considerably larger than on the left (marked) as a result of hemispheric atrophy.

sive angiopathy. They also occur, but very rarely, in infants and young children (Aram et al, 1983; Young et al, 1983). The onset of weakness is sudden and may occur during sleep or wakefulness.

Clinical Features. The face and limbs are involved and a typical hemiplegic posture and gait develop. Hypalgesia and decreased position sense are difficult to demonstrate in infants, but can be observed in older children. Larger infarcts affecting the striatum as well as the internal capsule of the dominant hemisphere produce speech disturbances. At the onset of hemiplegia, the child is mute and lethargic. As speech returns, there is evidence of dysarthria and aphasia. Eventually, speech becomes normal. Hemiplegia may clear completely in the following year, but some children have residual weakness of the hand.

Diagnosis. Capsular infarcts can be demonstrated by CT. However, a cause is rarely determined despite extensive study (see Table 11.3).

Treatment. Treatment is not available.

Idiopathic Cerebral Artery Infarction

Acute infantile hemiplegia may result from infarction in the distribution of the middle cerebral artery or one of its branches, the posterior cerebral artery, or the anterior cerebral artery.

Clinical Features. Sudden hemiplegia is the typical clinical presentation. Hemianesthesia, hemianopia, and aphasia (with dominant hemisphere infarction) are present as well. Some children are lethargic at the onset of symptoms, but consciousness generally is not lost completely.

In approximately one third of cases, epilepsia partialis continua precedes the hemiplegia (Gastaut et al, 1979). Such children do poorly; permanent hemiplegia is constant and epilepsy is usual. In contrast, when hemiplegia occurs without seizures, half of patients recover completely and the remainder are left with partial paralysis.

Diagnosis. Complete middle cerebral artery occlusion produces a large area of lucency on CT involving the cortex, underlying white matter, basal ganglia, and internal capsule. Occlusion of superficial branches of the middle cerebral artery produces a wedge-shaped area of lucency extending from the cortex into the subjacent white matter.

Treatment. Seizures should be treated with anticonvulsant drugs (see Chapter 1). When

seizures are intractable, hemispherectomy or commissurotomy should be considered (Goodman, 1986; Goodman et al, 1985).

Moyamoya Disease

Moyamoya disease is a slowly progressive, bilateral occlusion of the internal carotid arteries starting at the carotid siphon. The basilar artery is sometimes occluded as well. Because the occlusion is slowly progressive, there is time for multiple anastomoses to form between the internal and external carotid arteries. The result is a new vascular network at the base of the brain composed of collaterals from the anterior or posterior choroidal arteries, the basilar artery, and the meningeal arteries. These telangiectasias produce a hazy appearance on angiography—"like a puff of smoke," from which the Japanese word *moyamoya* is derived (Fig. 11.4). The disorder is worldwide in distribution with a female to male bias of 3:2. The underlying cause or causes have not been identified.

Clinical Features. The initial symptoms vary from recurrent headache to abrupt hemiparesis. Infants and young children tend to have an explosive onset characterized by the sudden onset of complete hemiplegia affecting face and limbs. The child is at least lethargic and sometimes comatose. When sufficiently alert to be examined, hemianopia, hemianesthesia, and aphasia may be present. Recovery follows, but before it is complete, new episodes of focal

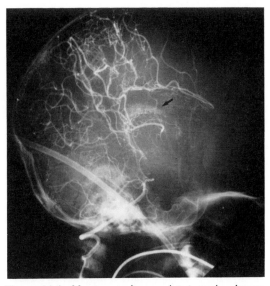

Figure 11.4 Moyamoya disease. Arteriography demonstrates occlusion of the carotid artery at the siphon and new anastomotic vessel formation (arrow).

neurologic dysfunction occur on either the same or the opposite side (Carlson et al, 1973). These episodes include hemiparesis, hemianesthesia, or aphasia, alone or in combination. The outcome is generally poor. Most children are left with chronic weakness of one or both sides, epilepsy, and mental retardation. Some have died.

Recurrent transient ischemic attacks are an alternate presentation (Fukuyama and Umezu, 1985). These are characterized by episodic hemiparesis and dysesthesias lasting for minutes or hours. Consciousness is retained. Attacks are frequently triggered by hyperpnea or excitement and may recur daily. After four or five years, the attacks cease but the child may be left with residual deficits.

Repeated episodes of monoparesis or symptoms of subarachnoid hemorrhage are other possible presenting features of moyamoya disease. Monoparesis generally occurs after infancy and subarachnoid hemorrhage after age sixteen.

Diagnosis. CT is likely to be the first diagnostic test performed in a child with acute hemiplegia. A large infarction is usually demonstrated because of stenosis in the internal carotid artery. Definitive diagnosis requires arteriographic demonstration of bilateral stenosis in the distal internal carotid arteries and the development of collaterals in the basal ganglia and meninges.

Treatment. Intravenous verapamil is effective acutely in providing return of function and radiographic evidence of increased perfusion (McLean et al, 1985). Temporal muscle graft, in which temporal muscle is placed over the arachnoid, has been attempted and is thought useful in providing better circulation to the superficial cortex (Takeuchi et al, 1983). However, it seems unlikely that this approach adds substantially to the natural development of arterial anastomoses.

Trauma to the Neck

Carotid Artery

In newborns, physical injury to the cervical portion of the carotid artery may occur during a difficult delivery owing to either misapplication of obstetric forceps or hyperextension and rotation of the neck with stretching of the artery over the lateral portion of the upper cervical vertebrae.

Older children may experience carotid thrombosis and dissection from rather trivial injuries sustained during exercise and sports. The carotid artery may be injured in the tonsillar fossa during

a tonsillectomy or when a child falls with a blunt object (pencil, lollipop) in the mouth.

Clinical Features. The onset of symptoms is usually delayed for several hours and sometimes days (Yamada et al, 1967). The delay probably represents the time needed for thrombus formation within the artery. Clinical features usually include hemiparesis, hemianesthesia, hemianopia, and aphasia when the dominant hemisphere is affected. Deficits may be transitory or permanent, but some recovery always occurs. Seizures are uncommon.

Diagnosis. Carotid occlusions in the neck may be demonstrated by ultrasonic imaging, but arteriography is essential for diagnosis.

Treatment. Neither anticoagulation nor surgical repair has proved useful in reversing hemiplegia.

Vertebral Artery

Vertebral artery thrombosis or dissection may follow minor neck trauma, especially rapid neck rotation (Katirji et al, 1985).

Clinical Features. The usual features of vertebral artery injury are headache and brainstem dysfunction. Repeated episodes of hemiparesis associated with bitemporal throbbing headache and vomiting are reported as well (Lewis and Berman, 1986). Episodes are provoked by exercise, last up to four hours, and are readily misdiagnosed as basilar artery migraine.

Diagnosis. The clue to diagnosis is the presence of one or more areas of infarction on CT scan. This should raise the possibility of stroke and lead to arteriography. Occlusion of the basilar artery is then visualized.

Treatment. Aspirin, 300 mg twice daily, was found effective in preventing further attacks in one patient (Lewis and Berman, 1986).

Cervical Infections

Unilateral and bilateral occlusions of the cervical portion of the internal carotid arteries may occur in children with a history of chronic tonsillitis and cervical lymphadenopathy (Tagawa et al, 1985). Whether this is cause and effect or coincidence is uncertain. It is speculated that tonsillitis produces carotid arteritis.

Unilateral cerebral infarction may occur in the course of cat-scratch disease (Selby and Walker, 1979) and mycoplasmal pneumonia (Parker et al, 1981). In cat-scratch disease, there is a clear association between the presence of submandibular lymph node involvement and arteritis of the adjacent carotid artery. A similar mechanism may account for cerebral infarction in mycoplasmal infection as well.

Necrotizing fasciitis is a serious cause of inflammatory arteritis with subsequent occlusion of one or both carotid arteries (Bush et al, 1984). The source of parapharyngeal space infection is usually chronic dental infection. Mixed aerobic and anaerobic organisms are cultured.

Clinical Features. Fever and neck tenderness followed by sudden hemiplegia is the usual sequence in cervical arteritis. Alternating hemiplegia may occur when both sides are involved.

Diagnosis. The offending organism or organisms must be identified by culture of the throat or lymph nodes in appropriate situations. Carotid occlusion is identified by arteriography.

Treatment. Aggressive therapy with antibiotics, especially for necrotizing fasciitis, is indicated. The outcome is variable and recovery may be partial or complete.

Fibromuscular Dysplasia

This is an idiopathic segmental nonatheromatous disorder of the internal carotid artery. The cervical portion of the artery is most often affected.

Clinical Features. Transient ischemic attacks and stroke are the only clinical features. Fibromuscular dysplasia occurs most often in women over the age of fifty but also has been reported in children (Llorens-Terol et al, 1983).

Diagnosis. Arteriography reveals an irregular contour of the internal carotid artery in the neck likened to "a string of beads." Concomitant fibromuscular dysplasia of the renal arteries should be suspected if hypertension is present.

Treatment. The occlusion may be treated by operative transluminal balloon angioplasty (Smith et al, 1985) or by carotid endarterectomy. The long-term prognosis in children is not known.

Congenital Heart Disease

Cerebrovascular complications of congenital heart disease are most likely to occur in children with cyanotic disorders. The usual complications are venous sinus thrombosis in infants and embolic arterial occlusion in children. Emboli may occur from valvular vegetations or from bacterial endocarditis. In either case, the development of cerebral abscess is a major concern. Cerebral abscess of embolic origin is exceedingly uncommon in children with congenital heart disease

younger than two years and occurs only as a complication of meningitis or surgery.

Venous Sinus Thrombosis

Venous thrombosis occurs most often in infants with cyanotic heart disease who are dehydrated and polycythemic. One or more sinuses may become occluded. Failure of venous drainage always leads to increased intracranial pressure.

Clinical Features. Hemiparesis is a major clinical feature and may alternate between the two sides when the sagittal sinus is obstructed. Seizures and states of decreased consciousness are almost always associated. Mortality is considerable in infants with thrombosis of major venous sinuses, and neurologic morbidity among survivors is almost constant.

Diagnosis. A CT scan demonstrates a pattern of hemorrhagic infarction adjacent to the site of venous thrombosis. Definitive diagnosis requires demonstration of venous occlusion by arteriography.

Treatment. Treatment is primarily supportive and directed toward correcting dehydration and controlling increased intracranial pressure. Dexamethasone can be used to decrease cerebral volume, but osmotic diuretics are contraindicated and may cause further thrombosis. The infarction is usually hemorrhagic and anticoagulants are contraindicated. It is impossible to determine if a thrombosis is septic or sterile and all infants should be treated with antibiotics.

Arterial Embolism and Abscess

Children with cyanotic heart disease are at risk for arterial embolism when vegetations are present within the heart or if a right-to-left shunt is present that allows peripheral emboli to bypass the lungs and reach the brain. This can occur spontaneously or at the time of cardiac surgery. The potential for cerebral abscess formation is increased in children with right-to-left shunt because decreased arterial oxygen saturation lowers cerebral resistance to infection.

Clinical Features. The initial feature is sudden onset of hemiparesis associated with headache, seizures, and loss of consciousness. Seizures may at first be focal and recurrent, but then become generalized.

Diagnosis. The CT appearance can be normal during the first twelve to twenty-four hours following embolization. By the next day, a low-intensity lesion with contrast enhancement can be observed. Although the sequence is consistent with a sterile embolus, the possibility of subsequent abscess formation still must be considered (Kurlan and Griggs, 1983). An enhanced CT scan should be repeated within one week to search for ring enhancement as a sign of abscess development.

Treatment. Children with arterial emboli, but without evidence of hemorrhagic ·infarction, should undergo anticoagulation to prevent further embolization. If the infarction is associated with cerebral edema and a mass effect, dexamethasone should be administered as well. In addition, it is reasonable to place all such children on antibiotic therapy to prevent cerebral abscess formation. If abscess formation does not occur, antibiotics can be stopped after one week. If abscess is demonstrated, therapy must be continued for six to eight weeks.

Rheumatic Heart Disease

The frequency and severity of rheumatic fever and rheumatic heart disease in North America have been decreasing for several decades. The mitral valve is involved in 85 percent of patients, the aortic valve in 54 percent, and the tricuspid and pulmonary valves in less than 5 percent (Kaplan, 1983).

Clinical Features. The cardinal features of mitral valve disease are cardiac failure and arrhythmia. Aortic valve disease is often asymptomatic. Neurologic manifestations are always due to bacterial endocarditis or embolism from a valvular vegetation during surgery. Symptoms are much the same as in congenital heart disease, except that cerebral abscess is less common.

Diagnosis. Children are known to have rheumatic heart disease long before they suffer a first stroke. The onset of neurologic abnormalities, except in the period following cardiac surgery, should suggest bacterial endocarditis as the underlying cause. Embolization is a more likely explanation in the postoperative period. Multiple blood cultures may be needed to identify the organism and select the best drug for intravenous antibiotic therapy.

Mitral Valve Prolapse

Mitral valve prolapse is a familial disorder that is present in 5 percent of all children (Greenwood, 1984). It is almost always asymptomatic but can be a rare cause of recurrent attacks of cerebral ischemia (Jackson et al, 1984). The attacks are attributed to sterile emboli from thrombus formation on the abnormal valve.

Clinical Features. The initial manifestation is usually a transitory ischemic attack in the distribution of the carotid circulation producing partial or complete hemiparesis. Weakness usually clears within twenty-four hours, but recurrent episodes, not necessarily in the same arterial distribution, are the rule. Basilar insufficiency is less common and usually results in visual field defects. The interval between recurrences varies from weeks to years. Fewer than 20 percent of individuals are left with permanent neurologic deficits.

Diagnosis. Only 25 percent of patients have late systolic murmurs or a midsystolic click. The remainder have a normal cardiac examination. Two-dimensional echocardiography is required to establish the diagnosis.

Treatment. Treatment is not needed for asymptomatic children with auscultatory or electrocardiographic abnormalities, nor is there specific treatment for a transient ischemic attack. However, once a child has suffered a transient ischemic attack, daily aspirin should be administered to reduce the likelihood of further thrombus formation in the heart.

Sickle Cell Anemia

Sickle cell anemia is a genetic disorder of black children transmitted by autosomal recessive inheritance. Neurologic manifestations occur in up to 25 percent of homozygotes and may occur at times of stress, such as surgery, in heterozygotes. The abnormal erythrocytes clog large and small vessels, causing a decrease in total, hemispheral, or regional blood flow (Huttenlocher et al, 1984).

Clinical Features. The major systemic manifestations are jaundice, pallor, weakness, and fatigability due to chronic hemolytic anemia. Half of homozygotes are symptomatic by one year, and all have symptoms by five years of age.

Strokes occur at the time of a thrombotic, vaso-occlusive crisis. Such crises are frequently precipitated by dehydration or anoxia and are characterized by fever and pain in the abdomen and chest. Focal or generalized seizures are the initial neurologic manifestation in 70 percent of patients. After the seizures have ended, hemiplegia and other focal neurologic deficits are noted (Portnoy and Herion, 1972). Some recovery follows, but there is a tendency for recurrent strokes and epilepsy. Strokes affecting both hemispheres produce a pseudobulbar palsy with brainstem dysfunction.

The worst case is a child who presents with coma and meningismus. This is usually caused by a diffuse decrease in cerebral blood flow associated with subarachnoid or intracerebral hemorrhage (Van Hoff et al, 1985). The mortality rate is high.

Diagnosis. The abnormal hemoglobin can be diagnosed at birth with acid agar gel electrophoresis or microcolumn chromatography. Most affected children have been diagnosed with sickle cell anemia long before their first stroke. The extent of cerebral infarction and hemorrhage during a cerebral vaso-occlusive crisis can be documented by CT. After several such crises, cortical atrophy may be present.

Cerebral arteriography should be avoided. It offers little additional information and carries the risk of increasing ischemia.

Treatment. A vaso-occlusive crisis requires prompt hydration, oxygen administration, and transfusions of packed red cells. Hydration should not occur to the point of increasing cerebral edema. Recurrent strokes may be prevented by a regimen of regular transfusions designed to keep the level of hemoglobin A above 60 percent (Russell et al, 1976).

Systemic Lupus Erythematosus

Several collagen vascular disorders can cause neurologic disturbances in adults, but systemic lupus erythematosus is the only important cause in children.

Clinical Features. Lupus is a systemic disorder in which 90 percent of children have fever, 88 percent have joint complaints, and 74 percent have skin rash at the time of diagnosis (Meislin and Rothfield, 1968). Neurologic complaints are present in a quarter of children at time of diagnosis and, unlike systemic complaints, are likely to progress or develop anew even after treatment is initiated. Thirty-eight percent of children will develop neurologic dysfunction sometime during the course of disease. Seizures, cranial neuropathies, and mental disorders are common features. Hemiplegia usually follows a seizure and may be caused by cerebral infarction or hemorrhage.

Diagnosis. The diagnosis of lupus requires a compatible clinical syndrome and the detection of positive antinuclear antibody. A CT scan is useful to determine the presence of hemorrhage or infarction. Cerebral arteriograms may be normal.

Treatment. Large doses of corticosteroids are the mainstay of therapy, but mortality in children is higher than in adults.

Takayasu Arteritis

This is an arteritis of unknown etiology involving the aorta and its major branches.

Clinical Features. Age at onset is usually between fifteen and twenty years, but may be as early as infancy (Kohrman and Huttenlocher, 1986). Ninety percent of patients are female. The most common manifestations are hypertension, absent pulses, and vascular bruits. Stroke occurs in only 5 to 10 percent of patients and is usually characterized by focal seizures and sudden hemiplegia.

Diagnosis. A CT scan reveals a focal hypodense area indicating infarction. Arteriography demonstrates involvement of the ascending aorta and its major branches. Cardiac catheterization is necessary to define the full extent of arteritis. Some vessels have a beaded appearance; others terminate abruptly and have prestenotic dilation.

Treatment. Aggressive immunosuppressive therapy with prednisone, 2 mg/kg/day, and azathioprine, 1 mg/kg/day is indicated. If patients remain untreated, the mortality rate is 75 percent. Early diagnosis and treatment can lead to full recovery.

Hypersensitivity Vasculitis

This term is used to include several disorders with a known underlying cause (drugs, infection) characterized by purpura of the legs and venulitis. Neurologic manifestations occur only in *Henoch-Schönlein purpura*, for which the cause has not been established but is thought to be an antecedent infection.

Clinical Features. The systemic features of Henoch-Schönlein purpura are fever, a purpuric rash on the extensor surfaces of the limbs, and abdominal pain with nausea and vomiting. Joint and renal disturbances may be present as well. Almost half of affected children have states of decreased consciousness and generalized seizures (Belman et al, 1985). Focal neurologic deficits occur in a third of patients, with hemiplegia accounting for half of these cases. Hemiplegia may or may not be preceded by a seizure, and can be associated with hemianesthesia, hemianopia, and aphasia. These deficits may be permanent.

Diagnosis. Infarction or hemorrhage, or both, may be demonstrated by CT.

Treatment. Corticosteroids are used to treat the underlying disease.

Mitochondrial Encephalopathy, Lactic Acidosis, and Stroke-Like Syndrome

MELAS is an acronym that stands for mitochondrial encephalopathy, lactic acidosis, and stroke-like syndrome (Pavlakis et al, 1984). Decreased concentrations of respiratory complex I (NADH [reduced form of nicotinamide adenine dinucleotide]-coenzyme Q reductase) have been identified in some patients (Fig. 8.5) (Kobayashi et al, 1987).

Clinical Features. Affected children are normal at birth and may develop normally. Mental deterioration, when present, occurs anytime during childhood. Growth retardation is common, and progressive deafness may be associated as well. The cardinal neurologic features are seizures (myoclonic, focal, generalized), the sudden onset of focal neurologic defects (hemiplegia, hemianopia, aphasia), and encephalopathy. Neurologic abnormalities are initially intermittent and then become progressive, leading to coma and death.

Diagnosis. The CT scan reveals single or multiple areas of infarction of the cerebral hemispheres. Basal ganglia calcification is occasionally present. The concentration of lactate in the blood and cerebrospinal fluid is elevated. Ragged red fibers are noted on muscle biopsy (see Fig. 7.6).

Treatment. Treatment is not available.

Lipoprotein Disorders

Familial lipid and lipoprotein abnormalities may cause premature cerebrovascular disease in infants and children (Glueck et al, 1982). These disorders are transmitted by autosomal dominant inheritance.

Clinical Features. Ischemic episodes produce transitory or permanent hemiplegia, sometimes associated with hemianopia, hemianesthesia, and aphasia. Family history is positive for cerebrovascular and coronary artery disease at an early age.

Diagnosis. Most children have low plasma concentrations of high-density lipoprotein (HDL) cholesterol, others have high plasma concentrations of triglycerides, and some have both. The mechanism of arteriosclerosis is lipoprotein-mediated endothelial damage with secondary thrombus formation.

Treatment. Dietary treatment and daily aspirin administration are indicated.

Cancer

Cerebrovascular accidents occur in 4 percent of children with cancer (Packer et al, 1985). Two thirds occur in children with lymphoreticular cancers and the other third in children with solid tumors. Four syndromes have been delineated: (1) vascular thrombosis due to disseminated intravascular coagulation, (2) acute arterial or sagittal sinus thrombosis due to L-asparaginase, (3) infarction due to methotrexate therapy, and (4) sinus thrombosis due to metastatic neuroblastoma.

Disseminated Intravascular Coagulation

Clinical Features. This syndrome occurs in children with leukemia, either as an initial manifestation or during therapy. Some have infarction and others have hemorrhage. Multiple infarctions and hemorrhages may be present. Hemiparesis and obtundation are major clinical features.

Diagnosis. The diagnosis is suspected in any child with coagulopathy who develops hemiparesis. The CT scan reveals infarction or hemorrhage, or both. The mortality rate in children with leukemia who have intracranial hemorrhages is high.

Treatment. Treatment is not available.

L-Asparaginase-Induced Thrombosis

This syndrome occurs in children with acute lymphocytic leukemia. L-asparaginase is believed to induce a coagulopathy.

Clinical Features. The clinical features of arterial thrombosis are hemiparesis and focal seizures. Full neurologic recovery is possible. In contrast, sagittal sinus thrombosis presents with marked increased intracranial pressure, hemiparesis, and seizures. There is progressive obtundation, coma, and death.

Diagnosis. The CT scan demonstrates multiple small areas of infarction.

Treatment. Treatment is not available.

Methotrexate-Induced Infarction

This condition occurs in children with osteogenic sarcoma that is treated with high-dose methotrexate. The time of occurrence is usually between the third and seventh courses. The mechanism of infarction is uncertain. Clinical features include acute hemiparesis, hemianesthesia, and focal seizures. Full recovery is the rule.

Metastatic Neuroblastoma

Metastases to the sagittal sinus produce increased intracranial pressure, obtundation, seizures, and alternating hemiplegia. Infarction subsequent to metastatic disease can be hemorrhagic and is readily identified on CT.

Venous Thrombosis

Venous thrombosis in children is usually due to a hypercoagulable state, polycythemia, or dehydration. Congenital heart disease and cancer, two of the leading causes, have been discussed in previous sections. Partial thrombosis of the sagittal sinus may also occur in young women taking oral contraceptives and during pregnancy (Imai et al, 1982).

Clinical Features. The typical clinical presentation is headache and obtundation due to increased intracranial pressure, seizures, and alternating hemiplegia.

Diagnosis. Venous thrombosis should be suspected in children who suddenly develop hemiplegia associated with increased intracranial pressure. Sagittal sinus thromboses can be suspected on CT by the presence of parasagittal hemorrhage or infarction. Definitive diagnosis requires cerebral arteriography.

Treatment. Treatment is directed at decreasing intracranial pressure and rehydrating the patient without increasing cerebral edema.

Intracerebral Hemorrhage

Nontraumatic intracerebral hemorrhage in childhood is usually caused by blood dyscrasias, especially idiopathic thrombocytopenic purpura, hemorrhagic infarction, and arteriovenous malformations. In newborns, and less often in infants, it may not be possible to determine a cause.

Neonatal Hemorrhage

Small unilateral parietal or temporal hemorrhages occur almost exclusively in term newborns and are not associated with either trauma or asphyxia (Cartwright et al, 1979; Leblanc and O'Gorman, 1980). Larger hemorrhages into the temporal lobe are sometimes caused when excessive force is applied with obstetric forceps, but more often they are idiopathic (Bergman et al, 1985). Intraventricular hemorrhage may be associated.

Clinical Features. Newborns with small hemorrhages are normal at birth and appear well until the onset of seizures anytime during the first week. Larger hemorrhages may present as apneic spells or seizures, or both. Seizures may be focal or generalized, and hemiplegia or hypotonia is present on examination. Some infants recover completely, whereas others are left with hemiplegia and mental retardation.

Diagnosis. Seizures and apneic spells usually prompt lumbar puncture in order to exclude the possibility of sepsis. The cerebrospinal fluid is found to be grossly bloody. The initial CT scan demonstrates hemorrhage (see Fig. 11.2), and follow-up studies reveal focal encephalomalacia.

Treatment. Treatment is available for seizures, but not for hemorrhage.

Arteriovenous Malformations

Clinical Features. The presenting feature of a vascular malformation confined to one hemisphere is either a seizure or an intracranial hemorrhage. Some children have a prior history of migraine-like headaches (see Chapter 4) or signs of undergrowth or paresis of the contralateral limbs (Kelly et al, 1978). Malformations must also be considered in the differential diagnosis of chronic, progressive hemiplegia.

Acute hemiplegia usually results from intraparenchymal hemorrhage. The risk of bleeding is considerably greater from a small malformation than from a large one (Graf et al, 1983). The major clinical manifestations of intrahemispheric hemorrhage are loss of consciousness, seizures, and hemiplegia. Large hematomas cause a shift of midline structures and increased intracranial pressure.

Diagnosis. Malformations are readily diagnosed by enhanced CT scans and are fully identified by arteriography.

Treatment. The immediate treatment for an acute hemorrhage is supportive care, especially measures to manage increased intracranial pressure (see Chapter 3). Large hematomas causing midline shift should be surgically evacuated. Options for management of the malformation include (1) doing nothing, (2) surgical excision, (3) embolization, (4) proton beam therapy, or (5) some combination of Nos. 2, 3, and 4 (Drake, 1983).

EPILEPSY

Hemiconvulsions-Hemiplegia Syndrome

Explosive and intractable focal motor seizures followed by hemiplegia in an infant or child without prior history of epilepsy is sometimes caused by infarction and was described in the preceding section on cerebrovascular disease (Gastaut et al, 1979). An additional small percentage are caused by focal "inflammatory disease" (Rasmussen, 1978) or viral infections such as herpes. No cause can be identified in the majority of cases.

Clinical Features. Jerking in part of the face or in a limb develops in an infant or young child who was previously healthy. At onset, the movements may be infrequent and of low amplitude, but they become continuous and involve the eyes, face, and both limbs within hours or days. Anticonvulsant therapy may stop the seizures temporarily or permanently. Afterwards, the affected limbs are hemiparetic. Some children develop hemianopia as well. Permanent hemiplegia and mental retardation can be expected in every case, and most patients will continue to have epilepsy.

Diagnosis. An electroencephalogram (EEG) demonstrates a continuous spike discharge on a background of polymorphic slowing in the hemisphere contralateral to the hemiparesis. Occasional spike discharges may be seen in the other hemisphere as well. An enhanced CT scan is indicated to search for infarction, hemorrhage, or arteriovenous malformation. The initial CT scan is usually normal, but a year later it will demonstrate atrophy of the hemisphere with dilation of the ipsilateral ventricle (see Fig. 11.3). The cerebrospinal fluid is usually normal, although a few monocytes may be present secondary to the prolonged convulsion.

Treatment. An intravenous load of phenytoin or phenobarbital should be administered first and may prove effective in stopping, or at least decreasing, the frequency of seizures. Unfortunately, most cases are refractory and complete control is not the rule. Several standard anticonvulsants (see Chapter 1), alone or in combination, may be tried before acceptable control is established.

Uncontrolled focal seizures may evolve into intractable tonic-clonic seizures. In such cases, interhemispheric commissurotomy is recommended (Goodman et al, 1986). This procedure prevents the development of a mirror focus and progression to generalized tonic-clonic seizures, and allows easier management of focal seizures with anticonvulsant drugs.

Hemiparetic Seizures

Todd paralysis is a term used to describe transitory hemiparesis, lasting minutes or days, following a focal or generalized seizure. It most often occurs when seizures are prolonged or caused by an underlying structural abnormality. An ischemic mechanism has been suggested, and radioisotope studies demonstrate focal uptake in the contralateral hemisphere during the paralysis in support of that notion (Yarnell, 1975).

Hemiparesis may be a seizure manifestation as well as a postictal event. They are called "hemiparetic" or "focal inhibitory" seizures (Hanson and Chodos, 1978). Todd paralysis may be difficult to distinguish from hemiparetic seizures, since it is not always clear if a seizure preceded the hemiparesis or if the hemiparesis is ictal or postictal.

Clinical Features. The initial manifestation may be a brief focal seizure followed by flaccid hemiparesis or the abrupt onset of flaccid monoparesis or hemiparesis. Consciousness is not impaired and the child seems well otherwise. The severity and distribution of weakness fluctuates, affecting one limb more than the other and sometimes the face. Tendon reflexes are normal in the hemiparetic limbs, but the plantar response may be extensor.

Diagnosis. The EEG reveals recurrent spike and slow-wave discharges in the contralateral hemisphere. A radioisotope scan demonstrates increased focal uptake in the affected hemisphere. The CT scan and cerebral arteriogram are normal.

Treatment. Seizures respond to standard anticonvulsant drugs (see Chapter 1).

Absence Status

Absence attacks in children are characterized by brief episodes of staring or eyeblinking associated with 3 Hz generalized spike-wave complexes on the EEG (see Chapter 1). Prolonged absence attacks are characterized by confusion and automatisms similar to complex partial seizures. In addition, a variant form of absence status has been described with hemiparesis as the primary feature (Niedermeyer et al, 1979).

Clinical Features. Some patients have a prior history of generalized tonic-clonic seizures but are not known to have a prior history of absence.

The patient seems confused, has poor motor performance, and is unable to carry on a conversation. Transient hemiparesis or face-hand weakness is noted and aphasia may be present as well. The attack ends spontaneously or with the intravenous administration of diazepam.

Diagnosis. An EEG is essential for diagnosis. Several different epileptiform patterns may be seen. Most constant are 3 Hz spike-wave complexes from the frontal region during an attack. These complexes are often generalized but always have a unilateral predominance.

Treatment. Standard anticonvulsants provide seizure control. However, it is difficult to know which class of drugs to use in any individual. Some respond to phenytoin or carbamazepine, whereas others respond to ethosuximide, valproic acid, or clonazepam.

MIGRAINE

Migraine is a hereditary disorder characterized by paroxysmal alterations in cerebral blood flow (see Chapter 3). Studies of regional blood flow during a classic migraine attack demonstrate an anterior spread of oligemia from the occipital to the parietal lobes (Lauritzen et al, 1983). The location and rate of spread suggest that the reduction in cerebral blood flow is secondary to changes in neuronal function: the spreading depression of Leao. The oligemia reaches the sensorimotor cortex during the headache phase and after the prodrome. This observation supports the concept that focal neurologic disturbances in migraine are caused by neuronal depression and not by ischemia.

Hemiplegic Migraine

The occurrence of focal motor deficits, usually hemiplegia or ophthalmoplegia (see Chapter 15), during a classic migraine attack is called "complicated migraine."

Clinical Features. Family history is positive for migraine, but other family members may not have experienced hemiplegia during an attack. The evolution of symptoms is variable but usually includes scintillating or simple scotomas, unilateral dysesthesias of the hand and mouth, and unilateral weakness of the arm and face. The leg is usually spared. Coincident with hemiparesis is a throbbing frontotemporal headache contralateral to the affected hemisphere (Heyck, 1973). Nausea and vomiting follow. The patient falls asleep and has usually recovered upon awakening. Hemiparesis lasts less than twenty-four hours.

Diagnosis. Migraine is a clinical diagnosis that relies heavily upon a positive family history. During an attack of hemiplegic migraine, an EEG focus of polymorphic *delta* activity is present in the hemisphere contralateral to weakness. Arteriography is contraindicated and may prolong the attack.

Small infarcts may be present on a CT scan (Broderick and Swanson, 1987). These are usually in the distribution of the posterior cerebral artery.

Treatment. The management of migraine is summarized in Chapter 3.

Familial Hemiplegic Migraine

This disorder differs from complicated migraine because all family members with migraine have at least one hemiplegic attack. The trait is transmitted by autosomal dominant inheritance.

Clinical Features. Attacks are stereotyped, occur primarily in childhood or adolescence, are precipitated by trivial head trauma, and rarely occur more often than once a year (Glista et al, 1975). The hemiplegia, though usually more severe in the face and arm, affects the leg as well. Hemianesthesia of the hemiplegic side is a prominent feature. Aphasia is present when the dominant hemisphere is affected. Confusion, stupor, or psychosis may be present during an attack. The psychosis includes both auditory and visual hallucinations as well as delusions (Feely et al, 1982). Occasionally, patients have fever and a stiff neck.

Symptoms last for two or three days. When the attack is over, the neurologic deficits usually resolve completely; however, permanent sequelae are possible. Recurrent hemiplegic attacks may occur on either the same or the opposite side.

Diagnosis. A positive family history of hemiplegic migraine is essential for diagnosis.

Treatment. Patients with familial hemiplegic migraine should be treated with a prophylactic agent such as propranolol to prevent recurrences (see Chapter 3).

DIABETES MELLITUS

Acute but transitory attacks of hemiparesis occur in children with insulin-dependent diabetes mellitus (MacDonald and Brown, 1979). Complicated migraine is a suggested mechanism

(Korobkin, 1980), but the pathophysiology remains uncertain.

Clinical Features. Attacks frequently occur during sleep, concurrent with a respiratory illness. Hemiparesis is present upon awakening; the face and arm are more affected than the leg. Sensation is intact, but aphasia is present if the dominant hemisphere is affected. Tendon reflexes may be depressed or brisk in the affected arm and an extensor plantar response is usually present. Headache is a constant feature and may be unilateral or generalized. Some patients are nauseated as well. There is no family history of migraine.

Attacks last for three to twenty-four hours and recovery is complete. Recurrences are common.

Diagnosis. Stroke is not a complication of juvenile insulin-dependent diabetes, except during episodes of ketoacidosis (see Chapter 2). A CT scan in children with transitory hemiplegia does not demonstrate infarction. An EEG reveals a focus of polymorphic *delta* activity that returns to normal after several days.

Treatment. Although some children have further attacks, there is no established method to prevent recurrences. Prophylactic phenobarbital was useful in one child.

INFECTIONS

Hemiplegia occurs during the course of bacterial meningitis, resulting from vasculitis or venous thromboses, and during the course of viral encephalitis, especially herpes simplex, resulting from parenchymal necrosis. In both bacterial and viral infections, hemiplegia is usually preceded by prolonged or repetitive focal seizures.

Brain abscess may cause hemiplegia, but its evolution is usually slowly progressive rather than acute (see Chapter 4).

TRAUMA

Trauma accounts for half of all deaths in children. Approximately 10 percent of traumatic injuries in children are not accidental. Head injury is the leading cause of death from child abuse, and half of survivors are left with permanent neurologic handicaps (McClelland et al, 1980).

Epidural hematoma, subdural hematoma, cerebral laceration, and intracerebral hemorrhage can produce focal signs such as hemiplegia. However, brain swelling is such a prominent

Table 11.5 PROGRESSIVE HEMIPLEGIA

Arteriovenous malformation (see Chapter 4)
Brain abscess (see Chapter 4)
Cerebral hemisphere tumor (see Chapter 4)
Demyelinating disease
  Adrenoleukodystrophy (see Chapter 5)
  Late onset globoid leukodystrophy (see Chapter 5)
  Multiple sclerosis (see Chapter 10)

feature of even trivial head injury in children (Snoek et al, 1984) that states of diminished consciousness and seizures are the typical clinical manifestations (see Chapter 2).

TUMORS

Primary tumors of the cerebral hemispheres are more likely to present as chronic progressive hemiplegia than acute hemiplegia and are discussed in Chapter 4. However, tumors may present as acute hemiplegia when they bleed or provoke seizures and must be considered in the evaluation of acute hemiplegia.

■ Chronic Progressive Hemiplegia

The important causes of chronic progressive hemiplegia are brain tumor, brain abscess, and arteriovenous malformations. All three frequently present with symptoms and signs of increased intracranial pressure and are discussed in Chapter 4. Less often, progressive hemiplegia is an initial feature of demyelinating diseases, which are discussed in Chapters 5 and 10 (Table 11.5).

References

1. Aram DM, Rose DF, Rekate HL, et al: Acquired capsular/striatal aphasia in childhood. Arch Neurol 40:614, 1983.
2. Barmada MA, Moosey J, Shuman RM: Cerebral infarcts with arterial occlusion in neonates. Ann Neurol 6:495, 1979.
3. Belman AL, Leicher CR, Moshe SL, et al: Neurologic manifestations of Schönlein-Henoch purpura: Report of three cases and review of the literature. Pediatrics 75:687, 1985.
4. Bergman I, Bauer RE, Barmada MA, et al: Intracerebral hemorrhage in the fullterm neonatal infant. Pediatrics 75:488, 1985.
5. Broderick JP, Swanson JW: Migraine-related strokes. Clinical profile and prognosis in 20 patients. Arch Neurol 44:868, 1987.

6. Bush JK, Giunere LB, Whitaker S, et al: Necrotizing fasciitis of the parapharyngeal space with carotid artery occlusion and acute hemiplegia. Pediatrics 73:343, 1984.

7. Carlson CB, Harvey FH, Loop J: Progressive alternating hemiplegia in early childhood with basal arterial stenosis and telangiectasia (moyamoya syndrome). Neurology 23:734, 1973.

8. Cartwright GW, Culbertson K, Schreiner RL, et al: Changes in clinical presentation of term infants with intracranial hemorrhage. Dev Med Child Neurol 21:730, 1979.

9. Clancy R, Malin S, Laraque D, et al: Focal motor seizures heralding stroke in full-term neonates. Am J Dis Child 139:601, 1985.

10. Drake CG: Arteriovenous malformations of the brain. The options of management. N Engl J Med 309:308, 1983.

11. Feely MP, O'Hara J, Veale D, et al: Episodes of acute confusion or psychosis in familial hemiplegic migraine. Acta Neurol Scand 65:369, 1982.

12. Fenichel GM, Webster DL, Wong WKT: Intracranial hemorrhage in the term newborn. Arch Neurol 41:30, 1984.

13. Fukuyama Y, Umezu R: Clinical and cerebral angiographic evolutions of idiopathic progressive occlusive disease of the circle of Willis ("Moyamoya" disease) in children. Brain Dev 7:21, 1985.

14. Gastaut H, Pinsard N, Gaustaut JL, et al: Acute hemiplegia in children. In Goldstein M, ed. Advances in Neurology. Raven Press, New York, 1979, p 329.

15. Glista GG, Mellinger JF, Rooke ED: Familial hemiplegic migraine. Mayo Clin Proc 50:307, 1975.

16. Glueck CJ, Daniels SR, Bates S, et al: Pediatric victims of unexplained stroke and their families: Familial lipid and lipoprotein abnormalities. Pediatrics 69:308, 1982.

17. Goodman R: Hemispherectomy and its alternatives in the treatment of intractable epilepsy in patients with infantile hemiplegia. Dev Med Child Neurol 28:251, 1986.

18. Goodman RN, Williamson PD, Reeves AG, et al: Interhemispheric commissurotomy for congenital hemiplegics with intractable epilepsy. Neurology 35:1351, 1985.

19. Graf CJ, Perret GE, Torner JC: Bleeding from cerebral arteriovenous malformations as part of their natural history. J Neurosurg 58:331, 1983.

20. Greenwood RD: Mitral valve prolapse. Incidence and clinical course in a pediatric population. Clin Pediatr 23:318, 1984.

21. Hanson PA, Chodos R: Hemiparetic seizures. Neurology 28:920, 1978.

22. Heyck H: Varieties of hemiplegic migraine. Headache 12:135, 1973.

23. Huttenlocher PR, Mohr JW, Johns L, et al: Cerebral blood flow in sickle cell cerebrovascular disease. Pediatrics 73:615, 1984.

24. Imai WK, Everhart FR, Sanders JM: Cerebral venous sinus thrombosis: Report of a case and review of the literature. Pediatrics 70:965, 1982.

25. Jackson AC, Boughner DR, Barnett HJM: Mitral valve prolapse and cerebral ischemic events in young patients. Neurology 34:784, 1984.

26. Kaplan S: Chronic rheumatic heart disease. In Adams FH, Emmanoullides GC, eds. Heart Disease in Infants, Children, and Adolescents. Williams and Wilkins Co, Baltimore, 1983, p 552.

27. Katirji MB, Reinmuth OM, Latchaw RE: Stroke due to vertebral artery injury. Arch Neurol 42:242, 1985.

28. Kelly JJ, Mellinger JF, Sundt TM: Intracranial arteriovenous malformations in childhood. Ann Neurol 3:338, 1978.

29. Kobayashi M, Morishita H, Sugiyama N, et al: Two cases of NADH-coenzyme Q reductase deficiency: Relationship to MELAS syndrome. J Pediatr 110:223, 1987.

30. Kohrman MH, Huttenlocher PR: Takayasu arteritis: A treatable cause of stroke in infancy. Pediatr Neurol 2:154, 1986.

31. Korobkin R: Active hemiparesis in juvenile insulin-dependent diabetes mellitus (JIDDM). Neurology 30:220, 1980.

32. Kotlarek F, Rodewig R, Brull D, et al: Computed tomographic findings in congenital hemiparesis in childhood and their relation to etiology and prognosis. Neuropediatria 12:101, 1981.

33. Kurlan R, Griggs RC: Cyanotic congenital heart disease with suspected stroke. Should all patients receive antibiotics? Arch Neurol 40:209, 1983.

34. Lauritzen M, Olsen TS, Lassen NA, et al: Changes in regional cerebral blood flow during the course of classic migraine attacks. Ann Neurol 13:633, 1983.

35. Leblanc R, O'Gorman AM: Neonatal intracranial hemorrhage: A clinical and serial computerized tomographic study. J Neurosurg 53:642, 1980.

36. Levy SR, Abroms IF, Marshall PC, et al: Seizures and cerebral infarction in the full-term newborn. Ann Neurol 17:366, 1985.

37. Lewis DW, Berman PH: Vertebral artery dissection and alternating hemiparesis in an adolescent. Pediatrics 78:610, 1986.

38. Llorens-Terol J, Sole-Llenas J, Tura A: Stroke due to fibromuscular hyperplasia of the internal carotid artery. Acta Paediatr Scand 72:299, 1983.

39. MacDonald JT, Brown DR: Acute hemiparesis in juvenile insulin-dependent diabetes mellitus (JIDDM). Neurology 29:893, 1979.

40. McClelland CQ, Rekate H, Kaufman B, et al: Cerebral injury in child abuse: A changing profile. Child Brain 7:225, 1980.

41. McLean MJ, Gebarski SS, Van Der Spek AFL, et al: Response of moyamoya disease to verapamil. Lancet 1:163, 1985.

42. Meislin AG, Rothfield N: Systemic lupus erythematosus in childhood. Analysis of 42 cases, with comparative data on 200 adult cases followed concurrently. Pediatrics 42:37, 1968.

43. Niedermeyer E, Fineyre F, Riley T, et al: Absence status (petit mal status) with focal characteristics. Arch Neurol 36:417, 1979.

44. Packer RJ, Rorke LB, Lange BJ, et al: Cerebrovascular accidents in children with cancer. Pediatrics 76:194, 1985.

45. Parker P, Puck J, Fernandez F: Cerebral infarction associated with mycoplasma pneumonia. Pediatrics 67:373, 1981.

46. Pavlakis SG, Phillips PC, DiMauro S, et al: Mitochondrial myopathy, encephalopathy, lactic acidosis, and strokelike episodes: A distinctive clinical syndrome. Ann Neurol 16:481, 1984.

47. Portnoy BA, Herion JC: Neurologic manifestations in sickle cell disease with a review of the literature and emphasis on the prevalence of hemiplegia. Ann Intern Med 76:643, 1972.

48. Rasmussen T: Further observations on the syndrome of chronic encephalitis and epilepsy. Appl Neurophysiol 41:1, 1978.

49. Roessmann U, Miller RT: Thrombosis of the middle

cerebral artery associated with birth trauma. Neurology 30:889, 1980.

50. Russell MO, Goldberg HI, Reis L, et al: Transfusion therapy for cerebrovascular abnormalities in sickle cell disease. J Pediatr 88:382, 1976.

51. Schoenberg BS, Mellinger JF, Schoenberg DG: Cerebrovascular disease in infants and children: A study of incidence, clinical features and survival. Neurology 26:358, 1976.

52. Selby G, Walker GL: Cerebral arteritis in cat-scratch disease. Neurology 29:1413, 1979.

53. Smith DC, Smith LL, Hesso AN: Fibromuscular dysplasia of the internal carotid artery treated by operative transluminal balloon angioplasty. Radiology 155:645, 1985.

54. Snoek JW, Minderhoud JM, Wilmink JT: Delayed deterioration following mild head injury in children. Brain 107:15, 1984.

55. Solomon GE, Hilal SK, Gold AP, et al: Natural history of acute hemiplegia of childhood. Brain 93:107, 1970.

56. Tagawa T, Mimaki T, Yabuuchi H, et al: Bilateral occlusions in the cervical portion of the internal carotid arteries in a child. Stroke 6:896, 1985.

57. Takeuchi S, Tsuchida T, Kobayashi K, et al: Treatment of Moyamoya disease by temporal muscle graft "encephalo-myo-synangiosis." Child Brain 10:1, 1983.

58. Van Hoff J, Ritchey K, Shaywitz BA: Intracranial hemorrhage in children with sickle cell disease. Am J Dis Child 139:1120, 1985.

59. Yamada S, Kindt GD, Youmans JR: Carotid artery occlusion due to non-penetrating injury. J Trauma 7:333, 1967.

60. Yarnell PR: Todd's paralysis: A cerebrovascular phenomenon? Stroke 6:301, 1975.

61. Young RSK, Coulter DL, Allen RJ: Capsular stroke as a cause of hemiplegia in infancy. Neurology 33:1044, 1983.

12 Paraplegia and Quadriplegia

The term paraplegia is used in this text to denote partial or complete weakness of both legs, therefore obviating the term paraparesis. Many conditions described fully in this chapter are abnormalities of the spinal cord. The same spinal abnormality can cause paraplegia or quadriplegia, depending upon the location of injury. Therefore, quadriplegia as an initial clinical manifestation is covered in this chapter as well. Here again, the term quadriplegia will be used to denote partial or complete weakness of all limbs and the term quadriparesis is not used.

■ Approach to Paraplegia

Weakness of both legs, without any involvement of the arms, should suggest an abnormality of either the spinal cord or the peripheral nerves. Ordinarily, peripheral neuropathies are readily identified on examination by the pattern of distal weakness and sensory loss, atrophy, and loss of tendon reflexes (see Chapters 7 and 9). In contrast, spinal paraplegia causes spasticity, exaggerated tendon reflexes, and a dermatomal level of sensory loss. Disturbances in the conus medullaris and cauda equina, especially congenital malformation, may produce a complex of signs in which spinal cord or peripheral nerve localization is difficult. Indeed, both may be involved. Spinal paraplegia may be asymmetric at onset and present as monoplegia (see Chapter 13). When there is difficulty in anatomic localization between spinal cord and peripheral nerves, electromyography (EMG) and nerve conduction studies are useful in making the distinction.

Paraplegia is sometimes caused by cerebral abnormalities. In such children, the arms as well as the legs are usually weak. However, leg weakness is so much greater than arm weakness that paraplegia is the chief complaint. Finally, it is important to remember that the brain and spinal cord may both be abnormal and that the abnormalities can be in continuity (syringomyelia) or separated (Arnold-Chiari malformation).

■ Spinal Paraplegia and Quadriplegia

There are only a few different pathologic processes that cause spinal paraplegia (Table 12.1). In the absence of trauma, the acute onset or rapid progression of paraplegia is caused by either spinal cord compression or myelitis. Spinal cord compression, from any cause, is a medical emergency requiring rapid diagnosis and therapy to avoid permanent paraplegia. Corticosteroids have the same dehydrating effect on the spinal cord as on the brain and provide transitory decompression prior to surgery.

Several techniques are now available to visualize the spinal cord. The advantages and disadvantages of each are summarized in Table 12.2. All have their place, and sometimes more than one technique must be used to achieve a comprehensive picture of the disease process.

SYMPTOMS AND SIGNS

Clumsiness of gait, refusal to stand or walk, and loss of bladder or bowel control are the common presenting complaints of spinal para-

Table 12.1 SPINAL PARAPLEGIA

Congenital
1. Dysraphic states
    a. Myelomeningocele
    b. Tethered spinal cord
2. Syringomyelia (see Chapter 9)
3. Arteriovenous malformations
4. Atlanto-axial dislocation

Tumors
1. Ependymoma
2. Astrocytoma
3. Neuroblastoma
4. Other

Acute Transverse Myelitis
1. Idiopathic
2. Devic syndrome
3. Encephalomyelitis

Infections
1. Diskitis
2. Polyradiculoneuropathy (see Chapter 7)
3. Epidural abscess
4. Tuberculous osteomyelitis

Trauma in Newborn
1. Transection (see Chapter 6)
2. Infarction

Trauma in Childhood
1. Concussion
2. Fracture dislocation
3. Epidural hematoma

Familial Spastic Paraplegia

plegia. Clumsiness of gait is the usual feature of slowly progressive disorders. The decline in function can be sufficiently insidious to be overlooked for years. Refusal to stand or walk is a symptom of an acute process. In young children who refuse to support weight, it is frequently difficult to distinguish weakness from pain as the underlying cause. Sometimes both are present.

Scoliosis is a constant feature of many spinal cord disorders. It is seen with neural tube defects (Park et al, 1985; McMaster, 1984), spinal cord tumors (Citron et al, 1984; McMaster, 1984), and several degenerative disorders. The pres-

ence of scoliosis prior to puberty in females and in males of all ages should strongly suggest either a spinal cord disorder or a neuromuscular disease (see Chapters 6 and 7).

The presence of abnormalities in the skin overlying the spine, such as an abnormal tuft of hair, pigmentation, a sinus opening, or a mass, may indicate an underlying dysraphic state. Spina bifida is almost always associated.

Foot deformities and especially stunted growth of a limb are malevolent signs of lower spinal cord dysfunction. The usual deformity is foreshortening of the foot, pes cavus. In such cases, disturbances of bladder control are often associated.

Spinal myoclonus is often misdiagnosed as seizure activity or fasciculations. It is characterized by brief, irregular contractions of small groups of muscles and persists in sleep. Myoclonus is caused by irritation to pools of motor neurons and interneurons, usually by an intramedullary tumor or syrinx. The dermatomal distribution of the myoclonus localizes the site of irritation within the spinal cord.

CONGENITAL MALFORMATIONS

Dysraphia comprises all defects in the closure of the neural tube and its coverings. Closure occurs during the third and fourth weeks of gestation. The mesoderm surrounding the neural tube gives rise to dura, skull, and vertebrae, but not to the skin. Therefore, defects in the final closure of the neural tube and its mesodermal case do not preclude the presence of a dermal covering.

Myelomeningocele

Despite extensive epidemiologic studies, the cause of myelomeningocele remains unknown.

Table 12.2 IMAGING THE SPINAL CORD

Myelography
   Advantages: Allows visualization of entire spinal cord at one time and demonstrates blockage of cerebrospinal fluid flow.
   Disadvantages: Invasive, requires the use of contrast media (metrizamide), which may cause allergic reactions or seizures. Two-dimensional, does not allow reconstruction in other planes.

Computerized Tomography
   Advantages: Noninvasive, allows reconstruction in many planes. Demonstrates bone–spinal cord relationship.
   Disadvantages: Allows only limited portion of spinal cord to be visualized at one time.

Magnetic Resonance Imaging
   Advantages: Noninvasive, no exposure to radiation, allows good cerebrospinal fluid–spinal cord contrast, ease of multiplanar imaging, improved discrimination of extramedullary and intramedullary masses, better definition of cavities.
   Disadvantages: Does not show bone, limited clinical-pathologic correlations.

Causes are likely to be multifactorial, including both genetic and environmental factors. Because women who have previously had a child with dysraphia have about a 2 percent risk of recurrence in future pregnancies, prenatal diagnosis can be offered to prevent repetition.

Alpha-fetoprotein is the principal plasma protein of the fetus and is present in amniotic fluid. When the fetus has a defect of the skin that allows the exudation of plasma proteins, the concentration of alpha-fetoprotein in the amniotic fluid is increased. Prenatal diagnosis is possible in about 95 percent of cases by amniocentesis performed at fourteen to sixteen weeks' gestation. The maternal serum concentration of alpha-fetoprotein is elevated as well and can be used as a screening test to determine the need for amniocentesis (Adams et al, 1984).

The incidence of dysraphic defects has been declining in the United States (Adams et al, 1985) and the United Kingdom (Carstairs and Cole, 1984). This decline cannot be explained by antenatal screening alone and may be due in part to changes in critical environmental factors.

Clinical Features. Spina bifida cystica, the protrusion of a cystic mass through the defect, is an obvious deformity of the newborn's spine. More than 90 percent are thoracolumbar in location. Among newborns with spina bifida cystica, the protruding sac is a meningocele without neural elements in 10 to 20 percent, and is a myelomeningocele in the remainder of patients. Meningoceles tend to have a partial dermal covering and are often pedunculated, with a narrow base connecting the sac to the underlying spinal cord. Myelomeningoceles usually have a broad base, are poorly epithelialized, and ooze a combination of cerebrospinal fluid and serum. Remnants of the spinal cord are fused to the exposed portion of the dome.

In newborns with spina bifida cystica, it is important to determine the extent of neurologic dysfunction caused by the myelopathy, the potential for the development of hydrocephalus, and the presence of other malformations in the nervous system and in other organs. When myelomeningocele is the only deformity, the newborn is alert and responsive, and there is no difficulty in feeding. States of diminished consciousness or responsiveness and difficulty in feeding should suggest perinatal asphyxia or cerebral malformations such as hydrocephalus. Cyanosis, pallor, or dyspnea may be due to associated malformations in the cardiovascular system. Multiple major defects are present in 27 percent of cases (Adams et al, 1985).

The Arnold-Chiari malformation is commonly associated. The essential feature of the Arnold-Chiari malformation is elongation of the cerebellar vermis with herniation of its caudal extreme through the foramen magnum. The herniated portion may become ischemic and necrotic and can cause compression of the brainstem and upper cervical spinal cord. Some displacement of the cerebellar vermis is present in most children with myelomeningocele; usually it is asymptomatic. Hydrocephalus is a common feature and may result from aqueductal stenosis or obstruction of the outflow of cerebrospinal fluid from the fourth ventricle resulting from herniation. Respiratory distress is the most important feature of the Arnold-Chiari malformation and the usual cause of death (Papasozomenos and Roessmann, 1981). Rapid respirations, episodes of apnea, and Cheyne-Stokes respirations may be observed. Other evidence of brainstem compression includes poor feeding, vomiting dysphagia, and paralysis of the tongue. Sudden cardiorespiratory failure is the usual cause of death.

Location of the myelomeningocele with reference to the ribs and iliac crest provides reasonably accurate information concerning the spinal segments involved. Several patterns of motor dysfunction may be observed depending upon the location of the cyst. Motor dysfunction results from interruption of the corticospinal tracts and from dysgenesis of the segmental innervation. At birth, the legs are flaccid and the hips are dislocated. Spastic paraplegia, a spastic bladder, and a level of sensory loss develop in infants with a thoracic lesion. Segmental withdrawal reflexes below the level of the lesion, which indicate the presence of an intact but isolated spinal cord segment below the cyst, can be demonstrated in 50 percent of cases. Infants with deformities of the conus medullaris maintain a flaccid paraplegia, have lumbosacral sensory loss, lack a withdrawal response in the legs, and have a distended bladder with overflow incontinence.

Only 15 percent of newborns with myelomeningocele have clinical evidence of hydrocephalus at birth (Stein et al, 1979), but hydrocephalus can be detected in 60 percent of affected newborns by ultrasound (Adams et al, 1985). Eighty percent of these newborns will eventually develop hydrocephalus. The first clinical manifestation frequently follows the repair of the myelomeningocele, but the two are not related. In 73 percent of newborns with myelomeningocele, hydrocephalus is caused by aqueductal stenosis.

Diagnosis. The diagnosis of spina bifida cystica is made by examination alone. An EMG may be useful to clarify the distribution of segmental dysfunction. Ultrasound should be performed on every newborn to look for hydrocephalus. Computerized tomography (CT) and magnetic resonance imaging (MRI) are useful to define malformations of the brain, especially the Arnold-Chiari malformation (see Fig. 10.5). This information may be needed in making therapeutic decisions. Even when hydrocephalus is not present at birth, ultrasound should be repeated in two to four weeks to evaluate ventricular size.

Treatment. It is clear that the chance of surviving the first year is poor unless the back is closed (Adams et al, 1985; Charney et al, 1985). However, the time of closure is not a "surgical emergency" and can be delayed for a week or longer without having an impact on survival rates (Charney et al, 1985). Other factors associated with an increased mortality are a high spinal location of the defect and clinical hydrocephalus at birth.

During the decade of the 1960s, an aggressive approach to the treatment of myelomeningocele was pursued in the United Kingdom. The results were not encouraging; only 2 percent of patients were free of any handicap and 80 percent were severely impaired (Lorber, 1971). Better results have been reported from the United States in the decade of the 1970s (McLone, 1983). Of one hundred newborns with myelomeningocele who were transferred to one medical center between 1975 and 1978, eighty-nine had closure of the back defect within twenty-four hours and eleven procedures were delayed. Hydrocephalus requiring a shunt developed in eighty patients; half of these children required at least one shunt revision. Shunt infection occurred in eight children. The incidence of shunt infection was higher in children who had delayed closure of the back. Fourteen children died, half because of the Arnold-Chiari malformation. Of eighty-six survivors who are older than four-and-a-half, 47 percent are intellectually normal and continent of urine but are not community ambulators.

There are probably several reasons for the difference between the experience in the United States and that in the United Kingdom, not the least of which being a decade of improvement in medical and surgical care. In the United States, survival rates improved in the last half of the 1970s when compared with the first half.

Newborns with respiratory distress due to the Arnold-Chiari malformation are often treated with posterior fossa decompression. Unfortunately, the results have not been encouraging.

Tethered Spinal Cord

The conus medullaris is sometimes anchored to the base of the vertebrae by a thickened filum terminale, a lipoma, a dermal sinus, or a diastematomyelia. Spina bifida occulta is usually associated, and for this reason these anomalies are considered part of the spectrum of dysraphia (Anderson, 1975). The result of the tether is that as the child grows, the spinal cord is stretched and the lumbosacral segments become hypoxic. The mitochondrial oxidative metabolism of neurons is impaired and neurologic dysfunction follows (Yamada et al, 1981).

Dermal sinus is a midline opening of the skin usually marked by a tuft of hair or port wine stain. It is caused by an abnormal invagination of ectoderm into the posterior closure site of the neural tube. Most sinuses terminate subcutaneously as a blind pouch or dermoid cyst. Others extend through a spina bifida to the developing neuraxis, at which point they attach to the dura or the spinal cord as a fibrous band or dermoid cyst. Such sinuses tether the spinal cord and may also serve as a route for bacteria from the skin to reach the subarachnoid space and cause meningitis.

Diastematomyelia consists of a bifid spinal cord (also diplomyelia) that is normal in the cervical and upper thoracic regions and then divides into lateral halves. Two types of diastematomyelia occur with equal frequency. In one type, each half of the cord is surrounded by its own dural sheath and the two halves are separated by a fibrous or bony septum. Once the cord separates, it never rejoins. In the other type, the two halves are surrounded by a single dural sheath, no septum is present and the two halves rejoin after one or two segments. Therefore, splitting of the spinal cord is not caused by the presence of a septum, but is instead a primary disturbance in the formation of luminal borders due to faulty closure of the neural tube. It is usually associated with other dysraphic disturbances such as spina bifida occulta or cystica (Dryden, 1980).

Clinical Features. The initial manifestations of a tethered spinal cord occur at any age from infancy to young adult life. The clinical features vary with age. External signs of spinal dysraphism (tuft of hair, subcutaneous lipoma, dermal sinus) are present in more than half of patients, and spina bifida occulta or sacral deformity is present in almost 90 percent (Anderson, 1975; Fitz and Harwood-Nash, 1975).

Infants and young children are most likely to present with clumsiness of gait, stunted growth or deformity of one foot or leg, and disturbances in bladder function. These symptoms may occur alone or in combination. Consequently, the first specialist consulted may be an orthopedic surgeon, a urologist, a neurologist, or a neurosurgeon. The progression of symptoms and signs is insidious, and at first most children are believed to have a static problem. Children presenting only with a clumsy gait or disturbances in urinary control tend to have normal or exaggerated tendon reflexes and a Babinski sign. At times the ankle tendon reflex is diminished or absent on one or both sides. Children presenting with foot deformity usually have pes cavus and stunted growth of the entire leg. The other leg may appear normal or have a milder deformity without a growth disturbance. Tendon reflexes are usually brisk at the knees, sometimes with crossed adductor responses, and may be either increased or diminished at the ankles. The tendon reflexes in the deformed foot are more likely to be diminished than increased.

The initial manifestation of tethered spinal cord in older children and adolescents is either increased clumsiness of gait or scoliosis. Bilateral, but mild, foot deformities are sometimes present and urinary incontinence and constipation may be reported as well. Tendon reflexes in the legs are usually exaggerated at the knees and ankles and the Babinski sign is frequently present.

Diagnosis. Radiographs of the lumbosacral spine are an excellent initial screening technique. The presence of spina bifida occulta or a sacral deformity should always lead to further imaging of the spine. Normal radiographs of the spine should not dissuade further investigation if the index of suspicion is high. An EMG is almost always normal and not useful as a screening procedure.

High-resolution real-time ultrasound can be used to screen infants less than one year of age (Scheible et al, 1983). The important feature is lack of normal pulsation of the spinal cord. In older children MRI is the appropriate next test. It is particularly useful in the detection of lumbosacral lipoma (Fig. 12.1). However, in the absence of lipoma, definitive diagnosis requires the combination of direct sagittal CT and metrizamide myelography (Altman et al, 1985).

The essential feature of a tethered spinal cord is a low-lying conus medullaris. At twenty-eight weeks' gestational age, the tip of the conus is at the L3 vertebral level. After forty weeks' gestation (Fitz and Harwood-Nash, 1975), a conus tip below the L2 to L3 interspace in children five years and older is always abnormal.

Treatment. Surgical relief of the tethering always prevents further deterioration of neurologic function. However, improvement of preexisting deficits is recorded in only 25 percent of patients with lipoma and in 50 percent of patients with a thickened filium terminale (James et al, 1984; Linder et al, 1982).

Arteriovenous Malformations

Arteriovenous malformations of the spinal cord are uncommon in childhood. The youngest patient reported was one year old, and only 14 percent of childhood onset cases are before age five (Scarff and Reigel, 1979).

Figure 12.1 Tethered cord. A lipoma (arrow) is seen as a low-density area beneath a myelomeningocele. (Courtesy of Drs. Partain, Heller, and Kessler, Department of Radiology and Radiological Sciences, Vanderbilt University, Nashville.)

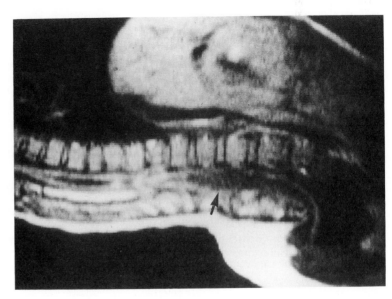

Clinical Features. The progression of symptoms is usually insidious. The average time from onset to diagnosis is approximately five years. Subacute or chronic pain is the initial feature in 38 percent of patients, and subarachnoid hemorrhage presents first in 26 percent. Paraplegia is an early feature in only 34 percent, but monoplegia or paraplegia is present in 92 percent of children at the time of diagnosis. The majority of patients demonstrate a slowly progressive spastic paraplegia with loss of bladder control.

When subarachnoid hemorrhage is the initial manifestation, the malformation is more likely to be in the cervical portion of the spinal cord. Blunt trauma to the spine may be a precipitating factor. The onset of paraplegia or quadriplegia is acute and is associated with back pain.

Back pain and episodic weakness that improves completely or in part may be initial features in some children. With time there is progressive impairment. This type of presentation is misleading and diagnosis may be delayed for several years.

Diagnosis. Myelography had been used previously as the first step in diagnosis but is being replaced by MRI (Doppman et al, 1987). It distinguishes intramedullary from dural and extramedullary locations of the malformation and even allows recognition of thrombus formation (DiChiro et al, 1985). At the present time, arteriography is still required to demonstrate the intramedullary extent of the malformation and all of the feeding vessels.

Treatment. The potential approaches to therapy of intraspinal and intracranial malformations are similar (see Chapter 11). They include embolization, arterial ligation, and excision.

Atlanto-axial Dislocation

The odontoid process is the major factor preventing dislocation of C1 onto C2. Aplasia of the odontoid process can occur alone or as part of mucopolysaccharidosis IV, the Klippel-Feil syndrome, and some chromosomal abnormalities (Greenberg, 1968; Roach et al, 1984).

Clinical Features. Congenital atlanto-axial dislocation produces an acute or slowly progressive quadriplegia that may begin anytime from the neonatal period to adult life. When the onset is in the newborn, the clinical features resemble an acute infantile spinal muscular atrophy (see Chapter 6). There is generalized hypotonia with preservation of facial expression and extraocular movement. The tendon reflexes are absent at first but then become hyperactive.

Mucopolysaccharidoses IV (Morquio syndrome) is primarily a disease of the skeleton with only secondary abnormalities of the spinal cord. In affected children, beginning in the second year and thereafter, there is development of prominent ribs and sternum, knock-knees, progressive shortening of the neck, and dwarfism. The odontoid process is aplastic or absent. Acute, subacute, or chronic cervical myelopathy develops, sometimes precipitated by a fall.

The essential feature of the Klippel-Feil syndrome is a reduced number and abnormal fusion of cervical vertebrae. As in Morquio syndrome, the head appears to rest directly upon the shoulders, the posterior hairline is low, and there is limited movement in all directions (Nagib et al, 1985). Elevation of the scapulae and deformity of the ribs (Sprengel deformity) is frequently present as well. Weakness and atrophy of the arm muscles and mirror movements of the hands are associated with the paraplegia. Associated abnormalities may be present in several different organ systems.

Diagnosis. Lateral radiographs of the cervical portion of the spine in extension and flexion may demonstrate atlanto-axial instability, but CT scans of the cervical vertebrae provide better documentation of the instability and of the spinal cord compression. When Morquio syndrome is suspected, the urine should be checked for the excretion of keratan sulfate.

Treatment. Surgical stabilization of the atlanto-axial junction must be undertaken in any child with evidence of spinal cord compression.

SPINAL CORD TUMORS

Astrocytoma, ependymoma, and neuroblastoma are the common spinal cord tumors of childhood. Sarcomas are next in frequency, followed by neurinoma and then by several different secondary tumors such as teratoma, dermoid, chondroma, and so forth. Motor deficits, usually paraplegia, are an early feature in 86 percent of all spinal cord tumors, and back pain presents early in 63 percent.

Ependymoma

Ependymomas are composed primarily of ependymal cells and arise from the lining of the ventricular system or central canal. They are more often intracranial than intraspinal in children. When intraspinal, they tend to be located in the lumbar region or in the cauda equina, but may occur anywhere along the neuraxis (Dohrmann et al, 1976; Fischer and Mansuy, 1980).

Clinical Features. Clinical features vary with the location of the tumor. The initial manifestation may be scoliosis, pain in the legs or back, paresthesia, or weakness in one or both legs. Diagnosis may be delayed for years when scoliosis is the only sign. Eventually, all children develop difficulty in walking and it is this symptom that usually leads to appropriate diagnostic testing.

Cervical ependymoma presents with stiff neck and cervical pain that is worse at night. Tumors of the cauda equina may sometimes rupture and produce meningismus, fever, and pleocytosis mimicking bacterial meningitis.

Spastic paraplegia is the usual finding on examination. Cervical tumors cause weakness of one arm as well. Tumors of the cauda equina produce flaccid weakness and atrophy of leg muscles associated with loss of tendon reflexes.

Diagnosis. Myelography had been the primary modality for demonstrating tumors of the spinal cord, but it is being replaced by MRI. Ependymomas frequently produce a complete block to the flow of contrast media when myelography is performed. The protein content of the cerebrospinal fluid is markedly elevated.

Treatment. Microsurgical techniques make possible the complete removal of intramedullary ependymoma (Fischer and Mansuy, 1980). The role of postoperative local radiotherapy for treating benign tumors is uncertain. Malignant ependymomas of the spinal cord are unusual in children, but require total neuraxis radiation when present.

Astrocytoma

The problem of differentiating cystic astrocytoma of the spinal cord from syringomyelia is discussed in Chapter 9 (see "syringomyelia").

Clinical Features. Astrocytomas are usually long and may extend from the lower brainstem to the conus medullaris. Two distinct syndromes are associated with holocord astrocytoma (Epstein and Epstein, 1982). The first is characterized primarily by weakness of one arm as the initial manifestation. Pain in the neck may be associated, but bowel and bladder function are normal. Examination reveals mild spastic weakness of the legs. In this group of patients, the solid portion of the tumor is in the neck and its caudal extension is cystic.

The second syndrome is characterized by progressive, spastic paraplegia, sometimes associated with thoracic pain. Scoliosis may be present as well. In these patients, the solid portion of the tumor is in the thoracic or lumbar region. When solid tumor extends into the conus medullaris, tendon reflexes in the legs may be diminished or absent and bowel and bladder function is impaired.

Diagnosis. Plain radiographs of the spine may reveal erosion of pedicles and scalloping of vertebral bodies. When present, these features accurately identify the location of the solid portion of the tumor. MRI is the definitive diagnostic procedure. It allows visualization of both the solid and cystic portions of the tumor (Fig. 12.2).

Treatment. Complete resection should be attempted whenever possible. A laminectomy is performed over the solid portion of the tumor. Using microsurgical technique, the solid portion is removed and the cystic portion is aspirated. MRI should be repeated one, six, and twelve months after surgery. If tumor remains or recurs, local radiation is indicated.

Neuroblastoma

Neuroblastoma is the most common extracranial solid tumor of infancy and childhood. It

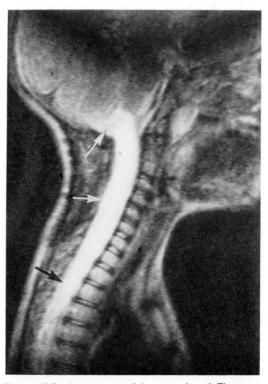

Figure 12.2 Astrocytoma of the cervical cord. The tumor demonstrates an intense signal (arrow) on T2 weighted images. (Courtesy of Drs. Partain, Heller, and Kessler, Department of Radiology and Radiological Sciences, Vanderbilt University, Nashville.)

produces neurologic dysfunction by direct invasion, by metastasis, and by distant "humeral" effects (see Chapter 10). Half of cases occur before two years of age and 60 percent occur before one year (Jaffe, 1976). Neuroblastoma is derived from cells of the sympathetic chain and cranial ganglia. Tumors in a paraspinal location may extend through a neural foramen and compress the spinal cord.

Clinical Features. Paraplegia is the initial manifestation of neuroblastoma extending into the epidural space from a paravertebral origin. Since most affected children are infants, the first symptom is usually refusal to stand or walk. Mild weakness may progress to complete paraplegia over a period of hours or days. Examination generally reveals a flaccid paraplegia, distended bladder, and exaggerated tendon reflexes in the legs. Sensation may be difficult to test.

Diagnosis. Radiographs of the chest usually reveal the extravertebral portion of the tumor. Myelography demonstrates a block to the flow of contrast medium at the level of the tumor in the chest. A CT scan of the spine is also useful in delineating the extent of spinal cord compression.

Treatment. Tumors causing an acute spinal cord compression syndrome must be surgically debulked and then irradiated. The survival rate in infants with neuroblastoma confined to a single organ is greater than 60 percent.

Other Tumors

Other spinal cord tumors of infancy and childhood include sarcoma, neurinoma, dermoid, teratoma, and epidermoid. Meningioma almost never occurs before the third decade.

The clinical features of spinal cord tumors are very much alike from tumor to tumor. Paraplegia and back pain are prominent. Sensory deficits and sphincter disturbances are less common and depend upon tumor location. Some combination of the studies listed in Table 12.2 is always diagnostic, and excision of the tumor is ordinarily the first step in treatment.

TRANSVERSE MYELITIS

Transverse myelitis is an acute demyelinating disorder of the spinal cord that evolves in hours or days. It may occur alone or in combination with demyelination in other portions of the nervous system. The association of transverse myelitis and optic neuritis is called Devic disease; acute demyelination throughout the neuraxis is called acute encephalomyelitis. These terms are descriptive and do not suggest an underlying cause.

Adults with transverse myelitis are usually suspected of having multiple sclerosis, although only 15 percent eventually have other demyelinating lesions disseminated in time (Ropper and Poskanzer, 1978). Multiple sclerosis is exceedingly uncommon in childhood and when it occurs usually presents as ataxia (see Chapter 10).

Transverse myelitis, and especially encephalomyelitis, in children is frequently blamed on a preceding viral infection or immunization. There is currently no basis to support such a notion. School-aged children average six "viral" episodes annually. Therefore, half of children with any illness may give a history of a viral infection within the preceding thirty days. Similarly, despite several case reports there is no epidemiologic evidence supporting a cause-and-effect relationship between presently licensed vaccines and demyelinating disorders of the central nervous system.

Devic Disease (Neuromyelitis Optica)

Clinical Features. A history of anorexia or a flu-like syndrome a few days or a week prior to the onset of neurologic symptoms is common. The anorexia may be part of the acute demyelinating illness rather than a viral infection. Myelitis precedes optic neuritis in 13 percent of patients, follows in 76 percent, and they occur simultaneously in 10 percent (Whitham and Brey, 1985). Optic neuritis and transverse myelitis generally occur within one week of each other. The child remains irritable while the neurologic symptoms are evolving.

Bilateral optic neuritis occurs in 80 percent of patients. Both eyes may be affected at onset, or one eye may become affected before the other. Loss of vision is acute, and blindness is often complete within hours. Results of the initial ophthalmoscopic examination are normal; with time, there is pallor of the disk, the pupils are dilated, and the response to light is sluggish.

Myelitis is heralded by back pain and discomfort in the legs. The legs become weak and there is difficulty standing and walking. Paraplegia becomes complete; first it is flaccid and then becomes spastic. Tendon reflexes may be diminished at first, but later become exaggerated and are associated with extensor plantar responses. The bladder is spastic and there is overflow incontinence. A sensory level may be detected, but more often the sensory deficit is patchy and difficult to delineate in an irritable child.

The course of Devic disease syndrome is variable. Approximately one quarter of cases evolve into an encephalomyelitis (see "Diffuse Encephalomyelitis"), another quarter remain stationary, and the other half demonstrate some recovery that is usually incomplete (Cloys and Netsky, 1970). In contrast, the outcome in children with acute transverse myelitis alone is somewhat better (Dunne et al, 1986). Fifty percent of these children make a full recovery, 10 percent have no recovery, and 40 percent recover incompletely.

Diagnosis. Any child who presents with acute transverse myelitis could also have a spinal cord compression syndrome. A space-occupying mass must be excluded by myelography or MRI. If optic neuritis precedes or occurs simultaneously with transverse myelitis, myelography is not needed and MRI of the head and spine should be performed to delineate the extent of demyelination.

Adrenoleukodystrophy should be considered in boys with Devic disease or encephalomyelitis. Carrier females may have paraparesis alone (Moser et al, 1984). This disorder may be explosive in onset and simulate an acute, acquired demyelinating disease (see Chapter 5). An adrenocorticotropic hormone (ACTH) stimulation test is a useful screening mechanism, but definitive diagnosis requires measuring the serum concentration of very-long-chain fatty acids.

The cerebrospinal fluid in children with Devic disease is usually abnormal. The protein content is mild to moderately elevated and there is a mixed pleocytosis of neutrophils and mononuclear cells.

Treatment. A course of corticosteroids is usually suggested for children with Devic disease. Their value has never been established, but most physicians feel more comfortable using them than doing nothing. Bladder care with intermittent catheterization is imperative, as are measures to prevent bed sores and infection. Psychologic counseling is often needed for the child and the family.

Diffuse Encephalomyelitis

This condition has been discussed in part in the section on Devic syndrome and in Chapter 2. The major clinical difference is that the cerebral hemispheres are affected as well as the spinal cord. Cerebral demyelination may precede, may follow, or may coincide with the myelitis.

Clinical Features. The child is devastated. In addition to the myelitis there is also an encephalopathy characterized by states of decreased consciousness, irritability, and spastic quadriparesis. If the brainstem is affected, there is also dysphagia, fever, cranial nerve palsies, and irregular respiration.

Diagnosis. The full extent of demyelination can be appreciated only by MRI (Perdue et al, 1985). Multiple white matter lesions are noted in the cerebral hemispheres that become confluent (see Fig. 2.4), in the cerebellum, and in the brainstem. Adrenoleukodystrophy must be excluded by measuring very-long-chain fatty acids.

Treatment. Most authorities agree that corticosteroids should be administered (Pasternak et al, 1980). Prednisone, 2 mg/kg/day, or its equivalent in a parenteral form is the initial dose, which is then tapered over a four-week period depending upon the response. The benefit of such a course of therapy is not established, but there are individual patients who become corticosteroid-dependent and relapse when prednisone is discontinued. Such children require long-term alternate-day therapy, which emphasizes the fact that encephalomyelitis is a syndrome due to multiple causes, none of which is fully understood.

INFECTIONS

Diskitis

Diskitis is a relatively common disorder of children in which there is inflammation of one disk space; adjacent vertebral bodies may be affected as well. The cause is uncertain, but bacterial infection, viral infection, and trauma have been suspected. *Staphylococcus aureus* is the organism most often cultured from disk material removed by needle biopsy and is probably the major cause (Wenger et al, 1978). The same organism is sometimes cultured from the blood of these patients.

Clinical Features. The initial manifestation is either difficulty walking or pain. Difficulty walking occurs almost exclusively in children less than three years of age. The typical child has a low-grade fever, is observed to be limping, and then refuses to stand or walk. This symptom complex evolves over twenty-four to forty-eight hours. Affected children prefer to lie on their sides rather than to rest supine, resist being brought to standing, and then seem uncomfortable and walk with a shuffling gait. Examination reveals loss of lumbar lordosis. Tenderness over the hips or back is sometimes present.

Pain as an initial feature occurs more often after the age of three. The pain may be abdominal or vertebral. When abdominal, the pain gradually increases in intensity and may radiate from the epigastrium to the umbilicus or pelvis. Abdominal pain in association with low-grade fever and an elevated peripheral white blood cell count invariably suggests the possibility of appendicitis or other intra-abdominal disease. Fortunately, abdominal pain is the least common presenting complaint.

Back pain is the most common complaint. Older children may indicate a specific area of pain and tenderness. Younger children may have only an abnormal posture intended to splint the painful area. Back pain usually leads to prompt diagnosis because attention is immediately directed to the spine. Examination reveals point tenderness, loss of lumbar lordosis, and decreased movement of the spine.

Diagnosis. Diskitis should be considered in all children who have a sudden onset of back pain or refuse to walk and have normal neurologic examination results. Strength, tone, and tendon reflexes in the legs are normal. Radiographs of the spine reveal narrowing of the affected intervertebral space, most often in the lumbar region, but sometimes as high as the C5 to C6 positions. The inflammation within the disk can be demonstrated by technetium bone scan or by MRI. The MRI is especially good at demonstrating the osteomyelitis of the surrounding vertebrae as well as of the disk space (Fig. 12.3).

Treatment. There is some controversy as to whether or not antibiotics are effective. However, it seems reasonable to provide a course of treatment directed at *S. aureus*, especially if the organism can be cultured from the blood. Immobilization is important, as much to reduce pain as to encourage healing. Bed rest is the only immobilization required for most children.

Epidural Abscess

Most epidural abscesses result from hematogenous spread of bacteria, most often hemolytic *S. aureus*, rather than direct extension from vertebral osteomyelitis. The abscess is usually located on the dorsal surface of the midthoracic or lower lumbar spine, at which point the epidural space is large. The source of infection may

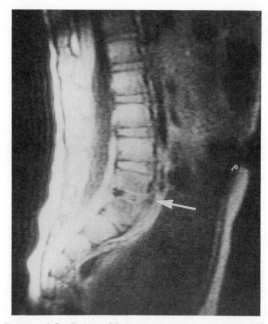

Figure 12.3 Diskitis. Magnetic resonance image reveals collapse of the disk space (arrow) and demineralization of the adjoining vertebral bodies. (Courtesy of Drs. Partain, Heller, and Kessler, Department of Radiology and Radiological Sciences, Vanderbilt University, Nashville.)

be cutaneous or intra-abdominal, and often a source cannot be identified. Despite occasional reports of epidural abscess in infancy, it rarely occurs in children less than ten years of age.

Clinical Features. A preceding bacterial infection or trauma to the back is described as an antecedent event in some children. The initial manifestation is usually back pain, which increases in severity and localizes at the site of the abscess. An effort is made to splint the trunk in extension; flexion and coughing intensify the pain. Fever is often present at the onset of pain, but may be delayed for days. Headache, vomiting, and stiff neck often develop and suggest the diagnosis of meningitis. At this stage, examination reveals a rigid spine with tenderness to percussion over the involved area (Bell and McCormick, 1981).

Symptoms of root irritation and spinal cord compression develop three to six days after the onset of localized back pain. Because the abscess is usually thoracic in location, root irritation is characterized by radiating pain around the chest or into the groin. Spinal cord compression is characterized by progressive paraplegia and bladder dysfunction. Back pain intensifies and is more severe than the pain associated with spinal cord compression by tumor. The presence of fever is an additional feature suggesting abscess.

Epidural abscess in the thoracic region may produce flaccid or spastic paraplegia with hyperreflexia in the legs. An abscess in the lumbar region produces flaccid paraplegia and diminished tendon reflexes.

Diagnosis. Most children with spinal epidural abscess will undergo lumbar puncture because meningitis is suspected. If the abscess is lumbar in location and is pierced by the spinal needle, meningitis will follow. The cerebrospinal fluid is ordinarily sterile, with an increased concentration of protein and a mixed pleocytosis in which lymphocytes predominate. The concentration of glucose is normal. Definitive diagnosis requires myelography or CT of the painful area.

Treatment. Intravenous antibiotics directed against S. aureus should be started immediately when spinal epidural abscess is suspected. As with other causes of spinal cord compression, early surgical decompression is essential. The likelihood of recovery is diminished with each day that paraplegia is allowed to persist.

Tuberculous Osteomyelitis

Vertebral infection is due to hematogenous dissemination. Any level of the vertebral column may be affected. The infection usually begins in one vertebral body and then spreads to adjacent vertebrae and the surrounding soft tissue. Less than 20 percent of patients with tuberculous osteomyelitis develop symptoms of spinal cord dysfunction. The pathophysiologic mechanisms include epidural abscess, arteritis, and vertebral collapse. In addition, tuberculous granuloma of the spine may occur in the absence of vertebral disease.

Clinical Features. Tuberculosis of the vertebrae and spine is primarily a disease of children and young adults. Young children with vertebral osteomyelitis without extension to the spinal cord may refuse to walk because of pain, and their presentation may mimic paraplegia. The prominent features are fever, anorexia, and back pain. In children less than ten years of age, infection is generally diffuse, affecting several vertebral and adjacent tissues (Hsu and Leong, 1984). Older children tend to have localized infection, but with a higher incidence of spinal cord compression.

The symptoms and signs of spinal cord compression from tuberculosis are similar to those described for epidural abscess except that progression is slower.

Diagnosis. The cerebrospinal fluid is usually under pressure and demonstrates a pleocytosis with polymorphonuclear leukocytes predominating early in the course and lymphocytes predominating in the later stages. The total cell count rarely exceeds 500 cells/mm³. Protein concentrations are elevated and glucose concentrations are depressed. Acid-fast organisms can be seen on stained smear and can be cultured from the cerebrospinal fluid.

Early stages of vertebral osteomyelitis can be demonstrated by technetium bone scan or plain radiographs. As the disease progresses, radiographs reveal collapse of adjacent vertebrae and gibbus formation.

Treatment. Tuberculous osteomyelitis and meningitis should be treated in a similar fashion. The current recommended drug combinations are oral isoniazid, 20 mg/kg/day (up to 500 mg/day); intramuscular streptomycin, 20 mg/kg/day (up to 1 g/day); and oral rifampin, 15 mg/kg/day (up to 15 mg/kg). Streptomycin and rifampin are continued for eight weeks following clinical improvement and isoniazid is continued for two years (Bell and McCormick, 1981).

TRAUMA IN THE NEWBORN

Physical injuries to the spinal cord during delivery are discussed in Chapter 6.

Infarction of the spinal cord is a potential hazard in newborns undergoing umbilical artery catheterization (Haldeman et al, 1983). The artery of Adamkiewitz arises from the aorta at the level of T10 to T12 and is the major segmental artery to the thoracolumbar spinal cord. Embolization of the artery may occur if the catheter tip is placed between levels T8 and T11. The result is acute, and sometimes irreversible, paraplegia.

TRAUMA IN CHILDHOOD

Spinal cord injuries are relatively rare in children, especially before adolescence. The major cause is motor vehicle accidents, followed by sports-related injuries (Zabramski et al, 1986). Cervical spinal cord injuries account for 65 percent of cases before age fifteen, and 71 percent of cases before age nine. Fifteen percent of patients have injuries at multiple levels. Children who are neurologically intact at presentation will remain intact afterward. Even those with incomplete function are likely to recover completely. Evidence of complete transection on initial examination indicates that paralysis is permanent.

Spinal Cord Concussion

A direct blow on the back may produce a transitory disturbance in spinal cord function similar to cerebral concussion (see Chapter 2). It is assumed that dysfunction is caused by edema (spinal shock) and that the structural integrity of the spinal cord is intact.

Clinical Features. The major clinical features are flaccid paraplegia with loss of tendon reflexes and urinary retention. Recovery begins within a few hours and is complete within a week.

Diagnosis. At the onset of weakness, it is not possible to exclude a spinal cord compression syndrome such as epidural hematoma, and myelography or MRI is necessary.

Treatment. Management is supportive.

Compressed Vertebral Body Fractures

Clinical Features. Compression fractures of the thoracolumbar region occur when a child jumps or falls from a height greater than ten feet and lands in a standing or sitting position. The spinal cord itself is not transected, but paraplegia may occur secondary to spinal cord concussion. Back pain at the site of fracture is immediate and intense. Nerve roots are compressed, causing radiating pain into the groin and legs.

Diagnosis. Thoracolumbar radiographs reveal the fracture, but when paraplegia is present, myelography is usually performed as well and the results prove to be normal.

Treatment. Immobilization relieves the back pain and promotes healing of the fracture.

Fracture Dislocation and Spinal Cord Transection

These are the most serious vertebral injuries and are usually associated with motor vehicle accidents, especially when the child is thrown from a motorcycle or has a sports injury. A forceful flexion of the spine fractures the articular facets and allows the vertebral body to move forward or laterally, with consequent contusion or transection of the spinal cord. The common sites of traumatic transection are the levels C1 to C2, C5 to C6, C6 to C7, T12 or L1, and L1 to L2.

Clinical Features. Neurologic deficits at and below the level of spinal cord contusion or transection are immediate and profound. Many children with fracture dislocations have sustained head injuries at the time of trauma and are unconscious as well.

Immediately after the injury there is flaccid weakness of the limbs below the level of the lesion associated with loss of tendon and cutaneous reflexes (spinal shock). In high cervical spinal cord lesions, the knee and ankle tendon reflexes may be elicited during the initial period of spinal shock, as may the anal reflex and the plantar response. Spinal shock lasts for approximately one week in infants and young children and up to six weeks in adolescents.

First the superficial reflexes return, then the plantar response becomes one of extension, and finally massive withdrawal reflexes (mass reflex) appear. The mass reflex is triggered by trivial stimulation of the foot or leg, usually in a specific zone unique to the patient. The response at first is dorsiflexion of the foot, flexion at the knees, and flexion and adduction at the thighs. Later, there is also contraction of the abdomen, sweating, piloerection, and emptying of the bladder and bowel. During this time of heightened reflex activity, the tendon reflexes return and become exaggerated.

Below the level of injury, sensation is lost to a variable degree, depending upon the completeness of the transection. When the injury is incomplete, sensation begins to return within weeks and many continue to improve for up to two years. Patients with partial or complete transections may complain of pain and tingling below the level of injury.

In addition to the development of a small spastic bladder, autonomic dysfunction includes constipation, lack of sweating, orthostatic hypotension, and disturbed temperature regulation.

Diagnosis. Fracture dislocation is readily identified by radiographs of the vertebrae. Imaging procedures of the spinal cord produce further information on the presence of compressive hematomas and the structural integrity of the spinal cord (see Fig. 12.4). The presence of a complete block on myelography indicates a poor prognosis for return of function (Bracken et al, 1985).

Treatment. The immediate care of fracture dislocation is to reduce the dislocation and prevent further damage to the cord. This is accomplished by surgery and immobilization. Corticosteroids, even when given immediately at very high doses, do not significantly alter outcome (Bracken et al, 1984; Bracken et al, 1985). Long-term management of spinal cord injuries is beyond the scope of this text, but is best accomplished at specialized centers.

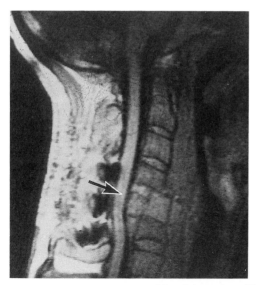

Figure 12.4 Fracture dislocation. C4 is dislocated on C5, causing compression (arrow) of the cord. (Courtesy of Drs. Partain, Heller, and Kessler, Department of Radiology and Radiological Sciences, Vanderbilt University, Nashville.)

Spinal Epidural Hematoma

Spinal epidural hematoma usually results from direct vertebral trauma and is especially common in children with an underlying bleeding tendency. The hematoma causes symptoms by progressive compression of the cord and presents like any other extradural mass lesion. Diagnosis is usually accomplished by myelography. Treatment is surgical evacuation.

FAMILIAL SPASTIC PARAPLEGIA

This is a heterogeneous group of genetic disorders in which the prominent clinical manifestation is a progressive spastic paraplegia. Degeneration occurs in the lateral and posterior columns of the spinal cord and for this reason these disorders are classified in the broader category of spinocerebellar degenerations. Some families have pure spastic paraplegia without clinical evidence of degeneration in the posterior columns or cerebellar pathways. Pure spastic paraplegia may be transmitted by autosomal dominant or recessive inheritance. Even within the dominant and recessive forms there is still genetic heterogeneity.

Autosomal Dominant Inheritance

Two types have been identified: type I designates cases with onset in childhood and type II

is composed of cases with onset in adult life (Harding, 1981). Only type I is discussed here.

Clinical Features. The mean age at onset is eleven years in boys and sixteen years in girls. Onset may be as early as infancy. Such infants present with toe-walking, and their condition is frequently misdiagnosed as cerebral palsy, especially if the affected parent is asymptomatic or has only a mildly stiff gait. Increased tone is more prominent than weakness. Tone increases slowly for a period of ten years and then stabilizes. At this point, the child may have minimal stiffness of gait or be entirely unable to stand or walk.

Tendon reflexes are usually increased in the legs and arms and ankle clonus may be present. Occasionally, patients have diminished or absent tendon reflexes at the ankle. Increased reflexes are usually the only sign of involvement of the arms, but almost 20 percent of patients have mild arm ataxia as well. One third of patients have urinary symptoms, usually in the form of frequency and urgency, and one third have a pes cavus deformity.

Diagnosis. This disorder is difficult to diagnose in the absence of a positive family history. It should be suspected in any child with very slowly progressive spastic paraplegia. Laboratory studies are not helpful except to exclude other conditions.

Treatment. Treatment is not available.

Autosomal Recessive Inheritance

Families with autosomal recessive inheritance are less common than those with autosomal dominant inheritance, and their condition may be associated with a sensory neuropathy (Cavanagh et al, 1979).

Clinical Features. In cases of pure spastic diplegia, the onset is in the first decade and the clinical features are similar to the early onset type with autosomal dominant transmission.

Those children with spastic paraplegia and sensory neuropathy have the onset of spasticity during infancy or early childhood. In many, development is delayed and bladder control is never achieved. Tendon reflexes in the legs, but not necessarily the arms, are exaggerated and ankle clonus is present. Contractures form at the hip, knees, and ankles.

Progressive sensory loss follows the onset of spastic paraplegia and affects the hands as well as the feet. The symptoms and signs are identical to the familial sensory neuropathies described in Chapter 9. Of all sensory modalities, pain and temperature are most severely affected. The anesthetic limb is repeatedly injured, with ulcers forming in the fingers and toes. Recurrent infection and osteomyelitis often result in loss of digits.

Diagnosis. The onset of paraplegia in infancy, in the absence of a positive family history, is likely to suggest cerebral palsy until the progressive nature of the spasticity is recognized. Sensory neuropathy with mutilation of digits may lead to the erroneous diagnosis of syringomyelia. Laboratory tests are useful only to exclude other diagnoses.

Treatment. Treatment for the underlying defect is not available, but supportive care for the sensory neuropathy to prevent further mutilation is needed (see Chapter 9).

■ Cerebral Paraplegia and Quadriplegia

Almost all progressive disorders of the brain that result in quadriplegia also have dementia as an initial or prominent feature (see Chapter 5). Pure paraplegia of cerebral origin is unusual. At the very least, there is impairment of fine finger movements and increased tendon reflex activity in the arms. Pure paraplegia should always direct attention to the spinal cord.

CEREBRAL PALSY

Cerebral palsy is a chronic disability of cerebral origin characterized by aberrant control of movement or posture, appearance during the neonatal period, and absence of progressive disease.

Many slowly progressive disorders are mistakenly diagnosed as cerebral palsy (Table 12.3). Perinatal asphyxia is a known cause of cerebral palsy but accounts for only a minority of cases. Among children with cerebral palsy, 55 percent have Apgar scores of 7 to 10 at one minute and 73 percent score 7 to 10 at five minutes (Nelson and Ellenberg, 1981). Most cerebral palsy is due to prenatal factors that are difficult to identify with precision in an individual case. Among the many factors that increase the relative risk of cerebral palsy, but are not absolute indicators, are low birth weight, maternal mental retardation and epilepsy, and the administration of estrogen and thyroid hormones during pregnancy (Nelson and Ellenberg, 1985, 1986).

Table 12.3 SLOWLY PROGRESSIVE DISORDERS SOMETIMES MISDIAGNOSED AS CEREBRAL PALSY

Condition	Chapter
Polyneuropathy	
1. Metachromatic leukodystrophy	5
2. GM$_1$ gangliosidosis II	5
3. Infantile neuroaxonal dystrophy	5
4. Hereditary motor and sensory neuropathies	7
Ataxia	
1. Ataxia-telangiectasia	10
2. Freidreich ataxia	10
3. Abetalipoproteinemia	10
Spasticity-Chorea	
1. Lesch-Nyhan syndrome	5
2. Pelizaeus-Merzbacher disease	5
3. Rett syndrome	5
4. Familial spastic paraplegia	12
5. Sea-blue histiocytosis	11

Cerebral palsy is not always a permanent condition. Many infants with only mild motor impairments improve and achieve normal motor function in childhood (Nelson and Ellenberg, 1982). Unfortunately, up to 25 percent of such children will be retarded or will have some behavioral or cognitive disturbance.

It has been traditional to classify the cerebral palsies by the pattern of motor impairment. The spastic types are paraplegia or diplegia, quadriplegia, and hemiplegia (see Chapter 11). The hypotonic types are ataxic (see Chapter 10) and athetoid (see Chapter 14).

Spastic Diplegia (Paraplegia)

Diplegia means that all four limbs are affected, but that the legs are more severely affected than the arms. The motor impairment in the arms may be limited to increased responses of tendon reflexes; such children are classified as paraplegic.

Clinical Features. Many children with spastic diplegia have normal tone, or even hypotonia, during the first four months. The onset of spasticity in the legs is insidious and slowly progressive during the first year. Four-point creeping is impossible because of leg extension, and early ambulation is usually achieved by either rolling or crawling on the floor, with the belly on the ground, using the arms to pull the body forward.

Sitting up alone is delayed or never achieved. From the supine position, the infant pulls to standing rather than to sitting. Sitting is later made possible by bending forward at the waist, to compensate for the lack of flexion at the hip and knee, and placing one hand on the floor for balance. Most children with spastic diplegia stand on their toes, with flexion at the knees and an increased lumbar lordosis. Walking is difficult because of the stiffness in the legs and can be accomplished only by throwing the body forward or side to side in order to transfer weight.

Examination always reveals spasticity of the legs and little or no spasticity of the arms. The tendon reflexes are exaggerated in all limbs. Reflex sensitivity and responsiveness are increased; percussion at the knee causes a crossed adductor response. Ankle clonus and a Babinski sign are usually present. When the infant is suspended vertically there are strong contractions of the adductor muscles, causing the legs to cross at the thigh (scissoring).

Subluxation or dislocation of the hips is relatively frequent in children with severe spasticity; this is caused in part by the constant adduction of the thighs and also by insufficient development of the hip joint because of delayed or absent standing.

Diagnosis. Spastic diplegia is a clinical diagnosis. The important consideration is to be certain that the child does not have a progressive disease of the brain or cervical portion of the spine. Features that suggest a progressive disease are a positive family history of "cerebral palsy," deterioration of mental function, loss of motor skills previously obtained, atrophy of muscles, and sensory loss.

Treatment. There are probably as many "methods" to manage spastic diplegia and quadriplegia as there are children with cerebral palsy. No one method can be endorsed on the basis of controlled clinical trials. In general, a multidisciplinary approach is used to help the child achieve an adequate functional status by physical and occupational therapy. Drugs to relieve spasticity are generally of no value unless doses that produce unacceptable sedation are used. Surgery is useful to relieve contractures, but should be carefully planned so that it is performed only once and is then followed by a program of physical therapy that maintains the desired range of motion.

Spastic Quadriplegia

The whole body is affected in spastic quadriplegia, but not symmetrically. One side is usually worse than the other, and the arms are affected more than the legs. For this reason, the condition is sometimes called *double hemiplegia*. If asymmetry is considerable, the child may be thought to have a hemiplegia.

Clinical Features. Developmental delay is profound and the infant is quickly identified as being neurologically abnormal. Failure to meet motor milestones and abnormal posturing of the head and limbs are the common reasons for neurologic evaluation.

In severely affected children, the supine posture is characteristic. The head and neck are retracted, the arms are flexed at the elbows with the hands clenched, and the legs are held in extension. Infantile reflexes (Moro and tonic-neck) are obligatory and stereotyped and persist after six months of age. Microcephaly is frequently associated.

Because both hemispheres are damaged, supranuclear bulbar palsy (dysphagia and dysarthria) is common. Disturbances in vision and ocular motility are frequently associated and seizures occur in 50 percent of affected children.

Diagnosis. This is a clinical diagnosis. Laboratory studies are useful in selected cases to establish a diagnosis when the underlying cause is not obvious or the possibility exists of a genetically transmitted defect.

Treatment. See "Spastic Diplegia (Paraplegia)."

References

1. Adams MJ, Windham GC, James LM, et al: Clinical interpretation of maternal serum a-fetoprotein concentrations. Am J Obstet Gynecol 148:241, 1984.
2. Adams MM, Greenberg F, Khoury MJ, et al: Trends in clinical characteristics of infants with spina bifida—Atlanta, 1972–1979. Am J Dis Child 139:514, 1985.
3. Altman N, Harwood-Nash DC, Fitz CR, et al: Evaluation of the infant spine by direct sagittal computed tomography. AJNR 6:65, 1985.
4. Anderson FM: Occult spinal dysraphism: A series of 73 cases. Pediatrics 55:826, 1975.
5. Bell WE, McCormick WF: Neurologic infections in children. In Markowitz M, ed. Major Problems in Clinical Pediatrics. Volume 12. WB Saunders Co, Philadelphia, 1981, p 244.
6. Bracken MB, Colleris WF, Freedman DF, et al: Efficacy of methylprednisolone in acute spinal cord injury. JAMA 251:45, 1984.
7. Bracken MB, Shepard MJ, Hellenbrand KG, et al: Methylprednisolone and neurological function 1 year after spinal cord injury. J Neurosurg 63:704, 1985.
8. Carstairs V, Cole S: Spina bifida and anencephaly in Scotland. Br Med J 289:1182, 1984.
9. Cavanagh NPC, Eames RA, Galvin RJ, et al: Hereditary sensory neuropathy with spastic paraplegia. Brain 102:79, 1979.
10. Charney EB, Weller SC, Sutton LN, et al: Management of the newborn with myelomeningocele: Time for a decision-making process. Pediatrics 75:58, 1985.

11. Citron N, Edgar MA, Sheeny J, et al: Intramedullary spinal cord tumors presenting as scoliosis. J Bone Joint Surg 66:513, 1984.

12. Cloys DE, Netsky MG: Neuromyelitis optica. In Vinken PJ, Brun GW, eds. Handbook of Clinical Neurology. Volume 9. North Holland Pub Co, Amsterdam, 1970, p 426.

13. DiChiro G, Doppman JL, Dwyer AJ, et al: Tumors and arteriovenous malformations of the spinal cord: Assessment using MR. Radiology 156:689, 1985.

14. Dohrmann GJ, Farwell JR, Flannery JT: Ependymomas and ependymoblastomas in children. J Neurosurg 45:273, 1976.

15. Doppman JL, Di Chiro G, Dwyer AJ, et al: Magnetic resonance imaging of spinal arteriovenous malformations. J Neurosurg 66:830, 1987.

16. Dryden RJ: Duplication of the spinal cord: A discussion of the possible embryogenesis of diplomyelia. Dev Med Child Neurol 22:234, 1980.

17. Dunne K, Hopkins IJ, Shield LK: Acute transverse myelopathy in childhood. Dev Med Child Neurol 28:198, 1986.

18. Epstein F, Epstein N: Surgical treatment of spinal cord astrocytomas of childhood. A series of 19 patients. J Neurosurg 57:685, 1982.

19. Fischer G, Mansuy L: Total removal of intramedullary ependymomas: Follow-up study of 16 cases. Surg Neurol 14:243, 1980.

20. Fitz CR, Harwood-Nash DC: The tethered conus. AJR 125:515, 1975.

21. Greenberg AD: Atlanto-axial dislocation. Brain 91:655, 1968.

22. Haldeman S, Fowler GW, Ashwal S: Acute flaccid neonatal paraplegia: a case report. Neurology 33:93, 1983.

23. Harding AE: Hereditary "pure" spastic paraplegia: a clinical and genetic study of 22 families. J Neurol Neurosurg Psychiatry 44:871, 1981.

24. Hsu LC, Leong JC: Tuberculosis of the lower cervical spine (C2 to C7). A report on 40 cases. J Bone Joint Surg 66:1, 1984.

25. Jaffe N: Neuroblastoma: Review of the literature and an examination of factors contributing to its enigmatic character. Cancer Treat Rev 3:61, 1976.

26. James HE, Williams J, Brock W, et al: Radical removal of lipomas of the conus and cauda equina with laser microneurosurgery. Neurosurgery 15:340, 1984.

27. Linder M, Rosenstein J, Sklar FH: Functional improvement after spinal surgery for the dysraphic malformations. Neurosurgery 11:622, 1982.

28. Lorber J: Results of treatment of myelomeningocele: An analysis of 524 unselected cases with special reference to possible selection for treatment. Dev Med Child Neurol 13:279, 1971.

29. McLone DG: Results of treatment of children born with a myelomeningocele. In Weiss ME, ed. Clinical Neurosurgery Volume 30. Williams & Wilkins, Baltimore, 1983, pp 407–412.

30. McMaster MJ: Occult intraspinal anomalies and congenital scoliosis. J Bone Joint Surg 66:588, 1984.

31. Moser HW, Moser AE, Singh I, et al: Adrenoleukodystrophy: Survey of 303 cases; biochemistry, diagnosis, and therapy. Ann Neurol 16:628, 1984.

32. Nagib MG, Maxwell RE, Chou SN: Klippel-Feil syndrome in children: clinical features and management. Child Nerv Syst 1:255, 1985.

33. Nelson KB, Ellenberg JH: Apgar scores as predictors of chronic neurologic disability. Pediatrics 68:36, 1981.

34. Nelson KB, Ellenberg JH: Children who "outgrew" cerebral palsy. Pediatrics 69:529, 1982.

35. Nelson KB, Ellenberg JH: Antecedents of cerebral palsy. Am J Dis Child 139:1031, 1985.

36. Nelson KB, Ellenberg JH: Antecedents of cerebral palsy. Multivariate analysis of risk. N Engl J Med 315:81, 1986.

37. Papasozomenos S, Roessmann U: Respiratory distress in Arnold-Chiari malformation. Neurology 31:97, 1981.

38. Park TS, Cail WS, Maggio WM, et al: Progressive spasticity and scoliosis in children with myelomeningocele. Radiological investigation and surgical treatment. J Neurosurg 62:367, 1985.

39. Pasternak JF, DeVivo DC, Prensky AL: Steroid-responsive encephalomyelitis in childhood. Neurology 30:481, 1980.

40. Perdue Z, Bale JF, Dunn VD, et al: Magnetic resonance imaging in childhood disseminated encephalomyelitis. Pediatr Neurol 1:370, 1985.

41. Roach JW, Duncan D, Wenger DR, et al: Atlanto-axial instability and spinal cord compression in children—diagnosis by computerized tomography. J Bone Joint Surg 66:708, 1984.

42. Ropper AH, Poskanzer DC: The prognosis of acute and subacute transverse myelopathy based on early signs and symptoms. Ann Neurol 4:51, 1978.

43. Scarff TB, Reigel DH: Arteriovenous malformations of the spinal cord in children. Child Brain 5:341, 1979.

44. Scheible W, James HE, Leopold GR, et al: Occult spinal dysraphism in infants: Screening with high-resolution real-time ultrasound. Radiology 145:743, 1983.

45. Stein S, Schut L, Borns P: Hydrocephalus in myelomeningocele. Child Brain 5:413, 1979.

46. Wenger DR, Bobechko WP, Gilday DL: The spectrum of intervertebral disc-space infection in children. J Bone Joint Surg 60:100, 1978.

47. Whitham RH, Brey RL: Neuromyelitis optica: Two new cases and review of the literature. J Clin Neuroophthalmol 5:263, 1985.

48. Yamada S, Zinke DE, Sanders D: Pathophysiology of "tethered cord syndrome." J Neurosurg 54:494, 1981.

49. Zabramski JM, Hadley MN, Browner CM, et al: Pediatric spinal and vertebral column injuries. Barrow Neurol Inst Q 2:11, 1986.

13 Monoplegia

Flaccid weakness of one limb is usually caused by abnormalities of the spine of proximal portion of the nerves. Many conditions that result in paraplegia or quadriplegia may begin as monoplegia. Therefore, the differential diagnosis of spinal paraplegia provided in Table 12.1 must also be consulted for monoplegia. In addition, several cerebral disorders that cause hemiplegia may present initially as a monoplegia and the tables in Chapter 11 must be consulted as well.

■ Approach to Monoplegia

If a child refuses to use a limb, the problem may be caused by either pain or weakness. Painful limbs are usually caused by injury, but they may also be caused by arthritis, infection, or tumor. Pain and weakness together are a feature of plexitis.

The differential diagnosis of acute monoplegia is summarized in Table 13.1. Plexopathies and neuropathies are the leading causes of pure monoplegia. Stroke often affects one limb, usually the arm, more than the other. The presentation suggests monoplegia, but careful examination reveals increased tendon reflexes and an extensor plantar response in the seemingly unaffected leg. Any suggestion of hemiplegia, rather than monoplegia, or increased tendon reflexes in the paretic limb should focus attention on the brain and cervical cord as the site of pathology.

Chronic progressive brachial monoplegia is uncommon. When present, syringomyelia and tumors of the cervical cord or brachial plexus should be suspected. Chronic progressive weakness of one leg suggests a congenital malformation or tumor of the spinal cord.

PLEXOPATHIES

Acute Idiopathic Plexitis

Acute plexitis is a demyelinating disorder of the brachial or lumbar plexus thought to be autoimmune-mediated. Brachial plexitis is far more common than lumbar plexitis and occurs with an annual incidence of 1.64/100,000 (Beghi et al, 1985).

Brachial Plexitis

Brachial plexitis (brachial neuritis, neuralgic amyotrophy) occurs from infancy (Charles and Jayam-Trouth, 1980) to adult life with the peak incidence in the fifth and sixth decades (Tsairis et al, 1972). An antecedent infectious disease is recorded in 25 percent of patients; this is not greater than the baseline of "viral" disease in the United States. Prior immunization with tetanus toxoid is recorded in 10 to 20 percent of cases, and this is probably a significant association. The site of immunization does not correlate with the arm involved.

Clinical Features. The onset of symptoms is usually explosive. Pain is the initial manifestation in 95 percent of patients. It is frequently localized to the shoulder, but may be more diffuse or limited only to the lower arm. Pain is severe, may awaken the patient, and is described as sharp, stabbing, throbbing, or aching. The duration of pain, which is frequently constant, varies from several hours to three weeks. As the pain subsides, weakness appears. Weakness is in the distribution of the upper plexus in 56 percent, the lower plexus in 6 percent, and the entire plexus in 38 percent. Although the initial pain has abated, paresthesias may be present concurrent with the weakness.

279

Table 13.1 ACUTE MONOPLEGIA

Plexopathy/Neuropathy
1. Acute neuritis
   a. Idiopathic plexitis
   b. Osteomyelitis plexitis
   c. Tetanus toxoid (?) plexitis
   d. Poliomyelitis (see Chapter 7)
2. Hereditary
   a. Hereditary brachial neuritis
   b. Hereditary recurrent pressure palsy
3. Injury
   a. Traction injuries
   b. Pressure injuries
   c. Lacerations

Stroke (see Table 11.2)

Complicated Migraine (see Chapter 11)

"Hemiparetic" Seizures (see Chapter 11)

Two thirds of patients report an improvement in strength during the first month after onset. Upper plexus palsies improve faster than do lower plexus palsies. Among all patients, 36 percent recover within one year, 75 percent by two years, and 89 percent by three years. The remainder may show continuing improvement after three years, but many will be left with permanent residua.

Recurrences are unusual and less severe than the initial episode.

Diagnosis. Pain and weakness in one arm are also symptoms of spinal cord compression, and an imaging study of the spinal cord is often needed. However, when the onset is characteristic of brachial plexus neuritis, the diagnosis can be established on clinical grounds and diagnostic tests deferred.

The cerebrospinal fluid is usually normal. A slight lymphocytosis and mild elevation in protein content is sometimes noted.

Electromyography (EMG) and nerve conduction studies are helpful in demonstrating the extent of plexopathy. Electrical evidence of bilateral involvement is often present in patients with unilateral symptoms.

Treatment. Corticosteroids have not been demonstrated to affect outcome. Range of motion exercises are recommended.

Lumbar Plexitis

Lumbar plexitis occurs at all ages and is similar to brachial plexitis, except that the leg is affected instead of the arm. An autoimmune mechanism is suspected, but an association with antecedent viral infection or immunization has not been established.

Clinical Features. Pain of one or both legs is the initial symptom in every case (Evans et al, 1981; Sander et al, 1981). The onset of pain is abrupt and may follow a femoral or sciatic distribution. Sciatica, when present, suggests disk disease. Young children will refuse to stand or walk, and older children develop a limp.

Weakness may develop concurrent with pain or may be delayed for as long as three weeks. The onset of weakness is insidious and often difficult to date, but usually begins eight days after the onset of pain. Weakness progresses for a week and then stabilizes. Tendon reflexes are absent in the affected leg, but are present in other limbs.

Recovery is characterized first by abatement of pain and then by increasing strength. The average time from onset of pain to maximal recovery is eighteen weeks, with a range of eight weeks to several years. Functional recovery is almost universal, but mild residual weakness may persist.

Diagnosis. The sudden onset of pain and weakness of one leg suggests spinal cord or disk disease. Many patients undergo myelography, the results of which are invariably normal. Examination of the cerebrospinal fluid is normal except for a mild elevation of protein concentration. An EMG performed three weeks after onset demonstrates patchy denervation.

Treatment. Corticosteroids have not been demonstrated to affect outcome. Range of motion exercises are recommended.

Osteomyelitis-Neuritis

Apparent limb weakness that is due to pain is a well-recognized phenomenon. However, a true brachial neuritis may occur in response to osteomyelitis of the shoulder (Clay, 1982). The mechanism is thought to be ischemic nerve damage due to vasculitis.

Clinical Features. The condition occurs predominantly during infancy. The initial manifestation is a flaccid arm without pain or tenderness. Body temperature may be normal at first but soon becomes elevated. Pain develops on movement of the shoulder, and finally there is tenderness to palpation. Swelling is not present. Both the biceps and triceps reflexes may be depressed or absent.

Diagnosis. Osteomyelitis of the proximal humerus should be suspected when brachial plexitis neuritis develops during infancy. Radiographs of the humerus do not become abnormal until the end of the first week and then reveal destruction of the lateral margin of the humerus. Radioisotope bone scan demonstrates a focal area of uptake in the proximal humerus, the scapula, or both shortly after onset. After three weeks, the EMG demonstrates patchy denervation in the muscles innervated by the upper plexus. The EMG supports the notion that this is a true plexitis and not just a painful limb.

Identification of the organism can be accomplished by aspiration of the shoulder joint or by blood cultures. Group B streptococcus is often isolated in very young infants, and other species of bacteria are isolated in older children.

Treatment. Intravenous antibiotics, usually penicillin, must be administered for three to four weeks. Recovery of arm strength may be incomplete.

Asthmatic Amyotrophy

Sudden flaccid paralysis of one or more limbs, resembling poliomyelitis, may occur after an asthmatic attack (Hopkins syndrome). All affected children had been previously immunized against poliomyelitis. The syndrome is believed to be caused by anterior horn cell infection by a neurotropic virus other than poliovirus (Masson and Thong, 1980). Adenovirus, echovirus, and coxsackievirus have been isolated from stool, throat, or cerebrospinal fluid in some cases.

Clinical Features. Age at onset is from two to eleven years and both sexes are involved. The interval between the asthmatic attack and the paralysis is one to eleven days with an average of five days. Among twenty reported cases, monoplegia occurred in seventeen; the arm was involved in twelve children and the leg in five, hemiplegia in two, and diplegia in one (Nihei et al, 1987). Meningeal irritation is not present but muscle pain in the paralyzed limb is noted in half of cases. Recovery is incomplete, and all affected children have been left with some degree of permanent paralysis.

Diagnosis. Asthmatic amyotrophy is primarily a clinical diagnosis based upon the sequence of events. It must be distinguished from paralytic poliomyelitis and idiopathic brachial neuritis. The distinction from paralytic poliomyelitis is made on on the basis of normal cerebrospinal fluid in asthmatic amyotrophy. A few white blood cells may be present in the cerebrospinal fluid, but never to the extent encountered in poliomyelitis, and the protein concentration is normal.

An EMG during the acute phase demonstrates active denervation of the paralyzed limb, but the pattern of denervation does not follow the radicular distribution expected in a brachial neuritis.

Treatment. Treatment is symptomatic and includes analgesics for pain and physical therapy.

Hereditary Brachial Plexopathy

There are two major phenotypes of focal, familial, recurrent neuropathy: hereditary brachial plexopathy (Bradley et al, 1975; Dunn et al, 1978; Geiger et al, 1974) and hereditary recurrent pressure palsy (see "Mononeuropathies" later on). They are genetically distinct, but can be confused because isolated nerve palsies may occur in hereditary brachial plexopathy and brachial plexopathy is reported in patients with hereditary recurrent pressure palsy. Both disorders are transmitted by autosomal dominant inheritance.

Clinical Features. This disorder may be difficult to distinguish from idiopathic brachial plexitis in the absence of a family history or a past history of similar episodes.

Several different antecedent events are reported to trigger an attack in genetically predisposed individuals. These include infection, emotional stress, strenuous use of the affected limb, and parturition. Immunization has not been implicated.

The initial attack usually occurs during the second or third decade but may appear as early as the first decade and can be present at birth. When brachial plexus palsy is present at birth, it is generally misinterpreted as traumatic even if the positive family history is known. Weakness subsequently resolves completely, only to recur later in childhood.

Typical attacks are characterized first by severe arm pain that may be exacerbated by movement. Weakness follows in days to weeks and is usually maximal within a few days and always by one month. The entire plexus may be involved, but most often the upper trunk is affected alone or most severely. Examination demonstrates proximal arm weakness and sometimes distal weakness as well. Tendon reflexes cannot be elicited from affected muscles. Weakness persists for weeks to months, during which time atrophy and fasciculations are observed. Pain, which is frequently the only sensory finding, subsides after the first week.

Recovery begins weeks to months after maximal weakness is attained. Return of function is usually complete, although some residual weakness may persist after repeated attacks. The frequency of attacks is variable; several attacks may occur within a single year, but two or three attacks per decade is more usual.

Occasional patients experience an episode of lumbar plexopathy, which is characterized by pain in the thigh and by proximal weakness. Brachial and lumbar plexopathy are never concurrent, although bilateral brachial plexopathy is a relatively common event. Isolated cranial nerve palsies are reported in families with hereditary brachial plexopathy. The vagus is most often affected, causing hoarseness and difficulty in swallowing. Transitory facial palsies and unilateral hearing loss are reported as well.

Diagnosis. The family history, early age at onset, unique triggering events, recurrences, and involvement of other nerves differentiate hereditary brachial plexopathy from idiopathic brachial neuritis. The EMG demonstrates a diffuse axonopathy in the affected arm and some evidence of denervation in the asymptomatic arm. Asymptomatic legs are electrically normal.

Treatment. There is no evidence that corticosteroids are of any benefit. Analgesics may be needed at the onset of an attack. Range of motion exercises are recommended.

Neonatal Brachial Neuropathy

The most recent survey of brachial plexus injuries in the newborn was reported by Painter and Bergman in 1973. Data collected from 1959 to 1965 showed that the incidence was 0.7 per 1,000 live births. This is a decline from prior studies and is probably attributable to improved obstetric practices.

Brachial plexus injuries in the newborn are caused by excessive traction. Upper plexus injuries occur when the head is suddenly pulled away from the arm. There are several scenarios in which this may occur. In vertex position, the head may be forcefully pulled to deliver the after-coming shoulder or the head and neck may be forced downward by normal contractions, while the shoulder is caught by the pelvis. Injuries in breech position occur when the arm is pulled downward to free the after-coming head or when the head is rotated to occipitoanterior, but the shoulder is fixed. Lower plexus injuries occur during vertex deliveries when there is traction on a prolapsed arm and in breech deliveries when the trunk is pulled downward, but an after-coming arm is fixed.

Clinical Features. Most neonatal brachial plexus injuries occur in large term newborns of primiparous mothers, especially when the fetus is malpositioned and the delivery is long and difficult. Although it is traditional to divide brachial plexus injuries into those involving the upper roots (named for Erb and Duchenne) and those involving the lower roots (named for Klumpke), solitary lower root injuries do not occur. The fifth and sixth cervical roots are constantly affected, the seventh cervical root is additionally affected in 50 percent of injuries, and all roots from the fifth cervical to the first thoracic in 10 percent (Eng, 1971; Hardy, 1981). Bilateral, but not necessarily symmetric, involvement occurs in up to 23 percent of cases.

Because the upper plexus is always involved, the posture of the arm is typical and reflects weakness in the proximal muscles. The arm is tightly abducted and internally rotated at the shoulder and is extended and pronated at the elbow, so that the partially flexed fingers face backward. When the seventh cervical segment is also involved, extension of the wrist is lost and fisting of the fingers is more prominent. The biceps and triceps reflexes are absent. Injuries that extend higher than the fourth cervical segment result in ipsilateral diaphragmatic paralysis.

Newborns with a complete brachial plexus palsy have a flaccid, dry limb with neither proximal nor distal movement. A Horner's syndrome is sometimes associated. Sensory loss to pinprick is present with partial or complete palsies, but need not conform to the segmental pattern of weakness.

Diagnosis. Brachial plexus palsy is easily recognized by the typical posture of the arm and by failure of movement when the Moro reflex is tested. Because the injury often takes place during a long and difficult delivery, asphyxia may be present as well. In such cases, focal arm weakness may be missed because of generalized hypotonia. Approximately 10 percent of newborns with brachial plexus injuries have facial nerve palsy and fractures of the clavicle or humerus.

An EMG may be useful for determining precise segmental localization of injury and for prognosis (Eng, 1971). Reinnervation can be predicted by the appearance of small polyphasic motor units that precede clinical evidence of recovery by one month.

Treatment. Spontaneous recovery rates are good, and the only goal of therapy is to prevent contractures from developing. This is accomplished by range of motion exercises; splinting or other forms of immobilization should be avoided.

Complete recovery is reported in 70 to 95 percent of cases. Significant recovery occurs throughout the first year, only minor improvement occurs in the second year, and the deficit is fixed after the second year.

Postnatal Injuries

Brachial Plexus

Traction and pressure injuries of the brachial plexus are relatively common because of its superficial position. Motor vehicle and sports accidents account for the majority of severe injuries. However, mild injuries can occur when an adult suddenly yanks a child's arm, either protectively or to force movement; by a blow to the shoulder, such as a football scrimmage or the recoil of a rifle (Wanamaker, 1974); by prolonged wearing of a heavy knapsack; when the arm is kept hyperextended during surgery; and by pressure in the axilla from poorly positioned crutches.

Clinical Features. Mild injuries do not affect all portions of the plexus equally. Diffuse weakness is uncommon. Pain may be an important initial feature, and sensory loss is uncommon. Recovery begins within days or weeks and is complete. Atrophy does not occur.

More severe injuries are usually associated with fractures of the clavicle and scapula and dislocation of the humerus. The upper plexus is generally affected more severely than is the lower plexus, but complete paralysis may be present at the onset. Sensory loss is less marked than weakness, and the two may not correspond in distribution. Pain is common, not only from the plexopathy but also from the bone and soft tissue injuries. The most painful injuries are those associated with root avulsion (Wynn-Parry, 1980).

Tendon reflexes are absent, and atrophy develops in denervated muscle. Recovery progresses proximal to distal and can be plotted by Tinel's sign: tingling in the distal part of a limb caused by tapping over the regenerating segment of a nerve. Complete reinnervation, when it occurs, may take several months or years. The completeness of recovery depends upon the severity and nature of the injury. Pressure and traction injuries in which anatomic integrity is not disturbed recover best, whereas injuries that tear the nerve or avulse the root do not recover at all.

Diagnosis. The EMG is useful in identifying the pattern of nerve injury and in providing information on prognosis (Trojaborg, 1977). Even with mild traction injuries, there is attenuation of the amplitude of motor and sensory action potentials and slowing of motor and sensory conduction velocities.

Treatment. Mild injuries do not require treatment other than range of motion exercises. For more severe traction injuries, it is usually necessary to rest the limb for the first month. During that time, analgesia is needed for pain and the muscles can be stimulated electrically, away from the site of injury, to maintain tone. Range of motion exercises should be started after the pain subsides.

Fractures and dislocations causing pressure on the brachial plexus must be corrected promptly. Where nerves have been lacerated, anatomic integrity must be restored surgically.

Lumbar Plexus

The lumbar plexus is much less likely to be injured than is the brachial plexus, because it is surrounded by the pelvis and the very heavy muscles of the proximal leg.

Clinical Features. Lumbar plexus injuries are almost always associated with fracture-dislocation of the pelvis. Motor vehicle accidents or falls from considerable height are required to produce sufficient force. Therefore, the patient usually has multiple injuries and the lumbar plexus injury may not be identified early.

Lumbar plexus injuries produce a patchy weakness that is difficult to differentiate from mononeuritis multiplex.

Diagnosis. The EMG is critical in helping one to make the distinction between plexus injuries and nerve injuries.

Treatment. Fracture-dislocations must be treated to relieve pressure on the plexus. As with brachial plexus injuries, the completeness of recovery depends upon the anatomic integrity of the nerves.

Plexus Tumors

Brachial plexus tumors in childhood are rare; when they do occur, however, they are likely to be malignant. The important primary tumor is a malignant schwannoma, and the important secondary tumors are neuroblastoma and other primitive neuroectodermal tumors arising in the chest.

MONONEUROPATHIES

Radial Neuropathy

The radial nerve is most often injured in the spinal groove of the humerus, just below the take-off of the motor branch to the triceps muscle. This may occur with fractures of the humerus or by external pressure. Such pressure usually results when a sleeping or sedated patient is in a position that compresses the nerve between the humerus and a hard surface, such as an operating room table or chair.

Clinical Features. Radial nerve injuries in the spinal groove are characterized by wrist and finger drop. The brachioradialis muscle may be weak as well and its tendon reflex lost. Sensory disturbances are restricted to the back of the hand near the base of the thumb. With the wrist dropped, it is mechanically difficult to make a fist but the finger flexors are not weak.

Diagnosis. Electrophysiologic studies are very useful in locating the site of injury, the anatomic integrity of the nerve, and the prognosis for recovery (Trojaborg, 1977).

Treatment. Pressure injuries recover completely in six to eight weeks. During that time, a splint is useful for placing the wrist in extension and for allowing the patient to flex the fingers.

Ulnar Neuropathy

The commonest site of ulnar injury is at the elbow. This type of injury can result from external pressure, recurrent dislocation of the nerve from its groove, and fracture of the distal humerus.

Clinical Features. Paresthesias are noted on the ulnar side of the hand, the little finger, and the ring finger. Tapping the ulnar groove increases the discomfort. Hand strength is lost, and there is wasting of the intrinsic muscles. Sensation over the little finger and the adjacent side of the ring finger is diminished or absent.

Diagnosis. Precise localization of the injury along the course of the nerve is readily accomplished by electrophysiologic techniques.

Treatment. Minor pressure injuries do not require treatment, and recovery is complete within a few weeks. For injuries to the elbow causing fracture or nerve dislocation, surgical intervention is frequently needed.

Peroneal Neuropathy

The peroneal nerve lies in a superficial position adjacent to the fibula and is readily compressed against the bone by external force. This most often occurs in people who have undergone significant weight loss (Jones, 1986; Sotaniemi, 1984). Such individuals have a mild dietary polyneuropathy, and the peroneal nerve is selectively injured by the pressure of crossing the legs while sitting.

Clinical Features. The prominent feature is a painless footdrop. There is weakness both of dorsiflexion and eversion of the foot. Sensation is usually intact, but sometimes there is numbness over the lower lateral leg and dorsum of the foot. When only the deep branch of the peroneal nerve is involved, sensory loss is restricted to a small triangle between the first two toes.

Diagnosis. Electrodiagnosis is useful in discriminating peroneal nerve lesions from disturbances of the fifth lumbar root.

Treatment. A footdrop brace is a useful aid to walking until recovery is complete.

Hereditary Recurrent Pressure Palsy

Transmitted by autosomal dominant inheritance, hereditary recurrent pressure palsy is characterized by the development of a mononeuropathy following trivial trauma (Attal et al, 1975; Roos and Thygesen, 1972). At times, the brachial plexus may be affected (Bosch et al, 1980).

Clinical Features. The first episode usually occurs during the second or third decade. Typical precipitating factors include sleeping on a limb, body contact in sports, constrictive clothing, or positioning during surgery. Individuals quickly learn to avoid provocative activities. Superficial nerves (radial, ulnar, median, peroneal) are the ones most commonly affected. The resulting mononeuropathy is painless and affects both motor and sensory fibers. Tendon reflexes are lost. Recovery is complete in a period of days to weeks.

Diagnosis. Except for the positive family history, the first episode might suggest an ordinary pressure palsy, although the trivial nature of the trauma should alert the physician to the underlying neuropathy.

Electrophysiologic studies demonstrate slow conduction time, not only in the affected limb but in all limbs. Generalized slowing of conduction can be demonstrated in other family members between attacks.

Treatment. Treatment is not available for the underlying neuropathy. Lifestyle may need to be altered to avoid pressure palsies. Acute episodes should be treated with physical therapy. In some patients, a generalized motor and sensory neuropathy eventually develops.

References

1. Attal C, Robain O, Chaouis G: Familial nerve trunk paralyses. Dev Med Child Neurol 17:787, 1975.
2. Beghi E, Kurland LT, Mulder DW, et al: Brachial plexus neuropathy in the population of Rochester, Minnesota, 1970–1981. Ann Neurol 18:320, 1985.
3. Bosch EP, Chui HC, Martin MA, et al: Brachial plexus involvement in familial pressure-sensitive neuropathy: Electrophysiological and morphological findings. Ann Neurol 8:620, 1980.
4. Bradley WG, Madrid R, Thrush DC, et al: Recurrent brachial plexus neuropathy. Brain 98:381, 1975.
5. Charles LM, Jayam-Trouth A: Brachial plexus neuropathy. Three cases in children. Am J Dis Child 134:299, 1980.
6. Clay SA: Osteomyelitis as a cause of brachial plexus neuropathy. Am J Dis Child 136:1054, 1982.
7. Dunn HG, Daube JR, Gomez MR: Heredofamilial brachial plexus neuropathy (hereditary neuralgic amyotrophy with brachial predilection) in childhood. Dev Med Child Neurol 20:28, 1978.
8. Eng GD: Brachial plexus palsy in newborn infants. Pediatrics 48:18, 1971.
9. Evans BA, Stevens C, Dyck PJ: Lumbosacral plexus neuropathy. Neurology 31:1327, 1981.
10. Geiger LR, Mancall EL, Penn AS, et al: Familial neuralgic amyotrophy—Report of three families with review of the literature. Brain 97:87, 1974.
11. Hardy AE: Birth injuries of the brachial plexus: Incidence and prognosis. J Bone Joint Surg 63B:98, 1981.
12. Jones HR: Compressive neuropathy in childhood: A report of 14 cases. Muscle Nerve 9:720, 1986.
13. Masson JI, Thong YH: Immunological abnormalities in the syndrome of poliomyelitis-like illness associated with acute bronchial asthma (Hopkins' syndrome). Arch Dis Child 55:26, 1980.
14. Nihei K, Naitoh H, Ikeda K: Poliomyelitis-like syndrome following asthmatic attack (Hopkins syndrome). Pediatr Neurol 3:166, 1987.
15. Painter MJ, Bergman I: Obstetrical trauma to the neonatal central and peripheral nervous system. Semin Perinatol 6:89, 1973.
16. Roos D, Thygesen P: Familial recurrent polyneuropathy. Brain 95:235, 1972.
17. Sander JE, Sharp FR: Lumbosacral plexus neuritis. Neurology 31:470, 1981.
18. Sotaniemi KA: Slimmer's paralysis-peroneal neuropathy during weight reduction. J Neurol Neurosurg Psychiatry 47:564, 1984.
19. Trojaborg W: Rate of recovery in motor and sensory fibres of the radial nerve: clinical and electrophysiological aspects. J Neurol Neurosurg Psychiatry 33:625, 1970.
20. Trojaborg W: Electrophysiological findings in pressure palsy of the brachial plexus. J Neurol Neurosurg Psychiatry 40:1160, 1977.
21. Tsairis P, Dyck PJ, Mulder DW: Natural history of brachial plexus neuropathy. Report on 99 patients. Arch Neurol 27:109, 1972.
22. Wanamaker WM: Firearm recoil palsy. Arch Neurol 31:208, 1974.
23. Wynn-Parry CB: Pain in avulsion lesions of the brachial plexus. Pain 9:41, 1980.

14 Movement Disorders

Involuntary movements are usually associated with abnormalities of the basal ganglia and their connections and may occur in a variety of neurologic conditions. Abnormal movements can be the major or presenting feature of disease, or they can occur as a late manifestation. The former type is discussed in this chapter, and the latter type is discussed in several other chapters of the text.

■ Approach to the Patient

There is no substitute for observing the patient. Movement disorders cannot be adequately described; they must be seen. If abnormal movements are not present at the time of examination, instruct the parents to videotape the movements at home. Some relatively common movements are recognizable by description, but the rich variety of abnormal movements and postures that may occur defy classification. The most experienced observer will at times mistake one movement for another or will have difficulty conceptualizing the nature of an abnormal movement.

Many abnormal movements are paroxysmal or at least intermittent. In such cases, the possibility of epilepsy is frequently an issue. Indeed, many neurologic disorders of childhood are characterized by the concurrent presence of seizures and involuntary movements. The clinical and conceptual distinction between spinal myoclonus and spinal seizures remains a gray area. There are no absolute rules to distinguish involuntary movements from seizures, but in general the following apply: (1) involuntary movements disappear during sleep and seizures persist or may worsen; (2) involuntary movements have a more stereotyped appearance and

are more persistent than seizures; (3) seizures are often characterized by loss of consciousness or awareness, and involuntary movements are not; (4) seizures are accompanied by epileptiform activity on electroencephalogram (EEG), and involuntary movements are not.

Involuntary contraction of a muscle that does not move a joint may be a fasciculation, a focal seizure, or myoclonus. Low-amplitude jerking movements that move a joint or muscles may be focal seizures, chorea, myoclonus, tics, or hemifacial spasms. High-amplitude jerking movements that move a limb or limbs may be seizures, ballismus, or myoclonus. Slow, writhing movements and abnormal posturing may be due to athetosis, dystonia, continuous motor unit activity, or seizures. Rhythmic movements may be caused by tremors, seizures, or myoclonus.

■ Chorea and Athetosis

Chorea is a rapid jerk affecting any part of the body and may be incorporated into a voluntary movement to hide the jerk. The movements are repetitive, but are neither rhythmic nor stereotyped, and migrate from side to side and limb to limb. Because the involuntary movement flows into a voluntary movement, it gives the appearance of constant movement ("restlessness"). Depending upon the condition, chorea may be unilateral or bilateral and may affect the face and trunk as well as the limbs.

Chorea is more readily observed when separated from the superimposed voluntary movement that follows. This is achieved by asking the child to raise both hands upward beside the head with palms facing each other. Low-amplitude jerking movements that turn the arm into pronation are observed. When the child is asked to lightly grip the examiner's fingers, the grip alternately tightens and loosens, as if the patient is "milking" the examiner's hands. Hypotonia is common in many conditions causing chorea. Tendon reflexes may be normoreactive, but at times a choreic jerk occurs during the patellar response, producing an extra kick.

Athetosis is a slow, writhing movement of the limbs that may occur alone but is often associated with chorea (choreoathetosis). Athetosis without chorea is almost always due to perinatal brain injury. Kernicterus was the major cause, but perinatal asphyxia is now predominant. Many such children have atonic cerebral palsy and others have spastic diplegia.

Ballismus is a high-amplitude, violent flinging of a limb from the shoulder or pelvis. In adults, it may occur in limbs contralateral to a vascular lesion in the subthalamic nucleus; in children, it is almost always associated with chorea.

Tardive dyskinesia is a complex syndrome characterized by buccolingual masticatory movements that include tongue protrusion, lip smacking, puckering, and chewing. Its occurrence in children is always related to the use of psychotropic drugs. It may be considered a subtype of chorea, or at least a related disorder, and is sometimes associated with choreic movements of the limbs.

The differential diagnosis of chorea and cho-

Table 14.1 DIFFERENTIAL DIAGNOSIS OF CHOREA AS PRESENTING OR PROMINENT SYMPTOM

Genetic Disorders
1. Abetalipoproteinemia (see Chapter 10)
2. Ataxia-telangiectasia (see Chapter 10)
3. Benign familial chorea
4. Fahr disease
5. Familial paroxysmal choreoathetosis (see Chapter 1)
6. Hallervorden-Spatz disease
7. Hepatolenticular degeneration (Wilson disease)
8. Huntington disease (see Chapter 5)
9. Infantile bilateral striatal necrosis
10. Lesch-Nyhan syndrome (see Chapter 5)
11. Machado-Joseph disease (see Chapter 5)

Drug-Induced Movement Disorders
1. Anticonvulsants
2. Antiemetics
3. Oral contraceptives
4. Psychotropic agents
5. Stimulants

Systemic Disorders
1. Hyperthyroidism
2. Lupus erythematosus
3. Pregnancy (chorea gravidarum)
4. Sydenham (rheumatic) chorea

Tumors of Cerebral Hemisphere (see Chapter 4)

Table 14.2 CONDITIONS THAT MAY INCLUDE CHOREOATHETOSIS

Cerebral Palsy
1. Congenital malformations (see Chapters 5 and 18)
2. Kernicterus (see Chapter 1)
3. Perinatal asphyxia (see Chapter 1)
4. Unknown causes

Genetic Disorders
1. Ceroid lipofuscinosis (see Chapter 5)
2. Dystonia musculorum deformans
3. Incontinentia pigmenti (see Chapter 1)
4. Phenylketonuria (see Chapter 5)
5. Porphyria (see Chapter 7)
6. Pelizaeus-Merzbacher disease (see Chapter 5)
7. Rett syndrome (see Chapter 5)

Infectious Diseases
1. Bacterial meningitis (see Chapter 4)
2. Viral encephalitis (see Chapter 2)

Metabolic Encephalopathies (see Chapter 2)
1. Addison disease
2. Burn encephalopathy
3. Hypocalcemia
4. Hypernatremia
5. Hypoparathyroidism
6. Vitamin B_{12} deficiency

Vascular—Poststroke (Chapter 11)

reoathetosis is summarized in Tables 14.1 and 14.2. Chorea is a cardinal feature of the conditions listed in Table 14.1. Nevertheless, many are detailed elsewhere in the text because other concurrent features are more prominent. Familial paroxysmal choreoathetosis is described in Chapter 1, although abnormal movements are the only manifestation, because it is more likely to be confused with epilepsy than with other causes of chorea.

Table 14.2 contains a partial list of conditions in which chorea and choreoathetosis may occur, but in which they are are either late manifestations or at least not prominent in disease presentation. Movement disorders are relatively common in many progressive cerebral degenerations and are an expected part of the devastating illness. In contrast, chorea may be misinterpreted as seizures when it develops during acute illnesses such as bacterial meningitis (Burnstein and Breningstall, 1986), metabolic encephalopathies, or encephalitis. At times, the movement disorder is due to the underlying brain disorder and at times to drugs used in treatment.

GENETIC DISORDERS

Abetalipoproteinemia and ataxia-telangiectasia ordinarily present with cerebellar ataxia. Chorea may be present as well in both conditions, but only in ataxia-telangiectasia may chorea occur without ataxia. Huntington disease is an important cause of chorea and dystonia and is dealt with in most texts as a movement disorder. However, the presenting sign of the childhood form of Huntington disease is usually declining school performance and is therefore discussed in Chapter 5.

Benign Familial Chorea

This is a rare disorder transmitted by autosomal dominant inheritance (Chun et al, 1973).

Clinical Features. The onset of chorea is always in early childhood. Some children demonstrate delayed motor development; other associated symptoms may include intention tremor, dysarthria, hypotonia, and athetosis. Most children have only chorea, which becomes less pronounced by adolescence. Adults may be asymptomatic or may have mild hypotonia and ataxia.

Diagnosis. This syndrome may be difficult to distinguish from other causes of chorea in children, especially familial paroxysmal chorea. A positive family history is critical to diagnosis but can be overlooked because of incomplete expression in parents. Chorea is continuous and not episodic or paroxysmal. Computerized tomography (CT) and EEG results are both normal.

Treatment. Tetrabenazine or haloperidol should be tried and are beneficial in some individuals.

Fahr Syndrome

Progressive calcification of the basal ganglia is termed Fahr syndrome. It may be familial or sporadic. Familial cases are transmitted by autosomal recessive or autosomal dominant inheritance (Smits et al, 1983). Dominant inheritance is associated with hypoparathyroidism or pseudohypoparathyroidism. Some sporadic cases probably represent autosomal recessive inheritance and others are secondary to systemic disease.

Clinical Features. Onset may be anytime from childhood to adult life but is consistent within a family. It is likely that disorders occurring before age ten are different from those that occur in adulthood. Affected children may have a Cockayne syndrome phenotype (see Chapter 16): dwarfism, senile appearance, and retinitis pigmentosa. Mental deterioration and cho-

reoathetosis are constant features. Ataxia, dysarthria, spasticity, and seizures are variable. Progressive neurologic deterioration results in early disability and death.

Diagnosis. Plain radiographs of the skull demonstrate bilateral calcification in the region of the basal ganglia that can be localized more precisely by CT. Calcification appears first in the dentate nuclei and pons, then in the basal ganglia, and finally in the corpus callosum. Parathyroid function must be assessed in every child with basal ganglia calcification to exclude the possibility of either hyperparathyroidism or pseudohypoparathyroidism.

Treatment. Treatment is not available except in cases of parathyroid dysfunction.

Infantile Bilateral Striatal Necrosis

This disorder may present in infancy or early childhood, and familial cases are thought to be transmitted by autosomal recessive inheritance (Mito et al, 1986).

Clinical Features. Three clinical syndromes are described: (1) acute infantile, (2) gradual infantile, and (3) childhood. Several different genetic disorders probably share a common pathologic identity. Symptoms may first appear following a febrile illness characterized by nausea and vomiting. Encephalitis is frequently suspected in infants with an acute onset of symptoms. Neurologic disturbances include nystagmus, choreoathetosis, and seizures. There is marked developmental delay, progressive spasticity, a decline to a vegetative state, and death.

Patients with onset after age three are less likely to have familial transmission and the disorder may not be genetic in origin. Some cases are suspected to be "postinfectious," but a cause-and-effect relationship with a toxic or infectious cause has not been established.

Diagnosis. Diagnosis can only be suspected antemortem; pathologic confirmation is required. Postmortem examination reveals diffuse but patchy neuronal loss and marked gliosis in the striatum and globus pallidus.

Treatment. Treatment is not available.

Hallervorden-Spatz Disease

This rare disorder is transmitted by autosomal dominant inheritance.

Clinical Features. Onset of symptoms is towards the end of the first decade. The prominent features are choreoathetosis, dystonia, rigidity, and retinitis pigmentosa. Dystonia may be more prominent than chorea. Mental deterioration and spasticity follow, with progression to spastic immobility and death within five to ten years.

Diagnosis. Antemortem diagnosis is primarily based on the clinical presentation and is difficult to establish in the absence of a positive family history. The CT and EEG are normal early in the course. At onset, Hallervorden-Spatz disease may be difficult to distinguish from dystonia musculorum deformans, but the later development of mental deterioration and retinitis pigmentosa is diagnostic of Hallervorden-Spatz disease and is not expected in dystonia musculorum deformans.

Postmortem examination reveals degeneration of the pallidum and substantia nigra with deposition of iron-containing material.

Treatment. Levodopa is useful to reduce symptoms in some patients, but not in others. Agents that chelate iron have not proved effective. In two siblings, benztropine, 2 mg twice daily, was found to produce a dramatic remission that persisted during two years of observation (Torch and Humphreys, 1986).

DRUG-INDUCED CHOREA

Choreiform movements and akathisia (restlessness) or dystonic posturing may occur as untoward effects of drugs (Table 14.3). Chorea and akathisia are more likely to be dose-related effects and dystonia an idiosyncratic reaction (see "Dystonia"). Phenytoin and ethosuximide may induce chorea as a toxic or idiosyncratic manifestation. Phenothiazines and haloperidol are associated with idiosyncratic dystonic reactions and tardive dyskinesia, and stimulant drugs (dextroamphetamine and methylphenidate) are associated with chorea, akathisia, and tic (see "Tic and Tourette Syndrome").

Tardive Dyskinesia

The term dyskinesia is used to describe drug-induced choreiform movements. These movements are often limited to the lingual-facial-buccal muscles and appear late (tardive) in the course of drug therapy. Tardive dyskinesias are most often associated with drugs used to modify behavior (neuroleptics), such as phenothiazines or haloperidol (see "Neuroleptic Malignant Syndrome" in Chapter 8). The incidence is estimated at 1 percent (Silverstein and Johnston, 1985).

Clinical Features. Tardive dyskinesia is a

Table 14.3 GENERIC AND BRAND NAMES OF DRUGS

Generic Name	Brand Name and Manufacturer
Benztropine	Cogentin (Merck, Sharp and Dohme)
Carbamazepine	Tegretol (Geigy)
Clonazepam	Klonipin (Roche)
Clonidine	Catapres (Boehringer Ingelheim)
Dextroamphetamine	Dexedrine (Smith, Kline and French)
Diazepam	Valium (Roche)
Haloperidol	Haldol (McNeil)
Methylphenidate	Ritalin (CIBA)
Metoclopramide	Reglan (Robins)
Phenothiazines	
Chlorpromazine	Chlorpromazine
Fluphenazine	Permitil (Schering) Prolixin (Squibb)
Thioridazine	Mellaril (Sandoz)
Pimozide	Orap (McNeil)
Primidone	Mysoline (Ayerst)
Tetrabenazine	Nitoman (Roche)*
Trihexyphenidyl	Artane (Lederle)
Valproic acid	Depakene (Abbott)

*Not available in the United States.

complex of stereotyped movements. It usually affects the mouth and face, resembles chewing, and includes tongue protrusion and lip smacking; the trunk may be involved in rocking movements and the fingers in alternating flexion and extension resembling piano playing. Limb chorea, dystonia, myoclonus, tics, and facial grimacing may be associated. These movements are exacerbated by stress and relieved by sleep.

The onset of symptoms is anytime from months to years after initiating therapy and is not related to changes in dose. In children, the movements usually cease when the drug is discontinued, but they may remain unchanged in adults.

Diagnosis. Drug-induced dyskinesia should be suspected in any child who develops abnormal movements of the face or limbs while taking neuroleptic drugs. It is important to distinguish tardive dyskinesia from facial mannerisms that occur in children with schizophrenia.

Treatment. The risk of tardive dyskinesia in children may be reduced by intermittent interruption of therapy or scheduled exchange of drugs (Singer, 1986). All neuroleptic drugs should be discontinued as quickly as possible after symptoms of dyskinesia develop. This may not be possible when drugs are needed to treat psychosis. In such circumstances, the movements sometimes respond to reserpine or diazepam.

Emergent Withdrawal Syndrome

Chorea and myoclonus may appear for the first time after neuroleptic drugs are abruptly discontinued or greatly reduced in dose (Gualtieri et al, 1984). Lingual-facial-buccal dyskinesia may be present as well. The symptoms are self-limited and cease in weeks to months.

SYSTEMIC DISORDERS

Hyperthyroidism

The ocular manifestations of thyrotoxicosis are discussed in Chapter 15. Tremor is the most common associated movement disorder. Chorea is unusual, but when present it may affect the face, limbs, and trunk (Swanson et al, 1981). The movements cease when the child becomes euthyroid.

Lupus Erythematosus

Clinical Features. Lupus-associated chorea is uncommon but may be the first manifestation of disease (Groothuis et al, 1977). The time of onset of chorea is variable, ranging from seven years before to three years after the appearance of systemic features. It is indistinguishable from Sydenham chorea in appearance. Average duration is twelve weeks, but a quarter of patients will suffer recurrence. Additional neurologic manifestations of lupus (ataxia, psychosis, seizures) are common in children who manifest chorea, but occur only after the appearance of systemic symptoms. Therefore, chorea may be a solitary manifestation of disease.

Diagnosis. Diagnosis is clear in children with known lupus erythematosus. When chorea is an initial manifestation of lupus, it must be differentiated from Sydenham chorea. Obtaining an erythrocyte sedimentation rate is helpful for screening. It will be elevated in 85 percent of children with lupus-associated chorea and in only 30 percent of children with Sydenham chorea. An elevated antistreptolysin O titer is often observed in both conditions and not discriminatory. The presence of elevated titers of antinuclear antibodies is critical to diagnosis.

Treatment. Children with neurologic manifestations of lupus erythematosus should be treated with high doses of corticosteroids. The overall outcome is poor.

Pregnancy (Chorea Gravidarum)

Chorea should not be accepted as a complication of pregnancy. More likely, pregnancy has added one more stress to an underlying condition. The major considerations are an initial attack or recurrence of Sydenham chorea and lupus erythematosus.

Sydenham (Rheumatic) Chorea

Sydenham chorea had been the most common form of acquired chorea in children. Its incidence in the United States is now greatly diminished and is second to drug-induced chorea. Sydenham chorea is a cardinal manifestation of rheumatic fever and occurs primarily in populations with untreated streptococcal infections.

Clinical Features. The onset is frequently insidious and diagnosis is often delayed. Chorea, emotional lability, and hypotonia are cardinal features. Difficulty in school may first bring the child to medical attention. Chorea causes the child to be restless and discipline by the teacher results in emotional excess. The change in behavior is often thought to be a sign of mental illness.

Examination reveals a fidgeting child with migratory chorea of limbs and face. The limbs of only one side may be affected initially, but it eventually becomes generalized in most patients. Efforts to conceal chorea with voluntary movement only add to the appearance of restlessness.

Gradual improvement occurs over several months. Most patients recover completely, but some have persistent behavioral disturbances (Bird et al, 1976). One third of untreated patients develop rheumatic valvular heart disease (Aron et al, 1965).

Diagnosis. The differential diagnosis is mainly between Sydenham chorea and lupus-associated chorea. They are difficult to distinguish on clinical grounds alone.

An EEG is usually abnormal and is consistent with a generalized encephalopathy. The posterior rhythm is slow, and epileptiform activity is sometimes recorded (Ch'ien et al, 1978). Despite the high frequency of EEG abnormalities, clinical seizures are rare.

Treatment. The acute neurologic symptoms are treated with sedatives. Diazepam is generally favored over phenobarbital, phenothiazines, or haloperidol. Every child with Sydenham chorea must be treated as if they had acute rheumatic fever: high-dose penicillin for ten days to eradicate active streptococcal infection and lifelong prophylactic penicillin therapy.

■ Dystonia

Dystonia is a disturbance of posture caused by simultaneous contracture of agonist and antagonist muscles. The posturing is initiated by involuntary movement in the limbs, face, or trunk; the movement has a writhing quality. However, the overall appearance is not of an involuntary movement disorder, but rather of an abnormal posture of the limbs or trunk and grimacing of the face. There may be involvement of a single body part (focal dystonia), a single limb and contiguous part of the trunk (segmental dystonia), the arm and leg on one side of the body (hemidystonia), or concurrent involvement of limbs and face (generalized dystonia).

The differential diagnosis of abnormal posturing is summarized in Table 14.4. Continuous motor unit activity (Chapter 8) may be difficult to differentiate from dystonia by clinical inspection alone, especially when only one or two limbs are affected. The two disorders are readily differentiated by electromyography (EMG), which is recommended in most cases.

Persistent focal dystonias are relatively common in adults, but are unusual in children except when drug-induced. Most dystonias in children that begin focally will eventually become generalized. Children with focal, stereotyped movements of the eyelids, face, or neck are much more likely to have tic than focal dystonia. Only childhood onset forms of focal dystonia are listed in Table 14.5: the full spectrum includes neck turning (torticollis), eye closure (blepharospasm), face and jaw involvement (Meige syndrome), laryngeal tightening (spasmodic dysphonia), and writer's cramp.

Generalized dystonia usually begins in one limb. There is difficulty in performing an act rather than a movement, so that the foot be-

Table 14.4 DIFFERENTIAL DIAGNOSIS OF ABNORMAL POSTURING

Continuous motor unit activity
Dystonia
Hysteria
Myotonia
Rigidity
Spasticity
Stiffman syndrome

Table 14.5 DIFFERENTIAL DIAGNOSIS OF DYSTONIA IN CHILDHOOD

Generalized Dystonia
1. Drug-induced dystonia
2. Genetic disorders
   a. Ceroid lipofuscinosis (see Chapter 5)
   b. Dystonia musculorum deformans
      (1) Autosomal dominant
      (2) Autosomal recessive
      (3) X-linked
   c. Dystonia-parkinsonism syndrome
      (1) With diurnal variation
      (2) Exercise-induced
   d. Familial paroxysmal choreoathetosis (see Chapter 1)
   e. Hallervorden-Spatz disease (see "Chorea")
   f. Hepatolenticular degeneration (Wilson disease)
   g. Huntington disease (see Chapter 5)
   h. Leber disease (see Chapter 16)
   i. Machado-Joseph disease (see Chapter 10)
3. Symptomatic dystonia
   a. Perinatal cerebral injury (see Chapter 1)
   b. Postinfectious
   c. Poststroke
   d. Post-traumatic
   e. Toxins
   f. Tumor

Focal Dystonia
1. Blepharospasm
2. Drug-induced dystonia
3. Torticollis
4. Writer's cramp

comes dystonic when walking forward but not when sitting, standing, or running.

BLEPHAROSPASM

Blepharospasm is an involuntary spasmodic closure of the eyes (Jankovic et al, 1982). The differential diagnosis for children is summarized in Table 14.6. Essential blepharospasm, an incapacitating focal dystonia, is a disorder of middle or late adult life and never begins in child-

Table 14.6 DIFFERENTIAL DIAGNOSIS OF BLEPHAROSPASM IN CHILDHOOD

Continuous motor unit activity
Drug-induced
Encephalitis
Hemifacial spasm
Hepatolenticular degeneration (Wilson disease)
Huntington disease
Hysteria
Myokymia
Myotonia
Schwartz-Jampel syndrome
Seizures

hood. Tic accounts for almost all cases of involuntary eye closure in children. Eye fluttering occurs during absence seizures (see Chapter 1), but is never confused with dystonia. Focal dystonia involving eye closure in children is almost always drug-induced.

Blepharospasm and orofacial dystonia in adult patients may be helped by treatment with trihexyphenidyl, tetrabenazine, lithium (Jankovic and Ford, 1983), and subcutaneous injections of botulinum A toxin (Jankovic and Orman, 1987).

DRUG-INDUCED DYSTONIA

Focal or generalized dystonia may occur as an idiosyncratic reaction following a first dose of phenothiazine or haloperidol. Possible reactions include trismus, opisthotonos, torticollis, and oculogyric crisis. Difficulty with swallowing and speaking may occur as well. The highest frequency of drug-induced generalized dystonia and oculogyric crisis is in children less than fifteen years of age (Knight and Roberts, 1986).

Dystonia may occur secondary to treatment with neuroleptic drugs (tardive dystonia). Onset varies from three days to eleven years after treatment is initiated. The dystonia is usually generalized in children, but may be focal in adults (Burke et al, 1982). Spontaneous remissions are unusual. Tetrabenazine is helpful in 68 percent of patients, and anticholinergics help in 39 percent.

Metoclopramide, a nonphenothiazine antiemetic that blocks postsynaptic dopamine receptors, may produce acute and tardive dystonic reactions. The acute reactions are usually self-limited or respond to treatment with benztropine, but they may be prolonged and resistant to therapy (Leopold, 1984).

GENETIC DYSTONIA

Dystonia Musculorum Deformans

This term encompasses several genetic disorders characterized by generalized dystonia without other symptoms of neurologic deterioration. *Primary torsion dystonia* is a preferred term because dystonia is not always deforming and is not a disease of muscle (Fahn et al, 1987). The condition can be divided into the following groups: (1) an autosomal dominant form in Ashkenazi Jews, (2) an autosomal recessive form that occurs in Jewish and non-Jewish popula-

tions, (3) a sex-linked form with adult onset in natives of the Philippines, and (4) sporadic cases. The autosomal recessive form occurring in Jewish and non-Jewish populations and the sporadic cases may be the same.

Clinical Features. Onset of dystonia is often between the ages of six and fourteen, but may be anytime after infancy. The limbs are usually affected before the trunk.

Forty-three percent of cases present with dystonia of the hands or arm and 36 percent present with gait abnormalities (Marsden and Harrison, 1974). Leg involvement as an initial feature is more common in children than adults. Despite the focal features at onset, dystonia always becomes generalized in children, affecting the limbs and trunk. Spontaneous remission is unusual, and complete disability is expected in untreated cases.

Other clinical features include dysarthria, orofacial movements, dysphagia, postural tremor, and blepharospasm. Mental deterioration does not occur.

Diagnosis. Diagnosis depends upon the clinical features of (1) dystonic movements and postures, (2) normal perinatal history, (3) no exposure to drugs, (4) no evidence of intellectual or corticospinal deterioration, and (5) no demonstrable biochemical disorder.

Treatment. Trihexyphenidyl is an effective agent in the treatment of dystonia musculorum deformans (Fahn, 1983). High dosages are required, usually 30 mg/day in three divided doses. Daily doses as high as 80 mg/day are sometimes required. Such high dosages can be tolerated in children if built up slowly, but are rarely tolerated by adults. The response cannot be predicted from measurement of plasma concentrations (Burke and Fahn, 1985).

If trihexyphenidyl is not effective, diazepam should be added at low dosages and slowly increased as tolerated. Patients who do not respond to this combination may be tried on some combination of carbamazepine, levodopa, benztropine, tetrabenazine, pimozide, or bromocriptine (Gautier and Awada, 1983).

Dystonia-Parkinsonism Syndrome

Some cases of this syndrome are described as autosomal dominant with incomplete penetrance and others as autosomal recessive. There may be genetic heterogeneity, or all cases may actually be autosomal dominant with incomplete penetrance (Nygaard and Duvoison, 1986). Most cases of "juvenile parkinsonism" with onset in childhood probably belong to this group (Lima et al, 1987).

Clinical Features. Age at onset is usually between four and eight years, but may be as early as sixteen months. The initial feature is nearly always a gait disturbance due to leg dystonia. There is flexion at the hip and knee with plantar flexion of the foot causing toe-walking. Both flexor and extensor posturing of the arms develops, and finally there is the appearance of parkinsonian features: cogwheel rigidity, mask-like facies, and bradykinesia. Postural or intention tremor occurs in almost half of patients, but typical parkinsonian tremor is unusual.

Diurnal fluctuation in symptoms occurs in more than half of patients. Symptoms are considerably improved upon awakening and become worse later in the day. Movement and exercise exacerbate dystonia in some patients and it is not clear if other disorders with exercise-induced dystonia as the major or solitary feature are expressions of the same genetic error (Plant et al, 1984).

Diagnosis. This syndrome may be difficult to separate from other genetic disorders with dystonia because of phenotypic variation among family members. An effort should be made to personally examine as many close relatives as possible. Important clues to diagnosis are features of parkinsonism without other neurologic signs, diurnal variation in severity of symptoms, exacerbation of symptoms with exercise, and response to levodopa.

Treatment. A small dose of levodopa provides immediate and complete relief in most patients, even when treatment is initiated after a long delay following onset of symptoms. No other dystonia responds as well. An initial dose of 10 mg/kg should be followed by 10 mg/kg increments as needed. Most patients require less than 1 g and none require more than 3 g. Long-term therapy is required, as symptoms return when drug is discontinued.

Trihexyphenidyl, in doses lower than ordinarily needed to treat dystonia musculorum deformans, and bromocriptine are also effective.

Hepatolenticular Degeneration
(Wilson Disease)

This disorder is transmitted by autosomal recessive inheritance. It is caused by a disturbance in the biliary excretion of copper and its incorporation into ceruloplasmin. The defective gene is located on chromosome 13. Symptoms are secondary to the accumulation of copper in liver, brain, and cornea.

Clinical Features. Hepatic failure is the prominent clinical feature in children less than ten years of age, usually without neurologic symptoms or signs. Neurologic manifestations with only minimal liver disease are more likely when the onset of symptoms is in the second decade. A single symptom, such as a disturbance of gait or speech, is often the initial feature and may remain unchanged for years (Sternlieb et al, 1987). Eventually the initial symptom worsens and new features develop: dysarthria (97 percent), dystonia (65 percent), dysdiadochokinesia (58 percent), rigidity (52 percent), gait and postural abnormalities (42 percent), tremor (32 percent), and drooling (23 percent) (Starosta-Rubinstein et al, 1987).

Dystonia of bulbar muscles is responsible for three prominent features of the disease: (1) dysarthria, (2) a fixed pseudo-smile (risus sardonicus), and (3) a high-pitched whining noise on inspiration.

Psychiatric disturbances may precede the neurologic abnormalities in 20 percent of cases. They may range from behavioral disturbances to paranoid psychoses. Dementia is not an early feature of disease.

The Kayser-Fleischer ring, a yellow-brown granular deposit at the limbus of the cornea, is a hallmark of the disease. It is caused by copper deposition in the Descemet membrane and is present in all patients with neurologic manifestations, but may be absent in children with liver disease alone.

Diagnosis. Hepatolenticular degeneration should be considered in any child with dysarthria and dystonia. The further association of chronic liver disease increases the probability of hepatolenticular degeneration. The diagnosis is confirmed by demonstrating an increased copper content by liver biopsy or by the demonstration of a Kayser-Fleischer ring by slit-lamp examination. Ninety-six percent of patients will have a serum ceruloplasmin concentration of less than 20 mg/dl, corresponding to less than 56 µg/dl of ceruloplasmin copper (Sternlieb et al, 1987).

Magnetic resonance imaging demonstrates increased signal intensity and decreased size of the caudate, putamen, subcortical white matter, midbrain, and pons. Dystonia and bradykinesia correlate with lesions in the putamen, and dysarthria correlates with lesions of the putamen and caudate.

Treatment. The treatment of choice is the oral administration of D-penicillamine, 250 mg four times a day, for children more than ten years of age and half as much for children less than ten. Penicillamine must always be given on an empty stomach together with a daily dose of 25 mg pyridoxine. Twenty-four hour urinary copper secretion is then monitored and the dose is adjusted to produce urinary excretion of copper at a rate of 2 mg/day during the first year. Later, an excretion of 1 mg/day is considered satisfactory. Improvement is slow and several months are frequently necessary for recovery of neurologic function. Worsening may occur during the first months of therapy, but this should not be a cause for alarm. When treatment is started early, the results are quite satisfactory without excess morbidity and mortality.

Discontinuation of penicillamine results in rapid clinical deterioration, which may prove fatal (Scheinberg et al, 1987). The replacement of penicillamine with trientine, a new chelating agent, prevents the adverse course associated with penicillamine withdrawal.

Siblings of patients with Wilson disease should be carefully screened for disease and treated as early as possible (Strickland and Leu, 1975).

SYMPTOMATIC DYSTONIA

Dystonia may be caused by an underlying tumor or an active encephalopathy (hypoxic, infectious, metabolic) or from prior brain damage resulting from encephalopathy, trauma, or stroke.

Clinical Features. The onset of dystonia may be at the time of an acute encephalopathy, after the acute phase is over, or several years later when the encephalopathy is thought to be static (Burke et al, 1980). Delayed-onset chorea and dystonia in children with perinatal disturbances such as asphyxia or kernicterus usually begin by age two or three, but may be delayed for fourteen years. Once involuntary movements appear, they tend to become progressively severe⁻ but intellectual decline is not associated. Delayed-onset dystonia is usually generalized.

Hemidystonia most often occurs after stroke or head injury, but may be symptomatic of neuronal storage diseases or tumors of the basal ganglia (Narbona et al, 1984; Pettigrew and Jankovic, 1985). The dystonic limbs are contralateral to the damaged basal ganglia.

Diagnosis. Children with a known predisposing cause for the development of dystonia or chorea need not be studied extensively. The new symptoms are discouraging for patients and families who have adjusted to a fixed neurologic

deficit. They may be assured that this is not evidence of new degeneration in the brain, but only the appearance of new symptoms from old lesions. This sequence is most likely when injury is perinatal and brain maturation is required to manifest involuntary movements.

The appearance of hemidystonia, even when the predisposing event is known, requires CT scanning to look for localized changes that may require treatment, such as an expanding cyst. The possibility of tumor must be considered in children who had previously been neurologically intact.

Treatment. The treatment of symptomatic dystonia is no different from that of genetic dystonia. The same drugs are used, but the results may not be as favorable.

TORTICOLLIS

The differential diagnoses of torticollis and head tilt are summarized in Table 14.7. The first step in diagnosis is to separate fixed from non-fixed torticollis. In fixed torticollis, the neck cannot be readily moved back to the neutral position. This may be due to structural disturbance of cervical vertebrae, but more often the patient experiences pain and resists movement.

If there is also evidence of dystonia in the face or limbs, further evaluation should be directed at underlying causes of dystonia. Torticollis associated with hyperactive tendon reflexes, ankle clonus, or extensor plantar responses suggests a cervical spinal cord disturbance and is an indication for radiographs of the cervical vertebrae and magnetic resonance imaging (MRI) of the cervical portion of the spine (Fig. 12.2). Signs or symptoms of increased intracranial pressure indicate a posterior fossa tumor with early herniation. When torticollis is the only abnormal feature, the underly-

Table 14.7 DIFFERENTIAL DIAGNOSIS OF TORTICOLLIS AND HEAD TILT

Benign paroxysmal torticollis
Cervical cord tumors (see Chapter 12)
Cervical cord syringomyelia (see Chapter 12)
Cervicomedullary malformations (see Chapter 18)
Diplopia (see Chapter 15)
Dystonia
Familial paroxysmal choreoathetosis (see Chapter 1)
Juvenile rheumatoid arthritis
Posterior fossa tumors (see Chapter 10)
Sandifer syndrome
Spasmus nutans (see Chapter 15)
Sternocleidomastoid injuries
Tic and tourette syndrome

ing causes are focal dystonia, injuries to the neck muscles, and juvenile rheumatoid arthritis.

Nonfixed torticollis that occurs in attacks suggests benign paroxysmal torticollis or familial paroxysmal choreoathetosis. The combination of head tilt and nystagmus is termed spasmus nutans (see Chapter 15). Tic produces head turning, but is so spasmodic that it should not be confused with torticollis.

Benign Paroxysmal Torticollis

This is a migraine variant occurring in infants and small children (Deonna and Martin, 1981). It is closely related to benign paroxysmal vertigo (see Chapter 10).

Clinical Features. Onset is always in the first year and is characterized by episodes in which the head is tilted to one side (not always to the same side) and may be slightly rotated. Efforts to return the head to a neutral position may be resisted, but this can be overcome. Some children have no other symptoms, whereas others have pallor, irritability, malaise, and vomiting. Attacks last for minutes to days, end spontaneously, and tend to recur monthly. Children who are old enough to stand and walk become ataxic during attacks.

With time, the attacks may evolve into episodes characteristic of benign paroxysmal vertigo or classic migraine, or may simply cease without further symptoms of any kind. The disorder has been described in siblings, but more often family history is positive only for migraine.

Diagnosis. The disorder should be suspected in any infant with attacks of torticollis that remit spontaneously. A positive family history of migraine is critical to the diagnosis. Familial paroxysmal choreoathetosis and familial paroxysmal dystonia do not begin during early infancy. *Sandifer syndrome*, intermittent torticollis associated with hiatal hernia, is an alternate consideration. I personally doubt that hiatal hernia is a cause of torticollis and suspect that most, if not all, such cases are migraine. The demonstration of reflux in occasional infants is probably coincidental and not symptomatic. The EEG during and after attacks is normal.

Treatment. Treatment is not available or needed for the acute attacks.

WRITER'S CRAMP

Writer's cramp is a focal dystonia that may occur only when writing, when performing other specific manual tasks such as typing or playing the piano (occupational cramp), or with nonspecific use of the hands (Sheehy and Marsden, 1982). It is most often an isolated finding, but may be associated with other focal dystonias, such as torticollis, or with generalized dystonia.

Clinical Features. Onset is almost always after age twenty, but may be in the second decade. Initial features are any of the following: aching in the hand when writing, loss of handwriting neatness or speed, and difficulty in holding a writing implement. All three symptoms are eventually present. Dystonic postures occur when the patient attempts to write. The hand and arm lift from the paper and the fingers extend. An attempt is made to overcome forced finger extension by forced grasping. Writing becomes impossible with the affected hand and the patient learns to write with the nondominant hand.

Symptoms are at first intermittent and are especially severe when writing is observed by others. Later, the cramp becomes a constant feature with each attempt at writing. Some patients have lifelong difficulty with using the dominant hand for writing and may have difficulty with other manual tasks as well. Others experience remissions and exacerbations, and a minority of patients develop generalized dystonia.

Diagnosis. It is an unfortunate fact that most people with writer's or occupational cramp are thought to have psychiatric illness despite the lack of associated psychopathologic features. Early diagnosis can save considerable expense and concern. Isolated focal dystonia must be distinguished from generalized dystonia with focal onset. Family history should be explored thoroughly and examination repeated to determine the presence of dystonia in other body parts.

Treatment. The same medications used to treat generalized dystonia should be used in patients with focal dystonia (see "Dystonia Musculorum Deformans").

■ Hemifacial Spasm

Hemifacial spasm is characterized by involuntary, irregular contraction of the muscles innervated by one facial nerve. It is very rare in children (Ronen et al, 1986). The spasms may develop because of aberrant regeneration following facial nerve injury, secondary to posterior fossa tumor, or without apparent cause.

Clinical Features. Spasms are embarrassing and disturbing but not painful. The orbicularis oculi muscles are affected first and most frequently, causing forced closure of the eye. All facial muscles on one side are eventually affected, with pulling of the mouth to one side. Several spasms may occur every minute, especially during times of stress. The subsequent course depends upon the underlying cause.

Diagnosis. Hemifacial spasm in children may be mistaken for a focal seizure. The stereotyped appearance of the spasm and a concurrent normal EEG should differentiate them. Posterior fossa tumor must be suspected in every child with hemifacial spasm. A CT or MRI is always indicated unless symptoms can be explained by a known history of facial nerve injury.

Treatment. Some patients respond to treatment with carbamazepine at anticonvulsant doses (see Chapter 1), but most have no response to medical therapy. Surgical procedures to relieve pressure on the facial nerve from adjacent vessels are of questionable value.

■ Myoclonus

The term myoclonus encompasses several different involuntary movements characterized by rapid muscle jerks. They are less frequent and severe during sleep, but may not disappear completely. Myoclonus may be rhythmic or nonrhythmic; focal, multifocal, or generalized; or spontaneous or activated by movement (action myoclonus) or sensory stimulation (reflex myoclonus).

Nonepileptic myoclonus must be distinguished from tic, chorea, tremor, and seizures. Tics are usually more complex and stereotyped movements than myoclonus and can be briefly suppressed by voluntary effort; myoclonus cannot be suppressed. Chorea is more random than myoclonus and tends to be incorporated into voluntary movement; myoclonus is never part of a larger movement. Rhythmic myoclonus and tremor look very much alike and are distinguished with certainty only by special studies. Tremor is a continuous to-and-fro movement, whereas rhythmic myoclonus is characterized by a pause between movements.

Marsden and associates (1982) proposed an etiologic classification of myoclonus that has proved useful and is summarized in Table 14.8. Physiologic myoclonus occurs in normal people when they fall asleep, during sleep (nocturnal myoclonus), when they wake up, and during times of anxiety. Nocturnal myoclonus is a rhythmic jerking of the legs during sleep and is classified as an essential myoclonus by Marsden

Table 14.8 ETIOLOGIC CLASSIFICATION OF MYOCLONUS

Physiologic
1. Anxiety-induced
2. Exercise-induced
3. Sleep jerks and nocturnal myoclonus

Essential
1. Familial
2. Sporadic

Epileptic (see Chapter 1)

Symptomatic
1. Basal ganglia degenerations
   a. Dystonia musculorum deformans
   b. Hallervorden-Spatz disease
   c. Hepatolenticular degeneration (Wilson disease)
   d. Huntington disease (see Chapter 5)
2. Lysosomal storage diseases (see Chapter 5)
3. Metabolic encephalopathies (see Chapter 2)
   a. Dialysis syndromes
   b. Disorders of osmolality
   c. Hepatic failure
   d. Renal failure
4. Myoclonic encephalopathy (see Chapter 10)
   a. Idiopathic
   b. Neuroblastoma
5. Post–central nervous system injury
   a. Hypoxia (see Chapter 2)
   b. Trauma (see Chapter 2)
   c. Stroke (see Chapter 11)
6. Spinal cord tumor (see Chapter 12)
7. Spinocerebellar degenerations (see Chapter 10)
8. Toxic encephalopathies (see Chapter 2)
9. Viral encephalitis

and associates (1982). I believe it is normal in children and have classified it as a physiologic myoclonus (see Chapter 1). Essential myoclonus is abnormal, but it occurs in people who have no other neurologic abnormality. Epileptic myoclonus is associated with epileptiform activity on the EEG (see Chapter 1). Symptomatic myoclonus follows a cerebral injury or is part of a generalized, and usually progressive, encephalopathy.

ESSENTIAL MYOCLONUS

Essential myoclonus may be sporadic or familial. Familial cases are transmitted by autosomal dominant inheritance.

Clinical Features. Onset is in the first or second decade. Males and females are affected equally. The movements are predominantly in the face, trunk, and proximal muscles. They are usually generalized, but may be restricted to one side of the body. No other neurologic disturbances develop and life span is not affected.

Essential tremor may be present in the same family.

Diagnosis. A positive family history of isolated myoclonus limits the differential diagnosis. Unfortunately, sporadic cases are more common than familial cases. Symptomatic and epileptic myoclonus must be eliminated by careful neurologic examination, an EEG, and a CT scan. Even then, a period of observation and repeat laboratory investigations may be required to eliminate other causes.

Treatment. Mild essential myoclonus may not require treatment. Carbamazepine, clonazepam, tetrabenazine, and valproic acid have been found useful in symptomatic myoclonus and may be useful in generalized myoclonus as well. Benztropine produced complete relief of symptoms in one family and may become the drug of choice (Chokroverty et al, 1987).

SYMPTOMATIC MYOCLONUS

Myoclonus is often a symptom of an underlying neurologic disease. It tends to be generalized when caused by diffuse, progressive encephalopathies (such as lysosomal storage diseases) and segmental when there is a focal lesion of the brainstem or spinal cord.

Posthypoxic Myoclonus (Lance-Adams Syndrome)

This is a form of action myoclonus in patients who have suffered an episode of hypoxia. It does not follow hypoxic-ischemic encephalopathy of the newborn. Single or repetitive myoclonic jerks occur when voluntary movement is attempted. Facial and pharyngeal muscles may be affected, interfering with speech and swallowing. Cerebellar disturbances are usually associated.

Myoclonus usually begins during the phase of recovery from anoxic encephalopathy and is lifelong. It may respond to valproic acid (Rollinson and Gilligan, 1979), 5-hydroxytryptophan, or clonazepam (Chadwick et al, 1977).

Segmental (Focal) Myoclonus

Segmental myoclonus is an involuntary contraction of contiguous muscles innervated by the brainstem or spinal cord. It may be rhythmic or nonrhythmic. Rhythmic segmental myoclonus looks like a focal seizure. The underlying causes in children are limited mainly to demyelinating diseases and intrinsic tumors.

Palatal myoclonus is the most frequent segmental myoclonus of brainstem origin. Cystic astrocytoma of the spinal cord is the major cause of spinal myoclonus and may be a presenting feature (see Chapter 12).

Palatal myoclonus is a unilateral or bilateral rhythmic contraction of the palate (80 to 180/minute) that usually persists during sleep. It may be associated with rhythmic contractions of the eyes, larynx, neck, diaphragm, trunk, and limbs and results from lesions in the central tegmental tract or dentato-olivary pathways, which produce a denervation hypersensitivity and hypertrophy of the contralateral inferior olivary nucleus (Matsuo and Ajax, 1979). The median interval between the precipitating cause and the onset of palatal myoclonus is ten to eleven months.

Clonazepam and tetrabenazine are the most useful drugs in the treatment of segmental myoclonus (Jankovic and Pardo, 1986).

■ Tic and Tourette Syndrome

Tics or *habit spasms* are complex, stereotyped movements (motor tic) or utterances (verbal tic) that are sudden, brief, and purposeless. They may be confused with chorea, but should be readily distinguished by their stereotyped appearance. Tic is more readily suppressed by voluntary effort than is chorea, and no effort is made to incorporate tic into voluntary movement. Tic and chorea are both exacerbated by stress and disappear during sleep.

Simple Motor Tic

This term is used to describe a mild and transient tic disorder that may occur in up to 10 percent of children (Abe and Oda, 1980). Onset is anytime in childhood, and duration is less than one year. A positive family history is often present, and males are affected more often than females. One or two motor tics are present, but verbal tics are rare. Treatment is not required.

Tourette Syndrome

Tourette syndrome is any combination of verbal and motor tics. It should not be considered a separate disease, but rather part of a phenotypic spectrum that includes simple motor tic and obsessive-compulsive behavior. It is believed to be transmitted as a highly penetrant, sex-influenced (male bias), autosomal dominant trait (Pauls and Leckman, 1986). However, X-linked inheritance cannot be excluded.

Clinical Features. Affected children are not mentally disturbed prior to onset of symptoms. Although behavioral disturbances occur with increased frequency, the movement disorder and the behavioral disturbances should be thought of as an organic encephalopathy, probably caused by an abnormality in the dopaminergic systems.

Onset is anytime from two to fifteen years with the mean between six and seven. Neck muscles are often affected first, causing a head movement in which the child appears to be tossing hair back from the face. A haircut is frequently the first unsuccessful intervention. At this stage, it is impossible to differentiate Tourette syndrome from simple motor tic. New motor tics develop and either replace or are added to existing tics. They usually affect the head, eyes, or face. Common tics include eye blinking, grimacing, lip smacking, and shrugging of one or both shoulders.

The initial verbal tics are either a clearing of the throat or a cough-like noise. Many such children will undergo an extensive evaluation for allergy and will be found to be allergic. Desensitization is then the initial unsuccessful intervention. Other verbal tics include grunting, snorting, sniffing, and hissing. Coprolalia occurs in a minority of cases and is rarely an early or initial symptom. The profanity is quickly suppressed and replaced by barking or coughing noises.

Symptoms wax and wane spontaneously and in response to stress. As a rule, tics become less frequent and severe with time and tend to disappear. Some children have lifelong difficulty, and others have prolonged remissions with recurrence in middle age or later (Klawans and Barr, 1985).

Concomitant disorders in children with tic are attention deficit disorder (54 percent) and obsessive-compulsive states (33 percent) (Comings and Comings, 1985). Attention deficit disorder is characterized by hyperactivity, short attention span, restlessness, poor concentration, and impaired impulse control. This syndrome is often treated with dextroamphetamine or methylphenidate, and there is considerable concern that these drugs may precipitate Tourette syndrome in genetically predisposed children (Erenberg et al, 1985; Lowe et al, 1982).

Obsessive-compulsive behavior is characterized by ritualistic actions and thoughts; these include touching things repeatedly, placing objects in a certain place, washing and rewashing hands, obsessive thoughts about sex or violence, and counting objects.

Diagnosis. Tic and Tourette syndrome is diagnosed by history and observation. Laboratory tests are not helpful and need not be done in obvious cases. The EEG, CT, and psychologic testing results are normal (Lees et al, 1984).

Tics do not ordinarily occur in degenerative diseases of the nervous system or as an adverse reaction to drugs. Drug-induced tics should be considered the potentiation of Tourette syndrome in a genetically predisposed child. Carbamazepine, as well as amphetamine and methylphenidate, may trigger the disorder (Neglia et al, 1984). Withdrawal of the potentiating drug does not always stop the tics (Singer, 1986).

A degenerative disorder that begins as a spinal muscular atrophy during childhood has been described in two brothers of consanguineous parents. Tourette syndrome develops in adult life and is replaced by parkinsonism (Spitz et al, 1985). Acanthocytosis is associated. This is the only degenerative disease that includes Tourette syndrome and the tics are not present in childhood.

Treatment. Most children with tics and Tourette syndrome do not require drug treatment. The "litmus test" for prescribing medication is determining whether the tics bother the child. Drugs should not be used if the tics bother parents or teachers, but do not disturb the child's life. Parents must be told that tics (1) are not a sign of progressive neurologic or mental illness, (2) are made worse by stress, and (3) will diminish if ignored.

Drug treatment is often difficult to evaluate because the natural history of the disorder is one of exacerbation and remission. Haloperidol is the most widely used drug and provides some improvement in 80 percent of cases. Fluphenazine is equally effective and should be used before haloperidol because of a lower frequency of adverse reactions (Goetz et al, 1984; Singer et al, 1986). Clonidine is useful in less than 50 percent of patients and can be tried when fluphenazine and haloperidol fail (Leckman et al, 1985). Any of these drugs may lose their efficacy after prolonged use, but effectiveness may return after discontinued use. Interrupted therapy with one drug or alternating between two drugs is reasonable.

Haloperidol is started as a single dose of 0.5 mg at night and is slowly increased by 0.5 mg each week until tics are reasonably controlled or adverse reactions are noted. The usual maintenance dose is 1 to 3 mg/day in two divided doses. The major adverse toxic reactions are sedation, irritability, and depression of appetite. Dystonia and akathisia are idiosyncratic reactions.

Fluphenazine is started at 1 mg/day and increased 1 mg each week. The usual maintenance dose is 2 to 6 mg/day. Adverse reactions are the same as with haloperidol, but occur less frequently. Clonidine is started at a dose of 0.05 mg/day and is increased 0.05 mg each week. The usual maintenance dose is 0.1 to 0.6 mg/day.

Pimozide is a newer drug that has been used in several hyperkinetic disorders and is now approved for use in Tourette syndrome (Regeur et al, 1986). It is effective in 80 percent of cases, but should not be used as a primary drug because of a high incidence of adverse reactions. The initial dose is 1 mg/day in two divided doses and increased 1 mg each week. The maintenance dose is 0.2 mg/kg/day or 10 mg/day, whichever is less. It may be used in combination with clonidine or tetrabenazine. Adverse reactions are similar to those with haloperidol.

■ Tremor

Tremor is an involuntary oscillating movement with a fixed frequency. Shuddering, cerebellar ataxia or dysmetria, and asterixis are not tremors because they lack rhythm. Myoclonus may be rhythmic but is interrupted between oscillations.

All normal people have a low-amplitude *physiologic tremor* inherent to movement that is not ordinarily observed without instrumentation. Physiologic tremor may be enhanced to clinical awareness by situations (anxiety, excitement, exercise, fatigue, stress) and drugs (adrenergic agonists, nicotine, prednisone, thyroid hormone, xanthines). Hyperthyroidism is routinely associated with enhanced physiologic tremor.

Parkinsonism is a major cause of pathologic tremors in adults, but it does not occur in children except when drug-induced or as part of a complex degenerative disorder. Typical parkinsonian tremor is not usually associated in these situations. Essential (familial) tremor is the major cause of tremor in children.

Essential (Familial) Tremor

This is a monosymptomatic condition probably transmitted as an autosomal dominant trait. Sporadic cases are called essential tremor, and familial cases are called familial tremor. It is likely that they are the same condition with subclinical penetrance in the affected parent. The preva-

lence is 414/100,000 in Mississippi (Haerer et al, 1982), and 24/100,000 in a white Minnesota population (Rajput et al, 1984). Because the prevalence is relatively high in some populations, essential tremor may coexist with another genetic neurologic disturbance, such as hereditary motor-sensory neuropathy. However, the association is probably incidental. There is no evidence that essential tremor is part of a larger neurologic disturbance.

Clinical Features. Essential tremor occurs only in a limb being used (action tremor). The head, face, and neck are sometimes affected. Neck tremor gives the appearance of torticollis. The frequency of essential tremor is typically between 4 and 8 Hz (Findley and Koller, 1987).

Onset of tremor is usually in adult life, but can be as early as two years. Most childhood-onset cases are in adolescence. Essential tremor may impair function, especially school work, and is therefore disturbing to the patient. In young children, the tremor has the appearance of restlessness or clumsiness. Later, it is quickly appreciated as an action tremor.

Tremor is enhanced by greater precision of movement and therefore appears first and most prominently in the hands. It is further enhanced by anxiety, concentrated effort to stop the tremor, and fatigue. In such cases, the worsening of tremor may be due to enhanced physiologic tremor rather than enhanced essential tremor. The distinction is important in considering treatment options.

Essential tremor is generally lifelong.

Diagnosis. Essential tremor in children is often mistaken for cerebellar dysfunction because it occurs with action (intention). The two should be easily separated because essential tremor is rhythmic and not dysmetric (does not become worse at the end point) and is not associated with other signs of cerebellar dysfunction.

The distinction between essential tremor and enhanced physiologic tremor may be more difficult because the two are often concurrent. Enhanced physiologic tremor is always circumstantial, whereas essential tremor remains even when the patient is alone and relaxed.

Treatment. Not all patients with essential tremor require treatment. Medication should be reserved for situations in which tremor impairs function. Propranolol is the drug of choice and a daily regimen of 240 mg/day in adults is effective in controlling high-amplitude tremor but not usually low-amplitude tremor (Calzetti et al, 1987).

Daily use of clonidine, 0.1 to 1 mg/day (Caccia and Mangoni, 1985), and primidone, 250 mg three times each day (Gorman et al, 1986), has also been found useful in controlling essential tremor in adults and should be considered when propranolol fails.

References

1. Abe K, Oda N: Incidence of tics in the offspring of childhood tiquers: a controlled follow-up study. Dev Med Child Neurol 22:649, 1980.
2. Aron AM, Freeman JM, Carter S: The natural history of Sydenham's chorea. Review of the literature and long-term evaluation with emphasis on cardiac sequelae. Am J Med 38:83, 1965.
3. Bird MT, Palkes H, Prensky AL: A follow-up study of Sydenham's chorea. Neurology 26:601, 1976.
4. Burke RE, Fahn S: Pharmacokinetics of trihexyphenidyl after short-term and long-term administration to dystonic patients. Ann Neurol 18:35, 1985.
5. Burke RE, Fahn S, Gold AP: Delayed-onset dystonia in patients with "static" encephalopathy. J Neurol Neurosurg Psychiatry 43:789, 1980.
6. Burke RE, Fahn S, Jankovic J, et al: Tardive dystonia: Late-onset and persistent dystonia caused by antipsychotic drugs. Neurology 32:1335, 1982.
7. Burnstein L, Breningstall GN: Movement disorders in bacterial meningitis. J Pediatr 109:260, 1986.
8. Caccia MR, Mangoni A: Clonidine in essential tremor: Preliminary observations from an open trial. J Neurol 232:55, 1985.
9. Calzetti S, Findley LJ, Perucca E, et al: The response of essential tremor to propranolol: evaluation of clinical variables governing its efficacy on prolonged administration. J Neurol Neurosurg Psychiatry 46:393, 1983.
10. Chadwick D, Hallett M, Harris R, et al: Clinical, biochemical and physiological factors distinguishing myoclonus responsive to 5-hydroxytryptophan, tryptophan plus a monoamine oxidase inhibitor and clonazepam. Brain 100:455, 1977.
11. Ch'ien L, Economides AN, Lemmi H: Sydenham's chorea and seizures. Arch Neurol 35:382, 1978.
12. Chokroverty S, Manocha M, Duvoisin RC: A physiologic and pharmacologic study in anticholinergic-responsive essential myoclonus. Neurology 37:608, 1987.
13. Chun RWM, Daly RF, Mansheim BJ, et al: Benign familial chorea with onset in childhood. JAMA 225:1603, 1973.
14. Comings DE, Comings BG: Tourette syndrome: Clinical and psychological aspects of 250 cases. Am J Hum Genet 37:435, 1985.
15. Deonna T, Martin D: Benign paroxysmal torticollis in infancy. Arch Dis Child 56:956, 1981.
16. Erenberg C, Cruse RP, Rothner AD: Gilles de la Tourette's syndrome. Effect of stimulant drugs. Neurology 35:1436, 1985.
17. Fahn S: High dosage anticholinergic therapy in dystonia. Neurology 33:1255, 1983.
18. Fahn S, Marsden CD, Calne DB: Classification and investigation of dystonia. In Marsden CD, Fahn S, eds. Movement Disorders 2. Butterworth's International Medical Reviews: Neurology, Volume 6. Butterworth, London, 1987, p 332.
19. Findley LJ, Koller WC: Essential tremor: a review. Neurology 37:1194, 1987.
20. Gautier JC, Awada A: Dystonia musculorum deformans improved by bromocriptine. Rev Neurol 139:449, 1983.
21. Goetz CG, Tanner CM, Klawans HL: Fluphenazine and multifocal tic disorder. Arch Neurol 41:271, 1984.
22. Gorman WP, Cooper P, Popock P, et al: A comparison of primidone, propranolol, and placebo in essential tremor, using quantitative analysis. J Neurol Neurosurg Psychiatry 49:64, 1986.
23. Groothuis JR, Groothuis DR, Mukhopadhyay D, et al: Lupus-associated chorea in children. Am J Dis Child 131:1131, 1977.
24. Gualtieri CT, Quade D, Hicks RE, et al: Tardive dyskinesia and other clinical consequences of neuroleptic treatment in children and adolescence. Am J Psychiatry 141:20, 1984.
25. Haerer AF, Anderson DW, Schoenberg BS: Prevalence of essential tremor. Arch Neurol 39:750, 1982.
26. Jankovic J, Ford J: Blepharospasm and orofacial-cervical dystonia: Clinical and pharmacological findings in 100 patients. Ann Neurol 13:402, 1983.
27. Jankovic J, Havins WE, Wilkins RB: Blinking and blepharospasm. Mechanism, diagnosis, and management. JAMA 248:3160, 1982.
28. Jankovic J, Orman J: Botulinum A toxin for cranial-cervical dystonia: A double-blind, placebo-controlled study. Neurology 37:616, 1987.
29. Jankovic J, Pardo R: Segmental myoclonus. Clinical and pharmacologic study. Arch Neurol 43:1025, 1986.
30. Klawans HL, Barr A: Recurrence of childhood multiple tic in late life. Arch Neurol 42:1079, 1985.
31. Knight ME, Roberts RJ: Phenothiazine and butyrophenone intoxication in children. Pediatr Clin North Am 33:299, 1986.
32. Leckman JF, Detlor J, Harcherik DF, et al: Short- and long-term treatment of Tourette syndrome with clonidine: a clinical perspective. Neurology 35:343, 1985.
33. Lees AJ, Robertson M, Trimble MR, et al: A clinical study of Gilles de la Tourette syndrome in the United Kingdom. J Neurol Neurosurg Psychiatry 47:1, 1984.
34. Leopold NA: Prolonged metoclopramide-induced dyskinetic reaction. Neurology 34:238, 1984.
35. Lima B, Neves G, Nora M: Juvenile parkinsonism: clinical and metabolic characteristics. J Neurol Neurosurg Psychiatry 50:345, 1987.
36. Lowe TL, Cohen DJ, Detlor J, et al: Stimulant medications precipitate Tourette's syndrome. JAMA 247:1729, 1982.
37. Marsden CD, Hallett M, Fahn S: The nosology and pathophysiology of myoclonus. In Marsden CD, Fahn S, eds. Movement Disorders. Butterworth's International Medical Reviews: Neurology, Volume 2. Butterworth, London, 1982, p 196.
38. Marsden CD, Harrison MJG: Idiopathic torsion dystonia (dystonia musculorum deformans). A review of forty-two patients. Brain 97:793, 1974.
39. Matsuo F, Ajax E: Palatal myoclonus and denervation supersensitivity in the central nervous system. Ann Neurol 5:72, 1979.
40. Mito T, Tanaka T, Becker LE, et al: Infantile bilateral striatal necrosis. Clinicopathologic classification. Arch Neurol 43:677, 1986.
41. Narbona J, Obeso JA, Martinez-Lage, et al: Hemidystonia secondary to localized basal ganglia tumor. J Neurol Neurosurg Psychiatry 47:704, 1984.
42. Neglia JP, Glaze DG, Zion TE: Tics and vocalizations in children treated with carbamazepine. Pediatrics 73:841, 1984.

43. Nygaard TG, Duvoison RC: Hereditary dystonia-parkinsonism syndrome of juvenile onset. Neurology 36:1424, 1986.
44. Pauls DL, Leckman JF: The inheritance of Gilles de la Tourette syndrome and associated behaviors. N Engl J Med 315:993, 1986.
45. Pettigrew LC, Jankovic J: Hemidystonia: a report of 22 patients and a review of the literature. J Neurol Neurosurg Psychiatry 48:650, 1985.
46. Plant GT, Williams AC, Earl CJ, et al: Familial paroxysmal dystonia induced by exercise. J Neurol Neurosurg Psychiatry 47:275, 1984.
47. Rajput A, Pfford KP, Beard CM, et al: Essential tremor in Rochester, Minnesota: A 45-year study. J Neurol Neurosurg Psychiatry 47:466, 1984.
48. Regeur L, Pakkenberg B, Fog R, et al: Clinical features and long-term treatment with pimozide in 65 patients with Gilles de la Tourette's syndrome. J Neurol Neurosurg Psychiatry 49:791, 1986.
49. Rollinson RD, Gilligan BS: Postanoxic action myoclonus (Lance-Adams syndrome) responding to valproate. Arch Neurol 36:44, 1979.
50. Ronen G, Donat JR, Hill A: Hemifacial spasm in children. Can J Neurol Sci 13:342, 1986.
51. Scheinberg IH, Jaffe ME, Sternlieb, I: The use of trientine in preventing the effects of interrupting penicillamine therapy in Wilson's disease. N Engl J Med 317:209, 1987.
52. Sheehy MP, Marsden CD: Writer's cramp—a focal dystonia. Brain 105:461, 1982.
53. Silverstein F, Johnston MV: Risks of neuroleptic drugs in children with neurological disorders. Ann Neurol 18:392, 1985.
54. Singer HS: Tardive dyskinesia: A concern for the pediatrician. Pediatrics 77:553, 1986.
55. Singer HS, Gammon K, Quaskey S: Haloperidol, fluphenazine and clonidine in Tourette syndrome: Controversies in treatment. Pediatr Neurosci 12:71, 1986.
56. Smits MG, Gabeels FJM, Thijssen HOM, et al: Progressive idiopathic strio-pallido-dentate calcinosis (Fahr's disease) with autosomal recessive inheritance. Report of three siblings. Eur Neurol 22:58, 1983.
57. Spitz MC, Jankovic J, Killian JM: Familial tic disorder, parkinsonism, motor neuron disease, and acanthocytosis: a new syndrome. Neurology 35:366, 1985.
58. Starosta-Rubinstein S, Young AB, Kluin K, et al: Clinical assessment of 31 patients with Wilson's disease. Correlations with structural changes on magnetic resonance imaging. Arch Neurol 44:365, 1987.
59. Sternlieb I, Giblin DR, Scheinberg IH: Wilson's disease. In Marsden CD, Fahn S, eds. Movement Disorders 2. Butterworth's International Medical Reviews. Neurology, Volume 7. Butterworth, London, 1987, p 288.
60. Strickland GT, Leu M-L: Wilson's disease: Clinical and laboratory manifestations in 40 patients. Medicine 54:113, 1975.
61. Swanson JW, Kelley Jr JJ, McConahey WM: Neurologic aspects of thyroid dysfunction. Mayo Clin Proc 56:504, 1981.
62. Torch WC, Humphreys HK: Pharmacological therapy of Hallervorden-Spatz syndrome: Two cases responsive to benztropine. Ann Neurol 20:445, 1986.

15 Disorders of Ocular Motility

The maintenance of binocular vision by conjugate movement of the eyes is perhaps the most delicate feat of muscular coordination achieved by the nervous system. Disorders of the visual sensory system, ocular muscles, ocular motor nerves, neuromuscular transmission, or the gaze centers of the central nervous system may result in disturbed ocular motility. This chapter deals with nonparalytic strabismus, paralytic strabismus (ophthalmoplegia), gaze palsies (supranuclear palsies), ptosis, and nystagmus. Visual disorders and disorders of the pupil are discussed in Chapter 16.

■ Nonparalytic Strabismus

Strabismus (squint), or abnormal ocular alignment, affects 3 to 4 percent of preschool children (Nelson, 1983). Most individuals have a latent tendency for ocular misalignment, *heterophoria*, which becomes apparent only under conditions of stress or fatigue. During periods of misalignment, the child may experience diplopia or headache. Constant ocular misalignment is called *heterotropia*. Children with heterotropia suppress the image in one eye to avoid diplopia. If only one eye is used for fixation, visual acuity may be permanently lost in the other (developmental amblyopia). In nonparalytic strabismus, the amount of deviation in different directions of gaze is relatively constant (comitant). Each eye moves through a normal range when tested separately (ductions), but the eyes are disconjugate when used together (versions). Many children with chronic brain damage syndromes, such as malformations or perinatal asphyxia, have nonparalytic strabismus. This is due to faulty control of conjugate gaze mechanisms by the abnormal brain. In neurologically normal children, the most common cause of nonparalytic strabismus is either a genetic influence or intraocular pathology.

Ocular alignment in the newborn is usually poor. There are transitory shifts from alignment to convergence and divergence. Constant ocular alignment usually occurs after three months of age. Approximately 2 percent of newborns exhibit a tendency for chronic downward deviation of the eyes during the waking state. The eyes assume a normal position during sleep and are able to move upward reflexly (Hoyt et al, 1980).

ESOTROPIA

Esotropia is an inward deviation (convergence) of the eyes. Early-onset or infantile esotropia is noted between three and six months of age and accommodative esotropia is noted after the age of six months.

Clinical Features. Children with infantile esotropia often alternate fixation between eyes and may cross-fixate, i.e. looking to the left with the right eye and to the right with the left eye. The misalignment is sufficient to be noticed by family members. Some children fixate almost entirely with one eye and are at risk for permanent loss of visual acuity, *amblyopia,* in the other.

Accommodative esotropia occurs when the accommodative reflex is used to correct hyperopia. The blurred hyperopic image can be more sharply focused by accommodation. Because accommodation is accompanied by convergence, the eyes turn inward. In children with accommodative esotropia, one eye is more hyperopic than the other and the better eye is used for fixation. In such cases, the potential for amblyopia in the other eye is considerable.

Diagnosis. The eyes should be refracted to determine whether hyperopia is present.

Treatment. Hyperopic errors should be corrected with eye-glasses. Early-onset esotropia in which only one eye is used for fixation is treated with alternate patching of the eyes. Early corrective surgery is required for persistent esotropia. A recently introduced alternative to surgery is chemodenervation of overactive muscles by injection of botulinum toxin. The technique has proven effective in research trials but is not yet approved for regular use (Magoon and Scott, 1987).

Table 15.1   THE EXTRAOCULAR MUSCLES

Ocular Muscle	Innervation	Function
Lateral rectus	Abducens	Abduction
Medial rectus	Oculomotor	Adduction
Superior rectus	Oculomotor	Elevation
		Intorsion
		Adduction
Inferior rectus	Oculomotor	Depression
		Extorsion
		Adduction
Inferior oblique	Oculomotor	Extorsion
		Elevation
		Abduction
Superior oblique	Trochlear	Intorsion
		Depression
		Abduction

EXOTROPIA

Exotropia is an outward deviation of the eyes; it may be intermittent or constant.

Clinical Features. The onset of intermittent exotropia usually occurs before four years of age. It is relatively common and most often evident when the child is fatigued and fixating on a far object. The natural history of the condition is uncertain.

Constant exotropia may be congenital, but can also be caused by poor vision in the outward turning eye.

Diagnosis. The eyes must be examined for intraocular pathology.

Treatment. In children with intermittent exotropia, the decision to perform corrective surgery depends upon the frequency and degree of exotropia. When exotropia is constant, treatment depends upon the underlying cause of visual loss.

■ Ophthalmoplegia
(Paralytic Strabismus)

Ophthalmoplegia can be due to disorders of the ocular motor nerves, the ocular muscles, or neuromuscular transmission. The muscles, the nerves, and their functions are summarized in Table 15.1. The eye appears to deviate in the direction opposite to the field of action of the paralyzed ocular muscle, and diplopia is experienced. Strabismus and diplopia are made worse when the child gazes in the direction of action of the paralyzed muscle.

CONGENITAL OPHTHALMOPLEGIA

Ophthalmoplegia in the newborn is often missed because eye movements are infrequently tested. It is commonplace for strabismus to remain unnoticed for several months and then to be discounted as transient esotropia. Therefore, congenital ophthalmoplegia should be considered even when there is no history of ophthalmoplegia at birth.

Oculomotor Nerve Palsy

Clinical Features. Most cases of congenital oculomotor nerve palsy are unilateral and complete. Involvement of the pupillary reflex is variable (Victor, 1976). Only half are observed at birth. An occasional case is familial or due to trauma of the orbit at birth, but most are idiopathic. The affected eye is exotropic and usually amblyopic. Aberrant regeneration may be evidenced by lid retraction on attempted adduction or downward gaze.

Diagnosis. Computerized tomography (CT) is indicated to exclude the possibility of an intracranial mass compressing the nerve. Exophthalmus should suggest a tumor of the orbit. The presence of a dilated pupil excludes the possibility of myasthenia gravis, but an edrophonium chloride (Tensilon) test is indicated if the pupil is normal.

Treatment. Recession of the lateral rectus muscle and resection of the medial rectus muscle of the involved eye may improve the cosmetic appearance, but does not improve ocular motility or visual function.

Trochlear Nerve Palsy

Clinical Features. Congenital superior oblique palsy is unilateral in 94 percent of cases (von Noorden et al, 1986). Birth trauma is often suspected, but is rarely established. The majority of congenital cases are idiopathic.

Diplopia is not a common complaint and may be relieved by a compensatory head tilt away from the paralyzed side. The major features on examination include (1) noncomitant hypertropia, greatest in the nasal field of the involved eye; (2) underaction of the paretic superior oblique and overaction of the inferior oblique muscle; and (3) increased hypertropia when the head is tilted to the paralyzed side (positive Bielschowsky test).

Diagnosis. Many children present with head tilt or torticollis (see Chapter 14). Once a superior oblique palsy is confirmed by examination, important etiologic considerations other than congenital ones include trauma, myasthenia gravis, and brainstem glioma.

Treatment. Most patients require surgery. Several procedures are available to restore balance between the superior and inferior oblique muscles.

Abducens Nerve Palsy

Clinical Features. Congenital abducens nerve palsy may be unilateral or bilateral and is sometimes associated with other cranial nerve palsies. There is partial or complete limitation of lateral movement of the affected eye(s). Most infants use cross-fixation, and vision is thereby retained in both eyes. The few reported cases with pathologic correlation demonstrate absence of the abducens nerve and hypoplasia of its nucleus (Hickey and Wagoner, 1983). *Mobius syndrome* is the association of congenital facial diplegia and bilateral abducens nerve palsies (see Chapter 17). *Duane syndrome* is characterized by a lateral rectus palsy, some limitation of adduction, and narrowing of the palpebral fissure because of globe retraction on attempted adduction. Other ocular, ear, and systemic malformations may be present as well (Tachibana et al, 1984).

Diagnosis. A CT scan is indicated to exclude the possibility of an intracranial mass lesion. Hearing should be tested, and an electromyogram (EMG) of the face may be useful if there is facial weakness to determine facial nerve function.

Treatment. Surgical procedures may be useful to correct head turn and are sometimes useful for cosmetic purposes, but do not restore ocular motility.

Congenital Myasthenia Gravis

There are several different syndromes of myasthenia gravis in the newborn (see Chapter 6). Congenital myasthenia gravis is the only one in which ophthalmoplegia is the primary clinical feature.

Clinical Features. Although the disorder is transmitted by autosomal recessive inheritance, there is a male-female bias of 2:1. Symmetric ptosis and ophthalmoplegia are noted at birth or shortly thereafter. Mild facial weakness may be present as well, but is not sufficiently severe to impair feeding. If the ophthalmoplegia is not complete at birth, it will become complete during infancy or childhood. Generalized weakness sometimes develops.

Diagnosis. The diagnosis should be suspected in any newborn with bilateral ptosis or limitation of eye movement. Intramuscular injection of Tensilon produces a transitory improvement in ocular motility. Repetitive nerve stimulation of the limbs at a frequency of 13 Hz may reveal a decremental response, reversible with Tensilon (Gath et al, 1970). This suggests that the underlying defect, though only symptomatic in the eyes, is already generalized at birth.

Treatment. There is no evidence for an immunopathy or a rationale basis for immunosuppressive therapy. Thymectomy and corticosteroids have been tried and found ineffective (Fenichel, 1978). Anticholinesterases may be helpful in improving facial paralysis, but they have little or no effect on ophthalmoplegia.

Fibrosis of Extraocular Muscles

This is an ill-defined entity with partial (Prakash et al, 1985) or complete (Apt and Axelrod, 1978) paralysis of ocular motility at birth and is caused by maldevelopment of the ocular muscles, which are represented as fibrous bands. In some of these cases, the underlying pathophysiology may be hypoplasia of the ocular motor nerves.

Clinical Features. The only clinical feature is restricted ocular motility, usually bilateral, but unilateral occurrence is reported. Ptosis is almost always present.

Diagnosis. Other causes of congenital ophthalmoplegia must be excluded. Biopsy of the fibrotic muscle is essential for definitive diagnosis.

Treatment. Surgery may provide some cosmetic benefit and relief of ptosis, but does not correct the disturbed motility.

Brown Syndrome

Brown syndrome consists of mechanical limitation of elevation in adduction as a result of congenital shortening of the superior oblique muscle or tendon (Wang et al, 1984).

Clinical Features. Elevation is limited in adduction, but normal in abduction. Passive elevation (forced duction) is restricted as well. Other features include widening of the palpebral fissure on adduction and backward head tilt.

Diagnosis. Congenital Brown syndrome must be differentiated from acquired shortening of the superior oblique muscle caused by juvenile rheumatoid arthritis, trauma, and inflammatory processes affecting the top of the orbit (see "Orbital Pseudotumor" later on in this chapter).

Treatment. Surgical procedures that extend the superior oblique muscle can be useful in congenital cases.

Congenital Ptosis

Clinical Features. Congenital drooping of one or both lids is relatively common, and the drooping is unilateral in 70 percent. The cause is unknown, and it is rarely familial. Congenital ptosis is often not noticed until early childhood or even adult life and then presents as an "acquired" ptosis. Miosis is sometimes associated and suggests the possibility of a Horner syndrome, except that the pupil responds normally to pharmacologic agents. Occasional patients demonstrate a synkinesis between the oculomotor and the trigeminal nerves, so that movements of the jaw produce opening of the eye (Marcus-Gunn phenomenon).

Diagnosis. The essential point in diagnosis is to demonstrate that ptosis has been present from birth. This is best accomplished by examining baby pictures. If miosis is present, the eye must be tested with pharmacologic agents to determine whether sympathetic hypersensitivity is present. Concurrent paralysis of extraocular motility is evidence against the diagnosis of congenital ptosis.

Treatment. Corrective surgery is useful in elevating the lid for cosmetic appearances or when ptosis is sufficiently severe to impair vision.

ACUTE UNILATERAL OPHTHALMOPLEGIA

The causes of acquired ophthalmoplegia are summarized in Table 15.2. Many of the conditions are discussed in other chapters.

"Acute" is defined as reaching maximum intensity within one week of onset, and "ophthalmoplegia" includes partial and complete weakness (Table 15.3). Generalized increased intracranial pressure is always an important consideration in patients presenting with unilateral or bilateral abducens palsy (see Chapter 4).

Table 15.2 CAUSES OF ACQUIRED OPHTHALMOPLEGIA

Brainstem
1. Tumor
   a. Brainstem glioma
   b. Craniopharyngioma (see Chapter 16)
   c. Pineal region tumors
   d. Lymphoma
   e. Leukemia
   f. Metastases
2. Vascular
   a. Migraine
   b. Infarction
   c. Hemorrhage
   d. Vasculitis
   e. Arteriovenous malformation
3. Multiple sclerosis (see Chapter 10)
4. Brainstem encephalitis (see Chapter 10)
5. Intoxication
6. Subacute necrotizing encephalopathy (see Chapter 10)

Nerve
1. Increased intracranial pressure (see Chapter 4)
2. Postinfectious
   a. Idiopathic (postviral)
   b. Polyradiculoneuropathy (see Chapter 7)
   c. Miller Fisher syndrome (see Chapter 10)
3. Infectious
   a. Orbital cellulitis
   b. Diphtheria
   c. Gradenigo syndrome
   d. Meningitis (see Chapter 4)
4. Familial recurrent neuropathies (see Chapter 17)
5. Trauma
   a. Orbital
   b. Head
6. Vascular
   a. Migraine
   b. Aneurysm
   c. Cavernous sinus thrombosis
   d. Carotid-cavernous fistula
7. Tumor
   a. Orbital tumors
   b. Cavernous hemangioma
   c. Sellar and parasellar tumors (see Chapter 16)
   d. Sphenoid sinus tumors
8. Inflammatory
   a. Tolosa-Hunt syndrome
   b. Orbital pseudotumor
   c. Sarcoid

Neuromuscular Transmission
1. Myasthenia gravis
2. Botulism (see Chapter 7)

Myopathies
1. Fiber type disproportion myopathies (see Chapter 6)
2. Mitochondrial myopathies (see Chapter 7)
3. Oculopharyngeal dystrophy (see Chapter 17)
4. Vitamin E deficiency
5. Thyrotoxicosis

Table 15.3 ACUTE UNILATERAL
OPHTHALMOPLEGIA

1. Increased intracranial pressure (see Chapter 4)
2. Idiopathic (postviral)
3. Migraine*†
4. Myasthenia gravis*
5. Orbital tumors†
6. Gradenigo syndrome
7. Aneurysm*†
8. Brain tumors
   a. Brainstem glioma
   b. Parasellar tumors (see Chapter 16)
   c. Tumors of pineal region (see Chapter 4)
9. Multiple sclerosis* (see Chapter 10)
10. Brainstem stroke*
11. Recurrent familial* (see Chapter 17)
12. Inflammatory
    a. Tolosa-Hunt syndrome*†
    b. Orbital pseudotumor*†
14. Trauma
    a. Orbital
    b. Head

*May be recurrent.
†May be associated with pain.

Idiopathic (Postviral) Nerve Palsy

Clinical Features. The sudden onset of a single cranial neuropathy without apparent cause is frequently attributed to a viral infection occurring during the previous month. The mechanism is thought to occur on an autoimmune basis. However, the average American school-aged child experiences an average of six viral infections a year; therefore, 50 percent of children presenting with a cranial neuropathy will give a history of a preceding viral infection by chance alone.

The abducens nerve is more frequently affected than is either the oculomotor or trochlear nerve. Bilateral involvement is unusual. The child complains of painless diplopia, and paralytic strabismus is observed. Full motility is restored within six months to a year and recurrences are not expected (Knox et al, 1967).

Diagnosis. Other causes of isolated nerve palsy must be excluded. Examination of the cerebrospinal fluid and CT are warranted in every case to exclude the possibility of tumor and infection. Tumors in and around the orbit are sometimes difficult to demonstrate, and if ophthalmoplegia persists, it may be necessary to repeat the scan with special views of the orbit. Myasthenia gravis is always a consideration, and a Tensilon test should be performed even though the diagnosis is less likely when there is a fixed single nerve deficit.

Treatment. Corticosteroids are not recommended. It may be necessary to patch the normal eye intermittently if the affected eye is not used for fixation.

Ophthalmoplegic Migraine

Clinical Features. Transitory ocular motor palsy, lasting sometimes as long as four weeks, may occur as part of a migraine attack in children and adults. The palsy affects the oculomotor nerve alone in 83 percent of cases and all three nerves in the remainder (Vijayan, 1980). Ptosis usually precedes ophthalmoplegia. Partial or complete pupillary involvement is present in 60 percent. The average age of occurrence is fifteen years, but the onset may be as early as infancy. In infants, recurrent painless ophthalmoplegia or ptosis may be the only manifestation of the migraine attack (Durkan et al, 1981). In older children, ophthalmoplegia usually occurs during the headache phase and is ipsilateral to the headache.

The mechanism of ophthalmoplegia is uncertain, but has been attributed either to an ischemic neuropathy or compression of the nerve by a swollen carotid artery in the cavernous sinus. Although migraine is hereditary, the tendency for ophthalmoplegia is not.

Diagnosis. The diagnosis is obvious when ophthalmoplegia occurs during a typical migraine attack in a child previously known to have migraine. Diagnostic uncertainty is greatest in an infant who develops transitory strabismus or ptosis as an isolated sign. In such cases, a positive family history of migraine is essential for diagnosis. Even so, most infants with a first episode of ophthalmoplegia should be studied with CT to exclude other causes. The transitory nature of the palsy is comforting and indicates that a structural abnormality is unlikely.

Treatment. Children with ophthalmoplegic migraine should be treated in the same manner as other children with migraine (see Chapter 3).

Myasthenia Gravis

Some neonatal forms of myasthenia are discussed in Chapter 6; congenital myasthenia is included in the section on "Congenital Ophthalmoplegia" earlier in this chapter, and limb-girdle myasthenia is discussed in Chapter 7. This section deals with the autoimmune form of myasthenia that is encountered from late infancy through adult life. Two forms can be recognized:

1. *Ocular myasthenia.* The eyes muscles are primarily or exclusively affected, but facial and limb muscles may be mildly involved as well.

2. Generalized myasthenia. Weakness of bulbar and limb muscles is moderate to severe.

The term *juvenile myasthenia* is sometimes used to denote myasthenia gravis in children, but since the nongenetic forms of myasthenia in children are not different from myasthenia gravis in adults, the term should not suggest a separate disorder.

Clinical Features. The first symptoms always appear after six months of age; 75 percent of children first become symptomatic after age ten. Girls are more often affected than boys. The initial features of both the ocular and the generalized forms are usually ptosis, diplopia, or both. Myasthenia is the most common cause of acquired ptosis, unilateral or bilateral. Pupillary function is always normal. Forty to 50 percent of patients demonstrate weakness of other bulbar muscles or limb weakness at the time of onset. Ocular motor weakness is generally not constant initially but changes from examination to examination. Both eyes are usually affected, but one more than the other.

Children with ocular myasthenia may have facial weakness and complain of easy fatiguability of the limbs. However, they never have difficulty speaking or swallowing and never have respiratory distress. The subsequent course is frequently characterized by relapses and remissions (Rollinson and Fenichel, 1981). The relapses are of varying severity and last for weeks to years. Remissions are recorded for as long as fourteen years before another relapse. At least 20 percent have permanent remissions.

Those with generalized myasthenia will experience generalized weakness within one year of the initial ocular symptoms. Dysarthria, dysphagia, difficulty chewing, and limb muscle fatiguability can be observed. Spontaneous remissions are not expected. As many as 40 percent of patients will experience respiratory insufficiency, or *myasthenic crises*, if not treated.

Children with generalized myasthenia, but not those with ocular myasthenia, have a higher than expected incidence of other autoimmune disorders, especially thyroiditis and collagen vascular diseases. Thymoma is present in 15 percent of all patients with generalized myasthenia. Most of these are adults. The incidence in children is probably less than 5 percent.

Diagnosis. The gold standard of diagnosis for both the ocular and generalized forms of myasthenia gravis is the Tensilon test. Tensilon is a short-acting anticholinesterase available in a vial containing 10 mg/ml. Before the test is initiated, it is important to determine an endpoint for the study. The best endpoint is the resolution of ptosis or the restoration of ocular motility. Ptosis generally responds better to Tensilon than does ocular motor paralysis. In the absence of ptosis or strabismus, the test results are difficult to evaluate (Daroff, 1986).

Some patients with myasthenia are supersensitive to Tensilon, and fasciculations and sometimes respiratory arrest develop when a full dose is administered. For this reason, a test dose of 1 mg is injected first. Unfortunately, an occasional patient may develop respiratory embarrassment in response to the test dose and a hand ventilator should be readily available before any drug is given. Atropine is an effective antidote for the muscarinic side effects of Tensilon, but is of no value to counteract the nicotinic effects on the motor endplate that result in paralysis of the skeletal muscles.

After the test dose is given, the remainder should be injected in 3 mg increments, with up to one minute allowed after each injection to test the response. Interpretation is not always easy. The judgment of improved strength is always subjective and may be influenced by examiner bias. The test becomes more objective when combined with electrophysiologic studies.

Repetitive stimulation of the ulnar nerve is abnormal in 17 percent of patients with ocular myasthenia and 100 percent of patients with generalized myasthenia (Oh et al, 1982). In patients with mild myasthenia, a decremental response is recorded at low (2 to 5/sec) rates of stimulation, but not at high (50/sec) rates. In severe myasthenia, a decremental response is recorded both at low and high rates of stimulation.

The clinical manifestations of myasthenia gravis are attributed to the presence of antibodies against the acetylcholine receptor protein. Elevated concentrations of the antibody, greater than 10 nmol/L, are detected in the sera of 90 percent of patients with generalized myasthenia. Patients with ocular myasthenia demonstrate concentrations of 0 to 10 nmol/L. Individuals with thymoma usually have exceptionally high concentrations of antibody, not only against the receptor protein but also against striated muscle. Antibodies against striated muscle are not usually detected in myasthenic children who do not have thymoma. For this reason, antibody testing is a better screen for thymoma than are radiographs of the chest. Thymoma is ordinarily a microscopic tumor and cannot be detected on chest CT. In addition, overall thymic size is too variable in children to determine a mass effect by routine chest radiographs.

Patients with generalized myasthenia who do

not have detectable concentrations of antibody against acetylcholine receptor protein may have antibodies to another receptor site (Mossman et al, 1986). Such patients do not have thymic abnormalities.

Treatment. When a treatment program is being selected, it is important to make a distinction between children with ocular myasthenia and those with generalized myasthenia. The former have a reasonable hope of spontaneous remission, but the latter do not. Anticholinesterase therapy is the treatment of choice for ocular myasthenia. The initial dose of neostigmine is 0.5 mg/kg every four hours in children younger than five years of age and 0.25 mg/kg in older children not to exceed 15 mg. The equivalent dose of pyridostigmine is four times greater. After treatment is initiated, the dose is slowly increased as tolerated. Diarrhea and gastrointestinal cramps are the usual limiting factors. Tensilon should not be administered to determine whether the child would benefit from higher oral doses of anticholinesterases. It is not an accurate guide and may cause cholinergic crisis in children with generalized myasthenia.

The response to anticholinesterases is usually transitory. Ocular myasthenia is difficult to treat. The addition of corticosteroids may provide temporary relief, but their use is not recommended. It is difficult to assess the efficacy of any drug regimen in ocular myasthenia because of its fluctuating course.

Children with generalized myasthenia and increased concentrations of antibody against acetylcholine receptor protein should undergo thymectomy as quickly as possible after diagnosis. Thymectomy must be performed by thoracotomy and not by transcervical approach. Sixty-one percent of children will experience remission within three years of surgery if thymectomy is performed early in the course of disease (Rodriguez et al, 1983). Corticosteroids should be started immediately after surgery, preferably while the patient is still in the surgical intensive care unit. An equivalent dose to prednisone, 2 mg/kg/day, is given parenterally until the patient is able to take oral medication. After five days, an alternate-day regimen is used for the remainder of the month. The dose of prednisone is then tapered by 10 percent each month until a maintenance dose is reached that keeps the patient symptom-free. High-dose corticosteroids may make the patient weaker at first. It is for this reason that treatment is initiated while the patient is still in intensive care with ventilator support. Improvement usually begins after the first week and continues in the months that follow.

Anticholinesterase medication should not be given concurrently with corticosteroids at first, but may be used later if the patient weakens on days that corticosteroids are not taken.

Plasmapheresis is useful as an acute intervention in patients who are experiencing respiratory insufficiency (myasthenic crisis) or are so weak that strength must be restored prior to thymectomy.

Orbital Tumors

Clinical Features. The initial manifestation of intraorbital tumors is proptosis, ophthalmoplegia, or ptosis. When the globe is displaced forward, the palpebral fissure is widened and it may not be possible to fully close the eye. As a consequence, the exposed portion of the eye becomes erythematous and may suffer exposure keratitis. The direction of displacement of the globe is the best clue to the position of the tumor. Ophthalmoplegia may occur because the globe is displaced or because of direct pressure on one or more ocular nerves.

Diagnosis. The differential diagnosis of proptosis in children includes infection and inflammation (30 percent), hemorrhage and other vascular disorders (19 percent), orbital tumors (16 percent), hyperthyroidism and other metabolic disorders (14 percent), developmental anomalies (9 percent), Hand-Schüller-Christian disease and related disorders (7 percent), and the remainder are idiopathic (Crawford, 1967). The most common orbital tumors are dermoid cyst, hemangioma, metastatic neuroblastoma, optic glioma, and rhabdomyosarcoma (Youseffi, 1969).

Treatment. Treatment varies with tumor type, and surgical resection is indicated for many.

Gradenigo Syndrome

Clinical Features. The abducens nerve lies adjacent to the medial aspect of the petrous bone before entering the cavernous sinus. Infections of the middle ear sometimes extend to the petrous bone and cause thrombophlebitis of the inferior petrosal sinus. The infection involves not only the abducens nerve but also the facial nerve and the trigeminal ganglion. The resulting syndrome is characterized by ipsilateral paralysis of abduction, facial palsy, and facial pain.

Diagnosis. The combination of unilateral abducens and facial palsy can also be seen after closed head injuries. The diagnosis of Gradenigo syndrome requires the demonstration of middle ear infection. Radiographs of the mastoid and lumbar puncture are indicated in all such patients.

Treatment. Antibiotic therapy must be initiated early in order to prevent permanent nerve damage.

Aneurysm

Arterial aneurysms are discussed fully in Chapter 4, because the important clinical feature in children is hemorrhage rather than nerve compression. This section deals only with possible ophthalmoplegic features.

Clinical Features. Aneurysms at the junction of the internal carotid and posterior communicating arteries are an important cause of unilateral oculomotor palsy. The palsy is attributed to hemorrhage within the sac, to which the nerve is adherent, or to hemorrhage into the nerve. Intense pain in and around the eye is frequently experienced at the time of hemorrhage. Mydriasis is an almost constant feature of ophthalmoplegia as a result of aneurysms of the posterior communicating artery, because the parasympathetic fibers are at the periphery of the nerve. However, pupillary involvement may develop several days after the onset of an incomplete ophthalmoplegia (Kissel et al, 1983). A normal pupil with complete ophthalmoplegia effectively excludes the possibility of aneurysm.

The superior branch of the oculomotor nerve is sometimes affected earlier and more severely than is the inferior branch. Ptosis may precede the development of other signs by hours or days.

Diagnosis. Many aneurysms can be identified by contrasted CT, but arteriography is essential for diagnosis.

Treatment. Surgical resection is the treatment of choice whenever technically feasible. Oculomotor function often returns to normal after the aneurysm is removed.

Brainstem Glioma

Clinical Features. The onset of symptoms is between three and thirteen years with a peak at age five. Cranial nerve palsies, usually abducens and facial, are the initial features in most cases. These are later associated with contralateral hemiplegia and ataxia, dysphagia, and hoarseness. With time, cranial nerve and corticospinal tract involvement may become bilateral. In-

creased intracranial pressure is not an early feature, but vomiting may occur from direct irritation of the brainstem emetic center. Intractable hiccough, facial spasm, personality change, and headache may be presenting symptoms in occasional patients.

These tumors are associated with the worst prognosis of any childhood tumor. The course is one of steady progression with median survival rates of nine to twelve months (Cohen et al, 1986).

Diagnosis. The characteristic CT appearance of most brainstem gliomas is isodense and contrast-enhancing. Some extend into the fourth ventricle; and these, which are low-grade gliomas, are associated with the best prognosis following resection (Stroink et al, 1986). Tumors that demonstrate a cystic portion and ring enhancement are associated with a poor prognosis. Magnetic resonance imaging (MRI) provides optimal delineation of tumor and is preferable to CT (Fig. 15.1).

Treatment. Radical surgery may be beneficial for focal benign tumors located at the cervicomedullary junction, but is of no value for diffuse malignant gliomas extending above the medulla (Epstein and McCleary, 1986). Radiation therapy is the treatment of choice. In addition, several chemotherapeutic programs are under-

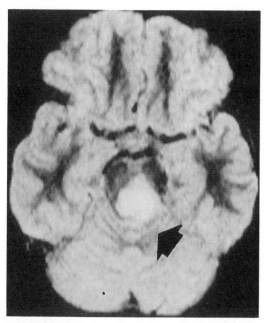

Figure 15.1 Brainstem glioma. T2 weighted magnetic resonance image (MRI) demonstrates an area of increased signal in the brainstem.

going experimental trials, but none are established as beneficial.

Brainstem Stroke

The causes of stroke in children are summarized in Table 11.2. Small brainstem hemorrhages due to emboli, leukemia, or blood dyscrasias have the potential of causing isolated ocular motor palsies, but this is not the rule. Other cranial nerves are also involved, and hemiparesis, ataxia, or states of decreased consciousness are typically associated.

Tolosa-Hunt Syndrome

This is a syndrome of painful ophthalmoplegia attributed to an idiopathic granulomatous disease of the cavernous sinus or superior orbital fissure. No other structure is involved.

Clinical Features. The pain is described as steady and boring, involving the entire hemicranium, but centered around the eye. It may precede the ophthalmoplegia by several days, may occur concurrently, or may appear later. The oculomotor nerve is ordinarily involved first and more severely than the others, but all three ocular motor nerves, as well as the first and second divisions of the trigeminal nerve, may be affected. Vision may be diminished; the pupil is usually small and may be reactive or nonreactive. Symptoms last for days or months. Spontaneous remissions occur, but partial neurologic deficits may persist.

Diagnosis. Tolosa-Hunt syndrome is easily confused with ophthalmoplegic migraine (Kandt and Goldstein, 1985). The major clinical points of differentiation are the following: (1) patients with ophthalmoplegic migraine also have nonophthalmoplegic migraine attacks; (2) they have a positive family history of migraine; and (3) they do not have trigeminal nerve involvement.

Tolosa-Hunt syndrome is differentiated from orbital pseudotumor by the absence of proptosis and the presence of trigeminal nerve involvement. Other diseases of the cavernous sinus, such as tumor or thrombosis, may mimic the Tolosa-Hunt syndrome.

The erythrocyte sedimentation rate is elevated in most, but not in all, cases. Radiographs of the orbit may demonstrate erosion of bone in the sellar and parasellar regions. Arteriography reveals irregular narrowing and displacement of the cavernous portion of the carotid artery, suggesting either a vasculitis or a mass lesion.

Treatment. Prednisone, 1 mg/kg/day, is both diagnostic and therapeutic. If pain subsides within two days, the diagnosis is likely but is not assured. Other lesions in the cavernous sinus or orbit may also respond to corticosteroids. Ophthalmoplegia may subside as well, but can take several days or weeks to clear completely. Alternatively, if prednisone has no effect on symptoms, Tolosa-Hunt syndrome can be excluded and other causes must be identified.

Orbital Pseudotumor

The term orbital pseudotumor encompasses a group of nonspecific inflammatory conditions involving the orbit. Some would include the Tolosa-Hunt syndrome as part the spectrum of orbital pseudotumor. Inflammation may be diffuse or localized to specific tissues within the orbit, *orbital myositis* (Kennerdell and Dresner, 1984).

Clinical Features. The disorder is unusual in those under twenty years of age, but has been recorded as early as three months. Males and females are affected equally. Acute and chronic forms are described.

The cardinal features of acute, diffuse orbital inflammation are pain, ophthalmoplegia, proptosis, and lid edema evolving over a period of several days or weeks. Unilateral involvement is the rule. The eye is usually pushed downward as well as outward and is painful when moved. Ocular motility is disturbed in part by the proptosis, but mainly by myositis. Some patients have only myositis, whereas others may have uveitis, papillitis, scleritis, and retinitis. Vision is initially preserved, but loss of vision is a threat in untreated cases. The chronic form has an insidious onset, progresses over several months, and results in complete ophthalmoplegia.

Diagnosis. The development of unilateral pain and proptosis in a child should suggest an orbital tumor. This possibility must be excluded by ultrasonography or CT of the orbit. Bilateral proptosis suggests thyroid myopathy.

A CT scan of the orbit demonstrates a soft tissue mass without sinus involvement or bone erosion. This radiographic picture may also be seen with orbital involvement by lymphoma or leukemia. The extraocular muscles may appear enlarged (Mauriello and Flanagan, 1984).

Treatment. Orbital pseudotumor has a self-limited course, but must be treated in order to prevent loss of visual acuity or permanent ophthalmoplegia. Prednisone, 1 mg/kg/day, should be administered for at least one month and then tapered. If there is a recurrence during the tapering process, the full dose should be reinitiated.

Cavernous Sinus Thrombosis

Cavernous sinus thrombosis may produce either unilateral or bilateral ophthalmoplegia. It is almost always caused by anterograde spread of infection from the mouth, face, or nose.

Clinical Features. A typical history is the development of fever, malaise, and frontal headache following dental infection. This is followed by proptosis, orbital congestion, ptosis, external ophthalmoplegia, and sometimes pupillary paralysis (Harbour et al, 1984). The infection begins in one sinus and then spreads to the other. If untreated, the infection may extend to the meninges. Even with vigorous antibiotic treatment, the mortality rate is 15 percent.

Diagnosis. The ocular signs may suggest orbital cellulitis or orbital pseudotumor. The cerebrospinal fluid is normal early in the course. A mixed leukocytosis develops, and the protein is moderately elevated even in the absence of meningitis. Once the meninges are involved, the pressure becomes elevated, the leukocytosis increases, and the concentration of glucose falls.

Radiographs of the skull may show clouding of infected paranasal sinuses. Angiography shows attenuation or complete blockage of the cavernous portion of the carotid artery.

Treatment. The infection must be vigorously treated with intravenous antibiotics as if one were treating meningitis. Surgical drainage of infected paranasal sinuses is sometimes necessary.

Trauma

Trauma is a common cause of isolated ocular motor nerve palsies and extraocular muscle damage. Hemorrhage and edema into the nerves or muscles may occur from closed head injuries even in the absence of direct orbital injury. When orbital fracture is present, the nerves and muscles may be lacerated, avulsed, or entrapped by bone fragments.

Clinical Features. Superior oblique palsy, secondary to trochlear nerve damage, is a relatively frequent consequence of closed head injuries. Usually the trauma is severe, often causing loss of consciousness, but may be mild. The palsy is unilateral in 62 percent and bilateral in 38 percent of cases (Sydnor et al, 1982). With unilateral superior oblique palsy, there is a marked hypertropia in primary position and a compensatory head tilt to preserve fusion. Sixty-five percent resolve spontaneously. When bilateral involvement is present, the hypertropia is milder and alternates between the two eyes.

Spontaneous recovery occurs in only 25 percent.

Transient lateral rectus palsy is a rare finding in newborns that has been attributed to birth trauma (de Grauw and Rotteveel, 1983). The palsy is unilateral and clears completely within six weeks.

Diagnosis. Direct injuries to the orbit with associated hemorrhage and swelling do not pose a diagnostic dilemma. A CT scan of the head with orbital views is needed to identify the extent of fracture in order to determine the need for surgical intervention and may also demonstrate a lateral midbrain hemorrhage as the cause of a trochlear nerve palsy.

A greater problem of diagnosis occurs when there is a delay between the time of injury and the onset of ophthalmoplegia. The possible mechanisms of delayed ophthalmoplegia following trauma to the head include (1) progressive local edema in the orbit, (2) progressive brainstem edema, (3) progressive increased intracranial pressure, (4) development of meningitis, mastoiditis or petrous osteomyelitis, (5) venous sinus or carotid artery thrombosis, and (6) carotid cavernous fistula (Marmor et al, 1982).

Treatment. Local trauma and fracture of the orbit may require surgical repair. Permanent ocular motor nerve palsies following head injury are sometimes improved by surgery directed at rebalancing the extraocular muscles.

Cavernous Sinus Fistula

Clinical Features. Arteriovenous communications between the carotid artery and the cavernous sinus may be congenital, but are usually traumatic. The injury may be closed or penetrating. The carotid artery or one of its branches ruptures into the cavernous sinus, causing increased pressure in the venous system. The result is a pulsating proptosis, redness and swelling of the conjunctiva, and ophthalmoplegia. A bruit, heard over the eye, is reduced in volume by compression of the ipsilateral carotid artery.

Diagnosis. A CT scan is always the first study in patients with the acute onset of proptosis. An enlarged superior ophthalmic vein is often visualized. Intravenous digital subtraction angiography demonstrates early filling of the cavernous sinus and retrograde filling of the superior ophthalmic vein.

Treatment. Several surgical procedures are recommended, including carotid ligation, injection of fibrin glue through the superior ophthalmic vein, transcavernous electrocoagulation, and intra-arterial occlusion with a balloon catheter.

ACUTE BILATERAL OPHTHALMOPLEGIA

Many of the conditions that cause acute unilateral ophthalmoplegia (Table 15.3) may cause bilateral ophthalmoplegia as well. The conditions listed in Table 15.4 are marked by a high incidence of bilateral involvement. Thyrotoxicosis could be added to this list as well; however it is discussed instead with the chronic conditions, as progression of ophthalmoplegia is likely to occur over a period greater than one week.

Intoxications

Clinical Features. Anticonvulsants, tricyclic antidepressants, and many other psychoactive drugs selectively impair ocular motility at toxic blood concentrations. The overdose may be accidental or intentional. A child is found unconscious and brought to the emergency room. The state of consciousness may vary from obtundation to stupor, but the eyes cannot be made to move either by the doll's-head maneuver or with ice water irrigation of the ears. Complete ophthalmoplegia may be expected in a comatose child in whom other brainstem function is impaired (see Chapter 2), but not in a noncomatose child with otherwise intact brainstem function. This should immediately suggest the ingestion of a drug that selectively impairs ocular motility.

Diagnosis. The family should be questioned with reference to the drugs available in the household and the blood and urine screened for toxic substances.

Treatment. Specific treatment depends upon the drug ingested. In most cases, supportive care is sufficient.

Botulism

Botulism is caused by a toxin elaborated by several strains of the bacterium *Clostridium bot-*

Table 15.4 ACUTE BILATERAL OPHTHALMOPLEGIA

---

1. Polyradiculoneuropathy (see Chapter 7)
2. Miller Fisher syndrome (see Chapter 10)
3. Myasthenia gravis
4. Basilar meningitis (see Chapter 4)
5. Brainstem encephalitis (see Chapter 10)
6. Intoxication
7. Botulism
8. Cavernous sinus thrombosis
9. Carotid-cavernous fistula

---

ulinum. The infantile form of botulism causes ptosis but not ophthalmoplegia and is discussed in Chapter 6. This section deals with cases of later onset.

Clinical Features. Most cases are caused by ingestion of toxin from home-canned food products. This is most likely to occur when canning is done at high altitudes where the boiling temperature is too low to destroy spores (Cherrington, 1974). Botulinal spores are ubiquitous in soil, and infection may also follow burns and wounds. The initial symptoms of blurred vision, diplopia, dizziness, dysarthria, and dysphagia begin twelve to thirty-six hours after ingestion of toxin. The pupillary response is usually normal. This is followed by an ascending paralysis that suggests acute inflammatory polyradiculoneuropathy (Guillain-Barré syndrome) that may lead to death from respiratory paralysis. Patients remain conscious and alert throughout. Most patients make a complete recovery within two to three months, but those with severe involvement may not return to normal for a year.

Diagnosis. The presence of ophthalmoplegia and a normal spinal fluid examination distinguishes botulism from acute inflammatory polyradiculoneuropathy. The EMG is very useful in suggesting the diagnosis (Swift, 1981). The motor and sensory nerve conduction velocities are normal, evoked muscle action potentials are usually reduced in amplitude, and a decremental response is not ordinarily present at low rates of stimulation, but facilitation may be present at high rates of stimulation.

Definitive diagnosis requires the demonstration of the organism or the toxin in food, stool, or wound.

Treatment. The administration of antitoxin, 20,000 to 40,000 units two or three times a day, is recommended. The stomach and intestinal contents should be emptied. Guanidine, 35 mg/kg, is effective in some patients and should be used for those with potential respiratory failure. Mechanical respiratory support must be immediately available to every patient as soon as the diagnosis is suspected.

CHRONIC BILATERAL OPHTHALMOPLEGIA

The conditions responsible for bilateral ophthalmoplegia developing over a period longer than one week are listed in Table 15.5. Most have been discussed in previous sections of this chapter or in other chapters.

Table 15.5 CHRONIC BILATERAL
OPHTHALMOPLEGIA

Myasthenia gravis
   Juvenile
   Congenital
Brainstem glioma
Myopathies
   Fiber type disproportion myopathy (see Chapter 6)
   Myotubular myopathy (see Chapter 6)
   Mitochondrial myopathies (see Chapter 6, 7, 8)
Thyrotoxicosis
Chronic meningitis (see Chapter 4)
Chronic orbital inflammation
Vitamin E deficiency

Thyrotoxicosis

Clinical Features. Disorders of ocular motility are present in the majority of patients with hyperthyroidism and may precede systemic features of nervousness, diaphoresis, weight loss, tachycardia, tremulousness, and weakness. The major pathology in the orbit is a myopathy of the extraocular muscles. They become swollen with edema and finally fibrotic. If the two eyes are affected equally, the patient may not complain of diplopia despite considerable limitation of ocular motility. Lid retraction (Dalrymple sign) occurs in more than 50 percent of cases, lid lag on downward gaze (von Graefe sign) in 30 to 50 percent, and proptosis (exophthalmos) in almost 90 percent. Severe exophthalmos is due to edema and infiltration of all orbital structures.

Diagnosis. Thyroid disease should be considered in any child with evolving ophthalmoplegia. A CT scan of the orbit demonstrates enlargement of the extraocular muscles. This must be followed by direct measurement of plasma thyroxine, triiodothyronine, and thyroid-stimulating hormone concentrations. If these are normal but the diagnosis remains suspect, a thyroid-releasing hormone stimulation test and a measure of the concentration of thyroid-stimulating immunoglobulin may be confirmatory.

Treatment. Treatment of the underlying thyroid problem does not necessarily cure the ophthalmopathy. If the exophthalmos progresses even after the patient is euthyroid, corticosteroids may be useful in preventing further proptosis, but surgical decompression is indicated if there is optic nerve compression.

■ Gaze Palsies

This section deals with supranuclear palsies. In order to verify that a palsy is supranuclear and not due to an abnormality of the ocular motor nuclei or nerves, ocular muscles, or myasthenia, it is necessary to demonstrate that the eyes move normally in response to brainstem reflexes, such as doll's-head maneuver, caloric testing, and Bell's phenomenon. The differential diagnosis of gaze palsies is listed in Table 15.6.

OCULAR MOTOR APRAXIA

Ocular motor apraxia is characterized by a deficiency in voluntary horizontal lateral fast eye movements (saccades) with retention of slow pursuit movements. Jerking movements of the head are used to bring the eyes to a desired position. The rapid phase of optokinetic nystagmus is absent.

Congenital Ocular Motor Apraxia

Clinical Features. Although congenital, the disorder is not usually noted until infancy. Blind-

Table 15.6 GAZE PALSIES

Ocular Motor Apraxia
1. Congenital
2. Ataxia telangiectasia (see Chapter 10)
3. Brainstem tumor
4. Gaucher disease III (see Chapter 5)
5. Niemann-Pick disease type C (see Chapter 5)

Internuclear Ophthalmoplegia (INO)
1. Multiple sclerosis (see Chapter 10)
2. Brainstem tumor
3. Toxic-metabolic
4. Brainstem stroke
5. Myasthenia gravis (pseudo-INO)
6. Exotropia (pseudo-INO)

Vertical Gaze Palsy
1. Tumor (see Chapter 4)
   a. Third ventricle
   b. Midbrain
   c. Pineal region
2. Aqueductal stenosis (see Chapter 18)
3. Hydrocephalus (see Chapter 4, 18)
4. DAF syndrome
5. Vitamin B_{12} deficiency
6. Miller Fisher syndrome (see Chapter 10)
7. Congenital vertical ocular motor apraxia

Horizontal Gaze Palsy
1. Destructive lesions of the frontal lobe (see Chapter 11)
2. Adversive seizures (see Chapter 1)
3. Brainstem tumors
4. Familial horizontal palsy

Convergence Palsy
1. Head trauma
2. Pineal region tumors (see Chapter 4)
3. Multiple sclerosis (see Chapter 10)
4. Idiopathic

ness may be suspected, because of failure of fixation. Instead, overshooting head thrusts, often accompanied by blinking of the eyes, are used instead for refixation. When the head is held immobilized, the child makes no effort at initiating horizontal eye movements (Zee et al, 1977).

Many children with ocular motor apraxia have other signs of cerebral abnormality, such as psychomotor retardation, learning disabilities, and clumsiness. When hypotonia is present, the child may have difficulty in making the head movements needed for refixation. Agenesis of the corpus callosum and agenesis of the vermis of the cerebellum have been described in several patients with congenital ocular motor apraxia. These malformations are more likely to be associated with, than responsible for, ocular motor apraxia.

Diagnosis. The possibility of ocular motor apraxia must be considered in any infant referred for evaluation of blindness. Once the presence of apraxia is established, CT is indicated to search for other cerebral malformations and studies should be performed to determine if the child has ataxia-telangiectasia (see Chapter 10) or a lysosomal storage disease (see Chapter 5).

Treatment. Treatment is not available.

INTERNUCLEAR OPHTHALMOPLEGIA

The medial longitudinal fasciculus (MLF) contains fibers that connect the abducens nucleus to the contralateral oculomotor nucleus for the purpose of performing horizontal conjugate lateral gaze. Unilateral lesions in the MLF disconnect the two nuclei, so that when the patient attempts lateral gaze, the adducting eye ipsilateral to the abnormal MLF is unable to move medially but the abducting eye is able to move laterally. Nystagmus is often present in the abducting eye. This symptom complex, which may be unilateral or bilateral, is called internuclear ophthalmoplegia (INO). Unilateral INO is most often caused by vascular occlusive disease. Bilateral INO usually results from demyelinating disease or toxic-metabolic causes.

Patients with myasthenia gravis sometimes have ocular motility dysfunction that resembles an INO, except that nystagmus is usually lacking. It is referred to as pseudo-INO, because the MLF is intact. Pseudo-INO can also be caused by exotropia (Ellenberger and Daroff, 1984). When the normal eye is fixating in full abduction,

there is no visual stimulus to bring the paretic eye into full adduction. Nystagmus is not present in the abducting eye.

The combination of an INO in one direction of lateral gaze and a complete gaze palsy in the other is called a one-and-a-half syndrome. The syndrome is caused by a unilateral lesion in the dorsal pontine tegmentum affecting the pontine lateral gaze center and the adjacent MLF. It is most often due to multiple sclerosis but may also be caused by brainstem glioma or infarction (Wall and Wray, 1980).

Toxic-Metabolic

Clinical Features. Toxic doses of several drugs may produce the clinical syndrome of INO. The patient is usually found comatose and may have complete ophthalmoplegia at first which then evolves into a bilateral INO, or the patient may demonstrate a bilateral INO at onset. The drugs that are reported to produce INO include amitriptyline, barbiturates, doxepin, phenothiazine, carbamazepine, and phenytoin. INO may also occur during hepatic coma.

Diagnosis. Drug intoxications are always a consideration in children who were previously well and then experience states of decreased consciousness. The presence of an INO following a drug ingestion limits the possibilities to anticonvulsant and psychotropic drugs.

Treatment. The INO resolves as the blood concentration of the drug falls.

VERTICAL GAZE PALSY

Children with supranuclear vertical gaze palsies are unable to look upward and/or downward fully; however, they retain reflex eye movements such as the Bell phenomenon. Disorders of upward gaze in children are generally due to lesions in the region of the dorsal midbrain and are almost always caused by tumors in the pineal region or aqueductal stenosis. The usual features are impaired upward and downward gaze, eyelid retraction, occasional disturbances in horizontal movement, convergence, and skew deviation. Mydriasis with light-near dissociation is an early feature of extrinsic compression of the dorsal midbrain. Isolated paralysis of upward gaze may be the initial feature of the Miller Fisher syndrome (Keane and Finstead, 1982) and of vitamin B_{12} or B_1 deficiency (Sandyk, 1984).

Isolated disturbances of downward gaze are caused by bilateral lesions in the midbrain reticular formation. They are rare in children, but may occur in neurovisceral lipid storage disease.

DAF Syndrome

The acronym DAF stands for the triad of downward gaze palsy, ataxia, and foam cells (Cogan et al, 1981). The disorder is generally regarded as a variant of either Niemann-Pick disease or sea-blue histiocytosis. Siblings are affected, and autosomal recessive inheritance is probable.

Clinical Features. Onset is usually between the ages of ten and twenty. Downward gaze palsy occurs first, followed by upward gaze palsy and then horizontal palsy. The end result is complete ophthalmoplegia. Saccadic movements are affected more than are pursuit movements, and head thrusting may be present to move the eyes in the vertical plane. The initial eye signs are followed by evidence of generalized cerebral disease (Ashwal et al, 1984). Prominent features are ataxia, dystonia, spasticity, and dementia. Seizures are sometimes associated. Splenomegaly is common, and hepatomegaly may be present as well. As a rule, visceromegaly is a more prominent feature when the onset of the disorder occurs in a child younger than two years of age.

Diagnosis. Characteristic storage cells are present in the bone marrow and resemble either the foamy histiocytes of Niemann-Pick disease or sea-blue histiocytes. When treated with Wright stain, foamy histiocytes have a foamy cytoplasm that is thought to be filled with ceramide or sphingolipids and sea-blue histiocytes that have a blue cytoplasm and blue granules that correspond to types of abnormal cytosomes.

Treatment. Treatment is not available.

Congenital Vertical Ocular Motor Apraxia

Clinical Features. This rare syndrome is similar to congenital horizontal ocular motor apraxia, except for the direction of gaze palsy. At rest, the eyes are fixed in either an upward or downward position with little random movement (Hughes et al, 1985). Initially, head flexion or extension is used to fixate in the vertical plane; later the child learns to use head thrusts. The Bell phenomenon is present.

Diagnosis. Vertical gaze palsy suggests the possibility of intracranial tumor, and CT must be performed. However, the presence of a gaze palsy from birth without the development of other neurologic signs usually indicates a nonprogressive process. Bilateral restriction of upward eye movement due to muscle fibrosis must be considered as well (Tychsen et al, 1986). However, in children with ocular motor apraxia, the eyes can move upward reflexly or by forced ductions; in children with muscle fibrosis, the eyes will not move upward by any means.

HORIZONTAL GAZE PALSY

Inability to look to one side is generally caused by a lesion in the contralateral frontal or ipsilateral pontine gaze center. In such cases, the eyes are tonically deviated towards the side of the lesion and contralateral hemiplegia is often present as well. The eyes can be made to move horizontally by stimulation of the pontine gaze center with ice water calorics.

In contrast, an irritative lesion, such as an epileptic seizure, generally causes the eyes to deviate in a direction opposite to the side with the seizure focus. Movements of the head and eyes during a seizure are called *adversive seizures* (see Chapter 1). The initial direction of eye movement is generally reliable in predicting a contralateral focus, especially if the movement is forced and sustained in a unilateral direction (Wyllie et al, 1986). Later movements that are mild and unsustained are not predictive.

CONVERGENCE PALSY

Convergence palsy, inability to adduct the eyes to focus on a near object in the absence of medial rectus palsies, can occur from pineal region tumors; in such cases, however, other signs of midbrain compression are usually present as well. Convergence palsy is sometimes factitious or due to lack of motivation or attention; this can be identified by the absence of pupillary constriction on attempted convergence.

Convergence insufficiency is frequently encountered after closed head injuries (Krohel et al, 1986). The head injury need not be severe to produce symptoms. Diplopia, headache, or eyestrain is reported during reading or other close work. Treatment consists of convergence exercises or prisms. Convergence insufficiency also occurs in the absence of prior head injury. The age of onset is fifteen or later, and women are affected more often than men.

■ Nystagmus

Nystagmus is an involuntary, rhythmic oscillation of the eyes in which at least one phase is slow. With *pendular nystagmus*, the movements in each direction are slow. The oscillations are in the horizontal plane even on upward and downward gaze. On lateral gaze, the oscillations may change to jerk nystagmus. *Jerk nystagmus* is characterized by movements that are unequal in speed. There is first a slow component in one direction, then a fast component in the other. Oscillation may be horizontal or vertical. The direction of nystagmus is named for the fast component. Nystagmus intensity increases in the horizontal plane when gaze is in the direction of the fast phase (Alexander law).

Table 15.7 describes other eye movements that cannot be classified as nystagmus but that have diagnostic significance. *Opsoclonus* consists of conjugate, rapid, chaotic movements in all directions of gaze, often referred to as "dancing eyes." It occurs in infants with occult and overt neuroblastoma and in idiopathic encephalopathy (see Chapter 10). *Ocular flutter* is a brief burst of conjugate, horizontal, saccadic eye movements that interrupt fixation. It may be seen in the recovery phase of opsoclonus or in association with cerebellar disease. *Ocular dysmetria* is either an overshoot of the eyes during refixation or an oscillation before the eyes come to rest on a new fixation target. *Ocular bobbing* is not downbeat nystagmus, but rather a sudden downward movement of both eyes with a slow drift back to midposition. It is most often seen in comatose patients with pontine dysfunction.

Congenital nystagmus and acquired nystagmus are best discussed separately because the differential diagnosis of each is different (Table 15.8).

Table 15.7 ABNORMAL EYE MOVEMENTS

Movement	Appearance	Pathology
Nystagmus	Rhythmic oscillation	Variable
Opsoclonus	Nonrhythmic, chaotic conjugate movements	Neuroblastoma, encephalitis
Ocular flutter	Intermittent bursts of rapid, horizontal, oscillations during fixation	Cerebellar disease
Ocular dysmetria	Overshooting or oscillation on refixation	Cerebellar disease
Ocular bobbing	Intermittent, rapid downward movement	Pontine lesions

Table 15.8 DIFFERENTIAL DIAGNOSIS OF NYSTAGMUS

Congenital
1. Associated with blindness
2. Familial
3. Idiopathic

Spasmus Nutans
1. Idiopathic
2. Tumors of optic nerve and chiasm (see Chapter 16)

Acquired Nystagmus
1. Pendular
   a. Spasmus nutans
   b. Multiple sclerosis (see Chapter 10)
   c. Brainstem infarction
   d. Oculopalatal syndrome
      (1) Spinocerebellar degeneration
      (2) Brainstem infarction
2. Jerk
   a. Horizontal
      (1) Drug induced
      (2) Vestibular nystagmus
      (3) Ictal
   b. Vertical
      (1) Upbeat
      (2) Downbeat
3. Dissociated
   a. Monocular
   b. Divergence
   c. See-saw
   d. Convergence

CONGENITAL NYSTAGMUS

Although congenital nystagmus is present at birth, it may not be noticed until infancy or childhood and then poses as acquired nystagmus. One reason why it may not be noticed is that the *null point*, the angle of ocular movement at which the nystagmus is minimal, may be very wide (Gresty et al, 1984). Often, the nystagmus is observed but is mistaken for normal movement.

The cause of congenital nystagmus is thought to be a defect in the slow eye movement system. There is considerable controversy between neurologists and ophthalmologists as to whether or not congenital nystagmus can be caused by diminished visual acuity (Dell'Osso, 1984). It had generally been held that loss of visual acuity, of any cause, before the age of two can produce nystagmus and that the nystagmus is reversed by correction of the visual disturbance. Recently, the thesis has been advanced that the visual defect is not causal, but associated, and serves to intensify the underlying defect in neural control.

Congenital nystagmus is sometimes inherited. The pattern of inheritance can be autosomal recessive, autosomal dominant, or X-linked.

Clinical Features. Both pendular and jerk nystagmus may be present. The jerk nystagmus can be unidirectional or bidirectional. A characteristic feature is an exponentially increasing, slow-phase velocity. Optokinetic nystagmus is almost always abnormal and usually demonstrates a reversed response; the fast phase is in the direction of rotation of the drum. A bidirectionally reversed optokinetic response is said to be pathognomonic of congenital nystagmus. The slow phase of pursuit is impaired in the majority of patients.

Two forms of head oscillation may be associated with congenital nystagmus. One is involuntary and does not improve vision. The other, also seen in spasmus nutans, is opposite in direction to the nystagmus and does improve vision. Many children have impaired vision from the nystagmus in the absence of a primary disturbance in visual acuity.

In addition to having tremor, the child may turn or tilt the head to the null zone where the nystagmus intensity is minimum. Periodic head turning may accompany periodic alternating nystagmus in an effort to maintain the direction of gaze in the null zone for optimal visual acuity.

Diagnosis. It is important, but not always possible, to determine that the nystagmus was present at birth. The eyes must be carefully examined for abnormalities in the sensory system that may be accentuating nystagmus. If the neurologic examination is otherwise normal, CT is not necessary.

Treatment. Nystagmus may be reduced by correcting a visual defect and by the use of prisms to move the eyes into the null zone without the head turning.

SPASMUS NUTANS

Spasmus nutans is difficult to classify as either a congenital or acquired nystagmus. It is probably never present at birth; the onset is early in infancy. It is a clinical entity characterized by nystagmus, head nodding, and abnormal head positioning.

Clinical Features. Onset typically occurs between six and twelve months of age. Nystagmus is characteristically binocular (but may be monocular), high-frequency and low-amplitude, and can be horizontal, vertical, or torsional in direction (King et al, 1986; Weissman et al, 1987). The head is held in a tilted position, and a titubation that resembles nodding is present. Head tilt and movement may be more promi-

nent than nystagmus, and torticollis is frequently the presenting complaint (see Chapter 14). The syndrome usually lasts one to two years, sometimes as long as five, and then resolves spontaneously. The incidence of later refractive errors may be higher in children with a history of spasmus nutans.

Diagnosis. Spasmus nutans is ordinarily a transitory, benign disorder of unknown cause. On rare occasions, the syndrome may be mimicked by a glioma of the anterior visual pathways (Albright et al, 1984), or by subacute necrotizing encephalopathy (see Chapter 10). The suspicion of tumor is greater if the nystagmus is monocular (Farmer and Hoyt, 1984). Therefore, CT of the head and orbit are recommended in most cases.

Treatment. Treatment is not available, nor is it needed.

ACQUIRED NYSTAGMUS

Pendular Nystagmus

Pendular nystagmus may be either congenital or acquired. In adults, the usual causes of acquired pendular nystagmus are brainstem infarction or multiple sclerosis. In children, pendular nystagmus in the absence of other neurologic signs is either congenital or the first sign of spasmus nutans. The development of optic atrophy in a child with pendular nystagmus indicates a glioma of the anterior visual pathway (Lavery et al, 1984).

A high-frequency (1 to 3 Hz), low-amplitude, pendular oscillation of the eyes occurs in normal people when lateral gaze is sustained to the point of fatigue (fatigue nystagmus). It has no clinical significance except its recognition as a normal phenomenon.

Vertical pendular nystagmus is unusual and sometimes occurs in association with rhythmic vertical oscillations of the palate (palatal myoclonus). This syndrome of oculopalatal oscillation is encountered in some spinocerebellar degenerations and ischemic disorders of the deep cerebellar nuclei and central tegmental tract.

Jerk Nystagmus

A physiologic jerk nystagmus is present at the endpoint of lateral gaze in many individuals (Abel et al, 1978). A few beats are usual, but even sustained nystagmus occurring at the endpoint should be considered normal unless it is associated with other signs of neurologic dysfunction or is distinctly asymmetric in right or left direction.

Drug-Induced Nystagmus

Clinical Features. Many psychoactive drugs, including tranquilizers, antidepressants, and anticonvulsants, produce nystagmus at high therapeutic or toxic blood concentrations. The nystagmus is horizontal or horizontal-rotary and is augmented by lateral gaze. Vertical nystagmus may be present on upward, but rarely on downward, gaze (Dell'Osso, 1984). Phenytoin and carbamazepine may occasionally produce downbeat nystagmus as well.

Diagnosis. Drug-induced nystagmus is very common and should be considered in any patient taking psychoactive drugs. Drug overdose should be suspected in patients with nystagmus and states of decreased consciousness. The diagnosis is confirmed by measuring the drug blood concentration.

Treatment. Nystagmus resolves when the drug blood concentration falls.

Vestibular Nystagmus

Vestibular nystagmus may occur with disorders of the labyrinth, vestibular nerve, vestibular nuclei of the brainstem, or cerebellum.

Clinical Features. Labyrinthine disease (especially labyrinthitis) is usually associated with severe vertigo, nausea, and vomiting. Deafness or tinnitus is frequently present as well. All symptoms and signs are enhanced by movement of the head, and motion may be more critical to the mechanism of nystagmus than the position obtained. Nystagmus is usually horizontal and torsional, with an initial slow component, followed by a rapid return. It is worse when gaze is in the direction of the fast phase. Fixation reduces nystagmus and vertigo.

Vertigo and nausea are mild when nystagmus is of central origin. Nystagmus is constantly present and not affected by head position. It may be horizontal or vertical and does not improve with fixation. Other neurologic disturbances referable to the brainstem or cerebellum are frequently associated.

Diagnosis. Vestibular nystagmus is readily identified by observation and is identical to the nystagmus provoked by caloric stimulation or rotation. Labyrinthine disorders in children are almost always infectious, sometimes viral, and sometimes secondary to otitis media. Central causes of vestibular nystagmus include spinocerebellar degenerations, brainstem glioma or infarction, subacute necrotizing encephalomyelitis, and demyelinating disorders.

Treatment. Vertigo and nausea associated with labyrinthine disease are appreciably improved by several different classes of drugs. Diazepam is especially effective. Other useful drugs include scopolamine, antihistamines, and tranquilizers.

Ictal Nystagmus

Clinical Features. Nystagmus as a seizure manifestation can be binocular or monocular (Jacome and FitzGerald, 1982); jerk, pendular or rotary; and may occur either alone or in association with other ictal manifestations. Pupillary oscillations synchronous with the nystagmus may be observed (Lavin, 1986). As a rule, concurrent epileptiform discharges are focal, contralateral to the fast phase of nystagmus, and frontal, parieto-occipital, or occipital in location. However, there are individual case reports of nystagmus accompanying generalized 3 Hz spike and wave discharges, ipsilateral focal discharges, and periodic lateralized epileptiform discharges.

Diagnosis. Ordinarily, other seizure manifestations are present that identify the nature of the nystagmus. The electroencephalogram (EEG) confirms the diagnosis by the presence of epileptiform activity concurrent with nystagmus.

Treatment. Ictal nystagmus responds to anticonvulsant drug therapy (see Chapter 1).

Upbeat Nystagmus

Clinical Features. In primary position, the eyes drift slowly downward and then spontaneously beat upward. A large and small-amplitude type are described (Daroff and Troost, 1973). Large-amplitude nystagmus increases in intensity during upward gaze and indicates a lesion in the anterior vermis of the cerebellum. Small-amplitude nystagmus decreases in intensity during upward gaze and indicates an intrinsic lesion of the medulla.

Diagnosis. Upbeat nystagmus is usually an acquired disorder caused by vascular lesions or tumors of the brainstem or cerebellum. Therefore, CT or MRI is indicated in every case. It is also reported with impairment of smooth pursuit movements in a familial cerebellar vermian atrophy transmitted by autosomal dominant inheritance (Furman et al, 1986).

Treatment. No specific treatment is available.

Downbeat Nystagmus

Clinical Features. In primary position, the eyes drift slowly upward and then spontaneously beat downward. The intensity of the nystagmus is usually greatest when the eyes are directed slightly downward and laterally (Daroff Rule). Downbeat nystagmus should be distinguished from *downward beating nystagmus* in which the nystagmus is present only on downward gaze. Downward beating nystagmus is usually caused by toxic doses of anticonvulsant and sedative drugs, while downbeat nystagmus indicates a structural abnormality of the brainstem, especially the cervicomedullary junction or cerebellum.

Patient complaints include oscillopsia, blurred vision, or difficulty reading. Approximately one third of patients are asymptomatic. Cerebellar ataxia is present in about half of patients and usually is the only associated neurologic sign (Halmagyi et al, 1983).

Diagnosis. Cerebellar degenerations, both congenital and acquired, are the most common identifiable cause. The Arnold-Chiari malformation must be considered as well. Metabolic disturbances include thiamine deficiency, phenytoin toxicity, and hypomagnesemia secondary either to dietary depletion or the use of lithium salts.

A congenital hereditary downbeat nystagmus was described in a mother and son (Bixenman, 1983). It was noted in the boy at birth, and by infancy he needed to keep his chin down in order to look at people. He had no other neurologic abnormalities, but the nystagmus caused difficulty in learning to read. His mother had a subclinical downbeat nystagmus evident only in oblique downward gaze.

Treatment. Oscillopsia can be improved in some individuals by the use of clonazepam (Currie and Matsuo, 1986). A single test dose of 1 to 2 mg can be tried to determine whether long-term therapy will be useful. Trihexyphenidyl may prove effective when clonazepam fails. Prisms that increase convergence may be useful as well.

Monocular Nystagmus

Monocular nystagmus may be congenital or acquired. The two most important diagnostic considerations in children are spasmus nutans and chiasmal tumors (Farmer and Hoyt, 1984). Although no clinical feature consistently separates the two groups, optic nerve anomalies, especially optic hypoplasia, are sometimes found in children with tumors but not in those with spasmus nutans.

A coarse, pendular, vertical nystagmus may develop in an amblyopic eye years after the visual loss (Smith et al, 1982). It is noted in the blind eye when distance fixation is attempted with the sighted eye and is inhibited by convergence.

Divergence Nystagmus

Divergence nystagmus is a rare condition in which each eye beats outward simultaneously. The mechanism is poorly understood, but suggests an abnormality in the posterior fossa and may be seen with spinocerebellar degenerations.

See-Saw Nystagmus

This unusual ocular movement is the result of two different oscillations. One is a pendular vertical oscillation, the other a torsional movement in which one eye rises and intorts while the other falls and extorts. It may be congenital or acquired. The congenital form is sometimes associated with a horizontal pendular nystagmus. Acquired cases are usually due to tumors of the sellar and parasellar regions.

References

1. Abel LA, Parker L, Daroff RB, et al: End-point nystagmus. Invest Ophthalmol Visual Sci 17:539, 1978.
2. Albright AL, Sclabassi RJ, Slamovits TL, et al: Spasmus nutans associated with optic gliomas in infants. J Pediatr 105:778, 1984.
3. Apt L, Axelrod RN: Generalized fibrosis of the extraocular muscles. Am J Ophthalmol 85:822, 1978.
4. Ashwal S, Thrasher TV, Rice DR, et al: A new form of sea-blue histiocytosis associated with progressive anterior horn cell and axonal degeneration. Ann Neurol 16:184, 1984.
5. Bixenman WW: Congenital hereditary downbeat nystagmus. Can J Ophthalmol 18:344, 1983.
6. Cherrington M: Botulism. Ten-year experience. Arch Neurol 30:432, 1974.
7. Cogan DG, Chu FC, Bachman DM, et al: The DAF syndrome. Neuroophthalmology 2:7, 1981.
8. Cohen ME, Duffner MD, Heffner RR, et al: Prognostic factors in brainstem gliomas. Neurology 36:602, 1986.
9. Crawford JS: Disease of the orbit. In Toronto Hospital for Sick Children, Department of Ophthalmology: The Eye in Childhood. Year Book Medical Publishers, Chicago, 1967, p 331.
10. Currie JN, Matsuo V: The use of clonazepam in the treatment of nystagmus-induced oscillopsia. Ophthalmology 93:924, 1986.
11. Daroff RB: The office Tensilon test for myasthenia gravis. Arch Neurol 43:843, 1986.
12. Daroff RB, Troost BT: Up-beat nystagmus. JAMA 225:312, 1973.
13. de Grauw AJC, Rotteveel JJ: Transient sixth cranial nerve paralysis in the newborn infant. Neuropediatrie 14:164, 1983.
14. Dell'Osso LF: Nystagmus and other ocular motor oscillations and intrusions. In Lessell S, van Dalen JTW,

eds. Neuro-ophthalmology 1984. Volume 3, Elsevier, Amsterdam, 1984.

15. Durkan GP, Troost BT, Slamovits TL, et al: Recurrent painless oculomotor palsy in children. A variant of ophthalmoplegic migraine? Headache 21:58, 1981.

16. Ellenberger C, Daroff RB: Neuro-ophthalmic aspects of multiple sclerosis. In Poser CM, ed. The Diagnosis of Multiple Sclerosis. Grune & Stratton, New York, 1984, p 49.

17. Epstein F, McCleary EL: Intrinsic brain-stem tumors of childhood: surgical indications. J Neurosurg 64:11, 1986.

18. Farmer J, Hoyt CS: Monocular nystagmus in infancy and early childhood. Am J Ophthalmol 98:504, 1984.

19. Fenichel GM: Clinical syndromes of myasthenia in infancy and childhood: A review. Arch Neurol 34:97, 1978.

20. Furman JMR, Baloh RW, Yee RD: Eye movement abnormalities in a family with cerebellar vermian atrophy. Acta Otolaryngol (Stockh) 101:371, 1986.

21. Gath I, Kayan A, Leegaard J, et al: Myasthenia congenita, electromyographic findings. Acta Neurol Scand 46:323, 1970.

22. Gresty ME, Page N, Barratt H: The differential diagnosis of congenital nystagmus. J Neurol Neurosurg Psychiatry 47:936, 1984.

23. Halmagyi GM, Rudge P, Gresty MA, et al: Downbeating nystagmus. A review of 62 cases. Arch Neurol 40:777, 1983.

24. Harbour RC, Trobe JD, Ballinger WE: Septic cavernous sinus thrombosis associated with gingivitis and parapharyngeal abscess. Arch Ophthalmol 102:94, 1984.

25. Hickey WF, Wagoner MD: Bilateral congenital absence of the abducens nerve. Virchows Arch 402:91, 1983.

26. Hoyt CS, Mousel DK, Weber AA: Transient supranuclear disturbances of gaze in healthy neonates. Am J Ophthalmol 89:708, 1980.

27. Hughes JL, O'Connor PS, Larsen PD, et al: Congenital vertical ocular motor apraxia. J Clin Neuro-ophthalmol 5:153, 1985.

28. Jacome DE, FitzGerald R: Monocular ictal nystagmus. Arch Neurol 39:653, 1982.

29. Kandt RS, Goldstein GW: Steroid-responsive ophthalmoplegia in a child. Diagnostic considerations. Arch Neurol 42:589, 1985.

30. Keane JR, Finstead BA: Upward gaze paralysis as the initial sign of Fisher's syndrome. Arch Neurol 39:781, 1982.

31. Kennerdell JS, Dresner SC: The nonspecific orbital inflammatory syndromes. Surv Ophthalmol 29:93, 1984.

32. King RA, Nelson LB, Wagner RS: Spasmus nutans. A benign clinical entity? Arch Ophthalmol 104:1501, 1986.

33. Kissel JT, Burde RM, Klingele TG, et al: Pupil-sparing oculomotor palsies with internal carotid-posterior communicating artery aneurysms. Ann Neurol 13:149, 1983.

34. Knox DL, Clark DB, Schuster FF: Benign VI nerve palsies in childhood. Pediatrics 40:560, 1967.

35. Krohel GB, Kristan RW, Simon JW, et al: Posttraumatic convergence insufficiency. Ann Ophthalmol 18:101, 1986.

36. Lavery MA, O'Neill JF, Chu FC, Martyn LJ: Acquired nystagmus in early childhood: A presenting sign of intracranial tumor. Ophthalmology 91:425, 1984.

37. Lavin PJM: Pupillary oscillations synchronous with ictal nystagmus. Neuro-ophthalmology 6:113, 1986.

38. Magoon E, Scott AB: Botulinum toxin chemodenervation in infants and children: An alternative to incisional strabismus surgery. J Pediatr 110:719, 1987.

39. Marmor M, Wertenbaker C, Berstien L: Delayed ophthalmoplegia following head trauma. Surv Ophthalmol 27:126, 1982.

40. Mauriello JA, Flanagan JC: Management of orbital inflammatory disease. A protocol. Surv Ophthalmol 29:104, 1984.

41. Mossman S, Vincent A, Newsome-Davis J: Myasthenia gravis without acetylcholine receptor antibody: A distinct disease entity. Lancet 1:116, 1986.

42. Nelson LB: Diagnosis and management of strabismus and amblyopia. Pediatr Clin North Am 30:1003, 1983.

43. Oh SJ, Eslami N, Nishihira T, et al: Electrophysiological and clinical correlation in myasthenia gravis. Ann Neurol 12:348, 1982.

44. Prakash P, Menon V, Ghosh G: Congenital fibrosis of superior rectus and superior oblique: a case report. Br J Ophthalmol 69:57, 1985.

45. Rodriguez M, Gomez MR, Howard FM, et al: Myasthenia gravis in children: Long-term follow-up. Ann Neurol 13:504, 1983.

46. Rollinson RD, Fenichel GM: Relapsing ocular myasthenia. Neurology 31:325, 1981.

47. Sandyk R: Paralysis of upward gaze as a presenting symptom of vitamin B12 deficiency. Eur Neurol 23:198, 1984.

48. Smith JL, Flynn JT, Spiro HJ: Monocular vertical oscillations of amblyopia: The Hermann-Bielschowsky phenomenon. J Clin Neuro-ophthalmol 2:85, 1982.

49. Stroink AR, Hoffman HJ, Hendrick AB, et al: Diagnosis and management of pediatric brain-stem gliomas. J Neurosurg 65:745, 1986.

50. Swift TR: Disorders of neuromuscular transmission other than myasthenia gravis. Muscle Nerve 4:334, 1981.

51. Sydnor CF, Sheaber JH, Buckley EG: Traumatic superior oblique palsies. Ophthalmology 89:134, 1982.

52. Tachibana M, Hoshino A, Nishimura H, et al: Duane's syndrome associated with crocodile tear and ear malformation. Arch Otolaryngol 110:761, 1984.

53. Tychsen L, Imes RK, Hoyt WF: Bilateral congenital restriction of upward eye movement. Arch Neurol 43:95, 1986.

54. Victor DI: The diagnosis of congenital unilateral third-nerve palsy. Brain 99:711, 1976.

55. Vijayan N: Ophthalmoplegic migraine: Ischemic or compressive neuropathy? Headache 20:300, 1980.

56. von Noorden GK, Murray E, Wong SY: Superior oblique paralysis. A review of 270 cases. Arch Ophthalmol 104:1771, 1986.

57. Wall M, Wray SH: The one-and-a-half syndrome. A unilateral disorder of the pontine tegmentum: A study of twenty cases and review of the literature. Neurology 33:971, 1980.

58. Wang FM, Wertenbaker C, Behrens MM, et al: Acquired Brown's syndrome in children with juvenile rheumatoid arthritis. Ophthalmology 91:23, 1984.

59. Weissman BM, Dell'Osso LF, Abel LA, et al: Spasmus nutans. A quantitative prospective study. Arch Ophthalmol 105:525, 1987.

60. Wyllie E, Luders H, Morris HM, et al: The lateralizing significance of versive head and eye movements during epileptic seizures. Neurology 36:606, 1986.

61. Youssefi B: Orbital tumors in children: A clinical study of 62 cases. J Pediatr Ophthalmol 6:177, 1969.

62. Zee DS, Yee RD, Singer HS: Congenital ocular motor apraxia. Brain 100:581, 1977.

16 Disorders of the Visual System

Congenital blindness and acquired visual loss in childhood are frequently associated with neurologic disorders. In newborns and infants, visual loss may be brought to neurologic, rather than ophthalmologic, attention because of nystagmus or abnormal development. Ophthalmologic abnormalities such as clouding of the cornea and cataracts are often the first clue to neurologic or systemic disorders. In older children, loss of visual acuity may present as strabismus, declining school performance, withdrawal and irritability, or clumsiness. The terms used in reference to disturbed vision are defined in Table 16.1 (Martyn, 1983).

■ Assessment of Visual Acuity

The assessment of visual acuity in preverbal children is difficult, and there are no universally accepted tests or norms of visual acuity for children under the age of six (Simons, 1983). Clinical assessment requires careful observation of the manner in which an infant or young child interacts with the environment (Hoyt et al, 1982).

CLINICAL ASSESSMENT

The pupillary light reflex is an excellent test of the functional integrity of the afferent and efferent pathways and is reliably present after 31 weeks' gestation. A blink response to light develops at about the same time, and the lid may remain closed for as long as light is present, i.e., *the dazzle reflex.* The blink response to threat is a learned response and may not be present until five months. These responses are integrated in the brainstem and do not provide information on the cognitive (cortical) aspects of vision.

Fixation and following are the principal means to assess visual function in newborns and infants. The human face, at a distance of approximately 30 cm, is the best target for fixation. After fixation is obtained, the examiner slowly moves laterally from side to side to test the following response. The child's head should be fixed to avoid eliciting a vestibulo-ocular reflex. After fixation and following are tested, the vestibulo-ocular reflex can be stimulated by rotating the child. Normal term newborns develop nystagmus, which is inhibited within three seconds by visual fixation. In blind children, nystagmus continues for up to fifteen seconds.

Visually directed grasping is always present in normal children by three months of age. How-

Table 16.1 DEFINITIONS

Amblyopia	Defective visual acuity after correction of refractive error, customarily reserved for visual loss associated with strabismus.
Amaurosis	Partial or total loss of vision.
Cortical blindness	Visual loss due to cerebral disease uncomplicated by abnormalities of the orbit or anterior visual pathways.
Obscurations	Transitory episodes of visual loss or blurring.
Photopsias	Abnormal visual sensations (hallucinations) such as flashing lights.
Scotoma	A visual field defect. *Central scotoma* involves the point of fixation and indicates macular or optic nerve disease. *Ceco-central scotoma* involves the blind spot and suggests optic nerve disease. *Arcuate scotoma* follows the pattern of the retinal fiber bundles and indicates retinal or optic nerve disease.

321

ever, it is difficult to test in children younger than six months of age and its absence may indicate motor rather than visual disturbances.

Optokinetic nystagmus can be used to demonstrate fixation in infants when observation alone provides inconclusive results. It is imperative that the stimulus be compelling by filling completely the visual field. Small hand-held tapes or drums may not be satisfactory for that purpose. When such small stimuli are used, the demonstration of optokinetic nystagmus is clear evidence of visual function, but its absence is not diagnostic.

Visual field may be evaluated in infants and young children by eliciting a fixation reflex when a stimulus is moved from the peripheral field onto the fovea.

VISUAL EVOKED RESPONSE

The visual evoked response to strobe light is an excellent technique to demonstrate the anatomic integrity of visual pathways without patient cooperation. A positive cortical wave with a peak latency of 300 ms is first demonstrated at thirty weeks' gestation. The latency linearly declines at a rate of 10 msec each week throughout the last ten weeks of gestation (Hrbek, 1973). In the newborn, the morphology of the visual evoked response is variable during wakefulness and active sleep and best studied just when the child goes to sleep. By three months of age, the morphology and latency of the visual evoked response are mature.

■ Congenital Blindness

Cortical blindness is the most common cause of congenital blindness, especially among children referred to a neurologist. The causes are numerous and include prenatal and perinatal disturbances. Optic nerve dysplasia, with or without other ocular malformations, is second in frequency, followed in order by congenital cataracts and corneal abnormalities. As a rule, corneal abnormalities are not a cause of visual loss unless clouding is extensive. Such extensive clouding may occur in mucopolysaccharidosis and Fabry disease. Table 16.2 lists those conditions in which corneal clouding is present during childhood.

CONGENITAL CATARACT

For the purpose of this discussion, congenital cataract includes cataracts discovered anytime within the first three months. The differential diagnosis is listed in Table 16.3 (Kohn, 1976).

The etiology of congenital cataracts cannot be determined in most cases. Approximately twenty-five percent are inherited. When cataract is the only abnormality, genetic transmission is usually by autosomal dominant inheritance; when hereditary cataracts are associated with other features comprising a syndrome, then the mode of genetic transmission is variable. In many hereditary syndromes, cataracts can either be congenital or delayed in appearance until infancy, childhood, or even adult life. Several of these syndromes are associated with dermatoses: Incontinentia pigmenti (irregular skin pigmentation), Marshall syndrome (anhidrotic ectodermal dysplasia), Schafer syndrome (follicular hyperkeratosis), congenital ichthyosis, and Siemens syndrome (cutaneous atrophy).

Congenital cataracts are present in approximately ten percent of children with trisomy 13 and trisomy 18. In the majority of children with Down syndrome, cataracts will develop, but these are not ordinarily present at birth. In up to forty percent of children with Turner syndrome, cataracts will develop by puberty.

Clinical Features. Small cataracts do not impair vision and may be difficult to detect by direct ophthalmoscopy. Large cataracts appear as a white mass in the pupil and, if left in place, can lead to loss of vision. The initial size of a cataract does not predict its future course; congenital cataracts may remain stationary or may become larger, but they never become smaller.

Forty to 50 percent of newborns with congenital cataracts have other congenital ocular abnormalities: aniridia, coloboma, and microphthalmos.

Diagnosis. Large cataracts are obvious on inspection. Smaller cataracts distort the normal red reflex when the direct ophthalmoscope is held at a distance from the eye.

Table 16.2 CORNEAL CLOUDING IN CHILDHOOD

1. Cerebrohepatorenal syndrome (Zellweger)
2. Congenital lues
3. Fabry disease (ceramide trihexosidosis)
4. Familial high-density lipoprotein deficiency (Tangier disease)
5. Generalized gangliosidosis GM$_1$
6. Juvenile metachromatic dystrophy
7. Marinesco-Sjögren disease
8. Mucolipidosis
9. Mucopolysaccharidoses
10. Pelizaeus-Merzbacher disease

Table 16.3 LENS ABNORMALITIES IN CHILDHOOD

Congenital Cataract	**Acquired Cataract**

Congenital Cataract

1. Idiopathic
2. Hereditary
   a. Autosomal dominant inheritance
      (1) Hereditary spherocytosis*
      (2) Incontinentia pigmenti*
      (3) Marshall syndrome*
      (4) Myotonic dystrophy*
      (5) Schafer syndrome*
      (6) Without other anomalies
   b. Autosomal recessive inheritance
      (1) Congenital ichthyosis*
      (2) Congenital stippled epiphyses (Conradi disease)
      (3) Marinesco-Sjögren syndrome*
      (4) Siemens syndrome*
      (5) Smith-Lemli-Opitz syndrome
   c. X-Linked inheritance oculocerebrorenal syndrome
      (Lowe syndrome)*
3. Chromosomal aberrations
   a. Down syndrome*
   b. Trisomy 13
   c. Trisomy 18
   d. Turner syndrome*
4. Syndromes of uncertain etiology
   a. Hallerman-Streiff
   b. Pseudo-Turner*
   c. With oxycephaly
   d. With polydactyly
5. Drug exposure during pregnancy
   a. Chlorpromazine
   b. Corticosteroids
   c. Sulfonamides
6. Other maternal factors
   a. Diabetes
   b. Radiation
   c. Malnutrition
7. Prematurity
8. Galactosemia
   a. Galactokinase deficiency
   b. Galactose-1-phosphate uridyl transferase deficiency
9. Intrauterine infection*
   a. Mumps
   b. Rubella
   c. Syphilis

Acquired Cataract

1. Hereditary
   a. Autosomal dominant inheritance (Alport syndrome)
   b. Autosomal recessive inheritance
      (1) Cockayne disease
      (2) Hepatolenticular degeneration (Wilson disease)
      (3) Laurence-Moon-Biedel syndrome
      (4) Rothmund-Thompson syndrome
      (5) Werner syndrome
   c. X-Linked inheritance (pseudo-pseudohypoparathyroidism)
   d. Chromosomal (Prader-Willi syndrome)
2. Metabolic disorders
   a. Cretinism
   b. Hypocalcemia
   c. Hypoparathyroidism
   d. Juvenile diabetes
   e. Pseudohypoparathyroidism
3. Drug induced
   a. Coticosteroids
   b. Long-acting miotics
4. Trauma
5. Acquired varicella

Dislocated Lens

1. Crouzon syndrome
2. Ehlers-Danlos syndrome
3. Homocystinuria
4. Hyperlysinemia
5. Marfan syndrome
6. Sturge-Weber syndrome
7. Sulfite oxidase deficiency

*Cataracts may not be noted until infancy or childhood.

Genetic disorders and maternal drug exposure should be considered when cataract is the only abnormality. Intrauterine disturbances, such as maternal illness and fetal infection, are usually associated with growth retardation and other malformations. Chromosome analysis should be performed in all children with dysmorphic features. Galactosemia is suspected in children with hepatomegaly and milk intolerance (see Chapter 5), but cataracts may be present even before the development of systemic features.

Treatment. Surgical removal of the cataract is the treatment of choice when vision is impaired.

CONGENITAL OPTIC NERVE HYPOPLASIA

Optic nerve hypoplasia is a developmental defect in the number of optic nerve fibers. Hypoplasia may be bilateral or unilateral and varies in severity. It may occur as an isolated defect, or it may be associated with other congenital anomalies. The most common association is with midline defects of the septum pellucidum and hypothalamus, *septo-optic dysplasia* (Margalith et al, 1985).

Clinical Features. When hypoplasia is severe, the child is blind and attention is drawn to the eyes at birth because of strabismus and nystagmus. Ophthalmoscopic examination reveals a small, pale nerve head (Fig. 16.1). A pigmented area is sometimes present between the nerve head and the disk margin, giving the appearance of a double ring.

The degree of hypothalamic-pituitary involvement is variable. Possible presenting symptoms include neonatal hypoglycemia and seizures, recurrent hypoglycemia in childhood, growth retardation, diabetes insipidus, and sexual infantilism. Some combination of mental retardation, cerebral palsy, and epilepsy is often present as well and indicates malformations in other portions of the brain.

Diagnosis. Computerized tomography (CT) of the head and an assessment of endocrine status should be performed in all infants with ophthalmoscopic evidence of optic nerve hypoplasia. The most common finding on CT is absence of the septum pellucidum, but other malformations may be present as well. Endocrine studies should include assays of growth hormone, antidiuretic hormone, and the integrity of hypothalamic-pituitary control of the thyroid, adrenal, and gonadal systems. Infants with hypoglycemia usually have growth hormone deficiency.

Treatment. Treatment is not available for optic hypoplasia, but endocrine abnormalities respond to appropriate replacement therapy.

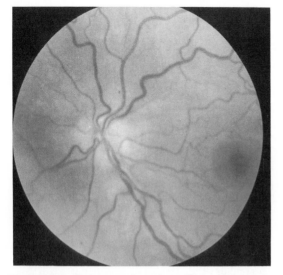

Figure 16.1 Optic nerve hypoplasia. The optic nerve is small and pale, but the vessels are of normal size.

OTHER DISK ANOMALIES

Morning glory disk is an enlarged disk, with a white excavated center, surrounded by an elevated annulus of pigmentary change. Retinal vessels enter and leave at the margin of the disk. The cause is not known, and a familial tendency has not been established. The majority of cases are unilateral, and visual acuity is decreased in the affected eye. The anomaly is sometimes associated with basal encephalocele (Steinkuller, 1980).

Congenital coloboma is a defect in embryogenesis that may affect only the disk or may include the retina, iris, ciliary body, and choroid as well. Colobomas isolated to the nerve head appear as deep excavations. They may be unilateral or bilateral and sometimes are transmitted as an autosomal dominant trait (Savall and Cook, 1976). Visual acuity is not affected unless there is an associated retinal detachment. Retinochoroidal colobomas are glistening white or yellow defects inferior or inferior-nasal to the disk. The margins are distinct and surrounded by pigment. The anomaly is sometimes inherited, but more often sporadic. It may be associated with some chromosomal disorders and with Aicardi syndrome. Visual acuity is not affected unless there is an associated retinal detachment.

LEBER CONGENITAL AMAUROSIS

A generalized retinal degeneration present at birth or early infancy, Leber congenital amaurosis accounts for 18 percent of blindness in children (Schappert-Kimmijser et al, 1959). It is usually transmitted as an autosomal recessive trait, but can be autosomal dominant in some families.

Clinical Features. Blindness is present at birth or shortly thereafter. Pendular nystagmus and photophobia may be associated. Ophthalmoscopic examination of the retina may be normal during infancy and early childhood. With time, progressive retinal stippling and pallor of the disk appear. Mental retardation and epilepsy are often associated.

Diagnosis. The diagnosis is not often considered during infancy because the retina appears normal. Electroretinography is the primary method for detecting the widespread retinal degeneration.

Treatment. Treatment is not available.

■ Acute Monocular or Binocular Blindness

There is considerable overlap in the differential diagnosis of acute and progressive blindness. Slowly progressive ocular disturbances may produce an asymptomatic decline in visual acuity until vision is severely disturbed. Then, the patient presents with "recent" loss of visual acuity. Visual disturbances are often noted first by a teacher or parent rather than by the child. Table 16.4 lists those conditions in which visual acuity is normal and then suddenly lost. Table 16.5 lists disorders in which the underlying pathologic process is progressive over time; in most of these conditions, the patient may perceive that visual loss has occurred acutely. Therefore, both tables should be consulted in the differential diagnosis of "acute blindness."

DEMYELINATING OPTIC NEUROPATHY

Demyelination of the optic nerve (optic neuritis) may occur as an isolated finding affecting

Table 16.4 CAUSES OF ACUTE LOSS OF VISION

Demyelinating Optic Neuropathy
1. Idiopathic optic neuritis
2. Neuromyelitis optica (see Chapter 12)
3. Multiple sclerosis (see Chapter 10)

Ischemic Optic Neuropathy
1. Retinal migraine
2. Retinal artery obstruction
   a. Embolism
   b. Hemoglobinopathy
   c. Coagulopathy

Cortical Blindness
1. Migraine (see Chapter 3)
2. Posttraumatic transient cerebral blindness
3. Benign occipital epilepsy (see Chapter 1)
4. Anoxic encephalopathy (see Chapter 2)
5. Occipital metastatic disease

Trauma
1. Posttraumatic transient cerebral blindness
2. Retinal injuries
3. Indirect optic neuropathy
4. Carotid dissection (see Chapter 11)

Pseudotumor Cerebri (see Chapter 4)

Toxic Optic Neuropathy

Measles Retinitis

Pituitary Apoplexy

Hysteria

Table 16.5 CAUSES OF PROGRESSIVE LOSS OF VISION

Disorders of the Lens
1. Cataract
2. Dislocation of the lens

Hereditary Optic Atrophy
1. Leber optic neuropathy
2. Dominant optic neuropathy
3. Juvenile diabetes mellitus–optic atrophy

Compressive Optic Neuropathies
1. Aneurysm (see Chapters 4 and 15)
2. Arteriovenous malformations (see Chapters 4, 10, and 11)
3. Craniopharyngioma
4. Hypothalamic and optic tumors
5. Pituitary adenoma
6. Pseudotumor cerebri (see Chapter 4)

Orbital Tumors

Tapetoretinal Degenerations
1. Abnormal lipid metabolism
   a. Abetalipoproteinemia (see Chapter 10)
   b. Hypobetalipoproteinemia (see Chapter 10)
   c. Neuronal ceroid lipofuscinosis (see Chapter 5)
   d. Niemann-Pick disease (see Chapter 5)
   e. Refsum disease (see Chapter 7)
2. Abnormal carbohydrate metabolism
   a. Mucopolysaccharidosis (see Chapter 5)
   b. Primary hyperoxaluria
3. Aminoacidopathies
   a. Cystinosis
   b. Cystinuria
   c. Gyrate atrophy of choroid and retina
4. Other syndromes of unknown etiology
   a. Cockayne syndrome
   b. Laurence-Moon-Biedel syndrome

Demyelinating Optic Neuropathy

one or both eyes, or it may be associated with demyelination in other portions of the nervous system. *Neuromyelitis optica*, the syndrome combining optic neuritis and transverse myelitis, is discussed in Chapter 12, multiple sclerosis in Chapter 10. Magnetic resonance imaging (MRI) is a useful technique for surveying the central nervous system for demyelinating lesions. Sixty to 70 percent of adults who present with optic neuritis have MRI evidence of disseminated lesions (Johns et al, 1986; Ormerod et al, 1986). Only a small number of children with optic neuritis have been studied, and the scans have been normal. Indeed, in one long-term follow-up study of children and adults who presented with bilateral optic neuritis, one third of the adults, but none of the children, later demonstrated clinical evidence of multiple sclerosis (Parkin et al, 1984).

Idiopathic Optic Neuritis

Clinical Features. Monocular involvement is the rule in adults, but binocular involvement occurs in over 50 percent of children (Kennedy and Carroll, 1960). Binocular involvement is often sequential, sometimes occurring over a period of weeks. The initial symptom is blurred vision, progressing within a few days to partial or complete blindness. Visual acuity is less than 20/200 in almost all patients. A history is often obtained of a preceding "viral" infection or immunization, but there is no evidence of a cause-and-effect relationship between optic neuritis and either of these events.

Ophthalmoscopic examination may be normal at the onset of symptoms, especially if neuritis is retrobulbar. Later, the nerve head becomes swollen and hemorrhages appear, mimicking papilledema. The two are readily distinguished because optic neuritis is characterized by early and severe visual loss with afferent pupillary defect and papilledema is not.

In the absence of myelitis, the prognosis in children is excellent; complete recovery occurs in 90 percent.

Diagnosis. Optic neuritis must be considered in any child with the sudden onset of monocular or binocular blindness. The diagnosis is often established by ophthalmoscopic or slit-lamp examination. Further confirmation, when necessitated by the suspicion of malingering or hysteria, can be accomplished by testing the visual evoked response; the latency of the major negative wave that ordinarily appears at 100 ms is invariably prolonged. Once optic neuritis is confirmed, MRI of the head is indicated to search for the development of diffuse encephalomyelitis because this may influence therapy. Peroneal-stimulated somatosensory evoked responses or MRI of the spine are indicated if spinal dysfunction is suggested by history or physical examination.

Examination of the cerebrospinal fluid is not indicated. When such examination is performed, a leukocytosis and increased concentration of protein are sometimes observed but results are not informative as to etiology or prognosis.

Demyelinating optic neuritis must be distinguished from *neuroretinitis*. Neuroretinitis is a condition of uncertain etiology in which the pathology is in the retina. Affected children present with sudden monocular blindness that resolves completely and is not associated with demyelination elsewhere in the nervous system. Ophthalmoscopic examination reveals disk swelling, peripapillary retinal detachment, and a macular star (Fig. 16.2).

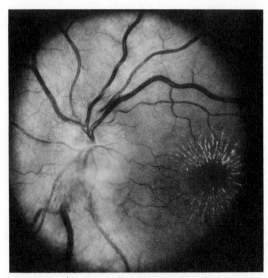

Figure 16.2 Neuroretinitis. The optic disk is swollen with peripapillary nerve fiber layer opacification. Exudates surround the macula in a star pattern. (Courtesy of Dr. Lavin and Mr. Adkins.)

Treatment. Corticosteroids are widely used in the treatment of optic neuritis, but there is no evidence that such a course of treatment is beneficial. However, most authorities would agree that corticosteroids are indicated in cases of acute, diffuse encephalomyelitis.

ISCHEMIC OPTIC NEUROPATHY

Infarction of the anterior portion of the optic nerve is rare in children and usually occurs on a background of systemic vascular disease or hypotension. In one series of retinal artery obstruction in children and young adults (Brown et al, 1981), a history of migraine was present in one third and a coagulopathy was present in a second third. Several different etiologic factors, including sickle cell disease, cardiac disorders, vasculitis, and pregnancy were present in the remainder. No cause could be determined in 15 percent.

Ischemic optic neuropathy usually occurs as a sudden loss of vision in one eye, but slow progression over several days is possible. Recurrent episodes are decidedly unusual except with migraine and some idiopathic cases (Dutton and Burde, 1983).

Retinal Migraine

Clinical Features. Visual symptoms are relatively common during an attack of classic migraine (see Chapter 3). The typical scintillating scotomata, or "fortification spectra," are field defects caused by altered neuronal function in the occipital cortex. The affected field is contralateral to the side of headache.

Monocular visual loss, a much less common phenomenon caused by retinal ischemia, is ipsilateral to the side of headache. Loss of vision is usually sudden, may be complete or partial, and often precedes headache. Rare attacks may be characterized by monocular blindness without headache.

Typical patients have a long history of classic migraine in which both field defects and monocular blindness are experienced separately or together during an individual attack. The visual aberrations ordinarily clear within minutes. Permanent monocular blindness is unusual and occurs mainly in adult females, some as young as adolescents (Coppeto et al, 1986). Many patients who develop persistent blindness have other risk factors for vascular disease, such as the use of oral contraceptives or vasculitis that may act synergistically with migraine to produce vaso-occlusive disease. In one patient, central retinal artery occlusion was coincident with starting propranolol therapy for migraine (Katz, 1986). Although propranolol can enhance adrenergically induced vasospasm, there is no evidence that it causes ischemia in migraineurs.

Diagnosis. The diagnosis can be considered only in patients with classic migraine. Ophthalmoscopic examination reveals retinal edema with scattered hemorrhages. Several different patterns of retinal vaso-occlusive disease may be observed by fluorescein angiography: branch retinal artery, central retinal artery, central retinal vein, and cilioretinal artery.

Treatment. Children who experience retinal ischemia during migraine attacks should be treated with agents that prevent further episodes. Propranolol remains the most effective drug for that purpose despite the theoretical fear that it might enhance vasospasm. Calcium channel blocking agents are an alternative.

Retinal Artery Obstruction

Congenital heart disease is the usual pre-existing condition causing emboli to the retinal artery in young people (Brown et al, 1981). Mitral valve prolapse is a potential cause, but is more likely to produce transient cerebral ischemia than transient monocular blindness (Jackson et al, 1984). Coagulopathies, especially when combined with other risk factors such as pregnancy or migraine, are more frequently associated with retinal artery obstruction than embolic disease. The more common coagulopathies are increased Factor VIII and increased platelet coagulant activity.

Clinical Features. In most patients, there is an abrupt loss of monocular vision of variable intensity without premonitory symptoms. Occasional patients describe spots, a shadow, or a descending veil prior to losing vision. The visual loss need not occur all at once, but may progress for a week or longer before stabilizing.

Altitudinal defects are present in 70 to 80 percent of cases. The severity of color vision loss is roughly equivalent to visual acuity loss. This is in contradistinction to demyelinating optic neuritis, which selectively affects color vision more than visual acuity (Miller, 1982).

Ophthalmoscopic examination reveals diffuse or partial swelling of the optic disk. When swelling is diffuse, it gives the appearance of papilledema and flame-shaped hemorrhages may be present adjacent to the disk margin. After acute swelling subsides, optic atrophy follows.

Bilateral retinal artery occlusion is uncommon in children.

Diagnosis. The diagnosis of retinal artery obstruction is usually based on the clinical history and ophthalmoscopic examination. Visual field examination and fluorescein angiography are helpful in some cases for confirmation. Once the diagnosis is established, a thorough evaluation of underlying causes must be undertaken. This should include auscultation of the heart, radiographs of the chest, echocardiography in selected cases, complete blood count with sedimentation rate, cholesterol and triglyceride screening, coagulation studies, hemoglobin electrophoresis, and antinuclear antibody levels.

Treatment. Treatment is determined by underlying cause. The management of idiopathic occlusion of the retinal artery is controversial in adults, with some authorities recommending the use of corticosteroids. In children, giant cell arteritis is not a consideration and corticosteroids are not indicated. As a rule, visual acuity is more likely to improve when the obstruction is in a branch artery rather than the central retinal artery.

CORTICAL BLINDNESS

Acquired cortical blindness in childhood is usually transitory and caused by migraine (see Chapter 3), head trauma, or benign occipital epilepsy (see Chapter 1). In addition, acute and sometimes permanent blindness may occur following anoxia, massive infarction of the visual cortex, and multifocal metastatic tumors or fungal abscesses in the occipital lobes.

The salient feature is loss of vision with preservation of the pupillary light response. Ophthalmoscopic examination is normal.

Transient Posttraumatic Cerebral Blindness

Clinical Features. This is a benign syndrome that most often occurs in children with a history of migraine or seizures (Greenblatt, 1982). The spectrum of visual disturbance is considerable, but a juvenile and an adolescent pattern have been delineated. In children younger than eight years of age, the precipitating trauma is usually associated with either a brief loss of consciousness or report that the "child was stunned." Blindness is noted almost immediately upon recovery of consciousness and lasts for an hour or less. During the episode, the child may be lethargic and irritable, but is usually coherent. Recovery is complete, and there may be amnesia for the event.

The syndrome in older children is characterized by blindness, confusion, and agitation several minutes or hours after trivial head trauma. Consciousness is not lost. All symptoms resolve after several hours, and there is complete amnesia for the event. These episodes share many features with acute confusional migraine and are probably a variant of that disorder (see Chapter 2).

Diagnosis. All children with blindness following head trauma, no matter how trivial the injury, will surely be studied by CT. In this condition, CT is normal. An electroencephalogram (EEG) performed within the first twenty-four hours is usually abnormal and may demonstrate occipital intermittent rhythmic delta (see Fig. 10.3), diffuse slowing, or epileptiform activity that may be generalized or restricted to the occipital region.

Recognition of the syndrome can spare the trouble and expense of other studies. Family history should be scrutinized for the possibility of migraine or epilepsy. The rapid and complete resolution of all symptoms confirms the diagnosis.

Another mechanism of blindness, monocular or binocular, following head injury is *indirect optic neuropathy*. The nerve is tethered along its course, not free to move, and subject to shearing forces with sudden acceleration or deceleration of the skull. Possible consequences include acute swelling, hemorrhage, or tear. It is easily distinguished from cortical blindness because the pupillary response is diminished and the blindness is longer-lasting.

Treatment. Treatment is not needed for transitory posttraumatic cerebral blindness because symptoms resolve spontaneously.

Cortical Blindness and Hypoglycemia

Repeated episodes of acute cortical blindness occurred in two children with different glycogen storage diseases at the time of mild hypoglycemia (Garty et al, 1987).

Clinical Features. Sudden blindness is associated with clinical evidence of hypoglycemia (sweating and confusion). Ophthalmoscopic examination and neurologic examination are normal. Recovery is complete in two to three hours.

Diagnosis. During the episode, EEG demonstrates high-voltage slowing over both occipital lobes. Afterward, the EEG returns to normal.

Treatment. Treatment is not available or needed.

RETINAL INJURIES

Direct blunt injury to the orbit may produce visual impairment by three mechanisms: retinal contusion, tear, and detachment. All three are characterized by diminished pupillary response. Contusion is associated with retinal edema. Visual loss is immediate, but the retina appears normal for the first few hours and only later becomes white and opaque. The severity of visual loss is variable, but complete recovery is the rule.

Retinal tear is often associated with vitreous hemorrhage. Visual loss is usually immediate and easily diagnosed by ophthalmoscopic appearance. Spontaneous recovery is the rule unless there is detachment, for which cryotherapy is required.

TOXIC OPTIC NEUROPATHIES

Toxic optic neuropathies may be due to drugs (Spiteri and James, 1983) or nutritional deficiency (Knox et al, 1982).

Clinical Features. Implicated drugs include chloramphenicol, isoniazid, streptomycin, sulfonamides, ethambutol, halogenated hydroxyquinolines, chemotherapeutic agents, digitalis, penicillamine, quinine, ergot, and chlorpropamide.

Clinical presentation varies with the specific drug, but progressive loss of central vision is typical. At times, visual loss is rapid and presents as acute monocular or binocular blindness. Many of the drugs produce optic neuropathy by interfering with the action of folic acid or vitamin B_{12}, causing a nutritional deficiency.

Diagnosis. Drug toxicity should be suspected whenever central and paracentral scotomas develop during the course of drug treatment. Optic nerve hyperemia may be an early feature with small paracentral hemorrhages. Later the disk becomes pale.

Treatment. Drug-induced optic neuropathy is dose-related. Reduction in dose may be satisfactory in some cases, especially if concurrent treatment with folic acid or vitamin B_{12} reverses the process. Some drugs must be discontinued completely.

MEASLES RETINITIS

Optic neuritis has been described as an immune-mediated response following natural infection and immunization against varicella, rubeola, rubella, and mumps (Selbst et al, 1983). A cause-and-effect relationship between naturally occurring or immunization-produced viral illness and optic neuritis has never been established. In contrast, retinitis is a known complication of natural measles infection, subacute sclerosing panencephalitis, and immunization with live-attenuated measles vaccine (Marshall et al, 1985).

Clinical Features. Sudden blindness occurs six to twelve days after appearance of the measles exanthem. Ophthalmoscopic examination reveals a diffuse chorioretinitis with perivascular retinal edema, mild papilledema, and a stellate macular configuration. A "salt-and-pepper" pigmentary pattern develops along the retinal veins in the following days. Recovery occurs over several months, but is frequently incomplete.

Diagnosis. The characteristic retinitis in temporal sequence with measles infection is diagnostic.

Treatment. Treatment is not available.

PITUITARY APOPLEXY

Pituitary apoplexy is a rare, life-threatening condition due to infarction of the pituitary (Reid et al, 1985).

Clinical Features. Pituitary infarction most often occurs when there is a pre-existing pituitary tumor but may also occur in the absence of tumor. Predisposing factors are summarized in Table 16.6.

A variety of clinical manifestations are possible, depending upon the structures compressed by the swollen gland. These include any of the following symptoms, alone or in combination: monocular or binocular blindness, visual field defects, proptosis, ophthalmoplegia, ptosis, facial paresthesias, and hemiplegia. Leakage of blood into the subarachnoid space is associated with headache, meningismus, and loss of consciousness.

Diagnosis. Computerized tomography with tomograms through the pituitary is diagnostic. Endocrine testing reveals deficiency of all pituitary hormones.

Treatment. Patients deteriorate rapidly and may die within a few days if corticosteroids are not administered promptly. Other hormones must be replaced as well, but are not life-saving. In patients who continue to do poorly, as evidenced by loss of consciousness or hypothalamic instability, surgical decompression of the expanding pituitary mass should be performed.

HYSTERICAL BLINDNESS

A claim of complete binocular blindness is easily identified as spurious. A pupillary response to light indicates that the anterior pathway is intact and only cerebral blindness is a possibility. Visual function can be assessed by using a full-field optokinetic tape or by moving a mirror in front of the patient to stimulate matching eye movements. When monocular blindness is claimed, the same tests can be performed with the good eye patched.

Table 16.6 PREDISPOSING FACTORS IN PITUITARY APOPLEXY

1. Acromegaly
2. Adrenalectomy
3. Anticoagulation
4. Bleeding disorders
5. Carotid angiography
6. Cushing syndrome
7. Diabetes
8. Increased intracranial pressure
9. Mechanical ventilation
10. Pituitary tumor
11. Pituitary radiation
12. Pregnancy
13. Sickle cell trait
14. Upper airway obstruction

Spurious claims of partial visual impairment are more difficult to challenge. Helpful tests include (1) failure of acuity to improve linearly with increasing test size; (2) inappropriate ability to detect small test objects on tangent screen; and (3) normal results on testing stereoscopic visual acuity or color perception (Keane, 1982).

■ Progressive Loss of Vision

HEREDITARY OPTIC ATROPHY

There are several hereditary optic neuropathies, some affecting only the visual system, others the visual system and central nervous system, and still others causing multisystem disease (Neetens and Martin, 1986). These disorders may produce acute, subacute, or chronic decline in visual acuity. Diagnosis relies heavily on a positive family history.

Leber Optic Neuropathy (Neuroretinopathy)

Eighty-five percent of cases of neuroretinopathy are men, and the trait was previously thought to be transmitted by X-linked inheritance. However, the condition is transmitted only through the female line, never by men, suggesting an abnormality in mitochondrial DNA (Egger and Wilson, 1983). The pathogenesis of the disorder is unknown, but there is some support for the notion of an inborn error in cyanide metabolism preventing its detoxification to thiocyanate and sulphite. Zinc deficiency has been implicated as well (Syme et al, 1983).

Clinical Features. The characteristic presentation is rapid loss of vision in young, otherwise healthy men. The peak age at onset is between eighteen and twenty-three years, but children younger than ten years of age may be affected. Age at onset may vary by several decades within a pedigree.

The initial complaint is usually painless blurred central vision in one eye, described as fogging of vision or central fading of color. The other eye ordinarily becomes symptomatic within days or weeks, but may remain unimpaired for several years. Examination of the visual fields reveals first central and then cecocentral scotomas.

The characteristic changes in the ocular fundus include circumpapillary telangiectatic microangiopathy, edema of the nerve fiber layer around the disk, and absence of peripapillary staining on fluorescein angiography. Telangiec-

tatic microangiopathy is the earliest feature and may be observed in presymptomatic family members (Lopez and Smith, 1986; Nikoskelainen et al, 1982). As the patient becomes symptomatic, the nerve fiber layer becomes swollen; retinal vessels on and around the disk become dilated, tortuous, and telangiectatic; and hemorrhages appear in the nerve fiber layer (Nikoskelainen et al, 1983). Atrophy appears first in the papillomacular bundle and then involves the rest of the retina. The vascular bed involutes, leaving a pale retina and optic atrophy.

Visual improvement occurs in perhaps 20 percent of patients one to five years after vision is lost. Ten percent are reported to regain full vision. Once vision is restored, relapses do not occur.

Although visual loss is the only symptom in most families, neurologic impairment may be associated in some kindreds. Commonly associated disturbances include dystonia, spastic paraplegia, and ataxia. Some family members may have neurologic impairment without optic atrophy, and some have optic atrophy with neurologic impairment.

Diagnosis. Leber optic neuropathy is a multisystem mitochondrial disease transmitted by mitochondrial DNA. It should be suspected in every kindred with optic neuropathy or with progressive neurologic impairment in which transmission is restricted to the maternal line. The optic fundus changes, especially the microangiopathy, are diagnostic in the context of a compatible family history. Fluorescein angiography definitively demonstrates the development and involution of the telangiectatic microangiopathy and is useful in the diagnosis of presymptomatic cases (Nikoskelainen et al, 1984).

Treatment. A proposed treatment protocol has been developed based on the concept that cyanide intoxication is critical to the mechanism of disease (Syme et al, 1983). A similar protocol is used for tobacco amblyopia. The elimination of cyanide is enhanced by the use of hydroxocobalamin, 1,000 mg, injected intramuscularly three times each week, and oral cystine, 4 to 8 mg daily. Smoking is discouraged. Using this protocol, the recovery rate is said to be higher than expected without treatment; however, further study is needed.

Dominant Optic Neuropathy

Clinical Features. The onset of symptoms is insidious, but most patients date the beginning of visual disturbances to the first decade, usually four to six years of age (Hoyt, 1980). Visual acuity is progressively reduced equally in both eyes and may be mild, remaining between 20/20 and 20/60 in 40 percent. Some cases are identified only because other family members are affected.

Visual fields show central, paracentral, or cecocentral scotomas, which are best delineated with red test objects. Optic atrophy primarily affects the temporal portion of the disk, which is pale in appearance.

Additional neurologic abnormalities are unusual.

Diagnosis. A positive family history is critical for diagnosis. It is easily distinguished from Leber optic neuropathy by the absence of microangiopathy.

Treatment. Treatment is not available.

Juvenile Diabetes Mellitus

Several kindreds have been reported with a combination of juvenile diabetes mellitus, optic atrophy, and other neurologic disorders (Lessell and Rosman, 1977). The disorder is thought to be transmitted as an autosomal recessive trait.

Clinical Features. The onset of diabetes is usually the first decade. Insulin therapy is required soon after diagnosis. Visual loss begins in the second decade. Pallor of the optic disk may be present immediately or may develop later. Hearing loss is present in all patients, and some have anosmia. The following features have been reported in some patients: ptosis, tremor, ataxia, nystagmus, seizures, diabetes insipidus, and endocrinopathies.

Diagnosis. Diagnosis depends upon the combination of juvenile onset diabetes mellitus and optic atrophy. Family history is not always present. Diabetes is not thought to cause optic atrophy. It is more likely that all features are due to a common underlying factor.

Treatment. Each of the clinical features is treated symptomatically.

COMPRESSIVE OPTIC NEUROPATHY

Compression of one or both optic nerves often occurs in the region of the chiasm. Visual loss may be confined to one eye or to a visual field. In children with tumors in and around the diencephalon, the most constant feature is growth failure. This is often not appreciated until other symptoms intervene.

Craniopharyngioma

Clinical Features. The common presenting features are growth retardation and visual disturbances in children and failure of sexual maturation in adolescents. Field defects are frequently asymmetric or unilateral. Bitemporal hemianopsia is present in 50 percent of children, and homonymous hemianopsia in 10 to 20 percent. Visual acuity is diminished in one or both eyes in every child (Hoffman et al, 1977).

Approximately 25 percent of children develop hydrocephalus and present with headache and papilledema. Hypothalamic involvement may produce diabetes insipidus or the *hypodipsia-hyponatremia syndrome* characterized clinically by lethargy, confusion, and hypotension. Other features depend upon the direction of tumor growth. Anterior extension may compress the olfactory tract, causing anosmia, whereas posterior extension may compress the third and fifth nerves.

Diagnosis. Craniopharyngiomas are readily visualized by CT. Calcification of the tumor is present in 80 percent of children. Arteriography must be performed prior to surgery in order to define the relationship of blood vessels to tumor.

Treatment. There is general agreement that subtotal resection followed by radiation therapy is the accepted standard of treatment. The extent of resection still remains an issue, but attempted total resection is discouraged (Baskin and Wilson, 1986; Fischer et al, 1985).

The recommended dose of local radiation is 5,000 rad with the dose per fraction not to exceed 200 rad per day. Hormone replacement therapy is needed in every case.

Hypothalamic and Optic Gliomas

Gliomas of the hypothalamus and optic nerves are difficult to distinguish by histologic criteria and share many clinical features. Optic gliomas represent 3 to 5 percent of all childhood brain tumors. Approximately half of children with optic gliomas have neurofibromatosis. The clinical presentation and prognosis are much the same whether or not neurofibromatosis is present (Stern et al, 1979).

Clinical Features. Initial symptoms depend on location, but hypothalamic tumors eventually affect the optic chiasm and optic chiasm tumors affect the hypothalamus. Under the age of three, tumors of the hypothalamus or optic chiasm frequently present as *the diencephalic syndrome.*

The diencephalic syndrome is characterized by marked loss of subcutaneous fat and total body weight with maintenance or acceleration of long-bone growth. Despite the appearance of cachexia, the infant is mentally alert and does not seem as "sick" as the appearance suggests. Pendular nystagmus is often present as well. The precise endocrine mechanism of the diencephalic syndrome has never been clarified. Precocious puberty, rather than the diencephalic syndrome, can be the initial manifestation of hypothalamic tumors in infants and children. Hamartomas of the tuber cinereum, astrocytomas, ependymomas, ectopic pinealomas, and craniopharyngiomas have all been associated.

Slowly progressive loss of vision is the most common presenting feature. Monocular visual loss suggests optic nerve involvement, but also may occur with tumors of the chiasm. Binocular involvement suggests involvement of the optic chiasm or tract. Visual field deficits are variable and may be congruous or incongruous. Tumors near the orbit may produce proptosis and papillitis, with blurring of the disk resembling papilledema, and central loss of vision. Ophthalmoplegia is unusual.

Increased intracranial pressure suggests extension of tumor from chiasm to hypothalamus. When this is the initial feature, it is difficult to know the site of tumor origin.

Diagnosis. Computerized tomography allows visualization of the optic nerves from orbit to chiasm. However, MRI is the preferred imaging modality because it provides the opportunity to visualize the hypothalamus in several different planes and identify brainstem extension of tumor (Fig. 16.3).

As a rule, optic nerve gliomas produce an enlarged, tubular appearance to the nerve and chiasm. Sometimes. the tumors are globular in shape and suprasellar in location and appear to compress the chiasm (Fletcher et al, 1986).

Intrinsic gliomas of the hypothalamus are identified by MRI as high-density signals on T2 weighted studies.

Treatment. Biopsy of hypothalamic tumors should be done to identify histologic type. The tumor is then radiated with doses of 5,000 to 6,000 rad. Five-year survivals of 70 percent and ten-year survivals of 50 percent are reported (Bloom, 1982). The value of chemotherapy is not established.

Management of optic gliomas is more problematic. Half of these tumors grow at a slow rate and have a relatively benign course. Unfortunately, it is difficult to differentiate slow- growing from aggressive tumors at the onset.

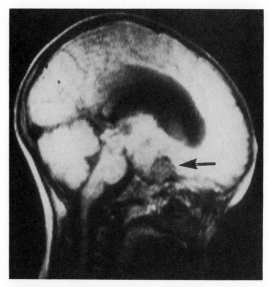

Figure 16.3 Optic nerve glioma identified by magnetic resonance image (arrow).

Biopsy of all tumors must be performed to identify tissue type. Several other tumors may mimic optic nerve gliomas both at the orbit and chiasm. Children with hydrocephalus require ventricular shunt to relieve symptoms of hydrocephalus. Surgical excision of the optic nerve, in order to accomplish complete tumor removal, should be considered if vision is already negligible. This is most often accomplished when the tumor is intraorbital. Those with chiasmatic tumors causing hypothalamic dysfunction require partial excision and radiation therapy. The benefits of radiation therapy are not established.

Pituitary Adenoma

Pituitary adenomas represent only 1 to 2 percent of intracranial tumors of childhood. Males and females are equally affected.

Clinical Features. Age at diagnosis is usually during adolescence (Mukai et al, 1986). Amenorrhea is the usual presenting symptom in females with prolactin-secreting tumors. Galactorrhea may be present as well. In males, the initial features are growth retardation, delayed puberty, and headache.

Papilledema is uncommon, but optic atrophy is present in 10 to 20 percent of cases. Visual field defects may be unilateral temporal, bitemporal, or homonymous (Richmond and Wilson, 1978).

Diagnosis. Visualization of the tumor and identification of its extrasellar extent can be accomplished by either CT or MRI. Measurement of hormone production is useful in distinguishing tumor type. Increased concentration of prolactin is recorded in 60 percent of adenomas, growth hormone in 15 percent, and adrenocorticotropic hormone (ACTH) in 12 percent; 12 percent of adenomas are nonfunctioning.

Treatment. Total resection can be accomplished when the tumor is restricted to the sella. In such cases, outcome is generally good, recurrence rate is low, and hormone replacement therapy is not always required. Radiation therapy should be used in patients with partial excision or recurrence.

INTRAOCULAR TUMORS

Although retro-orbital tumors generally present with strabismus and proptosis, intraocular tumors always result in diminished visual acuity. Retinoblastoma is the most common malignant intraocular tumor. Its prompt recognition can be life-saving.

The typical features of intraocular tumor in a young child are an abnormal appearance of the eye, loss of vision, and strabismus. Monocular blindness is usually not appreciated by parents. Older children may complain of visual blurring and floaters. Ocular pain is uncommon.

Leukokoria, a white pupillary reflex, is the initial symptom in most children with retinoblastoma. This is first noted in bright sunlight or in a flash photograph; the pupil does not restrict and has a white color. Misalignment of the eyes (strabismus) occurs when visual acuity is impaired (see Chapter 15). The sighted eye is used for fixation, and the other remains deviated outward in all directions of gaze.

Most children with intraocular tumors are referred directly to an ophthalmologist. A neurologist may be the primary consulting physician when the tumor is part of a larger syndrome that includes mental retardation. Such syndromes are (1) retinoblastoma associated with chromosome 13 long-arm deletion, (2) retinal astrocytoma associated with tuberous sclerosis, (3) choroidal hemangioma associated with Sturge-Weber disease, and (4) optic nerve glioma in children with neurofibromatosis.

TAPETORETINAL DEGENERATIONS

Most tapetoretinal degenerations are hereditary and due to inborn errors of lipid or carbohydrate metabolism. These disorders also cause dementia, peripheral neuropathy, and ataxia as initial features and are discussed in several chapters (see Table 16.5). The conditions discussed here are less common, but other neurologic features are not prominent initial complaints.

Aminoacidopathies

Cystinuria is transmitted as a recessive trait. There is impaired intestinal absorption and renal tubular reabsorption of cystine, lysine, arginine, and ornithine. The most common feature is renal stones, but retinal degeneration may be associated.

Cystinosis is a lysosomal storage disease transmitted by autosomal recessive inheritance. Cystine is stored in viscera, bone marrow, and eyes. The major clinical features are dwarfism, renal tubulopathy, vitamin-resistant renal rickets, and hepatosplenomegaly. In addition to cystine storage in the cornea, conjunctiva, and iris, there is pigmentary degeneration of the retina.

Gyrate atrophy of the choroid and retina is probably a disorder of ornithine metabolism (Francois, 1982). It may be the homozygote form of Alder anomaly, in which azurophilic granules are present in the cytoplasm of leukocytes. Visual function is adequate for many years, but eventually the patient becomes blind.

Cockayne Syndrome

Cockayne syndrome is transmitted by autosomal recessive inheritance with a male to female bias of 3:1. It is probably an inborn error of lipid metabolism and produces a leukodystrophy.

Clinical Features. Age at onset is during infancy. Primary pigmentary degeneration of the retina occurs early. Affected children appear cachectic, and a disproportionate dwarfism develops in which the limbs are large compared with the trunk. A characteristic facies includes lack of subcutaneous fat with prominence of facial bones, enophthalmos, a beaklike nose, large ears, and mental deficiency. Mental deficiency and microcephaly are constant features. Neurologic signs that may be associated include cerebellar ataxia, involuntary movements, spasticity, peripheral neuropathy, and sensorineural hearing loss.

Diagnosis. The constellation of clinical signs suggests the diagnosis. Hyperbetaglobulinemia, hyperinsulinemia, and hyperlipoproteinemia may be present in some cases.

Treatment. Treatment is not available.

Laurence-Moon-Biedel Syndrome

This syndrome comprises a heterogeneous group of disorders that share similar ocular and systemic features. It is transmitted by autosomal recessive inheritance.

Clinical Features. Pigmentary retinopathy usually becomes manifested in the second decade. It may be characterized by salt-and-pepper retinopathy, macular pigmentation, or macular degeneration. At times the retina may appear normal, but the electroretinogram is always abnormal. Other cardinal features include hypogenitalism, obesity, polydactyly, and mental retardation. Less common associated features are sensorineural deafness, cataract, external ophthalmoplegia, and diabetes mellitus.

Diagnosis. Diagnosis depends upon recognition of the clinical constellation of symptoms and signs.

Treatment. Treatment is not available for the underlying defect.

PROGRESSIVE OPTIC NEURITIS

Optic neuritis is generally regarded to be an acute process with sudden onset of blindness in one eye and then the other (see "Demyelinating Optic Neuropathy" earlier in this chapter). Occasional patients are seen who experience a slowly progressive optic neuritis (Roseman and Ellenberger, 1982). Those with adult onset usually have multiple sclerosis, but this may not be the case in children.

Clinical Features. Age at onset is adolescence or later. Initial symptoms may be transitory monocular blindness or blurring of vision during strenuous exercise. Disturbed color discrimination is an early feature. Vision worsens over a period of years, usually stepwise. Some patients report deterioration of vision in bright light. Recovery is not the rule.

Diagnosis. It is essential to exclude any possibility of compressive optic neuropathy. An MRI is helpful both to exclude a compressive lesion and to determine the presence of other foci of demyelination. Visual evoked response should demonstrate a prolonged latency of the major positive wave.

Treatment. There is no established treatment for this disorder.

■ Disorders of the Pupil

In the awake state, the size of the pupil is constantly changing in response to light and autonomic input. This pupillary unrest is called *hippus*. An isolated disturbance of pupillary size is never evidence of intracranial disease.

ESSENTIAL ANISOCORIA

Twenty percent of healthy people have an observable difference in the size of their pupils. Like congenital ptosis, it may not be noted until late in childhood or adult life and then thought to be a new finding. The difference is constant at all levels of illumination. The absence of other pupillary dysfunction or disturbed ocular motility suggests essential anisocoria, but old photographs are sometimes invaluable to confirm the diagnosis.

TONIC PUPIL SYNDROME
(Adie Syndrome)

Clinical Features. This syndrome is thought to be caused by a defect in the orbital ciliary ganglion. The age at onset is usually after childhood, but has been reported as early as five years. Women are more often affected than men.

It is usually monocular and presents as anisocoria. The abnormal pupil is slightly larger in bright light, but changes little, if at all, with alteration in illumination. In a dark room, the normal pupil dilates and then is larger than the tonic pupil. With accommodation, the pupil constricts slowly and incompletely and redilates slowly afterwards.

Binocular tonic pupils are seen in children with dysautonomia and in association with diminished tendon reflexes (the Holmes-Adie syndrome).

Diagnosis. The tonic pupil is supersensitive to parasympathomimetic agents, and constriction is achieved with 0.125 percent pilocarpine.

Treatment. The condition is benign. Treatment is not available and is not needed.

THE FIXED DILATED PUPIL

Clinical Features. A fixed dilated pupil is an ominous sign in unconscious patients because it suggests transtentorial herniation (see Chapter 4). However, a dilated pupil that does not respond to light or accommodation in a child that is otherwise well and has no evidence of ocular motor dysfunction can only result from the application of a pharmacologic agent. The application may by accidental, and careful history must be obtained of drugs and chemicals that may have been inadvertently wiped from hand to eye. Many cosmetics contain chemicals that can induce mydriasis.

Factitious application of mydriatics is relatively common as an attention-seeking device, and it is sometimes difficult to convince parents that the problem is self-inflicted.

Diagnosis. Pilocarpine, 1 percent, should be instilled in the dilated eye. Parasympathetic denervation produces prompt constriction. A slow or incomplete response indicates pharmacologic dilation.

Treatment. Most pharmacologic agents are long-acting, and there is no method that rapidly reverses their effect.

HORNER SYNDROME

This is a syndrome of sympathetic denervation. It may be congenital or acquired. When acquired, Horner syndrome may occur at birth as part of a brachial plexus injury, during infancy from neuroblastoma, or in childhood from tumors or injuries affecting the superior cervical ganglion or the carotid artery.

Clinical Features. Unilateral Horner syndrome consists of the following ipsilateral features: (1) mild to moderate ptosis, (2) miosis, which is best appreciated in dim light so that the normal pupil dilates, and (3) anhydrosis of the face. In addition, there will be apparent enophthalmos and heterochromia if the syndrome is congenital.

Diagnosis. Horner syndrome may be caused by disruption of the sympathetic system anywhere from the brainstem to the eye. Brainstem disturbances from stroke are common in adults, but peripheral lesions are more common in children. Topical instillation of norepinephrine produces immediate pupillary dilation when postganglionic denervation is present. Cocaine, 4 percent, produces little or no dilation regardless of the site of abnormality.

Treatment. Treatment depends upon the underlying cause.

ARGYLL ROBERTSON PUPIL

This pupillary disturbance is associated with tertiary syphilis and is almost never seen in children. Both pupils are irregular in shape and miotic. Iris atrophy may be present as well. The pupils respond poorly to light, but accommodation is present ("light-near dissociation").

ANIRIDIA

Hypoplasia of the iris may occur as a solitary abnormality or may be associated with mental retardation, genitourinary abnormalities, and Wilm tumor. In some cases, there is an abnormal short arm of chromosome 11.

References

1. Baskin DS, Wilson CB: Surgical management of craniopharyngiomas. A review of 74 cases. J Neurosurg 65:22, 1986.
2. Bloom HJG: Intracranial tumors: Response and resistance to therapeutic endeavors, 1970-1980. Int J Radiat Oncol Biol Phys 8:1083, 1982.
3. Brown GC, Magaral LE, Shields JA, et al: Retinal artery obstruction in children and young adults. Ophthalmology 88:18, 1981.
4. Coppeto JR, Lessell S, Sciarra R, et al: Vascular retinopathy in migraine. Neurology 36:267, 1986.
5. Dutton JJ, Burde RM: Anterior ischemic optic neuropathy of the young. J Clin Neuro-ophthalmol 3:137, 1983.
6. Egger J, Wilson J: Mitochondrial inheritance in a mitochondially mediated disease. N Engl J Med 309:142, 1983.
7. Fischer EG, Welch K, Belli JA, et al: Treatment of craniopharyngiomas in children: 1972-1981. J Neurosurg 62:496, 1985.
8. Fletcher WA, Imes RK, Hoyt WF: Chiasmal gliomas: appearance and long-term changes demonstrated by computerized tomography. J Neurosurg 65:154, 1986.
9. Francois J: Metabolic tapetoretinal degenerations. Surv Ophthalmol 26:293, 1982.
10. Garty B-Z, Dinari G, Nitzan M: Transient acute cortical blindness associated with hypoglycemia. Pediatr Neurol 3:169, 1987.
11. Greenblatt SH: Posttraumatic transient cerebral blindness. Association with migraine and seizure diathesis. JAMA 225:1073, 1982.
12. Hoffman HJ, Hendrick EB, Humphreys RP, et al: Management of craniopharyngioma in children. J Neurosurg 47:218, 1977.
13. Hoyt CS: Autosomal dominant optic atrophy: A spectrum of disability. Ophthalmology 87:245, 1980.
14. Hoyt CS, Nickel BL, Billson FA: Ophthalmological examination of the infant. Developmental aspects. Surv Ophthalmol 26:177, 1982.
15. Hrbek A, Karlberg P, Olsson T: Development of visual and somatosensory evoked responses in pre-term newborn infants. Electroencephalogr Clin Neurophysiol 34:225, 1973.
16. Jackson AC, Boughner DR, Barnett HJM: Mitral valve prolapse and cerebral ischemic events in young patients. Neurology 34:784, 1984.
17. Johns K, Lavin P, Elliot JE, et al: Magnetic resonance imaging of the brain in isolated optic neuritis. Arch Ophthalmol 104:1486, 1986.
18. Katz B: Migrainous central retinal artery occlusion. J Clin Neuroophthalmology 6:69, 1986.

19. Keane JR: Neuro-ophthalmic signs and symptoms of hysteria. Neurology 32:757, 1982.
20. Kennedy L, Carroll FD: Optic neuritis in children. Arch Ophthalmol 63:747, 1960.
21. Knox DL, Chen MF, Guilarte TR, et al: Nutritional amblyopia. Folic acid, vitamin B_{12}, and other vitamins. Retina 2:288, 1982.
22. Kohn BA: The differential diagnosis of cataracts in infancy and childhood. Am J Dis Child 130:184, 1976.
23. Lessell S, Rosman NP: Juvenile diabetes mellitus and optic atrophy. Arch Neurol 34:759, 1977.
24. Lopez PF, Smith JL: Leber's optic neuropathy. New observations. J Clin Neuro-ophthalmol 6:144, 1986.
25. Margalith D, Tze WJ, Jan JE: Congenital optic nerve hypoplasia with hypothalamic-pituitary dysplasia. Am J Dis Child 139:361, 1985.
26. Marshall GS, Wright PF, Fenichel GM, et al: Diffuse retinopathy following measles, mumps, and rubella vaccination. Pediatrics 76:989, 1985.
27. Martyn LJ: Pediatric neuro-ophthalmology. Ped Clin North Am 30:1103, 1983.
28. Miller NR: Anterior ischemic optic neuropathy. In Walsh and Hoyt's Clinical Neuro-ophthalmology. Volume I, 4th edition. Williams and Wilkins, Baltimore, 1982, p 212.
29. Mukai K, Seljeskog EL, Dehner LP: Pituitary adenomas in patients under 20 years old. A clinicopathological study of 112 cases. J Neuro-oncology 4:79, 1986.
30. Neetens A, Martin JJ: The hereditary optic atrophies. Neuroophthalmology 6:277, 1986.
31. Nikoskelainen E, Hoyt WF, Nummelin K: Ophthalmoscopic findings in Leber's hereditary optic neuropathy. I. Fundus findings in asymptomatic family members. Arch Ophthalmol 100:1597, 1982.
32. Nikoskelainen E, Hoyt WF, Nummelin K: Ophthalmoscopic findings in Leber's hereditary optic neuropathy. II. The fundus finding in the affected family members. Arch Ophthalmol 101:1059, 1983.
33. Nikoskelainen E, Hoyt WF, Nummelin K: Ophthalmoscopic findings in Leber's hereditary optic neuropathy. III. Fluorescein angiographic findings. Arch Ophthalmol 102:981, 1984.
34. Ormerod, IEC, McDonald WI, duBoulay GH, et al: Disseminated lesions at presentation in patients with optic neuritis. J Neurol Neurosurg Psychiatry 49:124, 1986.
35. Parkin PJ, Hierons R, McDonald WI: Bilateral optic neuritis: a long-term follow-up. Brain 107:951, 1984.
36. Reid RL, Quigley ME, Yen SSC: Pituitary apoplexy. A review. Arch Neurol 42:712, 1985.
37. Richmond IL, Wilson CB: Pituitary adenomas in childhood and adolescence. J Neurosurg 49:163, 1978.
38. Roseman R, Ellenberger C Jr: Slowly progressive optic neuritis. Neuro-ophthalmol 2:183, 1982.
39. Savall J, Cook JR: Optic nerve colobomas of autosomal dominant heredity. Arch Ophthalmol 94:395, 1976.
40. Schappert-Kimmijser J, Henkes HE, van den Borsch J: Amaurosis congenita (Leber). Arch Ophthalmol 61:211, 1959.
41. Selbst RC, Selhorst JB, Harbison JW, et al: Parainfectious optic neuritis. Report and review following varicella. Arch Neurol 40:347, 1983.
42. Simons K: Visual acuity norms in young children. Surv Ophthalmol 28:84, 1983.
43. Spiteri MA, James DG: Adverse ocular reactions to drugs. Postgrad Med J 59:343, 1983.
44. Steinkuller PG: The morning glory disc anomaly: Case report and literature review. J Pediatr Ophthalmol 17:81, 1980.
45. Stern J, DiGiacinto GV, Housepian AM: Neurofibromatosis and optic gliomas: Clinical and morphologic correlations. Neurosurgery 4:524, 1979.
46. Syme IG, Bronte-Stewart J, Foulds WS, et al: Clinical and biochemical findings in Leber's hereditary optic atrophy. Trans Ophthalmol Soc UK 103:556, 1983.

17 Lower Brainstem and Cranial Nerve Dysfunction

This chapter deals with disorders causing dysfunction of cranial nerves seven through twelve. Many such disorders disturb extraocular motility as well, and were discussed in Chapter 15. This assignment may seem arbitrary, but it is based upon the most common presenting feature. For example, myasthenia gravis is discussed in Chapter 15 because diplopia is much more frequent as an initial complaint than dysphagia.

An acute isolated cranial neuropathy, such as facial palsy, is usually a less ominous sign than multiple cranial neuropathies and is likely to have a self-limited course. However, an isolated cranial neuropathy may be the first sign of progressive cranial nerve dysfunction. Therefore, conditions causing isolated and multiple cranial neuropathies are discussed together because they may not be separable at the time of presentation.

■ Facial Weakness and Dysphagia

ANATOMIC CONSIDERATIONS

Facial Movement

The motor nucleus of the facial nerve forms a column of cells in the ventrolateral tegmentum of the pons. Nerve fibers leaving the nucleus take a circuitous path in the brainstem before emerging close to the pontomedullary junction, where they enter the internal auditory meatus with the acoustic nerve. After bending forward and downward around the inner ear, the facial nerve traverses the temporal bone in the facial canal and exits the skull at the stylomastoid foramen. Extracranially, the facial nerve passes into the parotid gland, where it subdivides into several branches and is distributed to all muscles of facial expression except the levator palpebrae superioris.

Sucking and Swallowing

The sucking reflex requires the integrity of the trigeminal, facial, and hypoglossal nerves. Stimulation of the lips produces coordinated movements of the face, jaw, and tongue. The automatic aspect of the reflex disappears after infancy, but returns when there is bilateral disease of the cerebral hemispheres.

The afferent arc of the swallowing reflex is formed by fibers of the trigeminal and glossopharyngeal nerves that end in the nucleus solitarius. The efferent arc is formed by the motor root of the trigeminal nerve, glossopharyngeal and vagus fibers from the nucleus ambiguus, and the hypoglossal nerves. A swallowing center to coordinate the reflex is located in the lower pons and upper medulla. A bolus of food stimulates the pharyngeal wall or back of the tongue, and food is moved into the esophagus by action of the tongue, palatine arches, soft palate, and pharynx.

APROACH TO DIAGNOSIS

Weakness of facial muscles may be caused by supranuclear palsy (pseudobulbar palsy), intrinsic brainstem disease, or motor unit disorders: facial nerve, neuromuscular junction, and facial muscles (Tables 17.1 and 17.2). The differential diagnosis of dysphagia is very similar

Table 17.1 CAUSES OF CONGENITAL FACIAL WEAKNESS

Aplasia of nuclei (Moebius syndrome)
Birth injury
Myasthenic syndromes
    Congenital myasthenia (see Chapter 15)
    Familial infantile myasthenia (see Chapter 6)
    Transitory neonatal myasthenia (see Chapter 6)

Table 17.2 CAUSES OF ACQUIRED FACIAL WEAKNESS

Autoimmune/Postinfectious
1. Bell's palsy
2. Idiopathic cranial polyneuropathy
3. Miller Fisher syndrome (see Chapter 10)
4. Myasthenia gravis (see Chapter 15)

Genetic
1. Muscular Disorders
    a. Facioscapulohumeral dystrophy, infantile form
    b. Fiber type disproportion myopathies (see Chapter 7)
    c. Myotonic dystrophy
    d. Oculopharyngeal dystrophy
2. Myasthenic syndromes
    a. Congenital myasthenia gravis (see Chapter 15)
    b. Familial infantile (see Chapter 6)
3. Recurrent facial palsy
    a. Melkerrson syndrome
    b. Multiple cranial neuropathies

Hypertension

Infectious
1. Diphtheria
2. Herpes zoster (Ramsay Hunt syndrome)
3. Infectious mononucleosis
4. Lyme disease (see Chapter 2)
5. Otitis media
6. Sarcoid
7. Tuberculosis

Juvenile Progressive Bulbar Palsy (Fazio-Londe)

Metabolic Disorders
1. Hyperparathyroidism
2. Hypothyroidism
3. Osteopetrosis (Albers-Schönberg disease)

Multiple Sclerosis (see Chapter 10)

Syringobulbia

Toxins

Trauma
1. Delayed
2. Immediate

Tumor
1. Glioma of brainstem (see Chapter 15)
2. Histiocytosis X
3. Leukemia
4. Meningeal carcinoma
5. Neurofibromatosis

(Table 17.3), except that isolated dysfunction of the nerves subserving swallowing is very uncommon.

Pseudobulbar Palsy

Because the corticobulbar innervation of most cranial nerves is bilateral, pseudobulbar palsy occurs only when there is bilateral hemispheric disease. Children with pseudobulbar palsy are likely to have cerebral palsy or a progressive degenerative disorder of gray or white matter. Most of these disorders are discussed in Chapter 5 because they usually present as dementia. In some, such as the juvenile form of Alexander disease, pseudobulbar palsy may be a presenting feature (Borrett and Becker, 1985). Bilateral stroke, simultaneous or in sequence, is a common cause of pseudobulbar palsy in adults, but not in children. The usual causes of bilateral stroke in children are coagulation defects, leukemia, and trauma (see Chapter 11).

Pseudobulbar palsy is characterized by inability to use bulbar muscles in voluntary effort, whereas reflex movements initiated at a brainstem level are performed normally. Extraocular motility is not affected. The child is able to suck, chew, and swallow but is unable to smile or make facial movements upon command. Severe dysarthria is often present (van Dongen et al, 1987). There is neither atrophy nor fasciculation of affected muscles. The gag reflex and jaw jerk are usually exaggerated, and emotional volatility is often associated.

Newborns with familial dysautonomia have difficulty in feeding, despite normal sucking and swallowing, because they fail to coordinate the two reflexes (see Chapter 6). The differential diagnosis of feeding difficulty in an alert newborn is summarized in Table 6.8. Children with cerebral palsy often have a similar disturbance in the coordination of chewing and swallowing that impairs feeding.

Motor Unit Disorders

Disorders of the facial nuclei and nerves always produce ipsilateral facial weakness and atrophy, but associated features vary with six possible anatomic sites of abnormality:

1. The motor nucleus. Hyperacusis is present, but taste, lacrimation, and salivation are normal.

2. The facial nerve between the pons and the internal auditory meatus. Taste is spared, but lacrimation and salivation are impaired and hyperacusis is present.

3. The geniculate ganglion. Taste, lacrimation, and salivation are impaired, and hyperacusis is present.

Table 17.3 NEUROLOGIC CAUSES OF DYSPHAGIA

Autoimmune/Postinfectious
1. Dermatomyositis (see Chapter 7)
2. Guillain-Barré syndrome (see Chapter 7)
3. Idiopathic cranial polyneuropathy
4. Myasthenia gravis (see Chapter 15)
5. Transitory neonatal myasthenia gravis (see Chapter 6)

Congenital/Perinatal
1. Aplasia of nuclei
2. Cerebral palsy (see Chapter 5)
3. Chiari malformation (see Chapter 10)
4. Syringobulbia

Genetic
1. Degenerative disorders (see Chapter 5)
2. Familial dysautonomia (see Chapter 6)
3. Familial infantile myasthenia (see Chapter 6)
4. Fiber type disproportion myopathies (see Chapter 6)
5. Myotonic dystrophy (see Chapters 6 and 7)
6. Oculopharyngeal dystrophy

Glioma of Brainstem

Infectious
1. Botulism (see Chapters 6 and 7)
2. Diphtheria
3. Poliomyelitis (see Chapter 7)

Juvenile Progressive Bulbar Palsy

4. The facial nerve from the geniculate ganglion to the stapedius nerve. Taste and salivation are impaired, hyperacusis is present, but lacrimation is normal.

5. The facial nerve from the stapedius nerve to the chorda tympani. Taste and salivation are impaired, hyperacusis is not present, and lacrimation is normal.

6. The facial nerve below the exit of the chorda tympani nerve. Only facial weakness is present.

Disturbances of cranial nerve nuclei do not usually occur in isolation; they are often associated with other features of brainstem dysfunction (bulbar palsy). There is usually some combination of dysarthria, dysphagia, and diplopia. Examination may reveal strabismus, facial diplegia, loss of gag reflex, atrophy of bulbar muscles, and fasciculations of the tongue.

The weakness of myasthenia gravis and facial myopathies is almost always bilateral, whereas brainstem disorders usually begin on one side but eventually cause bilateral impairment. Facial nerve palsies are usually unilateral. Recurrent facial palsy or dysphagia is characterized by a limited differential diagnosis (Table 17.4) confined to disorders of the facial nerve and neuromuscular junction.

CONGENITAL FACIAL WEAKNESS

Not all facial asymmetries observed at birth are traumatic in origin; some are due to congenital aplasia of muscle. Facial diplegia, whether complete or incomplete, suggests the Moebius syndrome or other congenital muscle aplasia. Complete unilateral palsies are likely to be traumatic in origin, whereas partial unilateral palsies may be either traumatic or aplastic. The term *neonatal facial asymmetry* is probably more accurate than *facial nerve palsy* to denote partial or complete unilateral facial weakness in the newborn and emphasizes the difficulty in differentiating traumatic nerve palsies from congenital aplasias.

Aplasia of Facial Muscles

Clinical Features. The Moebius syndrome is the best known congenital aplasia of facial nerve nuclei and facial muscles. It is not certain whether nerve or muscle aplasia is the primary event. Facial diplegia may occur alone, with bilateral abducens palsies, or with involvement of several cranial nerves (Sudarshan and Goldie, 1985). Congenital malformations elsewhere in the body—dextrocardia, talipes equinovarus, absent pectoral muscle, and limb deformities—may be associated as well. Unilateral facial weakness in the Moebius syndrome is unusual, but has been reported with documented evidence of nuclear hypoplasia (Richter, 1960).

Diagnosis. Congenital facial diplegia is by definition a Moebius syndrome. Imaging studies of the brain are indicated in all such cases to determine whether other cerebral malformations are associated. Causes other than primary malformation must be considered as well. Some cases are due to intrauterine toxins or structural disturbances of the brainstem, such as vascular malformation or infarction (Sudarshan and Goldie, 1985).

An electromyogram (EMG) can be helpful in determining the timing of injury. Denervation

Table 17.4 CAUSES OF RECURRENT CRANIAL NEUROPATHIES/PALSY

Familial
    Isolated facial palsy
    Melkerrson syndrome
Hypertensive facial palsy
Myasthenia gravis
Sporadic multiple cranial neuropathies
Toxins

potentials are present only if the facial nuclei or nerves have been injured two to six weeks prior to the study. Facial muscles that are aplastic as a result of Moebius syndrome or nerve injury occurring early in gestation would not demonstrate active denervation.

Treatment. Treatment is not available.

Depressor Anguli Oris Muscle Aplasia

Clinical Features. Isolated unilateral weakness of the depressor anguli oris muscle (DAOM) is the most common cause of facial asymmetry at birth (Nelson and Eng, 1972). One corner of the mouth fails to move downward when the child cries. All other movements of the face are symmetric. The lower lip on the paralyzed side feels thinner to palpation, even at birth, suggesting antepartum hypoplasia.

Diagnosis. Traumatic lesions of the facial nerve would never selectively injure fibers to the DAOM and spare all other facial muscles. Electrodiagnostic studies aid in differentiating aplasia of the DAOM from traumatic injury. In aplasia, the conduction velocity and latency of the facial nerve are normal. Fibrillations are not present at the site of the DAOM. Instead, there is a decreased number or a total absence of motor unit potentials.

Treatment. Treatment is not available and is not needed. The DAOM is not a significant component of facial expression in older children and adults, and its absence is never noted.

Birth Injury

The overall incidence of partial or complete facial paralysis in the newborn is approximately 0.3 per 1,000 live births (McHugh et al, 1969). A higher incidence of 60 per 1,000 births is obtained when prematures and breech deliveries are excluded (Hepner, 1951). These data suggest that facial palsy is most often encountered in term newborns delivered from cephalic presentation. The 6 percent incidence rate of facial nerve palsy among this group remains constant whether or not forceps are applied. There is a remarkably constant relationship between the side of the facial palsy and the obstetric position. Fetuses who lie in occipitoleft positions have left facial palsies; fetuses who lie in occipitoright positions have right facial palsies (Hepner, 1951). The implication of this relationship between occipital position and side of facial palsy is that traumatic facial nerve palsies in the newborn are the result of nerve compression against

the sacrum during labor and not of the misapplication of forceps. Although it is generally believed that the site of nerve compression is extracranial, beyond the point of emergence from the stylomastoid foramen, there is good evidence that the segment of nerve within the facial canal, without fracture of the thin overlying bone, can also sustain a compression injury (McHugh, 1963). Facial nerve injuries within the facial canal are associated with hemotympanum.

Clinical Features. The clinical expression of complete unilateral facial palsy in the newborn can be subtle and need not be apparent immediately after birth. Failure of eye closure on the affected side is the first sign that calls attention to the weakness. Only when the child cries does flaccid paralysis of all facial muscles become obvious. The eyeball rolls up behind the open lid, the nasolabial fold remains flat, and the corner of the mouth "droops" during crying. The normal side, which appears to pull and distort the face, may be thought to be paralyzed and the paralyzed side normal.

When there is partial paralysis of the facial nerve, the orbicularis oculi is the muscle most frequently spared. In these injuries, the site of compression is usually over the parotid gland with sparing of nerve fibers that course upward just after leaving the stylomastoid foramen.

Diagnosis. The diagnosis of facial asymmetry is made by observation of the crying newborn. The skin of the face must be carefully examined for laceration. Otoscopic examination is useful to establish the presence of hemotympanum, and electrodiagnosis is useful to demonstrate the severity of involvement of the facial nerve.

Treatment. Prospective studies are not available regarding the natural outcome of perinatal facial nerve injuries. Most authors are optimistic and indicate a high rate of spontaneous recovery. The optimism may be warranted, but it is based on anecdotal experience alone. In the absence of data on long-term outcome, it is impossible to evaluate the efficacy of suggested therapeutic measures. In most newborns, it is reasonable to caution against surgical intervention except when the nerve is lacerated. In that event, the best response is to reconstitute the nerve, if possible, or at least to allow the proximal stump a clear pathway towards regeneration by debridement of the wound.

CONGENITAL DYSPHAGIA

Congenital dysphagia is usually associated with infantile hypotonia and is therefore discussed in Chapter 6. Isolated aplasia of cranial nerve nuclei subserving swallowing has not been documented, but I have seen one infant with a clinical syndrome consistent with this.

AUTOIMMUNE/POSTINFECTIOUS DISORDERS

Most cases of acute unilateral facial neuritis (Bell palsy) or bilateral facial neuritis (Guillain-Barré syndrome) are attributed to postinfectious demyelination of the nerve. The distinction between Bell palsy and the Guillain-Barré syndrome is not clear; 75 percent of patients who present with Bell palsy are found to have electrophysiologic evidence of neuritis on the clinically unaffected side (Safman, 1971). The Guillain-Barré syndrome (acute polyradiculoneuropathy) is discussed in Chapter 7.

Bell Palsy

Bell palsy is an acute idiopathic paralysis of one side of the face and is due to dysfunction of the facial nerve. In adults, the pathogenesis is considered to be autoimmune demyelination or vascular insufficiency. Childhood cases are almost always considered to be autoimmune. The average annual incidence per 100,000 is 2.7 in the first decade and 10.1 in the second (Katusic et al, 1986).

Clinical Features. A history of prior viral infection, usually upper respiratory, is recorded in many cases, but is not proven to be significantly greater than expected by chance. The initial feature of neuritis is often pain or tingling in the ear canal ipsilateral to the subsequent facial palsy. Sensory symptoms, when present, are usually mild and do not demand medical attention.

The onset of palsy is explosive and becomes maximal within hours of onset. It may be noticed first by the child or the parents. All muscles on one side of the face are affected. Half the face sags, causing the palpebral fissure to be larger. Weakness of the levator palpebrae muscle prevents closure of the lid. Efforts to use muscles of expression cause the face to pull to the normal side. Eating and drinking become difficult, and the dribbling of liquids from the weak corner of the mouth causes embarrassment.

The portion of nerve affected is most often within the temporal bone: taste, lacrimation, and salivation are impaired and hyperacusis is pres-

ent. However, examination of all facial nerve functions is difficult to achieve in small children and precise localization is not critical to diagnosis or prognosis.

Weakness remains maximal for two to four weeks and then begins to recover spontaneously. There are no prospective studies on the natural history of Bell palsy in children, but experience would indicate that almost all patients recover completely.

Diagnosis. Every child who presents with acute unilateral facial weakness must be fully examined to determine whether or not the palsy is an isolated abnormality. The presence of mild facial weakness on the other side or the absence of tendon reflexes in the limbs suggests the possibility of a Guillain-Barré syndrome. Such children must be watched carefully for the development of progressive limb weakness.

Possible underlying causes (e.g., hypertension, infection, trauma) of facial nerve palsy should be excluded before there is satisfaction with the diagnosis of Bell palsy. A computerized tomogram (CT) of the head is not indicated in every child with acute, isolated facial palsy. A more reasonable approach is to watch the child and to recommend an imaging study if other neurologic disturbances develop or if the palsy does not begin to resolve within one month.

Treatment. If the blink reflex is absent, the cornea must be protected from injury. The eye should be patched when the child is outside of the home or at play, and artificial tears should be applied several times each day to keep the cornea moist.

The use of corticosteroids have been advocated on the basis of several controlled trials in adults (Brown, 1982; May et al, 1976; Wolf et al, 1978). All of these trials were flawed by faulty study design (Burgess et al, 1984). There is no scientific basis for the use of corticosteroids in children, in whom the prognosis for complete spontaneous recovery is excellent. If corticosteroid therapy is elected, it is imperative to exclude hypertension or infection as an underlying cause.

Idiopathic Cranial Polyneuropathy

As the name implies, idiopathic cranial neuropathy is of uncertain nosology, but is presumed to be a postinfectious syndrome and is considered by some to be an abortive form of the Guillain-Barré syndrome (Ropper, 1986).

Clinical Features. Onset usually occurs in adulthood (Juncos and Beal, 1987). Most childhood cases occur in adolescence. Similar cases have been described in infants; in many of these, however, limb weakness subsequently developed and may actually be unidentified cases of infant botulism (Grover et al, 1974).

Constant, aching facial pain precedes weakness by hours or days in most cases. It is usually localized to the temple or frontal region, but can be anywhere on the face. The progression of weakness may occur all in one day or may evolve over several weeks. Extraocular motility is usually affected. Facial and trigeminal nerve disturbances occur in half of cases, but lower cranial nerve involvement is uncommon. Occasional patients have transitory disturbances of vision, ptosis, pupillary abnormalities, and tinnitus. Tendon reflexes in the limbs remain active.

Recurrences, and even multiple recurrences, of idiopathic cranial neuropathies are reported in adults (Kansu et al, 1983). These are sporadic cases. Recurrent cranial neuropathies with childhood onset are more likely to be familial cases.

Diagnosis. The differential diagnosis includes the Guillain-Barré syndrome, infant and childhood forms of botulism, brainstem glioma, juvenile progressive bulbar palsy, pontobulbar palsy with deafness, and the Tolosa-Hunt syndrome. Preservation of tendon reflexes in idiopathic cranial polyneuropathy is the major distinguishing feature from the Guillain-Barré syndrome. Botulism can be separated clinically by its prominent autonomic dysfunction and limb weakness (see Chapters 6 and 7). Cranial nerve dysfunction in patients with brainstem glioma, juvenile progressive bulbar palsy, and pontobulbar palsy with deafness usually evolves over a longer period of time. The Tolosa-Hunt syndrome of painful ophthalmoplegia and idiopathic cranial polyneuropathy shares many features and may be a variant of the same disease process (see Chapter 15).

All laboratory investigations are normal. Computerized tomography or a magnetic resonance image (MRI) of the brainstem should be performed in all cases to exclude the possibility of a brainstem glioma. Examination of the cerebrospinal fluid occasionally reveals a mild elevation of protein concentration and five or six lymphocytes.

Treatment. The disease is self-limited, and full recovery is expected two to four months from onset. Corticosteroids are used routinely and believed to relieve facial pain and shorten the course. The relief of pain may be dramatic, but evidence documenting a shortened course is lacking.

GENETIC DISORDERS

Facioscapulohumeral (FSH) Dystrophy

This section brings attention to a rare infantile form of the disease that presents as facial diplegia. The more common childhood form is discussed in Chapter 7. All forms of the disease are transmitted by autosomal dominant inheritance.

Clinical Features. Onset usually occurs during infancy and no later than age five (Bailey et al, 1986). Facial diplegia is the first symptom and may be misdiagnosed as the Moebius syndrome when the onset is in infancy. Later, nasal speech and sometimes ptosis develop. Progressive proximal weakness begins one to two years after onset, first affecting the shoulders and then the pelvis. Pseudohypertrophy of the calves may be present as well. Tendon reflexes are depressed and then absent in weak muscle. Progression of weakness is rapid and unrelenting, leading to disability and death from respiratory insufficiency before age twenty.

Coats syndrome (retinal telangiectasia) and hearing impairment may be associated with infantile FSH dystrophy (Taylor et al, 1982; Voit et al, 1986). Such children present with the triad of hearing loss, visual impairment, and facial weakness.

Diagnosis. The diagnosis should be suspected in any child with progressive facial diplegia. A positive family history of FSH dystrophy cannot always be obtained because the defect may be only minimally expressed in the affected parent.

Myasthenia gravis and brainstem glioma are the major entities that produce progressive facial diplegia in this age group. The serum concentration of creatine kinase is helpful in distinguishing these disorders. It is usually elevated five to ten times the upper limit of normal in infantile FSH dystrophy and normal in myasthenia gravis and brainstem glioma.

Electrophysiologic studies reveal brief, small-amplitude polyphasic potentials in weak muscles and a normal response to repetitive nerve stimulation.

Treatment. Treatment is not available.

Oculopharyngeal Muscular Dystrophy

Oculopharyngeal muscular dystrophy is transmitted by autosomal dominant inheritance and is often described in families of French-Canadian descent (Little and Perl, 1982), but is not restricted to any ethnic group.

Clinical Features. Onset usually occurs in the fourth decade, but may begin as early as adolescence. The initial features are ptosis and dysphagia, followed later by proximal weakness in the legs and external ophthalmoplegia. Eventually, all skeletal muscle is affected but smooth muscle and cardiac muscle are spared.

Childhood onset cases are more likely to begin as ptosis and external ophthalmoplegia without dysphagia (Bray et al, 1965). Facial weakness may be present as well. It is not clear whether early-onset cases with pure ocular myopathy are genetically distinct from late-onset cases of oculopharyngeal dystrophy.

Diagnosis. Myasthenia gravis must be excluded by an edrophonium chloride (Tensilon) test and repetitive nerve stimulation. Serum concentration of creatine kinase is normal, but an EMG of affected muscles demonstrates brief, small-amplitude polyphasic potentials.

Treatment. Therapy is symptomatic. Ptosis can be corrected by levator palpebrae shortening, and dysphagia may be helped by constrictor/cricopharyngeal myotomy.

Recurrent Facial Palsy

At least 2 percent of facial palsies are recurrent (Yanagihara et al, 1984). Autosomal dominant inheritance with variable expression is suspected in most cases. One kindred may have some members with only recurrent facial nerve palsy, whereas others experience recurrent neuropathies of the facial and ocular motor nerves (Aldrich et al, 1984).

Melkerrson Syndrome

The Melkerrson syndrome may be genetically distinct from other recurrent facial palsies, but could also represent the concurrence of several linked genetic errors such as recurrent facial palsy, lingua plicata (deeply furrowed tongue), and migraine.

Clinical Features. This rare disorder is characterized by the triad of recurrent facial palsy, lingua plicata, and facial edema (Levenson et al, 1984). Attacks of facial palsy usually begin in the second decade, but the deeply furrowed tongue is present from birth.

The first attack of facial weakness is indistinguishable from Bell palsy, except that it may be preceded by a migraine-like headache. Subsequent attacks are associated with facial edema, which is soft, painless, nonerythematous, and nonpruritic. It is most often asymmetric, affecting only the upper lip on the paralyzed side, but may affect the cheek and eyelid of one or both sides. Attacks of facial swelling may be precipitated by cold weather or emotional stress and are not coincident with attacks of facial palsy.

Lingua plicata is present in 30 to 50 percent of cases. Furrowing and deep grooving on the dorsal surface of the tongue are permanent from birth. This feature is transmitted by autosomal dominant inheritance and occurs as an isolated finding in some families.

Diagnosis. Melkerrson syndrome can be diagnosed when any two features of the triad are present. It should be considered in any child with a personal or family history of recurrent facial palsy or recurrent facial edema. The presence of lingua plicata in any member of the kindred would confirm the diagnosis.

Treatment. There is no established treatment for this disease. Corticosteroids have not proved beneficial.

HYPERTENSION

Unilateral facial palsy may be a presenting feature of malignant hypertension in children (Lloyd et al, 1966). The palsy is caused by swelling and hemorrhage into the facial canal.

Clinical Features. The course of facial paralysis is indistinguishable from that in Bell palsy. Because the nerve is compressed in its proximal segment, lacrimation, salivation, and taste are all impaired. Time of onset coincides with a rise in blood pressure above 120 mm Hg, and recovery begins when pressure is reduced. The duration of palsy varies from days to weeks. Recurrences are associated with repeated episodes of hypertension.

Diagnosis. The occurrence of facial palsy in a child with known hypertension suggests that hypertension is out of control. Blood pressure should be measured in every child who develops Bell palsy.

Treatment. Control of hypertension is the only effective treatment.

INFECTION

The facial nerve is sometimes involved when there is spread of bacterial infection from the middle ear to the mastoid. External otitis may lead to facial nerve involvement by spread of infection from the tympanic membrane and then to the chorda tympani.

Diphtheria may cause single or multiple cranial neuropathies from a direct effect of its toxin. Facial palsy, dysarthria, and dysphagia are potential complications.

Basilar meningitis, from tuberculosis or other organisms, causes inflammation of cranial nerves as they leave the brain and enter the skull. Multiple and bilateral cranial nerve involvement is usually progressive.

Herpes Zoster Oticus (Ramsay Hunt Syndrome)

The Ramsay Hunt syndrome is a rare disorder caused by herpes zoster infection of the geniculate ganglion.

Clinical Features. The initial feature is pain in and behind the ear. This pain is more severe and persistent than that expected with Bell palsy. Unilateral facial palsy, which cannot be distinguished from Bell palsy by appearance, follows. However, examination of the ipsilateral ear, especially in the fossa of the helix and behind the lobule, demonstrates a vesicular eruption characteristic of herpes zoster (Aleksic et al, 1973).

Diagnosis. The only historical feature distinguishing herpes zoster oticus from Bell palsy is the severity of ear pain. Examination of the ear for vesicles is critical to the diagnosis. Herpes zoster is uncommon in childhood, and the possibility of an immunosuppressed state must be considered.

Treatment. Although herpes zoster oticus is a self-limited disease with full recovery expected, corticosteroids are useful to relieve pain.

Sarcoid

Cranial nerve dysfunction with sarcoidosis is usually due to basilar meningitis, but the facial nerve may also be involved when there is parotitis.

Clinical Features. Onset is usually in the third decade but may be as early as adolescence. Neurologic manifestations develop in only 5 percent of patients with sarcoidosis, but are a presenting feature in almost half. Facial nerve palsy, unilateral or bilateral, is the single most common manifestation (Delaney, 1977; Stern et al, 1985). Visual impairment or deafness is next in frequency. Single cranial neuropathies are present in 73 percent, and multiple cranial neuropathies occur in 58 percent. Any cranial nerve except the accessory nerve may be involved. Systemic features of sarcoidosis are demonstrable in almost every case: intrathoracic involvement is present in 81 percent and ocular involvement is present in 50 percent.

Uveoparotitis is an uncommon manifestation of sarcoidosis. The patient ordinarily comes to attention because of visual impairment and a painful eye. The mouth is dry and the parotid gland swollen. Facial nerve compression and palsy are present in 40 percent of cases.

Diagnosis. Sarcoidosis should be considered in any patient with single or multiple cranial neuropathies. The suspicion is confirmed by documentation of multisystem disease. Radiographs of the chest are diagnostic or at least compatible in 94 percent of patients with neurologic manifestations. The Kveim skin test is positive in almost all cases, but the antigen is not always readily available and interpretation requires experience (Sharma, 1983). Increased concentrations of serum angiotensin-converting enzyme are detected in approximately 75 percent of patients with active pulmonary disease. Biopsy of lymph nodes or other affected tissues provides histologic confirmation.

Treatment. Prednisone, 0.5 to 1 mg/kg/day, should be maintained until a clinical response is evident and then tapered at a slow enough rate to prevent relapse. The prognosis for neurologic complications of sarcoidosis is good without treatment, but corticosteroids appear to increase the speed of recovery.

JUVENILE PROGRESSIVE BULBAR PALSY

Also known as *Fazio-Londe disease*, juvenile progressive bulbar palsy is a motor neuron disease limited to bulbar muscles. Most cases are sporadic, but heredofamilial cases are reported (Albers et al, 1983; Gomez et al, 1962). No specific genetic mode of transmission has been identified.

Clinical Features. Age of onset is usually in the second decade. The initial feature may be facial weakness, dysphagia, or dysarthria. Eventually, all of the lower motor cranial nerve nuclei are affected and the ocular motor nerve nuclei spared. Fasciculations and atrophy of the arms are reported in some cases, but it is not clear whether such patients have a different disease. In most patients, bulbar atrophy is severe but limb muscles are spared and tendon reflexes are normal.

Diagnosis. The major diagnostic considerations are myasthenia gravis and brainstem glioma. These must be excluded with a Tensilon test and and MRI of the brainstem. Electrodiagnosis is useful to demonstrate active denervation of facial muscles with sparing of the limbs and normal repetitive stimulation of nerves.

Children with rapidly progressive motor neuron disease affecting the face and limbs should be considered to have a childhood form of amyotrophic lateral sclerosis.

Treatment. The disorder is often devastating. A previously normal child is no longer able to speak intelligibly or swallow. Feeding gastrostomy is often required for feeding. Considerable psychological support is required. Treatment is not available for the underlying disease.

METABOLIC DISORDERS

Hyperparathyroidism

The neurologic manifestations of primary hyperparathyroidism are usually characterized by headache and confusion (see Chapter 2). Occasionally, a syndrome similar to amyotrophic lateral sclerosis may develop that also includes ataxia and internuclear ophthalmoplegia (Patten and Pages, 1984). Dysarthria and dysphagia are prominent features.

Hypothyroidism

Cranial nerve abnormalities are unusual in hypothyroidism. Deafness is the most common manifestation, but acute facial nerve palsy, resembling Bell palsy, is occasionally described.

Osteopetrosis (Albers-Schönberg Disease)

Osteopetrosis is a genetic disease transmitted by autosomal recessive inheritance. The calvarium becomes thickened, and cranial nerves are compressed and compromised as they pass through the bone. Deafness and facial diplegia are common manifestations.

SYRINGOBULBIA

Syringobulbia is usually the medullary extension of a cervical syrinx (see Chapter 12), but may also originate in the medulla. It usually involves the nucleus ambiguus, and the spinal tract and motor nucleus of the trigeminal nerve. Swallowing and chewing are impaired.

TOXINS

Most neurotoxins produce either diffuse encephalopathy or peripheral neuropathy. Only ethylene glycol, trichlorethylene, and chlorocresol have been associated with selective toxicity to cranial nerves.

Ethylene glycol is used as an antifreeze. Accidental or suicidal ingestion produces facial diplegia, hearing impairment, and dysphagia (Mallya et al, 1986). Trichlorethylene intoxication may produce multiple cranial neuropathies, but has a predilection for the trigeminal nerve (Feldman et al, 1970) and was previously used in the treatment of tic douloureux.

Chlorocresol, a compound used in the industrial production of heparin, produced recurrent unilateral facial palsy, in an exposed worker (Dossing et al, 1986). Inhalation of the compound caused tingling of one side of the face followed by weakness of the muscles. The neurologic disturbance was brief, relieved by exposure to fresh air, and could be reproduced experimentally.

TRAUMA

Facial palsy following closed head injury is usually associated with bleeding from the ear and fracture of the petrous bone (Maiman et al, 1985; Puvanendren et al, 1977).

Clinical Features. The onset of palsy may be immediate or may be delayed for as long as three weeks. In most cases, the onset is between two and seven days. The mechanism of delay is unknown.

Diagnosis. Electrophysiologic studies are helpful in predicting prognosis. If the nerve is intact but demonstrates a conduction block, recovery usually begins within five days and is complete. If there is partial denervation, the majority of patients recover full facial movement but frequently have evidence of aberrant reinnervation. Full recovery is not expected when denervation is complete.

Treatment. The management of traumatic facial palsy is controversial. Surgical decompression and corticosteroids have been recommended by some, but evidence is not available to support either mode of therapy.

TUMORS

Tumors of the facial nerve are extremely unusual in children. Brainstem glioma is the major neoplastic cause of facial palsy (see Chapter 15), followed by tumors that infiltrate the meninges, such as leukemia, meningeal carcinoma, and histiocytosis X. Acoustic neuromas are unusual in childhood and are limited in occurrence to children with neurofibromatosis. These cause hearing impairment before facial palsy and are discussed in the next section.

■ Hearing Impairment and Deafness

ANATOMIC CONSIDERATIONS

Sound is funneled through the external auditory canal to the tympanic membrane, causing it to vibrate. The vibrations are transmitted by ossicles to the oval window of the cochlea, the sensory organ of hearing. The air-filled space from the tympanic membrane to the cochlea is the middle ear. The membranous labyrinth within the osseous labyrinth is the principal structure of the inner ear. It contains the cochlea, the semicircular canals, and the vestibule. The semicircular canals and vestibule are the sensory organs of vestibular function. The cochlea consists of three fluid-filled canals wound into a snail-like configuration.

The organ of Corti is the transducer within the cochlea that converts mechanical to electrical energy. Impulses are transmitted in the auditory portion of the eighth nerve to the ipsilateral cochlear nuclei of the medulla. The cochlear nuclei on each side transmit information to both superior olivary nuclei, causing bilateral representation of hearing throughout the remainder of the central pathways. From the superior olivary nuclei, impulses are transmitted by the lateral lemniscus to the inferior colliculus. Further cross-connections occur in collicular synapses. Rostrally directed fibers from the inferior colliculi ascend to the medial geniculate and auditory cortex of the temporal lobe.

SYMPTOMS OF AUDITORY DYSFUNCTION

The major symptoms of disturbance in the auditory pathways are hearing impairment, tinnitus, and hyperacusis. In infants, hearing impairment in infants is characterized by failure to develop speech (see Chapter 5), and in older children by inattentiveness and poor school performance.

Fifty percent of infants use words with meaning by twelve months and join words into sentences by twenty-one months. Failure to accomplish these tasks by twenty-one months and three years, respectively, is always abnormal (Neligan and Prudham, 1969).

Hearing Impairment

Hearing impairment is classified as (1) conductive, (2) sensorineural, or (3) central.

A *conductive hearing impairment* results from disturbances in the external or middle ear; the mechanical vibrations that comprise the sensory input of hearing are not faithfully delivered to the inner ear because the external canal is blocked or the tympanic membrane or ossicles are abnormal. The major defect in hearing is sound amplification. Patients with conductive hearing impairment are better able to hear loud speech in a noisy background than soft speech in a quiet background.

A *sensorineural hearing impairment* results from disturbances of the cochlea or auditory nerve. The frequency content of sound is improperly analyzed and transduced. High frequencies may be selectively lost. Individuals with sensorineural hearing have difficulty discriminating speech when there is background noise.

A *central hearing impairment* results from disturbance of the cochlear nuclei or their projections to the cortex. With lesions in the brainstem, hearing impairment is usually bilateral. Cortical lesions are characterized by difficulty in processing information. Pure tone audiometry is normal, but speech discrimination is impaired by background noise or competing messages.

Tinnitus

Tinnitus is the illusion of "noise" in the ear. The noise is usually high-pitched and constant. Tinnitus is usually caused by disturbances of the auditory nerve, but may also occur as a simple partial seizure originating from the primary auditory cortex. Sounds generated by the cardiovascular system, heartbeat and bruit, are sometimes audible, especially while a person is lying down, but should not be confused with tinnitus.

Hyperacusis

The term hyperacusis is sometimes used to denote an exaggerated startle response, but I believe that its use should be reserved for failure of the stapedius muscle to dampen sound by its effect on the ossicles. This occurs when the chorda tympani branch of the facial nerve is damaged (see Bell palsy earlier in this chapter).

APPROACH TO THE PATIENT

Hearing assessment in the office is satisfactory for severe hearing impairment but is unsatisfactory for detecting loss of specific frequency bands. The speech and hearing handicap generated by a high-frequency hearing impairment should not be underestimated.

In testing infants, the physician should stand behind the patient and provide interesting sounds to each ear. Such sounds could be produced by bells, chimes, rattles, or a tuning fork. Dropping a large object and watching the infant and parents startle from the noise is not a test of hearing. Once the infant sees the source of the interesting sound or hears it several times, interest is lost. Therefore, use different high-frequency and low-frequency sounds for each ear. The normal responses of the infant are to become alert and to attempt to localize the source of the sound.

Older children can be tested by observing their response to spoken words at different intensities and with tuning forks that provide pure tones of different frequencies. The *Rinne test* compares air conduction (conductive plus sensorineural hearing) with bone conduction (sensorineural hearing). A tuning fork is held against the mastoid process until the sound fades and is then held one inch from the ear. Normal children hear the vibration produced by air conduction twice as long as that produced by bone conduction. Impaired air conduction with normal bone conduction indicates a conductive hearing loss.

The *Weber test* compares bone conduction in the two ears. A tuning fork is placed at the center of the forehead, and the patient is asked whether sound is perceived equally in both ears. A normal response is to hear the sound in the center of the head. If bone conduction is normal in both ears, sound will be localized to an ear with impaired air conduction because the normal blocking response of air conduction is lacking. If a sensorineural hearing impairment is present in one ear, bone conduction is perceived in the good ear.

Otoscopic examination is imperative in every child with questionable hearing or tinnitus. The answer may be seen through the speculum in the form of impacted wax, otitis media, perforated tympanic membrane, or cholesteatoma.

TESTS OF HEARING

Pure Tone Audiometry

Selected frequencies are presented by earphones (air conduction) or by a vibrator applied to the mastoid (bone conduction), and the subject is asked to determine the minimum level perceived for each frequency. Normal hearing levels are defined by an international standard. The test can be performed adequately only in children who are old enough to cooperate. With conductive hearing impairment, air conduction is abnormal and bone conduction is normal; with sensorineural hearing impairment, both are abnormal; and with central hearing impairment, both are normal.

Speech Tests

The *speech reception threshold* measures the intensity at which a subject can correctly repeat 50 percent of presented words. The *speech discrimination test* measures the subject's ability to understand speech at normal conversational levels. Both tests are abnormal out of proportion to pure tone loss with auditory nerve disease, abnormal in proportion to pure tone loss with cochlear disease, and normal with conductive and central hearing loss.

Special Tests

Cochlear lesions may produce *diplacusis* and *recruitment*, auditory nerve lesions produce *tone decay*. Diplacusis is a distortion of pure tones so that the subject perceives a mixture of tones. With recruitment the sensation of loudness increases at an abnormally rapid rate as the intensity of sound is increased. Tone decay is diminished perception of a suprathreshold tone with time.

Brainstem Auditory Evoked Response (BAER)

The BAER (ABR) is used to test hearing and the integrity of the brainstem auditory pathways in infants and small children. No cooperation is required, and sedation improves the accuracy of results.

When each ear is stimulated with repetitive clicks and simultaneous recordings are made between the forehead and ipsilateral mastoid, five waves are recorded (Fig. 17.1). Wave I is generated by the acoustic nerve, wave II by the cochlear nerve, wave III by the superior olivary complex, wave IV by the lateral lemniscus, and wave V by the inferior colliculus. Normal values for the absolute latency of waves I and V have been published by several authors; the values of Despland and Galambos (1980) are summarized in Table 17.5.

The ABR first appears at a conceptional age of twenty-six to twenty-seven weeks. The absolute latencies of waves I and V and V-I interpeak interval decline progressively with advancing conceptional age. The latency of wave V bears an inverse relationship to the intensity of the stimulus and can be used to test hearing.

An initial test is performed using a stimulus intensity of 70 dB. If wave V is not produced, a hearing impairment is present and the test should be repeated at higher intensities until a response threshold is obtained. If wave V is present, the test is repeated at sequential reductions of 10 dB until the lowest intensity capable of producing wave V—the hearing threshold—is established. Because the latency of wave V is proportional to the intensity of the stimulus, a latency-intensity curve can be drawn (Fig. 17.2).

Table 17.5 BRAINSTEM AUDITORY EVOKED RESPONSE LATENCIES*

Conceptional Age		Wave I (ms)	Wave V (ms)	V-I Interval (ms)
30–31 weeks	Mean	3.50	9.10	5.60
	+3 SD	5.09	10.06	7.25
32–33 weeks	Mean	2.78	8.36	5.62
	+3 SD	3.44	9.98	6.52
34–35 weeks	Mean	2.56	8.00	5.44
	+3 SD	3.31	9.41	6.41
36–37 weeks	Mean	2.53	7.80	5.27
	+3 SD	3.10	9.42	6.41
38–39 weeks	Mean	2.30	7.42	5.09
	+3 SD	3.02	8.71	6.06
40–41 weeks	Mean	2.28	7.35	5.07
	+3 SD	3.09	8.73	6.30
42–43 weeks	Mean	2.28	7.17	4.89
	+3 Sd	2.88	7.47	5.49

*Stimulus intensity is 60 dB above adult threshold, stimulus frequency is 10 per second.

In normal newborns, the latency of wave V will decrease by 0.24 to 0.44 ms for each 10 dB in sound intensity between 70 and 110 dB (Stockard et al, 1983).

In children with conductive hearing impairment, the time required to transmit sound across the middle ear and activate the cochlea is prolonged and the total amount of sound energy is reduced. As a consequence, the latency of wave I is prolonged and the latency-intensity curve of wave V shifts to the right by an amount equiv-

Ipsilateral

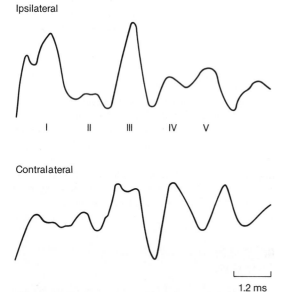

Contralateral

1.2 ms

Figure 17.1 Normal brainstem auditory evoked response (BAER, ABR). The generators of the five positive waves include the acoustic nerve (I), the cochlear nucleus (II), the superior olivary complex (III), the lateral lemniscus (IV), and the inferior colliculus (V). (From Fenichel GM: Neonatal Neurology. Churchill Livingstone, New York, 1985.)

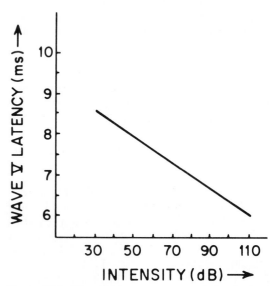

Figure 17.2 Wave V latency-intensity curve. In term newborns, the latency of wave V decreases about 0.3 ms for each intensity increase of 10 dB. (From Fenichel GM: Neonatal Neurology. Churchill Livingstone, New York, 1985.)

alent to the hearing impairment, without any alteration in the slope of the curve.

In those with sensorineural hearing impairment, the latency-intensity curve of wave V is shifted to the right because of the hearing impairment and in addition, the slope of the curve becomes steeper—exceeding 0.55 ms/dB.

CONGENITAL DEAFNESS

Congenital deafness is often missed in the newborn unless there is an obvious deformity of the external ear or a family history of genetic hearing loss. Congenital ear malformations are present in approximately 2 percent of newborns with congenital deafness (Fraser, 1964), and genetic factors are responsible for 35 percent of cases (Konigsmark and Gorlin, 1976). If one considers profound deafness of early onset, genetic causes account for 50 percent.

Aplasia of Inner Ear

Inner ear aplasia is always associated with auditory nerve abnormalities. There are three main types:

1. Michel defect, complete absence of the otic capsule and eighth cranial nerve.

2. Mondini defect, incomplete development of the bony and membranous labyrinths and dysgenesis of the spiral ganglion.

3. Scheibe defect, dysplasia of the membranous labyrinth and atrophy of the eighth nerve.

Chromosome Disorders

Hearing impairment is relatively uncommon in children with chromosomal disorders. Abnormalities of chromosome 18 are often associated with profound sensorineural hearing loss and malformations of the external ear.

Genetic Disorders

Isolated Deafness

Isolated deafness in newborns and infants is usually genetic and may be transmitted by autosomal dominant, autosomal recessive, or X-linked inheritance. In many sporadic cases, the hearing loss will prove to be transmitted by autosomal recessive inheritance.

The association of congenital deafness and external ear deformities is often caused by genetic disorders transmitted by autosomal dominant inheritance, but chromosomal disorders and fetal exposure to drugs and toxins must be considered as well. Maternal use of heparin during pregnancy produces an embryopathy characterized by skeletal deformities, flattening of the nose, cerebral dysgenesis, and deafness (Hall et al, 1980).

In the absence of external malformation, sporadic cases of deafness in infants may not be suspected until speech fails to be developed. Intrauterine infection with cytomegalovirus is an important cause of congenital deafness (see Chapter 5). Nearly 1 percent of newborns in the United States are infected with cytomegalovirus, and approximately 10 percent will develop sensorineural hearing loss (Bale, 1984). Rubella embryopathy had been an important cause as well, but has been almost eliminated in the United States by mass vaccination.

Pendred Syndrome

Pendred syndrome is a genetic defect in thyroxine synthesis transmitted by autosomal recessive inheritance (Konigsmark and Gorlin, 1976). It is characterized by goiter and sensorineural hearing impairment.

Clinical Features. Sensorineural hearing impairment is present at birth and is severe in 50 percent of cases. Milder hearing impairment may not be detected until the child is two years of age. Vestibular function may be impaired as well.

A diffuse, non-nodular goiter becomes apparent during the first decade, often in infancy. Clinical signs of hypothyroidism are not present. Growth and intelligence are usually normal.

Diagnosis. The laboratory method for assessing iodide organification is the perchlorate discharge test. It is a measure of thyroidal radioiodine content following the administration of potassium perchlorate. A decline from baseline levels of thyroidal radioiodine of 10 percent or more is considered a positive result.

Treatment. Goiter is best treated medically and not surgically. Exogenous hormone causes decreased production of thyroid-stimulating hormone (TSH) with subsequent reduction in goiter size. Hearing loss is not reversible.

Usher Syndrome

The Usher syndrome, characterized by congenital deafness and retinitis pigmentosa, is believed to be transmitted by autosomal recessive inheritance, but there is probably genetic heterogeneity (McLeod et al, 1971).

Clinical Features. Bilateral severe sensorineural deafness is present at birth. Slowly progressive loss of vision due to retinitis pigmentosa begins during the second decade, leading to blindness in the fifth decade or later. Vestibular responses to caloric testing are absent, and mild ataxia may be present. Mental retardation is present in 25 percent of cases.

Diagnosis. The combination of retinitis pigmentosa and hearing impairment is also present in other syndromes: (1) *Alstrom syndrome,* obesity and diabetes mellitus; (2) *Cockayne syndrome* (see Chapter 16); (3) *Laurence-Moon-Biedl syndrome,* mental deficiency, hypogonadism, obesity; and (4) *Refsum disease* (see Chapter 7). Usher syndrome is the only one in which profound deafness is present at birth.

Treatment. Deafness is too profound to be corrected with hearing aids. Treatment is not available.

ACQUIRED HEARING IMPAIRMENT

Drugs

Antibiotics are the most commonly used class of drugs with potential ototoxicity in children (Snavely and Hodges, 1984). The incidence of toxicity is greatest with amikacin, furosemide, and vancomycin and only a little less with kanamycin and neomycin. Permanent damage is unusual with any of these drugs. The characteristic syndrome consists of tinnitus and high-frequency hearing impairment. By contrast, aminoglycosides may produce irreversible cochlear toxicity, which begins as tinnitus, progresses to vertigo and high-frequency hearing impairment, and finally impairs all frequencies. Vancomycin produces hearing loss only when blood concentrations exceed 45 μg/ml.

Beta-adrenoceptor blocking drugs are a rare cause of hearing impairment and tinnitus (Faldt et al, 1984). Cessation of therapy reverses symptoms. Cis-platinum, an anticancer drug, produces ototoxicity in 30 percent of cases (Rozencweig et al, 1977). Tinnitus is the major feature. Hearing impairment occurs at frequencies above those used for speech.

Salicylates tend to concentrate in the perilymph of the labyrinth and are ototoxic. Tinnitus and high-frequency hearing impairment result from chronic exposure to high doses.

Genetic Neurologic Disorders

Several of the disorders listed in Table 17.6 are discussed in other chapters. Sensorineural hearing impairment occurs as part of several spinocerebellar degenerations, hereditary motor sensory neuropathies, and sensory autonomic neuropathies. It is a major feature of Refsum disease (HSM IV) and can be controlled by dietary measures to reduce serum concentrations of phytanic acid (Djupesland et al, 1983).

Pontobulbar Palsy with Deafness

A rare motor neuron disorder transmitted by autosomal recessive inheritance, pontobulbar palsy with deafness shares many clinical features with juvenile progressive bulbar palsy, and some cases may be variant expressions of the same genetic error (Brucher et al, 1981).

Clinical Features. Onset is most often during the second decade. Progressive sensorineural hearing loss is the initial symptom and may affect first one ear and then the other. Deafness is accompanied or quickly followed by facial weakness and dysphagia. Tongue atrophy occurs in the majority of cases, but masseter and ocular motor palsies are uncommon.

Approximately half of patients have evidence of pyramidal tract dysfunction, such as extensor plantar responses, and half have atrophy and fasciculations of limb muscle. Loss of tendon reflexes is an early feature of most cases.

Respiratory insufficiency is a common feature and a frequent cause of death.

Diagnosis. The presence of deafness and areflexia distinguishes this disorder from juvenile progressive bulbar palsy, but can also suggest a hereditary motor sensory neuropathy if symptoms of bulbar palsy are delayed. The diagnosis depends upon the clinical features and cannot be confirmed by laboratory tests. Magnetic resonance imaging or CT of the brainstem should be done to exclude the possibility of tumor.

Treatment. A feeding gastrostomy is needed in most patients. Treatment is not available for the underlying disease.

Infectious Diseases

Otitis media is a common cause of reversible conductive hearing impairment in children, but only rarely does suppurative infection spread to the inner ear (see ''Vertigo'' later on). Hearing impairment is a relatively common symptom of viral encephalitis (see Chapter 2) and may be a presenting feature (Rosenberg, 1984). Sudden hearing loss may also accompany childhood exanthems (chickenpox, mumps, measles), and in such cases virus can be isolated from the cochlear and auditory nerves.

The overall incidence of persistent unilateral or bilateral hearing loss in children with acute bacterial meningitis is 10 percent (Dodge et al, 1984). *Streptococcus pneumoniae* is associated with the highest incidence (31 percent) and *Haemophilus influenzae* with the lowest (6 percent). *S. pneumoniae* meningitis is also associated with a 20 percent incidence of persistent dizziness, gait ataxia, and other neurologic deficits (Bohr et al, 1984).

The site of disease is probably the inner ear or auditory nerve. Organisms may gain access to the inner ear from the subarachnoid space. Otitis media is the source of meningitis in many children and produces a transitory conductive hearing loss, but does not correlate with permanent sensorineural hearing loss.

Brainstem auditory evoked response audiometry should be performed to screen for hearing loss in all children with acute bacterial meningitis towards the end of their hospitalization.

Metabolic Disorders

Meniere disease is characterized by vertigo, tinnitus, and hearing impairment. Vertigo is often the presenting feature (see "Vertigo" later on).

Tinnitus and decreased hearing are common features of hypothyroidism and are reversible by thyroid replacement therapy (Swanson et al, 1981).

Skeletal Disorders

The combination of hearing impairment and skeletal deformities almost always indicates a genetic disease. Skeletal disorders may be limited, usually to the face and digits, or generalized. A partial list is provided in Table 17.6, which highlights the more common syndromes. Almost all are transmitted by autosomal dominant inheritance with variable expression. The exceptions are (1) osteopetrosis, which is transmitted by autosomal recessive inheritance; (2) craniometaphyseal dysplasia, which has both a dominant and recessive form; and (3) the Klippel-Feil anomaly, for which the pattern of transmission is uncertain.

Table 17.6 CAUSES OF HEARING IMPAIRMENT AND DEAFNESS

Congenital
1. Aplasia of inner ear
   a. Michel defect
   b. Mondini defect
   c. Scheibe defect
2. Chromosome disorders
   a. Trisomy 13
   b. Trisomy 18
   c. 18q- syndrome
3. Genetic disorders
   a. Isolated deafness
   b. Pendred syndrome
   c. Usher syndrome
4. Intrauterine viral infection (see Chapter 5)
5. Maternal drug use

Drugs
1. Antibiotics
2. Beta blockers
3. Chemotherapy

Genetic Neurologic Disorders
1. Facioscapulohumeral dystrophy (see Chapter 7)
2. Familial spastic paraparesis (see Chapter 12)
3. Hereditary motor sensory neuropathies (see Chapter 7)
4. Hereditary sensory autonomic neuropathies (see Chapter 9)
5. Pontobulbar palsy with deafness
6. Mitochondrial disorders (see Chapter 8)
7. Spinocerebellar degenerations (see Chapter 10)
8. Xeroderma pigmentosum (see Chapter 5)

Infectious Diseases
1. Bacterial meningitis
2. Otitis media (see "Vertigo")
3. Sarcoid (see "Facial Weakness")
4. Viral encephalitis (see Chapter 2)
5. Viral exanthems

Metabolic Disorders
1. Hypothyroidism
2. Meniere disease (see "Vertigo")

Skeletal Disorders
1. Apert acrocephalosyndactyly
2. Cleidocranial dysostosis
3. Craniofacial dysostosis (Crouzon disease)
4. Craniometaphyseal dysplasia (Pyle disease)
5. Klippel-Feil syndrome
6. Mandibulofacial dysostosis (Treacher-Collins syndrome)
7. Osteogenesis imperfecta
8. Osteopetrosis (Albers-Schönberg disease)

Trauma (see "Vertigo")

Tumor
1. Acoustic neuroma
2. Cholesteatoma (see "Vertigo")

Trauma

Acute auditory and vestibular injuries occur with fractures of the petrous portion of the temporal bone. Vestibular function is more likely to be impaired than auditory function (see "Vertigo" later on).

Tumor

Acoustic neuroma and cholesteatoma are the tumors most likely to cause hearing impairment in children. Other cerebello-pontine angle tumors are almost unheard of before the third or fourth decades. Cholesteatoma is discussed in the section on vertigo.

Acoustic Neuroma

Acoustic neuromas are more properly classified as schwannomas of the eighth nerve. Only 6 percent of acoustic neuromas present in the second decade, and even fewer are seen in the first decade. Children with acoustic neuroma almost always have a separate form of neurofibromatosis from the type that produces tumors of peripheral nerves. It is characterized by bilateral acoustic neuromas, the later development of other cerebral tumors such as meningioma, and fewer than five café-au-lait spots on the skin (Kaner et al, 1980).

Clinical Features. Deafness or tinnitus is the usual presenting complaint. Approximately one third of patients have nonaudiologic symptoms, such as facial numbness or paresthesia, vertigo, headache, and ataxia (Hart et al, 1983). Hearing impairment is present in almost every patient; ipsilateral diminished corneal reflex in half; and ataxia, facial hypesthesia or weakness, and nystagmus in 30 to 40 percent. Large tumors produce obstructive hydrocephalus with symptoms of increased intracranial pressure and brainstem compression.

Diagnosis. Every child with progressive hearing impairment or tinnitus should be carefully examined for café-au-lait spots on the skin and the family history explored for acoustic neuroma or other neurologic disturbance.

Abnormalities in pure tone audiometry and in the BAER results are present in almost every patient. Audiometry is consistent with a sensorineural hearing impairment. Small tumors produce ipsilateral prolongation of the V-I interval or absence of wave I of the BAER; large tumors cause absence of waves on the ipsilateral side and prolongation of the V-III interval on the contralateral side as a result of brainstem compression.

Computerized tomography provides excellent visualization of tumors larger than 1.5 cm (Fig. 17.3). The important CT findings are enlargement and erosion of the internal auditory canal and the presence of a mass in the cerebellopontine angle that is isodense with brain but that

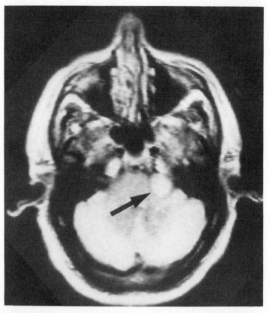

Figure 17.3 CT image of acoustic neuroma. A large tumor (arrow) is pressing upon and displacing the brainstem. (Courtesy of Dr. Mark Freeman, Department of Radiological Sciences, Vanderbilt University, Nashville.)

demonstrates contrast enhancement. Large tumors shift the brainstem and cause obstructive hydrocephalus.

Treatment. Acoustic neuromas must be surgically resected. Residual hearing is sacrificed; with care, however, facial nerve function may be preserved.

■ Vertigo

Vertigo is the sensation of rotation or spinning. It is very disturbing and can be terrifying to small children. Balance is lost, and posture is difficult to maintain, giving the appearance of ataxia (see Chapter 10). Nausea and nystagmus are often associated. When nystagmus is present, the fast phase is in the same direction as the perceived rotation. All symptoms are exacerbated by movement of the head.

ANATOMIC CONSIDERATIONS

The semicircular canals and the vestibule, within the labyrinth, are the sensory organs of the vestibular system. The stimulus for excitation of the semicircular canals is rotary motion of the head; for the vestibule it is gravity. Information from the sensory organs is transmitted by the vestibular portion of the eighth cranial nerve to the vestibular nuclei in the brainstem and the cerebellum. From the vestibular nuclei there are extensive connections to the cerebellum and medial longitudinal fasciculus. Cortical projections terminate in the superior temporal gyrus and frontal lobe.

APPROACH TO VERTIGO

History and Physical Examination

Patients complaining of dizziness or lightheadedness must be carefully questioned about the sensation of rotation. It is irrelevant whether the subject or the environment is perceived to rotate. The illusion of rotation separates vertigo from presyncope, ataxia, and other disturbances of balance and localizes the disturbance to the vestibular system. Vertigo always implies dysfunction of the labyrinth or vestibular nerve (peripheral vertigo) or the brainstem or temporal lobe (central vertigo).

Important historic points to document include (1) the course of vertigo (acute, recurrent, chronic), (2) precipitating events (trauma, infection, position change), (3) association of hearing impairment and tinnitus, (4) drug exposure, (5) cardiovascular disease, and (6) family history of migraine.

Acute, episodic attacks of vertigo, not induced by motion, are most often caused by migraine or epilepsy, with migraine as the more common of the two. A single, prolonged attack of vertigo, especially when combined with nausea and

Table 17.7 CAUSES OF VERTIGO

Drugs and toxins
Epilepsy
   Complex partial seizures
   Simple partial seizures
Infectious
   Otitis media
   Vestibular neuronitis
Meniere disease
Migraine
   Benign recurrent vertigo
   Benign paroxysmal vertigo (see Chapter 10)
Motion sickness
Multiple sclerosis (see Chapter 10)
Psychogenic (hyperventilation syndrome) (see Chapter 1)
Trauma
   Migraine
   Post-traumatic neurosis
   Temporal bone fracture
   Vestibular concussion
   Whiplash injury

Table 17.8 DISTINGUISHING PERIPHERAL AND CENTRAL VERTIGO

Peripheral Vertigo
Clinical Features
1. Hearing loss, tinnitus, and otalgia may be associated.
2. Past pointing and falling in direction of unilateral disease.
3. Ataxia with eyes closed in bilateral disease.
4. Vestibular and positional nystagmus.

Laboratory Features
1. Caloric testing reveals vestibular paresis, or directional preponderance, or both.
2. Pure tone audiometry reveals sensorineural hearing loss.
3. Recruitment is present with end organ disease and tone decay with nerve disease.

Central Vertigo
Clinical Features
1. Cerebellar and cranial nerve dysfunction are frequently associated.
2. Hearing is intact.
3. Loss of consciousness may be associated.

Laboratory Features
1. Pure tone audiometry and speech discrimination are normal.
2. Impaired comprehension of competing messages.
3. Caloric testing may reveal directional preponderance, but not vestibular paresis.
4. Possible abnormality of brainstem evoked response, electroencephalogram, computerized tomography, or magnetic resonance image.

vomiting, is usually due to infection of the labyrinth or vestibular nerve. Chronic vertigo often waxes and wanes in severity and may seem intermittent rather than chronic. Both central and peripheral causes must be considered (Table 17.7), but the two are readily distinguished by their clinical and laboratory features (Table 17.8).

Special Tests

Caloric and audiometric testing are indicated in most children with chronic vertigo. Caloric testing is described in this section and audiometric testing in the section on hearing impairment. The Nylen-Hallpike test is useful to define position-induced vertigo.

Caloric Testing

The simplest method of caloric testing is to instill small quantities of cool water into the external auditory canal using a rubber-tipped syringe. The canal must first be inspected to determine whether there is clear passage to an intact tympanic membrane. A sufficient quantity of water is used, depending upon the size of the child, to keep the tympanic membrane cooled for twenty seconds. The eyes are then observed for nystagmus. A normal response is slow deviation of the eyes to the side stimulated, followed by a fast component to the opposite side. If stimulation with cool water fails to produce a response, the procedure is repeated with ice water. Absence of nystagmus indicates absence of peripheral vestibular function. Partial dysfunction of one vestibular apparatus results in asymmetry of response, *directional preponderance*.

Electronystagmography

Electronystagmography is a technique that allows better quantification of caloric testing. A standard caloric stimulus is delivered into the ear, and the duration and velocity of nystagmus are recorded on paper. Commercial machines are available for this purpose.

Nylen-Hallpike Technique

From the sitting position, the patient is tilted back to the supine position so that the head hangs down below the level of the examining table. The head is then turned 45 degrees to the right, and the eyes are observed for position-induced nystagmus. Several minutes later, the maneuver is repeated with the head turned 45 degrees to the left, then repeated again with the head tilted 45 degrees backwards.

DISORDERS CAUSING VERTIGO

Drugs

Many drugs that disturb vestibular function disturb auditory function as well. This section deals only with drugs affecting vestibular function more than auditory function. Toxic doses of anticonvulsants and neuroleptics produce ataxia, incoordination, and measurable disturbances of vestibular function, but patients do not ordinarily complain of vertigo.

Antibiotics are the major class of drugs producing vestibular toxicity (Snavely and Hodges, 1984). Streptomycin, minocycline, and aminoglycosides are associated with a high frequency of toxicity, sulfonamides with a low frequency.

Streptomycin disturbs vestibular function, but has little effect on hearing. A milligram-per-kilogram dose that produces toxicity cannot be given because of variation in individual susceptibility. However, the vestibular toxicity of strep-

tomycin is so predictable at high doses that the drug has been used to destroy vestibular function in patients with severe Meniere disease. Dihydrostreptomycin affects auditory function and spares vestibular function. It is so ototoxic that its use has been abandoned.

Minocycline produces nausea, vomiting, dizziness, and ataxia at standard therapeutic doses. Symptoms begin two to three days after initiating therapy and cease two days after therapy is discontinued.

Gentamicin and other aminoglycosides have an adverse effect on both vestibular and auditory function. Some disturbance is noted in 2 percent of patients treated with gentamicin. Vestibular dysfunction, either alone or in combination with auditory dysfunction, occurs in 84 percent of cases, whereas auditory dysfunction alone occurs in only 16 percent. Ototoxicity develops when total dose exceeds 17.5 mg/kg (Gailiunas et al, 1978).

Epilepsy

Vertigo may be the only manifestation of a simple partial seizure or an initial feature of a complex partial seizure. Ten to 20 percent of people with complex partial seizures experience vertigo as an aura (Currie et al, 1971; Deonna et al, 1986).

Clinical Features. When vertigo is followed by a complex partial seizure, it is readily recognized as an aura. Diagnosis becomes problematic when vertigo is the solitary manifestation of a simple partial seizure. Activity stops, the child becomes pale, appears frightened, and then recovers. Unsteadiness and nausea may be associated.

Diagnosis. An electroencephalogram (EEG) is indicated in children with unexplained brief attacks of vertigo, especially when vestibular and auditory function are normal between attacks. Ambulatory EEG or twenty-four hour video monitoring may be needed to capture an attack if the interictal EEG is normal.

Treatment. Management of simple and complex partial seizures is discussed in Chapter 2.

Bacterial Infection

Otitis media and meningitis are leading causes of vestibular and auditory impairment in children. Syphilis had been a major cause before the antibiotic era, but is no longer a frequent cause.

Acute suppurative labyrinthitis secondary to extension of bacterial infection from the middle ear has become uncommon since the introduction of antibiotics. However, even without direct bacterial invasion, serous labyrinthitis may be caused by bacterial toxins.

Chronic otitic infections cause labyrinthine damage by the development of cholesteatoma. A cholesteatoma is a sac containing keratin, a silvery-white debris shed by squamous epithelium cells. Such cells are not normal constituents of the middle ear, but gain access from the external canal when the eardrum is repeatedly perforated by infection. Cholesteatomas erode surrounding tissues, including bone, and produce a fistula between the perilymph and the middle ear.

Clinical Features. Acute suppurative or serous labyrinthitis is characterized by the sudden onset of severe vertigo, nausea, vomiting, and unilateral hearing loss. Meningismus may be present as well. Chronic otitis produces similar symptoms. Fistula formation is identified when severe vertigo is provoked by sneezing, coughing, or merely applying pressure on the external canal.

Otoscopic examination reveals evidence of otitis media, tympanic membrane perforation, and allows visualization of cholesteatoma.

Diagnosis. In children with otitis media who develop vestibular dysfunction, radiographs or CT of the skull should be completed to visualize erosion of bone or mastoiditis. The presence of meningismus or increased intracranial pressure (see Chapter 4) necessitates CT to exclude the possibility of abscess and then examination of cerebrospinal fluid to exclude meningitis.

Treatment. Vigorous antibiotic therapy and drainage of the infected area is required in every case. Myringotomy and mastoidectomy may be needed for drainage. Cholesteatomas are always progressive and must be surgically excised.

Viral Infections

Viral infections may affect the labyrinth or vestibular nerve. The two are difficult to differentiate by clinical features, and the term vestibular neuritis or neuronitis is used to describe acute peripheral vestibulopathies. Vestibular neuritis may be part of a systemic viral infection, such as mumps, measles, and infectious mononucleosis, or it may occur in epidemics without an identifiable viral agent. Many cases of vestibular neuritis may be part of a postinfectious cranial polyneuritis (Adour et al, 1981).

Clinical Features. The major feature is the acute onset of vertigo. Any attempt to move the head is met with severe exacerbation of vertigo, nausea, and vomiting. Nystagmus is present on fixation and increased by head movement (Brandt, 1985). The patient is unable to maintain posture and lies motionless in bed. Recovery begins after three days. Spontaneous nausea diminishes, and nystagmus on fixation ceases. During the second week, vertigo decreases in severity but positional nystagmus is still present. Recovery is usually complete within three weeks.

Diagnosis. The diagnosis is often established by clinical features alone. Caloric testing reveals unilateral vestibular paresis, and hearing is normal.

Treatment. During the acute phase, the patient must be kept at bed rest and provided with vestibular sedation. Diazepam or dimenhydrinate is given orally, and scopolamine by transdermal absorption. Transdermal scopolamine should not be used in children, but may be used in adolescents. As recovery progresses, activity is gradually increased and sedation reduced.

Meniere Disease

Meniere disease is believed to be an overaccumulation of endolymph resulting in rupture of the labyrinth. It is uncommon in children, but can occur as early as the first decade.

Clinical Features. The clinical features of hearing impairment, tinnitus, and vertigo are attributed to rupture of the labyrinth. Hearing impairment fluctuates and may temporarily return to normal when the rupture heals. Tinnitus may be ignored, but vertigo demands attention and is often the presenting complaint.

A typical attack consists of disabling vertigo and tinnitus lasting one to three hours. The vertigo may be preceded by tinnitus, fullness in the ear, or increased loss of hearing. Tinnitus becomes worse during the attack. Pallor, sweating, nausea, and vomiting are often associated. Afterwards, the patient is tired and sleeps. Attacks occur at unpredictable intervals for years and then subside, leaving the patient with permanent hearing loss. Bilateral involvement is present in 20 percent of cases (Baloh and Honrubia, 1979).

Nystagmus is present during an attack. At first, the fast component is towards the abnormal ear (irritative); later, as the attack subsides, the fast component is away (paralytic). Between attacks, examination is normal with the exception of unilateral hearing impairment.

Diagnosis. Pure tone audiometry demonstrates threshold fluctuation. Speech discrimination is preserved, and recruitment is present on the abnormal side. Caloric stimulation demonstrates unilateral vestibular paresis or directional preponderance.

Treatment. The underlying disease cannot be reversed. Treatment is directed at management of the acute attack and attempts to increase the interval between attacks. The acute attack is treated with bed rest, sedation, and antiemetics. Maintenance therapy usually consists of a low-salt diet and diuretics; neither provides substantial benefit.

Migraine

Seventeen percent of migraineurs report vertigo at the time of an attack (Kayan and Hood, 1984). Such individuals have no difficulty in recognizing vertigo as a symptom of migraine. Another 10 percent experience vertigo in the interval between attacks and may have difficulty relating vertigo to migraine.

Brief (minutes), recurrent episodes of vertigo in infants and small children are recognized as a migraine equivalent, despite the absence of headache, because the attacks evolve into classic migraine. Affected children appear ataxic and for this reason the disorder is discussed in Chapter 10 (see "Benign Paroxysmal Vertigo").

Benign Recurrent Vertigo

This syndrome is similar to benign paroxysmal vertigo and is also believed to be a migraine equivalent (Slater, 1979).

Clinical Features. Children and adults are affected. The onset of vertigo is severe and without warning. Posture cannot be maintained. After a variable interval of minutes to hours, the spontaneous vertigo resolves, but positional vertigo persists for hours to days. Some attacks are associated with unilateral throbbing headache.

Diagnosis. Many patients have a positive family history for either benign recurrent vertigo or migraine. In the interval between attacks, audiometric and vestibular functions are normal. In some patients, permanent positional vertigo develops.

Treatment. No treatment has been established as beneficial, but prophylactic treatment with propranolol is suggested (see Chapter 3).

Motion Sickness

Motion sickness is induced by unfamiliar bodily accelerations or a mismatch between information provided by the visual and vestibular system to the brain on bodily acceleration (Brandt and Daroff, 1980). It is inhibited when motion in the visual field is in opposition to actual body movement. Therefore, looking out the window when driving reduces motion sickness. Small children in the back seat, where the only visual input is the car interior, are at the greatest risk for motion sickness.

The incidence of motion sickness depends upon "how hard you rock the boat" and approaches 100 percent in the worst case (Money, 1970). Twenty-five percent of a ship's passengers become sick during a two- to three-day Atlantic crossing, and 0.5 percent of commercial airline passengers are affected.

The first symptom is always pallor, followed by nausea and vomiting. It is unusual for vomiting to occur without the warning of nausea, thereby allowing time to prevent vomiting in some situations. Stopping the motion is the best way to abort an attack. Early attacks may be visually inhibited by watching the environment move opposite the direction of body movement. Individuals with known susceptibility to motion sickness should take an antihistamine, diazepam, or scopolamine prior to travel.

Trauma

Fifty percent of children complain of dizziness and headache during the first three days following a closed-head injury, with or without loss of consciousness (Eviatar et al, 1986). One third have persistent vertigo without hearing loss. These may be separated into those with direct trauma to the labyrinth (*vestibular concussion*), and those in which the vestibular apparatus is not injured (whiplash injury, migraine, and vertiginous seizures). Children with post-traumatic neurosis complain of dizziness or giddiness, but do not experience the illusion of rotation.

Vestibular Concussion

Clinical Features. Vestibular concussion follows blows to the parieto-occipital or temporoparietal region of the skull. Severe vertigo is present immediately after injury. The child is unsteady and sways toward the affected side. Symptoms persist for several days and then resolve completely, but recurrent episodes of vertigo and nausea lasting five to ten seconds are precipitated by specific movements of the head, *paroxysmal positional vertigo*.

Diagnosis. Radiographs of the skull with special attention to fractures through the petrous pyramid are indicated in all children with vertigo following head injury. Bleeding from the ear or a facial palsy should raise suspicion of such a skull fracture.

Positional nystagmus is induced by the Nylen-Hallpike technique when the injured ear is moved down. Caloric testing or electronystagmography demonstrates a reduced response from the injured ear.

Treatment. Immediately after injury, the patient should be treated with an antihistamine and diazepam until the acute phase is over.

Patients in whom paroxysmal positional vertigo develops are treated with *fatigue therapy*. This consists of tilting the patient to a position that reproduces symptoms. The patient remains in that position until the vertigo subsides for at least thirty seconds, then sits up for thirty seconds and repeats the procedure four times. This exercise is repeated several times each day until the patient is no longer sensitive to positional change.

Whiplash Injury

Whiplash injuries are frequently associated with vestibular and auditory dysfunction. Symptoms are probably caused by basilar artery spasm.

Clinical Features. Vertigo may be present immediately after injury and subsides within a few days. Brief attacks of vertigo and tinnitus, sometimes associated with headache or nausea, may develop months later in children who appear fully recovered from the injury. Many features of the attacks suggest basilar artery migraine (see Chapter 10) and probably represent a post-traumatic migraine.

Diagnosis. During the acute phase, vertigo may be induced by the Nylen-Hallpike technique and unilateral dysfunction documented by caloric testing. Vestibular function may also be abnormal in children who are experiencing basilar artery migraine, especially at the time of attack. The EEG is often abnormal and demonstrates occipital intermittent rhythmic *delta* activity (see Fig. 10.3).

References

1. Adour KK, Sprague MA, Hilsinger RL Jr: Vestibular vertigo. A form of polyneuritis? JAMA 246:1564, 1981.

2. Albers JW, Zimnowodski S, Lowrey CM, et al: Juvenile progressive bulbar palsy. Clinical and electrodiagnostic findings. Arch Neurol 40:351, 1983.

3. Aldrich MS, Beck RW, Albers J: Familial recurrent facial and ocular motor palsies. Neurology 34 (Suppl 1):165, 1984.

4. Aleksic SN, Budzilovich GN, Lieberman AN: Herpes zoster oticus and facial paralysis (Ramsay Hunt syndrome). Clinico-pathologic study and review of literature. J Neurol Sci 20:149, 1973.

5. Bailey RO, Marzulo DC, Hans MB: Infantile facioscapulohumeral muscular dystrophy: new observations. Acta Neurol Scand 74:51, 1986.

6. Bale JF Jr: Human cytomegalovirus infection and disorders of the nervous system. Arch Neurol 41:310, 1984.

7. Baloh RW, Honrubia V: Clinical Neurophysiology of the Vestibular System. Contemporary Neurology Series. FA Davis Co, Philadelphia, 1979, p 203.

8. Bohr V, Paulson OB, Rasamussen N: Pneumococcal meningitis. Late neurological sequelae and features of prognostic impact. Arch Neurol 41:1045, 1984.

9. Borrett D, Becker LE: Alexander's disease: A disease of astrocytes. Brain 108:367, 1985.

10. Brandt T: Episodic vertigo. In Rakel RE, ed. Conn's Current Therapy. WB Saunders Co, Philadelphia, 1985, p 741.

11. Brandt T, Daroff RB: The multisensory physiological and pathological vertigo syndromes. Ann Neurol 7:195, 1980.

12. Bray GM, Kaarsoo M, Ross RT: Ocular myopathy with dysphagia. Neurology 15:678, 1965.

13. Brown JS: Bell's palsy: A 5-year review of 174 consecutive cases: An attempted double-blind study. Laryngoscope 92:1369, 1982.

14. Brucher JM, Dom R, Lombaert A, et al: Progressive pontobulbar palsy with deafness. Clinical and pathological study of two cases. Arch Neurol 38:186, 1981.

15. Burgess LPA, Yim DWS, Lepore LM, et al: Bell's palsy: The steroid controversy revisited. Laryngoscope 94:1472, 1984.

16. Currie S, Heathfield KWG, Henson RA, et al: Clinical course and prognosis of temporal lobe epilepsy. A survey of 666 patients. Brain 94:173, 1971.

17. Delaney P: Neurologic manifestations in sarcoidosis. Review of the literature, with a report of 23 cases. Ann Int Med 87:336, 1977.

18. Deonna T, Ziegler A-L, Despland P-A, et al: Partial epilepsy in neurologically normal children: clinical syndromes and prognosis. Epilepsia 27:241, 1986.

19. Despland PA, Galambos R: Use of the auditory brainstem responses by prematures and newborn infants. Neuropediatrie 11:99, 1980.

20. Djupesland G, Flottorp G, Refsum S: Phytanic acid storage disease: Hearing maintained after 15 years of dietary treatment. Neurology 33:237, 1983.

21. Dodge PR, Davis H, Feigen RD, et al: Prospective evaluation of hearing impairment as a sequela of acute bacterial meningitis. N Engl J Med 311:869, 1984.

22. Dossing M, Wulff CH, Olsen PZ: Repeated facial palsies after chlorocresol inhalation. J Neurol Neurosurg Psychiatry 49:1452, 1986.

23. Eviatar L, Bergtraum M, Randel RM: Post-traumatic vertigo in children: A diagnostic approach. Pediatr Neurol 2:61, 1986.

24. Faldt R, Liedholm H, Aurnes J: Beta blockers and loss of hearing. Br Med J 289:1490, 1984.

25. Feldman RG, Mayer RM, Taub A: Evidence for a peripheral neurotoxic effect of trichlorethylene. Neurology 20:599, 1970.

26. Fraser GR: Profound childhood deafness. J Med Genet 1:118, 1964.

27. Gailiunas P, Dominguez-Moreno M, Lazarus M, et al: Vestibular toxicity of gentamicin. Arch Intern Med 138:1621, 1978.

28. Gomez M, Clermont V, Bernstein J: Progressive bulbar paralysis in childhood (Fazio-Londe disease). Arch Neurol 6:77, 1962.

29. Grover WD, Peckham GJ, Berman PH: Recovery following cranial nerve dysfunction and muscle weakness in infancy. Dev Med Child Neurol 16:163, 1974.

30. Hall JG, Pauli RM, Wilson KM: Maternal and fetal sequelae of anticoagulation during pregnancy. Am J Med 68:122, 1980.

31. Hart RG, Gardner DP, Howieson J: Acoustic tumors: Atypical features and recent diagnostic tests. Neurology 33:211, 1983.

32. Hepner WR Jr: Some observations on facial paresis in the newborn infant: Etiology and incidence. Pediatrics 8:494, 1951.

33. Juncos JL, Beal MF: Idiopathic cranial polyneuropathy. A fifteen year experience. Brain 110:197, 1987.

34. Kaner WR, Eldridge R, Fabricant R, et al: Central neurofibromatosis with bilateral acoustic neuroma: genetic, clinical and biochemical distinctions from peripheral neurofibromatosis. Neurology 30:851, 1980.

35. Kansu T, Us O, Sarpel G, et al: Recurrent multiple cranial nerve palsies (Tolosa-Hunt plus?). J Clin Neuroophthalmol 3:263, 1983.

36. Katusic S, Beard CM, Wiederholt WC, et al: Incidence, clinical features, and prognosis in Bell's palsy, Rochester, Minnesota, 1968–1982. Ann Neurol 20:622, 1986.

37. Kayan A, Hood JD: Neuro-otological manifestations of migraine. Brain 107:1123, 1984.

38. Konigsmark BW, Gorlin RJ: Genetic and Metabolic Deafness. WB Saunders Co, Philadelphia, 1976.

39. Levenson MJ, Ingerman M, Grimes C, et al: Melkersson-Rosenthal syndrome. Arch Otolaryngol 110:540, 1984.

40. Little BW, Perl DP: Oculopharyngeal muscular dystrophy. An autopsied case from the French-Canadian kindred. J Neurol Sci 53:145, 1982.

41. Lloyd AVC, Jewitt DE, Lloyd Still JD: Facial paralysis in children with hypertension. Arch Dis Child 41:292, 1966.

42. Maiman DJ, Cusick JF, Anderson AJ, et al: Nonoperative management of traumatic facial nerve palsy. J Trauma 25:644 1985.

43. Mallya KB, Mendis T, Guberman A: Bilateral facial paralysis following ethylene glycol ingestion. Can J Neurol Sci 13:340, 1986.

44. May M, Wette R, Hardin WB, et al: The use of steroids in Bell's palsy: A prospective controlled study. Laryngoscope 86:1111, 1976.

45. McHugh HE: Facial paralysis in birth injury and skull fractures. Arch Otolaryngol 78:445, 1963.

46. McHugh HE, Sowden KA, Levitt MN: Facial paralysis and muscle agenesis in the newborn. Arch Otolaryngol 89:157, 1969.

47. McLeod AC, McConnell F, Sweeney A, et al: Clinical variation in Usher syndrome. Arch Otolaryngol 94:321, 1971.

48. Money KE: Motion sickness. Physiol Rev 50:1,1970.

49. Neligan G, Prudham D: Norms for four standard developmental milestones by sex, social class and place in family. Dev Med Child Neurol 11:413, 1969.

50. Nelson KB, Eng GD: Congenital hypoplasia of the depressor anguli oris muscle: Differentiation from congenital facial palsy. J Pediatr 81:16, 1972.

51. Patten BM, Pages M: Severe neurological disease associated with hyperparathyroidism. Ann Neurol 15:453, 1984.

52. Puvanendran K, Vitharana M, Wong PK: Delayed facial palsy after head injury. J Neurol Neurosurg Psychiatry 40:342, 1977.

53. Richter RB: Unilateral congenital hypoplasia of the facial nucleus. J Neuropathol Exp Neurol 19:33, 1960.

54. Ropper AH: Unusual clinical variants and signs of Guillain-Barré syndrome. Arch Neurol 43:1150, 1986.

55. Rosenberg NL: Hearing loss as an initial symptom of the opsoclonus-myoclonus syndrome. Arch Neurol 41:998, 1984.

56. Rozencweig M, Von Hoff DD, Slavik M, et al: Cis-diamminedichloroplatinum (II). A new anticancer drug. Ann Intern Med 86:803, 1977.

57. Safman BL: Bilateral pathology in Bell's palsy. Arch Otolaryngol 93:55, 1971.

58. Sharma OP: Diagnosis of sarcoidosis. Arch Intern Med 143:1418, 1983.

59. Slater R: Benign recurrent vertigo. J Neurol Neurosurg Psychiatry 42:363, 1979.

60. Snavely SR, Hodges GR: The neurotoxicity of antibacterial agents. Ann Intern Med 101:92, 1984.

61. Stern BJ, Krumholz A, Johns C, et al: Sarcoidosis and its neurological manifestations. Arch Neurol 42:909, 1985.

62. Stockard JE, Stockard JJ, Kleinberg F, et al: Prognostic values of brainstem auditory evoked responses in newborns. Arch Neurol 40:360, 1983.

63. Sudarshan A, Goldie WD: The spectrum of congenital facial diplegia (Moebius syndrome). Pediatr Neurol 1:180, 1985.

64. Swanson JW, Kelly JJ Jr, McConahey WM: Neurologic aspects of thyroid dysfunction. Mayo Clin Proc 56:504, 1981.

65. Taylor DA, Carroll JE, Smith ME, et al: Facioscapulohumeral dystrophy associated with hearing loss and Coats syndrome. Ann Neurol 12:395, 1982.

66. van Dongen HR, Arts WFM, Yousef-Bak E: Acquired dysarthria in childhood: An analysis of dysarthric features in relation to neurologic deficits. Neurology 37:296, 1987.

67. Voit T, Lamprecht H-G, Goebel HH: Hearing loss in facioscapulohumeral dystrophy. Eur J Pediatr 145:280, 1986.

68. Wolf SM, Wagner JH Jr, Davidson S, et al: Treatment of Bell's palsy with prednisone: A prospective-randomized study. Neurology 28:158, 1978.

69. Yanagihara N, Mori H, Kozawà T, et al: Bell's palsy. Nonrecurrent v recurrent and unilateral v bilateral. Arch Otolaryngol 110:374, 1984.

18 Disorders of Cranial Volume and Shape

During infancy, the size of the cranium reflects the size of its contents. Normal contents are the brain, cerebrospinal fluid, and blood. These three compartments fill the calvarium, and the sum of their volumes determines head size. Expansion of one compartment is usually at the expense of another in order to maintain intracranial volume and pressure constant (see Chapter 4). The extracerebral spaces (epidural, subdural, and subarachnoid) may expand with blood and significantly affect cranial volume. Less important factors contributing to head size are the thickness of the skull bones and the rate of their fusion.

The shape of the skull is determined in part by its content, but external forces on the skull and the rate at which individual skull bones fuse are even more important factors.

■ Measuring Head Size

Head circumference is a time-honored and relatively accurate measure of cranial volume. It is determined by measuring the greatest occipital-frontal circumference. Two variables influence the accuracy of using head circumference to estimate cranial volume. One is fluid in and beneath the scalp, the other is head shape.

The scalp can be thickened from edema or blood following a prolonged and difficult delivery, and cephalohematoma may be present as well. Fluid that infiltrates from a scalp infusion is capable of markedly increasing head circumference.

A round head has a larger intracranial volume than an oval head of equal head circumference. A head with a relatively large occipital-frontal diameter measures larger than a head with a relatively large biparietal diameter.

Head circumference measurements are most informative when plotted over time. The head sizes of male and female infants are different, and head growth charts that provide median values for both sexes should not be used. The rate of head growth in prematures is considerably faster than in term newborns (Fig. 18.1). For this reason, head circumference must always be charted by conceptional age and not by postnatal age.

■ Macrocephaly

Macrocephaly means a large head, larger than two standard deviations from the normal distribution. This means that 2 percent of the "normal" population have macrocephaly. Investigation of such individuals usually reveals some "abnormality" that causes them to be in the top 2 percent for head size. Some are normal.

The causes of a large head include (1) *hydrocephalus*, excessive volume of cerebrospinal fluid in the skull; (2) *megalencephaly*, enlargement of the brain; (3) thickening of the skull; and (4) hemorrhage into the subdural or epidural spaces. Hydrocephalus is traditionally *communicating* (nonobstructive) or *noncommunicating* (obstructive), depending upon whether or not cerebrospinal fluid communicates between the ventricles and subarachnoid space (Table 18.1). Hydrocephalus is the only cause of macrocephaly at birth associated with increased intracranial pressure.

359

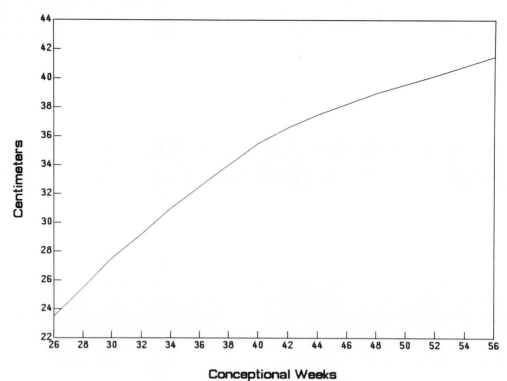

Conceptional Weeks

Figure 18.1 Normal growth of head circumference in boys. The rate of growth in the premature is greater than at term.

Megalencephaly has been divided into two major categories: *anatomic* and *metabolic* (DeMyer, 1986). Anatomic disorders include primary megalencephaly and neurocutaneous

Table 18.1 CAUSES OF HYDROCEPHALUS

Communicating
1. Achondroplasia
2. Basilar impression (see Chapter 10)
3. Benign enlargement of subarachnoid space
4. Choroid plexus papilloma (see Chapter 4)
5. Meningeal malignancy
6. Meningitis (see Chapter 4)
7. Posthemorrhagic (see Chapter 4)

Noncommunicating
1. Aqueductal stenosis
   a. Infectious
   b. X-linked
2. Chiari malformation (see Chapter 10)
3. Dandy-Walker malformation
4. Klippel-Feil syndrome
5. Mass lesions
   a. Abscess (see Chapter 4)
   b. Hematoma (see Chapters 1 and 2)
   c. Tumors and neurocutaneous disorders
   d. Vein of Galen malformation
6. Warburg syndrome

Hydranencephaly
1. Holoprosencephaly
2. Massive hydrocephalus
3. Porencephaly

disorders (Table 18.2). Children with anatomic megalencephaly often have macrocephaly at birth, but intracranial pressure is not increased. Those with metabolic megalencephaly have normal head size at birth, but cerebral edema and macrocephaly develop during the neonatal period.

Macrocephaly caused by increased thickness of the skull bones is not present at birth or in

Table 18.2 MEGALENCEPHALY

Anatomic Megalencephaly
1. Genetic megalencephaly
2. Megalencephaly with neurologic abnormality
3. Megalencephaly with achondroplasia
4. Megalencephaly with gigantism (Sotos syndrome)
5. Neurocutaneous disorders
   a. Hypomelanosis of Ito
   b. Incontinentia pigmenti (see Chapter 1)
   c. Linear nevus sebaceous syndrome
   d. Neurofibromatosis (see Chapter 5)
   e. Tuberous sclerosis (see Chapter 5)

Metabolic Megalencephaly
1. Alexander disease (see Chapter 5)
2. Canavan disease (see Chapter 5)
3. Galactosemia: transferase deficiency (see Chapter 5)
4. Gangliosidosis (see Chapter 5)
5. Globoid leukodystrophy (see Chapter 5)
6. Maple syrup urine disease (see Chapter 1)
7. Metachromatic leukodystrophy (see Chapter 5)
8. Mucopolysaccharidoses (Chapter 5)

the newborn period, but develops during infancy. The conditions associated with increased skull growth are summarized in Table 18.3 but are not discussed further in the text.

Intracranial hemorrhage in the newborn has been discussed in Chapter 1; intracranial hemorrhage in older children is detailed in Chapter 2.

COMMUNICATING HYDROCEPHALUS

Communicating hydrocephalus is usually caused by impaired absorption of cerebrospinal fluid secondary to meningitis or subarachnoid hemorrhage. Meningeal malignancy, usually resulting from leukemia or primary brain tumor, is a less common cause. The excessive production of cerebrospinal fluid by a choroid plexus papilloma is a rare cause of communicating hydrocephalus, because the potential rate of cerebrospinal reabsorption far exceeds the productive capacity of the choroid plexus (see Chapter 4). A more common mechanism of hydrocephalus with such tumors is obstruction of one or more ventricles.

Achondroplasia

Achondroplasia is a genetic disorder transmitted as an autosomal dominant trait that produces skeletal deformities resulting in dwarfism.

Clinical Features. The major features of achondroplasia are macrocephaly and rhizomelic shortening of the limbs: the proximal portion of the limbs is shorter than the distal portion. Enchondral bone formation at the base of the skull and in the face is stunted, causing the typical recessed appearance of the face.

Affected newborns have megalencephaly, but do not have hydrocephalus (Mueller, 1980). The

Table 18.3 CONDITIONS WITH A THICKENED SKULL CAUSING MACROCEPHALY*

   1. Anemia
   2. Cleidocranial dysostosis
   3. Craniometaphyseal dysplasia of Pyle
   4. Epiphyseal dysplasia
   5. Hyperphosphatemia
   6. Leontiasis ossea
   7. Orodigitofacial dysostosis
   8. Osteogenesis imperfecta
   9. Osteopetrosis
  10. Pycnodystosis
  11. Rickets
  12. Russell dwarf

*Modified from DeMyer W: Pediatr Neurol 2:321, 1986.

ventricles begin to enlarge during infancy because of impaired reabsorption of cerebrospinal fluid as a result of increased venous pressure (Mueller and Reinertson, 1980). Venous return from the brain is probably obstructed by the reduced size of venous sinuses in the small posterior fossa.

Despite considerable, and sometimes alarming, enlargement of head circumference, it is unusual for achondroplastic dwarfs to demonstrate clinical evidence of increased intracranial pressure or progressive dementia.

Respiratory disturbances occur in 85 percent of children with achondroplasia (Reid et al, 1987). Thirty-five percent are caused by cervicomedullary compression but the majority are the result of primary pulmonary problems, such as a small thoracic cage or an obstructed airway.

Diagnosis. The diagnosis of achondroplasia is established by clinical examination and positive family history. Computerized tomography (CT) reveals a small posterior fossa and enlargement of the sphenoid sinuses. Basilar impression is sometimes present. Ventricular size varies from normal in newborns and young infants to moderate or severe dilation in older children and adults.

Treatment. Ventricular size, after initial dilation, usually remains stable, and surgical diversion of cerebrospinal fluid is rarely required.

Benign Enlargement of Subarachnoid Space

This condition is described under several titles in the literature: *external hydrocephalus, extraventricular hydrocephalus, benign subdural effusions,* and *benign extracerebral fluid collections* (Hamza et al, 1987). It is a relatively common cause of macrocephaly in infants (16 percent), a fact not fully appreciated before the widespread use of CT (Nickel and Gallenstein, 1987). A genetic etiology of this condition is likely in some cases, with the infant's father often having macrocrania as well.

Clinical Features. The condition is more frequent in males than females. Macrocrania is the only feature. An otherwise normal infant is brought to attention because serial head circumference measurements reveal an enlarging skull. Circumference is usually above the 90th percentile at birth, grows to exceed the 98th percentile, and then parallels the normal curve (Fig. 18.2). The anterior fontanelle is large, but soft. Neurologic examination and developmental status are normal.

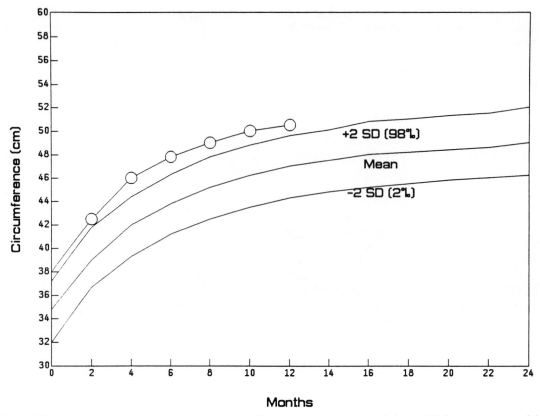

Figure 18.2 Benign enlargement of subarachnoid space. Head circumference is already large at birth, grows to exceed the 98th percentile, and then parallels the curve.

Diagnosis. Computerized tomography reveals an enlarged frontal subarachnoid space, widening of the sylvian fissures and other sulci, and normal or minimally enlarged ventricular size (Fig. 18.3). Normal ventricular size distinguishes this condition from cerebral atrophy. The upper limit of normal size for the frontal subarachnoid space in infants is 5.7 mm; for the sylvian fissure it is 7.6 mm (Fukuyama et al, 1979).

Treatment. Affected infants develop normally and do not require ventricular shunts. Head circumference measurements should be plotted monthly for the next six months to be certain that growth is paralleling the normal curve. Repeat CT is not needed unless (1) head growth deviates upward from the normal curve, (2) neurologic examination becomes abnormal, or (3) development is delayed.

Meningeal Malignancy

Tumors that infiltrate the meninges and subarachnoid space impair the reabsorption of cerebrospinal fluid and may produce communicating hydrocephalus. The primary site of tumor is usually established prior to its meningeal spread, but hydrocephalus may be the initial feature of diffuse meningeal gliomatosis (Whelan et al, in press).

Clinical Features. Tumors that infiltrate the meninges are usually aggressive, causing a rapid progression of symptoms and signs. Headache and vomiting are the presenting features and are followed by lethargy and personality change. Examination often reveals meningismus and papilledema, which suggest a bacterial meningitis. Multifocal neurologic disturbances may be present as well.

Diagnosis. Computerized tomography demonstrates dilation of the entire ventricular system, but not the subarachnoid space, which may appear obliterated. Some tumors cause contrast enhancement of the meninges (Jaeckle et al, 1985).

Examination of the cerebrospinal fluid demonstrates an increased pressure and protein concentration. Glucose concentration may be depressed or normal. Tumor cell identification in the cerebrospinal fluid is essential for early di-

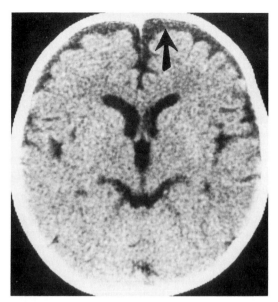

Figure 18.3 Benign enlargement of subarachnoid space. An enlarged frontal subarachnoid space, prominent sulci, and normal ventricular size are revealed on CT scan.

agnosis and treatment, but is rarely accomplished unless large volumes are examined. Meningeal biopsy is required for tissue diagnosis in many cases.

Treatment. Ventricular shunt is required to relieve symptoms of increased intracranial pressure. Radiotherapy and chemotherapy provide palliation and extend life in some cases, but the outcome is generally poor.

NONCOMMUNICATING HYDROCEPHALUS

Complete obstruction of the egress of cerebrospinal fluid from the ventricles to the subarachnoid space causes increased pressure and dilation of all ventricles proximal to the obstruction. The rate of cerebrospinal fluid production is reduced in response to the increased intraventricular pressure.

Noncommunicating hydrocephalus is the most common cause of hydrocephalus in the fetus, with aqueductal stenosis accounting for 20 percent of congenital hydrocephalus without other malformations (Burton, 1977). It becomes less common during infancy, but increases in frequency again during childhood. Childhood-onset cases are usually caused by mass lesions.

Aqueductal Stenosis

The mean length of the cerebral aqueduct at birth is 12.8 mm (Friede, 1975). At its smallest

cross-sectional diameter, the cerebral aqueduct of normal newborns is usually 0.5 mm. The small lumen of the cerebral aqueduct, in relation to its length, makes it especially vulnerable to internal compromise from infection and hemorrhage and external compression by tumors and venous malformations.

Congenital atresia or stenosis of the cerebral aqueduct can occur as a solitary malformation, but a familial form transmitted by X-linked inheritance accounts for 2 percent of all cases of congenital hydrocephalus.

Clinical Features. Hydrocephalus is present at birth. Head circumference ranges from 40 to 50 cm and may cause cephalopelvic disproportion and poor progress of labor. The forehead is bowed, the scalp veins are dilated, the skull sutures are widely separated, and the fontanelles are large and tense. These signs are exaggerated when the child cries, but are present in the quiet state as well. The eyes are deviated downward so that the sclera shows above the iris (setting-sun sign), and abducens palsies may be present.

Adduction and flexion of the thumbs are noted in approximately 20 percent of newborns with X-linked aqueductal stenosis (Kuzniecky et al, 1986). This phenomenon was thought to be an associated malformation, but probably represents a nonspecific sign of corticospinal tract compression by the dilated lateral ventricles.

Diagnosis. Antenatal diagnosis has been made possible by intrauterine sonography. When macrocephaly is present in the fetus, alpha-fetoprotein should be assayed in the amniotic fluid for the detection of neural tube defects (see Chapter 12) and chromosomal analysis performed. Information concerning the integrity of the fetal nervous system is needed to develop a management plan.

The postpartum diagnosis of aqueductal stenosis is readily accomplished by CT. The lateral and third ventricles are markedly enlarged, as is the cephalic end of the cerebral aqueduct. The remainder of the cerebral aqueduct and the fourth ventricle cannot be visualized (Fig. 18.4).

Treatment. Congenital hydrocephalus caused by aqueductal stenosis is always severe, does not respond to medical therapy directed at decreasing the volume of cerebrospinal fluid, and does not arrest at a stage that is less than harmful to the brain. Diversion of the cerebrospinal fluid from the ventricular system to an extracranial site is the only effective method of management.

The management of fetal hydrocephalus depends upon the presence of other malformations. Seventy to eighty percent of cases have other abnormalities, usually spina bifida (Cher-

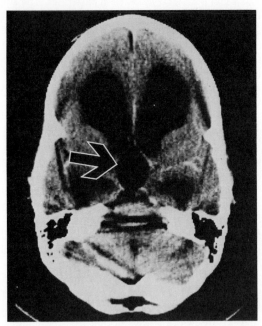

Figure 18.4 Aqueductal stenosis. Marked enlargement of the third ventricle (arrow) and the lateral ventricles is demonstrated on CT scan.

venak et al, 1985; Vintzileos et al, 1987). Many such pregnancies are terminated voluntarily. When aqueductal stenosis is the only identifiable malformation, ventriculoamniotic shunt may be considered to reduce pressure on the developing brain. Delivery by cesarean section is then planned at the earliest age consistent with lung maturity.

Ventriculoperitoneal shunt is generally considered the procedure of choice for newborns and small infants with aqueductal stenosis. It is easier to revise and better tolerated than is ventriculoatrial shunt. Mechanical obstruction and infection are the two most common complications of shunt placement at this age (see Chapter 4).

The relief of hydrocephalus increases the potential for normal development even when the cerebral mantle appears very thin preoperatively (Kovnar et al, 1984), but does not necessarily result in a normal child. The growth of intelligence is often uneven, with nonverbal skills being lower than verbal skills (Dennis et al, 1981). Motor deficits and seizures may be present as a result of associated anomalies.

Dandy-Walker Malformation

The Dandy-Walker malformation consists of cystic dilation of the fourth ventricle and agenesis (25 percent), or hypoplasia (75 percent), of the cerebellar vermis. Hydrocephalus is usually associated, but is not an essential feature. The size of the lateral ventricles does not correlate with the size of the cyst in the fourth ventricle (Hart et al, 1972). Other malformations are present in 68 percent of cases. The most common associated malformation is agenesis of the corpus callosum. Other malformations include heterotopia, abnormal gyral formation, dysraphic states, aqueductal stenosis, and congenital tumors.

Clinical Features. The onset of hydrocephalus is usually during infancy, but may be present at birth (Tal et al, 1980). Bulging of the skull is more prominent in the occipital than in the frontal region, and the rapidity of head growth is considerably slower than with aqueductal stenosis. Neurologic dysfunction is referable to compression of posterior fossa structures: apneic spells, nystagmus, truncal ataxia, cranial nerve palsies, and hyperreflexia in the legs.

Diagnosis. A CT scan is usually ordered because of macrocephaly or ataxia. Cystic dilation of the fourth ventricle and partial or complete agenesis of the cerebellar vermis are readily visualized (Fig. 18.5).

Treatment. Decompression of the cyst alone provides immediate relief of symptoms; however, hydrocephalus recurs and ventricular shunting is required in two thirds of affected children. Shunting of the lateral ventricle alone

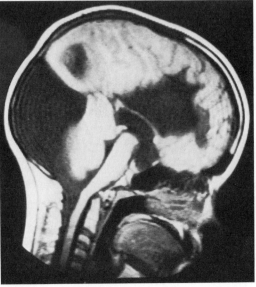

Figure 18.5 Dandy-Walker malformation. Cystic dilation of the fourth ventricle and partial agenesis of the cerebellar vermis are shown on CT scan. (From Fenichel GM: Neonatal Neurology. Churchill Livingstone, New York, 1985.)

provides immediate relief of hydrocephalus, but fails to relieve brainstem compression. The present procedure of choice is a dual shunt of both the lateral ventricle and the posterior fossa cyst.

Even after successful shunt placement, many children experience transitory episodes of lethargy, personality change, and vomiting. Shunt failure is suspected, but cannot be substantiated. The mechanism of such episodes, which may prove fatal, is unknown.

Klippel-Feil Syndrome

This malformation of the craniocervical skeleton may be associated with the Chiari malformation and basilar impression. Hydrocephalus is produced by obstruction of the egress of cerebrospinal fluid from the fourth ventricle to the subarachnoid space. The malformation is classified into three types: extensive fusion of thoracic and upper cervical vertebrae (type I), one or two interspace fusions with hemivertebrae and occipito-atlantal fusion (type II), and cervical and lower thoracic or lumbar fusion (type III). Type II is the most common form.

Clinical Features. The essential features of this syndrome are a low posterior hairline, short neck, and limitation of neck movement (Nagib et al, 1985). Head asymmetry, facial asymmetry, and scoliosis are common. Unilateral or bilateral failure of downward migration of the scapula (Sprengel deformity) is present in 25 to 35 percent of patients. Mirror movements of the hands are noted in the majority of patients. Malformations of the genitourinary system and deafness are also associated.

Hydrocephalus affects the fourth ventricle first and then the lateral ventricles. This results in symptoms of posterior fossa compression: ataxia, apnea, and cranial nerve dysfunction.

Diagnosis. Radiographs of the spine reveal the characteristic fusion and malformations of vertebrae. Magnetic resonance imaging (MRI) may demonstrate an associated Chiari malformation and dilation of the ventricles.

Treatment. Children with unstable cervical vertebrae require cervical fusion to prevent myelopathy. Those with symptoms of obstructive hydrocephalus require decompression to relieve pressure in the posterior fossa.

Congenital Brain Tumors

In the United States during the period 1960 to 1966, neonatal mortality attributable to intracranial tumors was 1/340,000 live births (Miller,

1969). There is considerable concurrence between congenital brain tumors and congenital brain malformations. Both are disorders of cellular proliferation, and a noxious agent active during early embryogenesis might stimulate either or both abnormalities. The relative oncogenicity or teratogenicity depends upon the virulence of the agent, the timing of the insult, the duration of exposure, and the genetic background and health of the fetus.

The tumors that occur most frequently during infancy are astrocytoma, medulloblastoma, teratoma, and choroid plexus papilloma (Jellinger and Sunder-Plassman, 1973; Tomita and Mc-Lone, 1985).

Clinical Features. Congenital tumors are more often supratentorial than infratentorial in location and more often in the midline than placed laterally. Newborns with hemispheric gliomas and teratomas may have intrauterine hydrocephalus, or hydrocephalus may develop in the first days or weeks post partum. The point of obstruction is usually at the cerebral aqueduct (see Chapter 4). Choroid plexus papillomas are usually located in one lateral ventricle and are more likely to present during infancy than the perinatal period. They produce hydrocephalus either by obstruction of the foramen of Monroe or by excessive production of cerebrospinal fluid (see Chapter 4). Medulloblastomas are located in the posterior fossa and obstruct the fourth ventricle and cerebral aqueduct (see Chapter 10).

The clinical features of all congenital tumors are those of increasing intracranial pressure: enlarging head size, separation of the sutures, lethargy, irritability, difficult feeding, and vomiting. Convulsions are unusual. Medulloblastoma, because of its posterior fossa location, also produces nystagmus, downward deviation of the eyes, opisthotonus, and apnea.

Diagnosis. All congenital tumors are readily visualized by CT or MRI performed to investigate hydrocephalus. Fetal teratoma has been identified by uterine sonography (Lipman et al, 1985).

Treatment. Complete resection of congenital brain tumors is unusual with the exception of choroid plexus papilloma. The management of individual tumors is discussed in Chapters 4 and 10.

Vein of Galen Malformation

A variety of arteriovenous malformations of the cerebral circulation may present during infancy and childhood (see Chapters 4 and 10), but the one associated with congenital hydro-cephalus is the vein of Galen malformation (Kelly et al, 1978; Norman et al, 1974). The vein of Galen is positioned just above the quad-rigeminal plate and, when dilated, compresses the cerebral aqueduct and causes dilation of the lateral ventricles. Macrocrania also occurs from the increased volume of blood in the skull.

Clinical Features. Eighty percent of new-borns with this malformation are males. The usual presentation is an enlarging head. Hem-orrhage almost never occurs as an initial feature. A cranial bruit is invariably present. Unex-plained, persistent hypoglycemia has been noted in some children. Some newborns present with high-output cardiac failure because of the vol-ume demands of the shunt.

Diagnosis. Vein of Galen malformations are readily visualized by contrast-enhanced CT (Fig. 18.6). The lateral and third ventricles are dilated behind the compressed cerebral aqueduct. Radiographs of the chest in newborns with high-output cardiac failure demonstrate an enlarged heart that has a normal shape.

Treatment. Several surgical approaches to the malformation have been considered. The overall results are poor; the mortality rate is high, as is neurologic morbidity in survivors.

Warburg Syndrome

The cause of Warburg syndrome, character-ized by congenital hydrocephalus and ocular

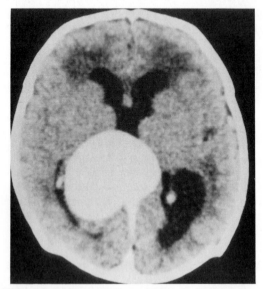

Figure 18.6 Vein of Galen malformation. The malforma-tion is visualized on a contrast-enhanced CT scan as a large aneurysmal sac compressing the midbrain and producing obstructive hydrocephalus.

abnormalities, is unknown (Bordarier et al, 1984; Williams et al, 1984). The risk of recur-rence among siblings exceeds 50 percent, but transmission does not occur from one generation to another. Some believe that this is a genetic disease transmitted by autosomal recessive in-heritance; others believe the disorder to be caused by an acquired agent transmitted trans-placentally through consecutive pregnancies.

Clinical Features. Hydrocephalus is usually present at birth. It may be caused by aqueductal stenosis or the Dandy-Walker malformation. Most cases of Dandy-Walker malformation with ocular abnormalities are probably cases of the Warburg syndrome. Some children are born with microcephaly, but still have enlarged ven-tricles.

Severe neurologic abnormalities are caused by partial or total agyria (lissencephaly) due to failure of neuronal migration. The pattern of architectural abnormalities present throughout the neuraxis suggests a disruption of cerebral maturation in the fourth conceptional month.

Several different ocular abnormalities may be present, usually in combination: hypoplasia of the iris, abnormal anterior chamber, microph-thalmus, cataracts, persistence of primary vitre-ous, optic disk coloboma, retinal detachment, retinal dysplasia, and hypoplasia of the optic nerve.

In addition to hydrocephalus and blindness, affected infants are hypotonic and have difficulty feeding. Some have a severe myopathy. Sei-zures are uncommon. Most children with War-burg syndrome die during the neonatal period or early infancy.

Diagnosis. This is a clinical diagnosis based on the characteristic combination of cerebral and ocular abnormalities. Congenital infections may produce similar disturbances and must be ex-cluded, but multisystem disease (visceromegaly and disturbed hematopoiesis), an expected fea-ture of most intrauterine infections, is lacking in the Warburg syndrome.

Cerebro-ocular abnormalities at birth are also encountered in septo-optic dysplasia (see Chap-ter 16) and oculocerebrorenal syndrome (see Chapter 6), but hydrocephalus is not a compo-nent of either syndrome.

The combination of cerebral malformations due to disturbed neuronal migration and con-genital myopathy occurs in the Fukuyama form of congenital muscular dystrophy (see Chapter 6). However, the clinical picture of Fukuyama dystrophy differs from the Warburg syndrome by the absence of hydrocephalus and prolonged survival.

Treatment. Hydrocephalus can be managed by ventricular shunt, but outcome is poor because of the severe cerebral malformations.

HYDRANENCEPHALY

The term hydranencephaly encompasses several conditions that result in the extensive replacement of brain by cerebrospinal fluid. This may result from failure of normal brain development or from an intrauterine disorder that destroys the brain parenchyma. Progressive obstructive hydrocephalus may result in hydranencephaly if left untreated. Excessive pressure within the lateral ventricles destroys the midline structures and reduces the cerebral mantle to a thin membrane.

Head circumference at birth is large when hydranencephaly is secondary to obstructive hydrocephalus, is small when secondary to intrauterine diseases, and may be large or small with primary malformations.

Holoprosencephaly

Holoprosencephaly is a primary malformation caused by failure of the forebrain to cleave into two hemispheres. The brain is a single fluid-filled sac, but the head is usually small in size and is therefore discussed in the section on microcephaly.

Porencephaly

Porencephaly is a term that is used loosely in the literature; originally, it was intended to describe circumscribed defects in one or both cerebral hemispheres, often the result of intrauterine or perinatal destructive lesions such as infarction or physical trauma. The immature brain suffers loss of brain, glia, and supporting structures. A fluid-filled cyst is formed in the injured area, which may or may not communicate with the ventricular system or subarachnoid space. Pressure within the cyst may become excessive and may cause compression of adjacent structures and macrocrania.

Congenital midline porencephaly is a distinct malformation characterized by congenital hydrocephalus, alopecia or cephalocele in the parietal midline, and a midline defect in the posterior cerebral mantle (Yokota and Matsukado, 1979). Midline porencephaly differs from holoprosencephaly, because the forebrain divides into two separate hemispheres. A possible mechanism is early hydrocephalus with upward outpouching

and destruction of adjacent structures: corpus callosum, cerebral mantle, skull, and scalp.

Clinical Features. The head is large in utero and may cause cephalopelvic disproportion. Possible defects in the parietal midline range from a small round area of alopecia to encephalocele. Affected children are severely retarded and blind. Most die during infancy or early childhood.

Diagnosis. A large dorsal cyst that has destroyed the septum pellucidum and corpus callosum is seen on CT. The cyst communicates with enlarged lateral ventricles and extends through a skull defect to produce an encephalocele.

Treatment. Shunting the cyst may improve ease of child care by reducing the size of the head or encephalocele, but does not prevent severe neurologic impairment from the underlying cerebral malformation.

ANATOMIC MEGALENCEPHALY

Anatomic megalencephaly includes those conditions in which the brain is enlarged as a result of an increased number or size of cells. There is no evidence of metabolic disease or acute encephalopathy.

Genetic Megalencephaly

Clinical Features. The term genetic megalencephaly describes families with normal neurologic and mental function whose head circumference measurement is larger than the 98th percentile in size. Head circumference may not be large at birth, but becomes large during infancy, usually 2 to 4 cm above the 98th percentile (Lorber and Priestly, 1981). Body size is normal, and there are no physical deformities.

Diagnosis. Such families are shown by examination to be indistinguishable from those with benign enlargement of the subarachnoid space, but they can be discriminated by CT, the results of which are normal in this condition.

Treatment. Treatment is not required.

Megalencephaly with Neurologic Disorder

This term is used to encompass all disorders, other than neurocutaneous syndromes, that present with megalencephaly and evidence of cerebral dysfunction.

Clinical Features. Head circumference may be large at birth or may become large during infancy. It is generally 2 to 4 cm greater than that described at the 98th percentile. Neurologic examination is otherwise normal, but the children have learning disabilities, mental deficiency, or seizures. There is never a progressive deterioration of neurologic status.

Diagnosis. The skin of the patient and other family members must be carefully examined, including the use of Wood's light, to exclude the possibility of a neurocutaneous disorder. Ophthalmoscopic examination of family members should be carried out as well.

Results of a CT scan may be normal or may reveal mild dilation of the ventricular system. Agenesis of the corpus callosum is described as the only abnormality in some families with macrocrania and borderline intelligence (Lynn et al, 1980).

Treatment. Seizures often respond to anticonvulsant therapy. Special education is usually required. Treatment is not available for the underlying disorder.

Megalencephaly with Gigantism

Megalencephaly with gigantism is also termed *cerebral gigantism* or *Sotos syndrome*. It probably encompasses several different disorders. Most are sporadic; some are clearly genetic and may be transmitted by autosomal recessive or dominant inheritance (Winship, 1985). Chromosome studies are normal.

Clinical Features. Affected children are large at birth (75th to 90th percentile) and demonstrate excessive growth with advanced height, weight, head circumference, and bone age up to the age of three (Sotos and Cutler, 1977). Afterwards, the rate of growth is normal. All children with the syndrome are large as adults, but they are not usually giants.

Prominent forehead, high arched palate, and hypertelorism are present in almost every case. Several other dysmorphic features are reported in small numbers of patients. Approximately 80 percent of cases demonstrate some degree of mental retardation.

Diagnosis. Cranial CT is usually normal except for mild ventricular widening. Extensive studies of endocrine function have failed to reveal a consistent abnormality other than glucose intolerance. Plasma somatomedin levels are elevated during the first year in some affected infants and then fall below normal during early childhood (Wit et al, 1985).

Treatment. Girls may benefit from high doses of estrogens to curtail excessive growth, but

treatment is not available for the underlying disorder.

Neurocutaneous Disorders

Seizures (see Table 1.10) or mental retardation (see Chapter 5) are the common presenting features of most neurocutaneous disorders. Some present at birth (incontinentia pigmenti) or during infancy (neurofibromatosis, tuberous sclerosis) with macrocrania due either to hydrocephalus or megalencephaly. Hemimegalencephaly, hemihypertrophy of the body, or hypertrophy of a single limb should always suggest the possibility of a neurocutaneous disorder.

Hypomelanosis of Ito

This rare syndrome, also called *incontinentia pigmenti achromians*, is believed to be transmitted by autosomal dominant inheritance. A small translocation between chromosome 2 and 8 has been detected in one case (Miller and Parker, 1985).

Clinical Features. The cutaneous manifestation is a large hypopigmented area that has a whorled or streaked appearance. It is a negative image of the hyperpigmented lesions of incontinentia pigmenti (see Chapter 1). Neurologic complications (mental retardation, seizures, and spastic diplegia) occur in 40 percent of cases. These are caused by disturbances of neuronal migration (Golden and Kaplan, 1986). Megalencephaly occurs in only a minority of cases.

Other possible abnormalities include strabismus, corneal opacities, limb hypertrophy or atrophy, facial hemiatrophy, hypertelorism, poorly formed ears, and dysplastic teeth.

Diagnosis. The presence of characteristic cutaneous lesions is critical to the diagnosis and should be looked for in the parents and siblings as well as the child. Chromosome studies with specific interest in chromosomes 2 and 8 are indicated in the child and parents.

Treatment. Treatment is not available.

Linear Nevus Sebaceous Syndrome

This syndrome is also called the *organoid nevus syndrome* (Clancy et al, 1985).

Clinical Features. The cutaneous manifestation is a unilateral linear nevus, usually on the face or scalp, that may not be visible at birth but becomes apparent during infancy. Hemihypertrophy of the face and limbs ipsilateral to the nevus may be present at birth or may develop during infancy.

The spectrum of neurologic disability is considerable. Most affected children experience developmental delay and seizures. Head size may be enlarged generally or unilaterally. Focal neurologic deficits, such as hemiplegia and hemianopia, contralateral to the nevus are relatively common.

Diagnosis. Diagnosis relies upon recognition of the dermatologic manifestations. Electroencephalography (EEG) frequently reveals unilateral slowing and epileptiform discharges ipsilateral to the nevus. Hypsarrhythmia is present when infantile spasms are the presenting feature (see Chapter 1). Hemihypsarrhythmia has been described as well (Tjiam et al, 1978).

Cranial CT reveals asymmetry of the cranial vault with enlargement of one hemisphere. The abnormal hemisphere has an enlarged lateral ventricle and a simplified convolutional pattern.

Treatment. Seizures may respond to standard anticonvulsant therapy (see Chapter 1), but treatment is not available for the underlying cerebral malformation.

METABOLIC MEGALENCEPHALY

Several inborn errors of metabolism produce megalencephaly because of the storage of abnormal substances or by producing cerebral edema (see Table 18.2). They are discussed elsewhere in the text because they usually present as developmental regression (see Chapter 5) or seizures (see Chapter 1). As a rule, affected infants have a normal head circumference at birth. Head enlargement parallels neurologic regression and clinical evidence of increased intracranial pressure. Ventricular size is often small.

■ Microcephaly

Microcephaly indicates a head circumference that is less than two standard deviations below the normal distribution. A small head circumference indicates a small brain. Almost every individual with microcephaly is mentally retarded, but there are occasional families of normal stature and intelligence in whom head circumference is microcephalic.

A small head circumference at birth establishes the antepartum timing of brain damage, but does not separate primary from secondary

microcephaly (Table 18.4). *Primary microcephaly* encompasses conditions in which the brain is small because it never formed properly because of genetic or chromosomal causes. *Secondary microcephaly* implies that the brain was forming normally but was severely injured by a disease process that impaired further growth. Normal head circumference at birth followed by failure of normal head growth almost always indicates a secondary microcephaly. Chromosomal disorders are an exception to that rule unless they produce defective prosencephalization or cellular migration.

Perinatal brain damage does not cause a recognizable decrease of head circumference until three to six months post partum. Failure of normal brain growth removes the force keeping the cranial bones separated, and they fuse prematurely. Premature closure of the cranial sutures may also occur as a result of a primary disorder of the skull (craniostenosis) even though the brain is attempting to grow normally. The distinction between the two is relatively simple: craniostenosis is always associated with an abnormal skull shape and heaping up of bone along the cranial sutures; failure of brain growth produces a relatively normal-shaped skull with some overlapping of skull bones.

Cranial CT may be informative in distinguishing primary from secondary microcephaly (Jaworski et al, 1986). In most children with pri-

Table 18.4 CONDITIONS CAUSING MICROCEPHALY

Primary Microcephaly
1. Microcephaly vera (genetic)
2. Chromosomal disorders
3. Defective neurolation
   a. Anencephaly
   b. Encephalocele
4. Defective prosencephalization
   a. Holoprosencephaly (arhinencephaly)
   b. Agenesis of the corpus callosum
5. Defective cellular migration

Secondary Microcephaly
1. Intrauterine disorders
   a. Infection
   b. Toxins
   c. Vascular
2. Perinatal brain injuries
   a. Hypoxic-ischemic encephalopathy
   b. Intracranial hemorrhage
   c. Meningitis and encephalitis
   d. Stroke
3. Postnatal systemic diseases
   a. Chronic cardiopulmonary disease
   b. Chronic renal disease
   c. Malnutrition

mary microcephaly, either CT results are normal or there is a recognizable pattern of cerebral malformation. In those with secondary microcephaly, usually CT results are abnormal, characterized by one or more of the following features: ventricular enlargement, cerebral atrophy, and porencephaly.

PRIMARY MICROCEPHALY

Many cerebral malformations are of uncertain cause and cannot be classified as primary or secondary. Morphogenetic errors, although lacking in the traditional stigmata of tissue injury, could result from exposure of the embryo to a noxious agent during the first weeks after conception. At this early stage, the delicate sequencing of neuronal development could be disorganized at a time when the brain is incapable of generating a cellular response.

Microcephaly Vera (Genetic)

Microcephaly vera is a term applied to genetic defects resulting in decreased bulk growth of the brain. Autosomal dominant and autosomal recessive transmission are described (Haslam and Smith, 1979).

Clinical Features. The autosomal dominant form is less disabling than the recessive form. Intelligence ranges from normal to mild mental retardation. Learning disabilities are a common presentation. The face is not usually dysmorphic, although some children have a receding forehead, upslanting of the palpebral fissures, and large prominent ears. Physical stature is normal. Seizures may be present during childhood, but tend to disappear by adult life.

Children with the autosomal recessive form of microcephaly vera are usually short of stature and have a characteristic disproportion between the size of the face and skull. The forehead slants backward, and the reduced size of the skull causes the scalp to wrinkle in the occipital region. The chin is small, and the ears and nose are prominent. Mental retardation is moderate to severe, and other neurologic abnormalities, such as spastic diplegia and seizures, may be present as well.

Diagnosis. A family history of microcephaly is critical to the diagnosis in the autosomal dominant form, but is often lacking in the autosomal recessive form. Results of CT are normal.

Treatment. Treatment is not available.

Chromosome Disorders

Chromosomal disorders are unlikely to present as microcephaly at birth unless cerebral aplasia, such as holoprosencephaly, is part of the syndrome. Hypotonia and dysmorphism are the prominent features of chromosomal disorders in the newborn (see Chapter 5), and microcephaly becomes evident during infancy.

Defective Neurolation

At the end of the first week, a rostrocaudal axis appears on the dorsal aspect of the embryo that is responsible for the subsequent induction of a neural plate, the anlage of the nervous system. The neural plate is converted into a closed neural tube during the third and fourth week. Defects in closure are called dysraphic states. The most rostral portion of the neural tube, the anterior neuropore, closes at about the twenty-fourth day.

Anencephaly

Anencephaly is the result of defective closure of the anterior neuropore, just as myelomeningocele is the result of defective closure of the posterior neuropore (see Chapter 12). The present prevalence rate for each is 5/10,000 live births in the United States and 10/10,000 live births in the United Kingdom (Windham and Edmonds, 1982).

Clinical Features. Less than half of anencephalics are born alive, and these rarely survive the first month (Raven et al, 1983). The scalp is absent, and the skull is open from the vertex to the foramen magnum. The brain, appearing hemorrhagic and fibrotic, is exposed to view. It consists mainly of the hindbrain and parts of the diencephalon; the forebrain is completely lacking.

The orbits are shallow, and the eyes protrude. The neck is held in retroflexion, and the proximal portion of the arms seem overgrown compared with the legs. The overall appearance of the anencephalic newborn is grotesque and described as "toad-like."

Diagnosis. Following the birth of a child with a neural tube defect, the chance of anencephaly or myelomeningocele in subsequent pregnancies increases twofold to fivefold. After two affected children have been born, the chance of having another affected child doubles again (McBride, 1979). The prenatal diagnosis of dysraphic states is discussed in the section on myelomeningocele (see Chapter 12).

Treatment. No effort should be made to prolong life.

Encephalocele

An encephalocele is a protrusion of cortex and meninges, covered by skin, through a defect in the skull. Encephaloceles may occur in any location; however, most are midline-occipital, except in Orientals, in whom the defects are usually midline-frontal.

Clinical Features. The size of the encephalocele may range from a small protrusion to a large cyst equal in size to the skull. When the protrusion is large, the skull is likely to be microcephalic. No conclusion can be drawn concerning the contents of the mass by its size, but an encephalocele with a sessile base is more likely to contain cerebral tissue than is one with a pedunculated base.

Encephaloceles rarely occur as a solitary cerebral malformation and are usually associated with abnormalities of the cerebral hemispheres, cerebellum, and midbrain (Friede, 1975).

Diagnosis. A CT scan is reasonably accurate in defining the contents of the encephalocele. Despite its midline location, the protruded material is usually derived from one hemisphere that is smaller than the other and is displaced across the midline by the larger hemisphere.

Treatment. The desire to remove the encephalocele surgically should be tempered by its contents and the extent of associated anomalies. Occipital meningocele, in which the sac contains no neural tissue, should be surgically removed, and the outcome is often excellent. Those with protruded brain material and associated malformations usually die during infancy.

Defective Prosencephalization

The forebrain develops between twenty-five and thirty days' gestation from a midline vesicle that is generated from the closed anterior neuropore. Between thirty and forty days' gestation, bilateral cerebral vesicles are formed by the cleavage and outpouching of the midline vesicle. The midline vesicle is the primordium of the third ventricle, and the bilateral cerebral vesicles are the primordia of the lateral ventricles.

Holoprosencephaly

A spectrum of malformations have been described as a result of defective cleavage of the embryonic forebrain. The term *arhinencephaly* is often used to describe the full spectrum of abnormalities (Kobori et al, 1987), but holoprosencephaly is a more accurate term.

Total failure of cleavage produces a small brain with a midline vesicle covered by a horseshoe of limbic cortex. With less severe defects, the third ventricle and diencephalon differentiate and partial cleavage of the hemispheres is present in the occipital lobe. The corpus callosum is hypoplastic or absent. The minimal defect (arhinencephaly) is the unilateral or bilateral absence of the olfactory bulbs and tracts associated with some degree of rhinic lobe aplasia. Hemispheric cleavage is complete, the ventricles are normal, and the corpus callosum is present in part or in total.

Chromosomal abnormalities are often demonstrable in newborns with holoprosencephaly. Trisomy, deletions, and rings of chromosome 13 account for most of the chromosomal abnormalities. The remainder are composed of trisomy, deletions, and rings of chromosome 18 and partial trisomy of chromosome 7.

Clinical Features. Holoprosencephaly is associated with craniofacial dysplasia in 92.8 percent of cases and with malformations in other organs in 53 to 67 percent (Jellinger et al, 1981). The facial deformities are primarily in the midline (cyclopia or ocular hypotelorism, flat nose, cleft lip, cleft palate), and their severity is often predictive of the severity of the brain malformation. Other associated malformations include congenital heart defects, clubbing of the hands or feet, polydactyly and syndactyly, hypoplasia of the genitourinary system, accessory spleen and liver, and malrotation of the intestine.

Most children with severe defects in cleavage of the forebrain are stillborn or die in the neonatal period. Microcephaly, hypotonia, apnea, and seizures are prominent features. Hypotonia is especially severe when the defect is associated with a chromosomal abnormality. Infants who survive have severe intellectual, motor, and sensory impairment.

Children with only arhinencephaly may appear physically normal and may display minor disturbances in neurologic function such as learning disabilities and seizures.

Diagnosis. Holoprosencephaly should be suspected in every child with midline facial deformities, especially when malformations are present in other organs. Excellent visualization of the malformation is provided by CT or MRI.

Treatment. If we consider the multiplicity of malformations, measures to extend life are inappropriate.

Agenesis of the Corpus Callosum

Anomalous development of the three telencephalic commissures, the corpus callosum, the anterior commissure, and the hippocampal commissure is an almost constant feature of defective prosencephalization, but it also occurs in association with many other malformations and as a solitary genetic defect (see "Megalencephaly" earlier in this chapter).

Solitary agenesis of the corpus callosum is clinically silent except for subtle disturbances in the interhemispheric transfer of information, for which special testing is required to document.

Defective Cellular Migration

When neurons destined to form the superficial layers of the cerebral cortex are unable to pass through the already established deeper layers of neurons, the result is a simplification of the cortical convolutional pattern (*agyria*) and an abnormal accumulation of neurons in the white matter (*heterotopia*). Complete absence of gyri causes a smooth cerebral surface (*lissencephaly*), whereas incomplete gyral formation causes the existing convolutions to be reduced in number and large in size (*pachygyria*).

Most cases are sporadic, and the etiologic mechanism is probably multifactorial but must be operative early in gestation. Several neurocutaneous disorders are characterized by disturbances of neuronal migration.

Clinical Features. Most children are referred for developmental delay or intractable myoclonic seizures. Microcephaly is present in only half of cases, but all are mentally retarded (Gastaut et al, 1987). Many infants have an infiltrated and swollen appearance of the face and palmar skin, but only a few have dysmorphic features: high forehead, dolichocephaly, anteverted nostrils, polydactyly, and syndactyly. Axial hypotonia is constant.

Diagnosis. The EEG is characteristic, but not specific. Fast, high-voltage dysrhythmic activity dominates the background. It does not react to eye opening or photic stimulation and resembles a fast hypsarrhythmia.

The CT abnormalities are diagnostic: a smooth cortical surface except for rudimentary sulci in the frontal region; a broad, triangular-shaped sylvian fissure; and a widened interhemispheric fissure. The ventricles may be enlarged and the corpus callosum absent.

Treatment. Seizures are usually intractable, but may be partially controlled by standard drugs for the management of infantile spasms or myoclonic seizures (see Chapter 1). Death often occurs during infancy, but long survivals are possible.

SECONDARY MICROCEPHALY

Intrauterine Disorders

Intrauterine infection is an established cause of microcephaly. Cytomegalovirus infection (see Chapter 5) can present as microcephaly, without any features of systemic disease. Because maternal infection is silent, such cases are difficult to identify as being caused by cytomegalovirus disease. However, surveys of cytomegalovirus antibody demonstrate a higher rate of seropositive individuals among microcephalic than normocephalic children (Hanshaw, 1966). This suggests that such cases do exist.

There has been only limited success in identifying environmental toxins that produce cerebral malformation (Kalter and Warkany, 1983). Drugs of abuse and several pharmaceutical agents have been implicated, but the evidence is rarely compelling. The only absolute conclusion that can be derived from an abundance of studies is that there is a real negative impact on fetuses of women whose life style includes some combination of heavy alcohol or drug use, poor nutrition, and inadequate health care. This negative impact is usually expressed as intrauterine growth retardation, dysmorphic features, and microcephaly.

Aplasia of major cerebral vessels is a rare malformation of unknown cause. Brain tissue that should have been supplied by the aplastic vessels either never forms or is infarcted and replaced by calcified cystic cavities. The cavities are present at birth, and the CT appearance suggests an intrauterine infection, except that the cysts conform to a vascular distribution.

Perinatal Brain Injuries

Perinatal brain injuries are the most frequent cause of failure of brain growth during infancy when head circumference is normal at birth. This group of disorders generally presents as neonatal seizures (see Chapter 1). Children with microcephaly and mental retardation from perinatal brain injuries always have cerebral palsy and often have epilepsy as well. Microcephaly and mental retardation in the absence of motor impairment are always of prenatal origin.

Postnatal Systemic Disease

Infants who are chronically ill and malnourished fail to thrive. All growth is retarded; however, as a rule, head circumference maintains itself better than length and weight. Therefore, if body size is below the third percentile, head circumference might be at the fifth or tenth percentile. If the systemic disturbance is not corrected, brain injury generally occurs, brain growth slows, and head circumference falls into the microcephalic range.

■ Abnormal Head Shape

Whereas the size of the skull is determined almost exclusively by its contents, the shape of the skull is the result of forces acting from within and without, and of the time of closure of the cranial sutures.

INTRACRANIAL FORCES

The shape of the brain contributes to the shape of the skull by influencing the time of closure of cranial sutures. Temporal lobe agenesis results in a narrower calvarium and cerebellar agenesis in a small posterior fossa. Hydrocephalus produces characteristic changes in skull shape. Large lateral ventricles cause bowing of the forehead, and the Dandy-Walker malformation causes bowing of the occiput. In infants with subdural hematomas, bitemporal widening may be seen because of separation of the sagittal suture.

EXTRACRANIAL FORCES

Head shape may be influenced in utero by constricting forces, such as a bicornuate uterus or multiple fetuses. Physical constraint of the skull in utero may contribute to premature closure of a cranial suture (Graham et al, 1980; Graham and Smith, 1980), but perinatal and postnatal constraints do not. Molding of the skull is common during a prolonged vaginal delivery, but the closure of cranial sutures is unaffected and eventual head shape is not influenced by the molding.

In prematures, scaphocephaly (Table 18.5) often develops because the poorly mineralized skull becomes flattened on one side and then the other as the child is turned back and forth.

Table 18.5 TERMS THAT DESCRIBE HEAD SHAPES

Acrocephaly	High, tower-like head with vertical forehead
Brachycephaly	Broad head with recessed lower forehead
Oxycephaly	Pointed head
Plagiocephaly	Flattening of one side of head
Scaphocephaly (dolicocephaly)	An abnormally long and narrow head
Trigonocephaly	Triangular-shaped head with a prominent vertical ridge in the midforehead

The shape of the skull becomes normal with maturity.

Plagiocephaly, or occipital flattening, is a frequent finding in hypotonic infants. This is caused by constantly lying in the same position. The hair over the flattened portion of skull is usually sparse from rubbing against the bed surface. A normal head shape is resumed if the infant's lying position can be changed.

Craniostenosis

Craniostenosis or *craniosynostosis* are terms used to describe premature closure of one or more cranial sutures that result in an abnormal skull shape. These terms should be applied only to infants in whom the sutures close while the brain is still growing. Early closure of sutures in infants with microcephaly is not premature, because the intracranial pressure required to keep sutures apart is lacking.

Most cases of craniostenosis are sporadic and of uncertain etiology. Autosomal dominant and recessive forms of single-suture closure are reported (Cohen, 1983). Autosomal dominant inheritance is more common than autosomal recessive inheritance but is also more easily identified as hereditary. Many sporadic cases could represent autosomal recessive inheritance.

Craniostenosis may be one feature of a larger recognized syndrome of chromosomal or genetic abnormality. Genetic disorders are often associated with syndactyly or polydactyly (see "Acrocephalosyndactyly" later on in this chapter), whereas chromosomal disorders are usually characterized by other limb malformations and growth retardation (Table 18.6).

Craniostenosis is also reported in association with other disorders (Table 18.7). Some of these associations are coincidental, but a cause-and-effect relationship probably does exist with metabolic disorders of bone.

Table 18.6 CHROMOSOMAL DISORDERS THAT INCLUDE CRANIOSTENOSIS*

1q− syndrome	Brachycephaly, facial asymmetry, shallow orbits, small low-set ears, broad proximally placed thumbs, clinodactyly, growth deficiency, and mental retardation
3q+ syndrome	Oxycephaly, low hairline, ocular anomalies, anteverted nostrils, cleft palate, micrognathia, cryptorchidism, talipes equinovarus, growth deficiency, and mental retardation
5p+ syndrome	Scaphocephaly, renal anomalies, short great toe, and mental retardation
6q+ syndrome	Acrocephaly, hypertelorism, low-set ears, micognathia, cleft lip and palate, and mental retardation
7p− syndrome	Craniostenosis and other anomalies; phenotype not fully established.
7p+ syndrome	Acrocephalodactyly; phenotype not fully established
9p− syndrome	Trigonocephaly, flat auricles, pointed eyebrows, upslanting palpebral fissures, epicanthal folds, short neck, micrognathia, elongated thorax, and long fingers
11q− syndrome	Trigonocephaly; upslanting palpebral fissures; epicanthal folds; broad, flat nasal bridge; low-set ears; micrognathia; congenital heart disease; growth deficiency; and mental retardation
12p− syndrome	Microcephaly, narrow forehead, protruding occipital bone, low-set ears, highly arched eyebrows, downslanting palpebral fissures, pointed nose, and mental retardation
13q− syndrome	Trigonocephaly; microcephaly; holoprosencephaly; microphthalmia; micrognathia; malformed ears; and anomalies of the renal, cardiac, and gastrointestinal systems
Triploidy	Acrocephalosyndactyly, anomalies of the cardiac and genitourinary system, facial dysmorphism, growth deficiency, and mental retardation

*Modified from Cohen MM Jr: In Emery AE, Rimoin DA, eds. Principles and Practice of Medical Genetics. Churchill Livingstone, London, 1983, p 576.

Clinical Features. The first, and usually the only, symptom is an abnormal head shape. Normal bone growth is impaired in a plane perpendicular to the fused suture, but is able to grow in a parallel plane. Scaphocephaly is caused by premature fusion of the sagittal suture, brachycephaly of both coronal sutures, plagiocephaly of one coronal or one lambdoid suture, trigonocephaly of the metopic suture, and oxycephaly of all sutures.

When several sutures close prematurely, the growing brain is constricted and symptoms of increased intracranial pressure develop. Hydro-cephalus occurs more frequently in children with craniostenosis than in normal children (Whittle et al, 1984). Several different forms of communicating and noncommunicating hydrocephalus are described. It seems more likely that both are caused by a common underlying factor rather than one causing the other.

Scaphocephaly accounts for 50 to 60 percent of all cases of craniostenosis. Seventy-five percent of infants with scaphocephaly are males. Brachycephaly and plagiocephaly each account for 10 percent of cases.

Diagnosis. Visual inspection of the skull and palpation of the sutures is sufficient for diagnosis in most cases of single-suture craniostenosis. Radiographs of the skull demonstrate a band of increased density at the site of the prematurely closed suture. A CT is indicated in all children with craniostenosis of multiple sutures and in children with craniostenosis of a single suture if there is a question of hydrocephalus.

Treatment. The two indications for surgery to correct craniostenosis are to improve the appearance of the head and to relieve increased intracranial pressure (Winston, 1985). The cosmetic indication should be used sparingly and only to make severe deformities less noticeable.

Crouzon Disease
(Craniofacial Dysostosis)

Crouzon disease is the combination of premature closure of any or all cranial sutures and maldevelopment of facial bones. It is transmitted by autosomal dominant inheritance.

Clinical Features. The facial deformity is present at birth and becomes worse during infancy. The skull is usually widened anteriorly as a result of premature closure of the coronal suture. The eyes are widely separated and prominent, but the lower face appears recessed because of maxillary hypoplasia and prognathism. Adding to the deformity are a beak-like nose

Table 18.7 DISORDERS ASSOCIATED WITH CRANIOSTENOSIS

1. Ataxia-telangiectasia
2. Familial hypophosphatemia
3. Hyperthyroidism
4. Idiopathic hypercalcemia
5. Mucopolysaccharidoses
6. Polycythemia vera
7. Rickets
   a. Renal rickets
   b. Vitamin D deficient
   c. Vitamin D resistant
8. Sickle cell disease
9. Thalassemia major

and a large protuberant tongue. Intracranial pressure is often increased because several cranial sutures are usually involved.

Diagnosis. The typical facies and genetic pattern of inheritance are diagnostic. Computerized tomography of the head is indicated in every case to follow the progression of cerebral compression.

Treatment. A sequential neurosurgical and plastic surgical approach has been successful in opening the sutures to relieve increased intracranial pressure and in advancing the facial bones forward to improve cosmetic appearance.

Acrocephalosyndactyly

Acrocephalosyndactyly is characterized by the combination of craniostenosis and fusion of fingers and toes. Some degree of mental retardation is often present. Several different syndromes with this basic combination have been described (Cohen, 1983).

Apert syndrome is characterized by syndactyly and premature closure of the coronal suture resulting in brachycephaly. The forehead is high and prominent, and the face is similar to, but less severe in deformity than, in Crouzon disease. Most cases are sporadic, but autosomal dominant inheritance is suspected. Agenesis of the corpus callosum and limbic structures may be associated (de Leon et al, 1987).

Carpenter syndrome differs from Apert syndrome because it is transmitted by autosomal recessive inheritance and there is polydactyly as well as syndactyly, premature closure of all sutures, obesity, and hypogonadism.

Chotzen syndrome is similar to Carpenter syndrome, but is transmitted by autosomal dominant inheritance and also is marked by a low-set frontal hairline, ptosis, and a deviated nasal septum.

References

1. Bordarier C, Aicardi J, Goutieres F: Congenital hydrocephalus and eye abnormalities with severe developmental brain: Warburg's syndrome. Ann Neurol 16:60, 1984.
2. Burton B: Recurrence risks for congenital hydrocephalus. Clin Genet 16:47, 1977.
3. Chervenak FA, Berkowitz RL, Tortora M, et al: The management of fetal hydrocephalus. Am J Obstet Gynecol 151:933, 1985.
4. Clancy RR, Kurtz MB, Baker D, et al: Neurologic manifestations of the organoid nevus syndrome. Arch Neurol 42:236, 1985.
5. Cohen MM Jr: Craniofacial disorders. In Emery AE,

Rimoin DA, eds. Principles and Practice of Medical Genetics. Churchill Livingstone, London, 1983, p 576.
6. de Leon GA, de Leon G, Grover WD, et al: Agenesis of the corpus callosum and limbic malformation in Apert syndrome (Type I acrocephalosyndactyly). Arch Neurol 44:979, 1987.
7. DeMyer W: Megalencephaly: Types, clinical syndromes, and management. Pediatr Neurol 2:321, 1986.
8. Dennis M, Fitz CR, Netley CT, et al: The intelligence of hydrocephalic children. Arch Neurol 38:607, 1981.
9. Friede RL: Developmental Neuropathology. Springer-Verlag, New York, 1975, p 315.
10. Fukuyama Y, Miyao M, Ishizu, et al: Developmental changes in normal cranial measurements by computed tomography. Dev Med Child Neurol 21:425, 1979.
11. Gastaut H, Pinsard N, Raybaud C, et al: Lissencephaly (agyria-pachygyria): Clinical findings and serial EEG. Dev Med Child Neurol 29:167, 1987.
12. Golden SE, Kaplan AM: Hypomelanosis of Ito: Neurologic complications. Pediatr Neurol 2:170, 1986.
13. Graham JM Jr, Badura RJ, Smith DW: Coronal craniostenosis: Fetal head constraint as one possible cause. Pediatrics 65:995, 1980.
14. Graham JM Jr, Smith DW: Metopic craniostenosis as a consequence of fetal head constraint: Two interesting experiments of nature. Pediatrics 65:1000, 1980.
15. Hamza M, Bodensteiner JB, Noorani PA, et al: Benign extracerebral fluid collections: a cause of macrocrania in infancy. Pediatr Neurol, 3:218, 1987.
16. Hanshaw JB: Cytomegalovirus complement-fixing antibodies in microcephaly. N Engl J Med 275:476, 1966.
17. Hart MN, Malamud N, Ellis WG: The Dandy-Walker syndrome: A clinicopathological study based on 28 cases. Neurology 22:771, 1972.
18. Haslam RHA, Smith DW: Autosomal dominant microcephaly. J Pediatr 95:701, 1979.
19. Jaeckle KA, Krol G, Posner JB: Evolution of computed tomographic abnormalities in leptomeningeal metastases. Ann Neurol 17:85, 1985.
20. Jaworski M, Hersh JH, Donat J, et al: Computed tomography of the head in the evaluation of microcephaly. Pediatrics 78:1064, 1986.
21. Jellinger K, Gross H, Kaltenback E, et al: Holoprosencephaly and agenesis of the corpus callosum: Frequency of associated malformations. Acta Neuropathol 55:1, 1981.
22. Jellinger K, Sunder-Plassman M: Connatal intracranial tumors. Neuropediatrie 4:46, 1973.
23. Kalter H, Warkany J: Congenital malformations. N Engl J Med 308:491, 1983.
24. Kelly JJ Jr, Mellinger JF, Sundt TM Jr: Intracranial arteriovenous malformations in childhood. Ann Neurol 3:338, 1978.
25. Kobori JA, Herrick MK, Urich H: Arhinencephaly. The spectrum of associated malformations. Brain 110:237, 1987.
26. Kovnar EH, Coxe WS, Volpe JJ: Normal neurologic development and marked reconstitution of cerebral mantle after postnatal treatment of intrauterine hydrocephalus. Neurology 34:840, 1984.
27. Kuzniecky RI, Watters GV, Watters L, et al: X-linked hydrocephalus. Can J Neurol Sci 13:344, 1986.
28. Lipman SP, Pretorius H, Rumack CM, et al: Fetal intracranial teratoma: US diagnosis of three cases and a review of the literature. Radiology 157:491, 1985.
29. Lorber J, Priestly BL: Children with large heads: a practical approach to diagnosis in 577 children, with special reference to 109 children with megalencephaly. Dev Med Child Neurol 23:494, 1981.

30. Lynn RB, Buchanan DC, Fenichel GM, et al: Agenesis of the corpus callosum. Arch Neurol 37:444, 1980.

31. McBride ML: Sib risks of anencephaly and spina bifida in British Columbia. Am J Med Genet 3:377, 1979.

32. Miller CA, Parker WD Jr: Hypomelanosis of Ito: Association with a chromosomal abnormality. Neurology 35:607, 1985.

33. Miller RW: Childhood cancer and congenital defects: A study of U.S. death certificates during the period 1960–1966. Pediatr Res 3:389, 1969.

34. Mueller SM: Enlarged cerebral ventricular system in infant achondroplastic dwarf. Neurology 30:767, 1980.

35. Mueller SM, Reinertson JE: Reversal of emissary vein blood flow in achondroplastic dwarfs. Neurology 30:769, 1980.

36. Nagib MG, Maxwell RE, Chou SN: Klippel-Feil syndrome in children: clinical features and management. Child Nerv Sys 1:255, 1985.

37. Nickel RE, Gallenstein JS: Developmental prognosis for infants with enlargement of the subarachnoid spaces. Dev Med Child Neurol 29:181, 1987.

38. Norman MG, Becker LE: Cerebral damage in neonates resulting from arteriovenous malformations of the vein of Galen. J Neurol Neurosurg Psychiatry 37:252, 1974.

39. Raven RH, Schoenberg BS, Bharucha NE, et al: Geographic distribution of anencephaly in the United States. Neurology 33:1243, 1983.

40. Reid CS, Pyeritz RE, Kopits SE, et al: Cervicomedullary compression in young patients with achondroplasia: Value of comprehensive neurologic and respiratory evaluation. J Pediatr 110:522, 1987.

41. Sotos JF, Cutler EA: Cerebral gigantism. Am J Dis Child 131:625, 1977.

42. Tal Y, Freigang B, Dunn HG, et al: Dandy-Walker syndrome: Analysis of 21 cases. Dev Med Child Neurol 22:189, 1980.

43. Tjiam AT, Stefanko S, Schenk VW, et al: Infantile spasms associated with hemihypsarrhythmia and hemimegalencephaly. Dev Med Child Neurol 20:779, 1978.

44. Tomita T, McLone DG: Brain tumors during the first twenty-four months of life. Neurosurgery 17:913, 1985.

45. Vintzileos AM, Campbell WA, Weinbaum PJ, et al: Perinatal management and outcome of fetal ventriculomegaly. Obstet Gynecol 69:5, 1987.

46. Whelan HT, Sung JH, Mastri AR: Diffuse leptomeningeal gliomatosis: report of three cases. Clin Neuropath, 6:164, 1987.

47. Whittle IR, Johnston IH, Besser M: Intracranial pressure changes in craniostenosis. Surg Neurol 21:367, 1984.

48. Williams RS, Swisher CN, Jennings M, et al: Cerebro-ocular dysgenesis (Walker-Warburg syndrome): Neuropathologic and etiologic analysis. Neurology 34:1531, 1984.

49. Windham GC, Edmonds LD: Current trends in the incidence of neural tube defects. Pediatrics 70:333, 1982.

50. Winship IG: Sotos syndrome—autosomal dominant inheritance substantiated. Clin Genet 28:243, 1985.

51. Winston KR: Craniosynostosis. In Wilkins RH, Rengachary SS, eds. Neurosurgery. McGraw-Hill Book Co, New York, 1985, p 2171.

52. Wit JM, Beemer FA, Barth PG, et al: Cerebral gigantism (Sotos syndrome). Compiled data of 22 cases. Analysis of clinical features, growth and plasma somatomedin. Eur J Pediatr 144:131, 1985.

53. Yokota A, Matsukado Y: Congenital midline porencephaly. A new malformation associated with scalp anomaly. Child Brain 5:380, 1979.

Index

Note: Page numbers in *italics* refer to figures; page numbers followed by t refer to tables.

Abducens nerve, congenital palsy of, 304
  idiopathic palsy of, ophthalmoplegia and, 306
Abetalipoproteinemia, chronic ataxia and, 243
Abscess, brain, acute hemiplegia and, 253–254
    increased intracranial pressure and, *111*,
      111–112
   epidural, 112
    paraplegia and, 272–273
   subdural, 112
Absence epilepsy, 26–27, *27*
Absence myoclonus, 28
Absence status, acute hemiplegia and, 258–259
Acanthocyte, in abetalipoproteinemia, 243
Acanthocytosis, 243
Acetazolamide, for posthemorrhagic hydrocepha-
  lus, 104
  for seizures, 35
Acetylcoenzyme A, in muscle activity, 204, *205*
Achondroplasia, communicating hydrocephalus
  and, 361
Acid maltase, deficiency of, infantile hypotonia
  and, 166
   proximal limb weakness and, 181–182
Acidemia, isovaleric, neonatal seizures and, 11, *11*
  methylmalonic, neonatal seizures and, 12
  propionic, neonatal seizures and, 12
Acoustic neuroma, acquired hearing impairment
  and, 352, *352*
Acquired immune deficiency syndrome, encepha-
  litis in, 53–54
Acrocephalosyndactyly, 375
Acrocephaly, 373t
ACTH. See *Adrenocorticotropic hormone.*
Adamkiewitz, artery of, embolization of, paraple-
  gia and, 273
Additives, food, vascular headache and, 81–82
Adenoma, pituitary, progressive vision loss and,
  332–333
Adie syndrome, 334
Adrenal cortex, failure of, central nervous system
  demyelination and, 143
Adrenal gland, hypersecretion of, altered states of
  consciousness and, 63
Adrenocorticotropic hormone (ACTH), for infan-
  tile spasms, 21

Adrenoleukodystrophy, chronic ataxia and, 245
  neonatal, cerebral hypotonia and, 152
  paraplegia and, 271
  progressive encephalopathy and, 143
Agitation, causes of, 43t
Agyria, 372
Albers-Schönberg disease, facial weakness and,
  345
Alcohol, abuse of, 66
  vascular headache and, 81
Alexander disease, progressive encephalopathy
  and, 137–138
Algodystrophy, 218–219
Alice-in-Wonderland syndrome, 77
Allergy, migraine and, 76
Alper disease, progressive encephalopathy and,
  133–134
Alpha-fetoprotein, amniotic fluid level of, 265
Altitude, high, hypoxia and, 47
Aluminum toxicity, dialysis dementia syndrome
  and, 60
  uremic encephalopathy and, 59
Amaurosis, 321
  congenital, Leber, congenital blindness and,
   324
Amblyopia, 302, 321
Amino acids, branched-chain, metabolism of, *11*
  excessive, encephalopathy and, 63
Aminoacidopathy, neonatal, seizures and, 10–13,
  11, *12*, 13t
  progressive vision loss and, 333
Aminoaciduria, progressive encephalopathy and,
  124–127, *125*, 125t, *126*
Aminoglycosides, vertigo and, 354
Ammonia, levels of, muscle biopsy and, 206
  neonatal seizures and, *12*, 12–13, 13t
  metabolism of, *12*
Amnesia, global, transient, 64
Amphetamine, abuse of, 66
Amphotericin B, for coccidioidal meningitis, 114
  for cryptococcal meningitis, 113, 113t
Amyloid neuropathy, hereditary, distal limb weakness and, 187
Amyotrophy, asthmatic, 281
  neuralgic, monoplegia and, 279–280

Anemia, sickle cell, acute hemiplegia and, 254–255

Anencephaly, 370–371

Anesthetics, local, fetal intoxication by, 14

Aneurysm, arterial, increased intracranial pressure and, 105

unilateral ophthalmoplegia and, 309

Aniridia, 335

Anisocoria, essential, 334

Anoxia-ischemia, acute, 47–48

Antibiotics, ototoxicity of, 350

vertigo and, 354

Anticonvulsant drugs, 33–38

in neonatal seizures, 8t

Antidepressants, tricyclic, overdose of, 65–66

Anxiety, chronic tension headache and, 85–86

Apert syndrome, 375

Aphasia, seizures and, 31–32

Apnea, heart rate and, 4

in infants, 17–18

in newborns, 2, 3–4, *4*

Apoplexy, pituitary, acute blindness and, 329, 329t

Apraxia, motor, ocular, 313–314

congenital, 313–314

vertical, congenital, 315

Aqueductal stenosis, noncommunicating hydrocephalus and, 363–364, *364*

Arachnoid cyst, intracranial, increased intracranial pressure and, 101

Arboviral encephalitis, 52–53

Arginase deficiency, neonatal seizures and, *12*, 12–13

Argininosuccinic acidemia, neonatal seizures and, 12–13

Argyll Robertson pupil, 335

Arhinencephaly, 371

Arms, weakness of. See *Limb weakness.*

Arnold-Chiari malformation, 265

Arteriovenous malformation, acute hemiplegia and, 257

increased intracranial pressure and, 105–107

midline, increased intracranial pressure and, 106

paraplegia and, 267–268

supratentorial, increased intracranial pressure and, 106–107

Arteritis, Takayasu, acute hemiplegia and, 255

Arthrogryposis, differential diagnosis of, 147, 148t

neurogenic, infantile hypotonia and, 158

Aseptic meningitis, 49–55

L-Asparaginase, thrombosis induced by, acute hemiplegia and, 256

N-Aspartyl-β-glucosaminidase, deficiency of, 140

Aspartylglycosaminuria, progressive encephalopathy and, 140

Asphyxia, fetal, 6–9, *8*, 8t

perinatal, jitteriness and, 5

Asthma, monoplegia after, 281

Astrocytoma, cerebellar, chronic ataxia and, 235–236

increased intracranial pressure and, 97–98, *98*

noncommunicating hydrocephalus and, 365

spinal paraplegia and, 269, *269*

Ataxia, 223–247

acute, 223t, 224–235, *225*

basilar migraine and, 229–230, *230*

benign paroxysmal vertigo and, 230–231

brain tumor and, 234

Ataxia *(Continued)*

acute, brainstem encephalitis and, 228

carnitine acetyltransferase deficiency and, 232

cerebellar hemorrhage and, 233

conversion reaction and, 234–235

diagnostic studies for, *225*

drug ingestion and, 224

epileptic, 234

genetic disorders and, 231–233

Hartnup disease and, 232–233

Kawasaki disease and, 234

lupus erythematosus and, 233–234

maple syrup urine disease and, 232

migraine and, 229–230, *230*

Miller Fisher syndrome and, 226

multiple sclerosis and, 227–228, *228*

myoclonic encephalopathy and, 226–227

postconcussion syndrome and, 228–229

postinfectious cerebellitis and, 225–226

postinfectious/immune disorders and, 224–228

pseudo-, 234

pyruvate decarboxylase deficiency and, 231

trauma and, 228–229

vascular disorders and, 233–234

vertebrobasilar occlusion and, 229

chronic, 235–246

basilar impression and, 239

brain tumors and, 235–238

cerebellar astrocytoma and, 235–236

cerebellar hemangioblastoma and, 237–238

cerebellar hypoplasia and, 238

Chiari malformation and, 239, *239*

congenital malformations and, 238–239

dementia with, 245–246

ependymoma and, 237

hereditary, 239–246

abetalipoproteinemia and, 243

adrenoleukodystrophy and, 245

dominant, 239–240

episodic dystonia and, 245

Friedreich, 240–241

Hartnup disease and, 245

hypobetalipoproteinemia and, 243–244

juvenile GM_2 gangliosidosis and, 244

juvenile sulfatide lipidosis and, 244

Leber optic neuropathy and, 245

Machado-Joseph disease and, 240

maple syrup urine disease and, 245

Marinesco-Sjögren syndrome and, 242–243

olivopontocerebellar degeneration and, 240

Ramsay Hunt syndrome of, 241–242

Ramsay Hunt variants of, 240

Refsum disease and, 245

sea-blue histiocytoses and, 244–245

X-linked, 245

medulloblastoma and, 236

vermal aplasia and, 238–239

von Hippel–Lindau disease and, 237–238

differential diagnosis of, 223t, 224t

hysterical, 234–235

progressive, 235–246

recurrent, dominant, 231

Ataxia telangiectasia, 242

Athetosis, 286–291, 287t

Atlanto-axial dislocation, paraplegia and, 268

Atrophy, optic, hereditary, progressive vision loss and, 330–333
Attention deficit disorder, Tourette syndrome and, 298
Audiometry, pure tone, 347
Auditory evoked response, brainstem, 347–348, *348*, 348t
Autism, infantile, language delay and, 120
Axonal neuropathy, chronic, distal limb weakness and, 190
Axonopathy, 184

Bacterial meningitis, 49
Bacterial sepsis, 55–56
Ballismus, 287
Basal ganglia, calcification of, chorea and, 288
Basilar impression, chronic ataxia and, 239
Bassen-Kornzweig syndrome, 243
Becker muscular dystrophy, 175–178
  vs. limb-girdle muscular dystrophy, 178
Bell palsy, facial weakness and, 341
  vs. herpes zoster oticus, 344
Beta-adrenoceptor blocking drugs, ototoxicity of, 350
Bielschowsky-Jansky ceroid lipofuscinosis, progressive encephalopathy and, 141–142
Biopsy, muscle, in infantile hypotonia, 156
  nerve, in infantile hypotonia, 156
Birth, breech presentation at, infantile hypotonia and, 154
  cervical presentation at, infantile hypotonia and, 154–155
  trauma of, 9
Blastomycosis, 115
Blepharospasm, 291t, 291–292
Blindness, acute, 325t, 325–330
  cortical, 327–328
    hypoglycemia and, 328
    demyelinating optic neuropathy and, 325–326
    hysterical, 329–330
    idiopathic optic neuritis and, 326
    ischemic optic neuropathy and, 326–327
    measles retinitis and, 329
    pituitary apoplexy and, 329, 329t
    posttraumatic, 328
    retinal artery obstruction and, 327
    retinal injury and, 328
    retinal migraine and, 326–327
    toxic optic neuropathies and, 328–329
  cerebral, posttraumatic, transient, 328
  congenital, 322t, 322–324, 323t, *324*
    congenital cataract and, 322–323, 323t
    congenital coloboma and, 324
    congenital optic nerve hypoplasia and, 323–324, *324*
    Leber congenital amaurosis and, 324
    morning glory disk and, 324
  cortical, 321
Bobbing, ocular, 316, 316t
Borrelia bergdorfei, 49
Botulism, bilateral ophthalmoplegia and, 312
  generalized weakness and, 194
  infantile, hypotonia and, 160
Brachial plexus, newborn injury to, monoplegia and, 282–283
  postnatal injury to, monoplegia and, 283
  tumor of, monoplegia and, 283

Brain, abscess of, increased intracranial pressure and, *111*, 111–112
  congenital tumor of, noncommunicating hydrocephalus and, 365
  cystic cavities of, secondary microcephaly and, 372
  malformation of, developmental delay and, 122
  perinatal injury to, secondary microcephaly and, 372
  tumor of, acute ataxia and, 234
    chronic ataxia and, 235–238
    congenital, noncommunicating hydrocephalus and, 365
    increased intracranial pressure and, 96–101, 97t
Brain death, 48, 48t
Brainstem, glioma of, progressive facial diplegia and, 342
  immaturity of, apnea and, 4
  lower, dysfunction of, 337–358
Brainstem auditory evoked response test, 347–348, *348*, 348t
Brainstem stroke, unilateral ophthalmoplegia and, 310
Breathholding, in infants, 18
Breathing, apneustic, 46
  ataxic, 46
  periodic, in newborn, 4
Breech presentation, infantile hypotonia and, 154
Brody disease, muscle cramps and, 211–212
Brown syndrome, ophthalmoplegia and, 304–305
Bulbar palsy, progressive, juvenile, facial weakness and, 344–345
Burns, metabolic encephalopathy and, 63

Caffeine, withdrawal from, vascular headache and, 81
Calcinosis universalis, in dermatomyositis, 180
Calcium channel blocking agents, for migraine prophylaxis, 79
California-LaCrosse encephalitis, 53
Caloric testing, 353–354
Cancer, acute hemiplegia and, 256–257
Candida, infection with, 114–115
Carbamyl phosphate synthetase deficiency, neonatal seizures and, *12*, 12–13
Carbohydrate, metabolism of, muscle activity and, *204*
  muscle utilization of, defects of, 206–207
Carnitine, deficiency of, differential diagnosis of, 58t
  infantile hypotonia and, 167
  primary, encephalopathy and, 58–59
  proximal limb weakness and, 182
  systemic, encephalopathy and, 58, 58t
Carnitine acetyltransferase, deficiency of, acute ataxia and, 232
Carnitine palmityltransferase, deficiency of, decreased muscle energy and, 207–208
Carotid artery, infection of, acute hemiplegia and, 252
  trauma to, acute hemiplegia and, 252
Carpenter syndrome, 375
Cataract, congenital, blindness and, 322–323, 323t
Cat-scratch disease, 54
  acute hemiplegia and, 252
Causalgia, 218–219

Cavernous sinus, fistula of, unilateral ophthalmoplegia and, 311
  thrombosis of, unilateral ophthalmoplegia and, 311
Celontin. See *Methsuximide.*
Central core disease, infantile hypotonia and, 163–164
Cephalic presentation, facial nerve injury and, 340
Cerebellitis, postinfectious, acute, ataxia and, 225–226
Cerebellum, herniation of, increased intracranial pressure and, 94
Cerebral aqueduct, stenosis of, noncommunicating hydrocephalus and, 363–364, *364*
Cerebral artery, idiopathic infarction of, acute hemiplegia and, 251
Cerebral blood flow, increased intracranial pressure and, 90
Cerebral gigantism, 368
Cerebral malformation, developmental delay and, 122
Cerebral palsy, 276t, 276–277
Cerebral perfusion pressure, 90
Cerebrohepatorenal syndrome, cerebral hypotonia and, 152
Cerebrospinal fluid, intracranial pressure and, 89–90
Cerebrotendinous xanthomatosis, progressive encephalopathy and, 143–144
Cerebrovascular disease, acute hemiplegia and, 248–257
  causes of, 249t
Ceruloplasmin, level of, in Wilson disease, 293
Cervical presentation, infantile hypotonia and, 154–155
Charcot-Marie-Tooth disease, 185
  neuronal type, 185–186
Chédiak-Higashi syndrome, progressive encephalopathy and, 136
Cherry-red spot, lysosomal enzyme disorders with, 130t
Cherry-red spot–myoclonus syndrome, 29–30
Cheyne-Stokes respiration, 46
Chiari malformation, chronic ataxia and, 239, *239*
Child abuse, conversion reaction and, 234–235
Chlorocresol, poisoning with, facial weakness and, 345
Chlorpromazine, for migraine, 79
Cholesteatoma, vertigo and, 355
Chorea, 286–291, 287t
  delayed-onset, 294
  differential diagnosis of, 287t
  drug-induced, 289t, 289–290
  Fahr syndrome and, 288
  familial, benign, 288
  genetic disorders with, 287–289
  Hallervorden-Spatz disease and, 288–289
  hyperthyroidism and, 290
  infantile bilateral striatal necrosis and, 288
  lupus erythematosus and, 290
  pregnancy and, 290
  rheumatic, 290
  Sydenham, 290
  systemic disorders and, 290
Chorea gravidarum, 290
Choreoathetosis, conditions with, 287t
  paroxysmal, familial, 25
Choriocarcinoma, 100

Choroid plexus, papilloma of, increased intracranial pressure and, 100–101
  noncommunicating hydrocephalus and, 365
Chotzen syndrome, 375
Chromosomes, abnormalities of, autosomal, 121t
  developmental delay and, 120–122, *121*, 121t
  analysis of, clinical indications for, 121t
Cis-platinum, ototoxicity of, 350
Citrobacter diversus, infection with, 108
Citrullinemia, neonatal siezures and, 12–13
Clonazepam, for seizures, 35–36
Clorazepate, for seizures, 36
Clostridium botulinum, 194, 312. See also *Botulism.*
Cluster headache, 77–78
  lithium carbonate for, 80
  methysergide maleate for, 80
  prednisone for, 80
  treatment of, 80
Coats syndrome, facioscapulohumeral dystrophy and, 342
  facioscapulohumeral syndrome and, 179
Cocaine, abuse of, 66
Coccidioidomycosis, increased intracranial pressure and, 113–114
Cockayne syndrome, distal limb weakness and, 187
  progressive vision loss and, 333
Cohen syndrome, cerebral hypotonia and, 153
Coloboma, congenital, congenital blindness and, 324
Coma, 42t
  barbiturate, in anoxia-ischemia, 48
  causes of, 42, 43t, 44t
  diagnostic approach to, 44, 46
  Glasgow scale for, 68t
  hepatic, 60–61
  irreversible, 48
  migraine, 64
  ocular motility in, 46
  patient history in, 44
  pentobarbital, for increased intracranial pressure, 95–96, *96*
Confusion, causes of, 43t
Connective tissue disorders, headache and, 83
Consciousness, altered states of, 42–72. See also specific states, e.g., *Coma.*
  aseptic meningitis and, 49–55
  bacterial sepsis and, 55–56
  drug poisoning and, 65–66
  endocrine disorders and, 63
  infectious disorders and, 48–55
  metabolic encephalopathies and, 58–63
  migraine and, 63–64
  osmolality disorders and, 61–63
  postimmunization encephalopathy and, 57–58
  postinfectious encephalomyelitis and, *56*, 56–57
  psychologic disorders and, 64–65
  trauma and, 67–70
  viral encephalitis and, 48–49
Conus medullaris, in tethered spinal cord, 267
Convergence palsy, 315
Conversion reaction, acute ataxia and, 234–235
Convulsion. See *Seizure(s).*
Copper, intestinal transport of, defect of, 134

Cornea, clouding of, 322, 322t
Corpus callosum, agenesis of, primary microcephaly and, 372
Corticosteroids, for increased intracranial pressure, 95
Coxsackievirus, infection with, generalized weakness and, 192–193
Cramps, 199, 209–212
  evaluation of, *206*
Cranial nerves, dysfunction of, 337–358
Cranial polyneuropathy, idiopathic, facial weakness and, 341–342
Craniofacial dysostosis, abnormal head shape and, 374–375
Craniopharyngioma, progressive vision loss and, 331
Craniostenosis, abnormal head shape and, 373–374
  chromosomal disorders with, 374t
Craniosynostosis, abnormal head shape and, 373–374
Craniovertebral junction, basilar impression of, chronic ataxia and, 239
Cranium. See also *Head.*
  shape disorders of, 373–375
  volume disorders of, 357–373
Creatine kinase, in Duchenne dystrophy, 177
  in infantile hypotonia, 155
  level of, muscle biopsy and, 205
Crouzon disease, abnormal head shape and, 374–375
Cryptococcus immitis, infection with, 113–114
Cryptococcus neoformans, infection with, 112–113, 113t
CSF. See *Cerebrospinal fluid.*
Cyanosis, infant syncope with, 18
Cyanotic syncope, in infants, 18
Cyproheptadine, for migraine prophylaxis, 80
Cyst, arachnoid, intracranial, increased intracranial pressure and, 101
Cystinuria, progressive vision loss and, 333
Cytochrome-*c*-oxidase deficiency, infantile hypotonia and, 166–167
Cytomegalic inclusion disease, developmental delay and, 122
Cytomegalovirus, intrauterine, deafness and, 349
  secondary microcephaly, 372

Dandy-Walker malformation, noncommunicating hydrocephalus and, *364,* 364–365
Daydreaming. See *Staring spells.*
Dazzle reflex, in visual acuity assessment, 321
Deafness, 346–352
  congenital, 349–350
    chromosome disorders and, 349–350
    genetic disorders and, 349
    inner ear aplasia and, 349–350
    isolated, 349
    Pendred syndrome and, 349
    thyroxine synthesis defect and, 349
    Usher syndrome and, 349–350
Death, brain, 48, 48t
Debrancher enzyme, deficiency of, proximal limb weakness and, 182
Decerebrate posturing, 3
Decerebrate rigidity, 46

Decorticate rigidity, 46
Déjérine-Roussy syndrome, sensory disturbance and, 221
Déjérine-Sottas disease, 186
Delirium, diagnostic approach to, 42–44
  eye examination in, 43
  laboratory investigations in, 43–44, *45*
  patient history in, 43
  physical examination in, 43
Dementia, chronic ataxia and, 245–246
  dialysis and, 60
  progressive, evaluation of, *139*
    of infancy, 123–138
  scapulohumeral syndrome with, distal limb weakness and, 192
Demyelination, cerebral, in Krabbe disease, *124*
  postinfectious, *56,* 56–57
Denver Developmental Screening Test, 118
Depakene. See *Valproic acid.*
Depression, chronic tension headache and, 85
Depressor anguli oris muscle, aplasia of, facial weakness and, 340
Dermal sinus, of spine, 266
Dermatomyositis, diagnosis of, 180
  perifascicular atrophy in, 181, *181*
  prednisone for, 180–181
  proximal limb weakness and, 179–181, *180*
  treatment of, 180–181
Developmental delay, 118t, 118–123, 119t, *121,* 121t
  cytomegalic inclusion disease and, 122
  diagnosis of, 118t
  global, 120–123, *121,* 121t
    cerebral malformations and, 122
    chromosomal disturbances and, 120–121, 121t
    evaluation of, *121*
  in histidinemia, 120
  in infantile autism, 120
  in language delay, 119–120
  intrauterine infections and, 122–123
  language delay and, 118–120
  motor, 120
  perinatal disorders and, 123
  rubella embryopathy and, 123
  toxoplasmosis and, 122
Devic disease, spinal paraplegia and, 270–271
Diabetes mellitus, acute hemiplegia and, 259–260
  juvenile, progressive vision loss and, 331
Dialysis, headache and, 82
  kidney, encephalopathy with, 60
Dialysis dementia syndrome, 60
Diamox. See *Acetazolamide.*
Diastematomyelia, 266
Diazepam, safety of, 65
Diencephalic syndrome, 331
Diet, migraine and, 76
DiGeorge syndrome, neonatal siezures and, 10
Dilantin. See *Phenytoin.*
Diplacusis test, 347
Diplegia, facial, congenital, 339–340
    progressive, brainstem glioma and, 342
      myasthenia gravis and, 342
  spastic, 276–277
Diplomyelia, 266
Diplopia, intracranial pressure increase and, 92
Diskitis, paraplegia and, 271–272, *272*
Disseminated intravascular coagulation, acute hemiplegia and, 256

Diuretic, osmotic, for increased intracranial pressure, 95
Divergence nystagmus, 319
Doliocephaly, 373t
Down syndrome, cataracts in, 322
Downbeat nystagmus, 318
Downward gaze palsy, ataxia, and foam cell syndrome, 315
Drug(s), acute ataxia and, 224
  intoxication with, bilateral ophthalmoplegia and, 312, 312t
    hearing impairment and, 350
    internuclear ophthalmoplegia and, 314
    nystagmus and, 318
    secondary microcephaly and, 372
    vertigo and, 354
  neonatal withdrawal from, 14
  neuropathies with, 188
  prescription, poisoning with, 65–66
  tardive dyskinesia with, 289, 289t
  vascular headache and, 81
  withdrawal syndrome with, 290
Duane syndrome, 304
Duchenne muscular dystrophy, 175–178, *176*, *177*
  carrier status in, 177
  diagnosis of, 176
  treatment of, 176–177
Dysautonomia, familial, 216
  cerebral hypotonia and, 153
Dyskinesia, tardive, 287
Dysmetria, ocular, 316, 316t
Dysostosis, craniofacial, abnormal head shape and, 374–375
Dysphagia, 337–346. See also *Facial weakness.*
  congenital, 340–341
  neurologic causes of, 339t
Dysplasia, cerebro-ocular, infantile hypotonia and, 165
  fibromuscular, acute hemiplegia and, 253
Dysraphia, paraplegia and, 264–266
Dyssynergia cerebellaris myoclonica, 241–242
Dystonia, 291t, 291–295, 294t
  benign paroxysmal torticollis and, 295
  blepharospasm and, 291t, 291–292
  delayed-onset, 294
  differential diagnosis of, 291t
  drug-induced, 292
  episodic, chronic ataxia and, 245
  focal, 291
  genetic, 292–294
  hepatolenticular degeneration and, 293–294
  symptomatic, 294
  torsion, primary, 292
  torticollis and, 294t, 294–295
  Wilson disease and, 293–294
  writer's cramp and, 295
Dystonia musculorum deformans, 292
Dystonia-Parkinsonism syndrome, 292–293
Dystrophy, facioscapulohumeral, facial weakness and, 342
  muscular, 148t
    Becker, 175–178
    clinical features of, 179t
    congenital, Fukuyama type of, 164–165
      hypotonia and, *164*, 164–166
    Duchenne, 175–178, *176*, *177*
    infantile hypotonia and, *164*, 164–166
    limb-girdle, 178, *178*

Dystrophy *(Continued)*
  muscular, oculopharyngeal, facial weakness and, 342–343
    proximal limb weakness and, 175–179, *176*, *177*
  myotonic, 165–166
    distal limb weakness and, 190–191
  neuroaxonal, infantile, 136

Ear, inner, aplasia of, congenital deafness and, 349
Eastern equine encephalitis, 52
Echovirus, infection with, generalized weakness and, 192–193
Edema, cerebral, diabetic ketoacidosis and, 61
    increased intracranial pressure and, 90
  cytotoxic, 90
  interstitial, 90
  of optic disk, intracranial pressure and, *92*, 92t, 92–93, *93*, 93t
  vasogenic, 90
Edrophonium chloride test, in infantile hypotonia, 156
Electronystagmography, 354
Embolism, arterial, acute hemiplegia and, 253–254
Embryonal cell carcinoma, 100
Emery-Dreifuss muscular dystrophy, distal limb weakness and, 191–192
Empyema, epidural, increased intracranial pressure and, 112
  subdural, increased intracranial pressure and, 112
Encephalitis, acquired immune deficiency and, 53–54
  arboviral, 52–53
  brainstem, 228
    vs. Miller Fisher syndrome, 226
  California-LaCrosse, 53
  cat-scratch disease and, 54
  definition of, 42
  equine, Eastern, 52
    Western, 52
  headache and, 83
  herpes simplex, 49–50
    EEG in, 50, *51*
    neonatal seizures and, 13–14
  Japanese B, 53
  measles, 50–52
  Reye syndrome and, 54–55
  St. Louis, 52
  viral, 48–49
Encephalocele, primary microcephaly and, 371
Encephalomyelitis, diffuse, paraplegia and, 271
  postinfectious, altered states of consciousness and, *56*, 56–57
Encephalomyelopathy, necrotizing, subacute, 133
Encephalomyopathy, mitochondrial, 142–143
Encephalopathy, bilirubin, neonatal, seizures and, 15
  definition of, 42
  dialysis, 60
  EEG in, *45*
  glycine, neonatal seizures and, 11
  hemorrhagic shock and, 56
  hepatic, 60–61
    EEG in, *45*

Encephalopathy *(Continued)*
  hypertensive, 59–60, 70
  hyponatremic, 62
  hypoxia and, 46–47
  hypoxic-ischemic, neonatal, 6–9, *8*, 8t
    burst suppression pattern of, *8*
    clinical features of, 6–7
    mannitol for, 9
    treatment of, 7, 9
  metabolic, altered states of consciousness and,
      58–63
    burn injury and, 63
    hypomagnesemia and, 63
    parenteral hyperalimentation and, 63
  myoclonic, acute ataxia and, 226–227
    neuroblastoma and, 227
  nonprogressive, chronic, cerebral hypotonia
      and, 151
  pertussis vaccine and, 57–58
  postanoxic, delayed, 47
  postimmunization, altered states of conscious-
      ness and, 57–58
  progressive, after age two, 119
    before age two, 119t
    childhood, 138–144, *139*
      adrenoleukodystrophy and, 143
      aspartylglycosaminuria and, 140
      Bielschowsky-Jansky ceroid lipofuscinosis
          and, 141–142
      cerebrotendinous xanthomatosis and, 143–
          144
      ceroid lipofuscinosis and, 141
      glucosylceramide lipidosis and, 140
      glycoprotein degradation disorders and,
          140
      gray matter genetic disorders and, 141–
          143
      Hunter syndrome and, 139
      Huntington disease and, 142
      infection and, 144
      juvenile type ceroid lipofuscinosis and, 142
      late infantile ceroid lipofuscinosis and,
          141–142
      late-onset globoid leukodystrophy and,
          140–141
      lysosomal enzyme disorders and, 139–141
      mannosidosis II and, 140
      mitochondrial encephalomyopathy and,
          142–143
      mucopolysaccharidoses and, 138–140
      mucopolysaccharidosis II and, 139
      mucopolysaccharidosis VII and, 139
      progressive rubella panencephalitis and,
          144
      Sly disease and, 139
      sphingomyelin lipidosis and, 140
      Spielmeyer-Vogt-Sjögren disease and, 142
      subacute sclerosing panencephalitis and,
          144
      type C Niemann-Pick disease and, 140
      white matter disease and, 143–144
      xeroderma pigmentosum and, 141
    Gaucher disease III and, 140
    infantile, 123–138
      Alexander disease and, 137
      aminoacidurias and, 124–127, *125*, 125t,
          126
      Chédiak-Higashi syndrome and, 136
      evaluation of, *124*

Encephalopathy *(Continued)*
  progressive, infantile, fucosidosis I and, 129
      fucosidosis II and, 129
      galactosemia and, 134–135
      Gaucher disease II and, 130–131
      globoid cell leukodystrophy and, 131
      glucosylceramide lipidosis and, 130–131
      GM_1 gangliosidosis I and, 132
      GM_1 gangliosidosis II and, 132
      gray matter disorders and, 136–137
      homocystinuria and, *126*, 126–127
      Hurler syndrome and, 128, 128t
      I-cell disease and, 128–129, *129*
      kinky hair disease and, 134
      Krabbe disease and, 131
      Leigh disease and, 133
      Lesch-Nyhan disease and, 135
      lysosomal enzymes and, 127–133, 128t,
          129, *130*, 130t
      Menkes syndrome and, 134
      metachromatic leukodystrophy and, 131–
          132
      mild maple syrup urine disease and, *126*,
          127
      mitochondrial enzyme disorders and, 133–
          134
      mucolipidosis type II and, 128–129, *129*
      mucolipidosis type IV and, 129
      neurocutaneous syndromes and, 135–136
      neurofibromatosis and, 135–136
      neuronal ceroid lipofuscinosis and, 137
      Niemann-Pick disease and, 130
      Pelizaeus-Merzbacher disease and, 137–
          138
      phenylketonuria and, *125*, 125t, 125–126
      pyruvate metabolism disorders and, 133–
          134
      Sandhoff disease and, 132–133
      Santavuori disease and, 137
      sialidosis II and, 129–130, 130t
      spongy degeneration of infancy and, 138
      sulfatide lipidosis and, 131–132
      Tay-Sachs disease and, 132
      tuberous sclerosis and, 135
      type I mucopolysaccharidosis and, 128,
          128t
      white matter genetic disorders and, 137–
          138
    Rett syndrome and , 136–137
    renal disorders and, 59–60
    toxic, 63–67
    uremic, acute, 59
      chronic, 59
      EEG in, *45*
Enterovirus, infection with, generalized weakness
      and, 192–193
Enzymes, mitochondrial, disorders of, progressive
      encephalopathy and, 133–134
Ependymoma, chronic ataxia and, 237
    increased intracranial pressure and, 99
    spinal paraplegia and, 268–269
Epilepsia partialis continua, 32
    idiopathic cerebral artery infarction and, 251
Epilepsy. See also *Seizure(s)*.
    absence, EEG pattern of, 27
      in children, 26–27, *27*
      vs. myoclonic absence, 28
    acute hemiplegia and, 258–259
    benign, 16, 30, *31*

Epilepsy *(Continued)*
  childhood risk of, 19
  continual, 32
  febrile seizures and, 19
  headache and, 86
  hypoxic-ischemic encephalopathy and, 7, 9
  in children, 25–26
  migraine and, 25–26
  myoclonic, absence type of, 28
    benign, in infants, 22
    juvenile, 28–29
    progressive, 29t, 29–30
    severe, in infants, 22
    vs. febrile seizures, 22
  myoclonic-astatic, 23
  posttraumatic, 69–70
  pseudoataxia and, 234
  rolandic, 30. *31*
  status, treatment of, 38–39
  vertigo and, 354
Ergotamine, for migraine, 79
Erythrocyte, acanthocyte transformation of, in
    abetalipoproteinemia, 243
Escherichia coli, in newborn meningitis, 107
Esotrophia, 302–303
  accommodative, 302
  early-onset, 303
Estrogen, migraine and, 76
Ethosuximide, for seizures, 36
Ethylene glycol, poisoning with, facial weakness
    and, 345
Exercise, benign headache and, 82
  migraine and, 75
Exercise intolerance, 199. See also *Muscle(s), de-
    creased energy of.*
  evaluation of, *206*
Exotrophia, 303
Eye(s), esotrophia of, 302–303
  examination of, in delirium, 43
  exotrophia of, 303
  extraocular muscles of, 303t
    fibrosis of, 304
  motility of, assessment of, in coma, 46
    disorders of, 302–320
  rolling of, EEG seizure monitoring and, *3*
  straining of, headache and, 84
  tonic lateral deviation of, 46
  trauma to, unilateral ophthalmoplegia and, 311
  venous pulsations of, intracranial pressure and,
    92
Eyestrain, headache and, 84

Face, movement of, 337
Facial muscles, aplasia of, facial weakness and,
    339–340
Facial nerve, birth injury to, 340
  motor unit disorders of, 338–339
Facial palsy, recurrent, 343
Facial weakness, 337–346
  Albers-Schönberg disease and, 345
  autoimmune disorders and, 341–342
  Bell palsy and, 341
  birth injury and, 340
  causes of, 338t
  chlorocresol and, 345
  congenital, 339–340
    causes of, 338t

Facial weakness *(Continued)*
  congenital, depressor anguli oris muscle aplasia
      and, 340
    facial muscle aplasia and, 339–340
    Moebius syndrome and, 339–340
  diagnostic approach to, 337–338, 338t
  ethylene glycol and, 345
  facioscapulohumeral dystrophy and, 342
  familial dysautonomia and, 338
  genetic disorders and, 342–343
  Guillain-Barré syndrome and, 341–342
  herpes zoster oticus and, 344
  hyperparathyroidism and, 345
  hypertension and, 343
  hypothyroidism and, 345
  idiopathic cranial polyneuropathy and, 341–
      342
  infection and, 343
  juvenile progressive bulbar palsy and, 344–345
  Melkersson syndrome and, 343
  metabolic disorders and, 345
  motor unit disorders and, 338–339
  oculopharyngeal muscular dystrophy and, 342–
      343
  osteopetrosis and, 345
  postinfectious disorders and, 341–342
  pseudobulbar palsy and, 338
  Ramsay Hunt syndrome and, 344
  recurrent facial palsy and, 343
  sarcoidosis and, 344
  syringobulbia and, 345
  toxins and, 345
  trauma and, 345
  tumors and, 346
Facioscapulohumeral dystrophy, facial weakness
    and, 342
Facioscapulohumeral syndrome, infantile form of,
    179
  proximal limb weakness and, 178–179
Fahr syndrome, chorea and, 288
Fainting, 17–18, 23–24
Falling, frequent, 170
Falx herniation, increased intracranial pressure
    and, 93
Familial dysautonomia, cerebral hypotonia and,
    153
Familial paroxysmal choreoathetosis, 25
Fasciculation, 200t
Fasciitis, necrotizing, acute hemiplegia and, 253
Fazio-Londe disease, 344–345
Feeding, newborn difficulty in, 151t
Fever, vascular headache and, 81
Fibrillation, 200t
Fibromuscular dysplasia, acute hemiplegia and,
    253
Fibrosis, of extraocular muscles, 304
Fingers, dysesthesias of, foramen magnum tumors
    and, 221
Fisting, infantile hypotonia and, 150
Fistula, of cavernous sinus, unilateral ophthalmo-
    plegia and, 311
Fixation and following, in visual acuity assess-
    ment, 321
Flutter, ocular, 316, 316t
Fontanelle, anterior, tension of, intracranial pres-
    sure and, 91
Food additives, vascular headache and, 81–82
Foot (feet), sensory loss in, hereditary sensory and
    autonomic neuropathy I and, 215

Foot (feet) *(Continued)*
    ulcers of, hereditary sensory and autonomic
        neuropathy I and, 215
Footdrop, 170
Foramen magnum, tumors of, sensory disturbance
    and, 220–221
Forearm ischemic exercise test, 206t
Fractures, skull, 69
    spinal, paraplegia and, 274–275, *275*
Fragile-X syndrome, 121
Friedreich ataxia, 240–241
Fucosidosis, type I, progressive encephalopathy
    and, 129
    type II, progressive encephalopathy and, 129
Furosemide, for posthemorrhagic hydrocephalus,
    104

Gait, abnormal, 170
    disturbance of. See *Ataxia.*
    steppage, 170, 223
Galactosemia, progressive encephalopathy and,
    134–135
Gangliosidosis, GM_1, progressive encephalopathy
    and, 132
    GM_2, chronic ataxia and, 244
        progressive encephalopathy and, 132
        proximal limb weakness and, 174
Gaucher cell, 131
Gaucher disease, type II, progressive encephalop-
    athy and, 130–131
    type III, progressive encephalopathy and, 140
Gaze palsy, 313t, 313–315
    horizontal, 315
    ocular motor apraxia and, 313–314
    vertical, 314–315
        congenital vertical ocular motor apraxia and,
        315
        DAF syndrome and, 315
Gentamicin, vertigo and, 354
Germinoma, 100
Giant axonal neuropathy, 189
Gigantism, megalencephaly with, 368
Glasgow coma scale, 68t
Glioma, brainstem, progressive facial diplegia and,
    342
        unilateral ophthalmoplegia and, *309*, 309–
        310
    complex partial seizures and, 28
    hypothalamic, progressive vision loss and, 331–
        332
    increased intracranial pressure and, 97–98, *98*
    optic, progressive vision loss and, 331–332,
        332
Globoid cell leukodystrophy, distal limb weakness
    and, 187
Globus pallidus, atrophy of, 240
Glucose, metabolism of, muscle activity and, 204,
    204
Glucosylceramide lipidosis, progressive encepha-
    lopathy and, 140
β-Glucuronidase, deficiency of, 139
Glutamic decarboxylase, impaired activity of, neo-
    natal seizures and, 15
Glycine encephalopathy, neonatal seizures and,
    11
Glycoprotein, degradation disorders of, progres-
    sive encephalopathy and, 140

Gower sign, *171*
Gradenigo syndrome, unilateral ophthalmoplegia
    and, 308–309
Gray matter, genetic disorders of, progressive en-
    cephalopathy and, 141–143
    idiopathic disorders of, progressive encephalop-
    athy and, 136–137
Great vein of Galen, malformation of, increased
    intracranial pressure and, 106
    noncommunicating hydrocephalus and, 365–
    366
Growing pains, 199
Guillain-Barré syndrome, abortive form of, 341–
    342
    CSF in, 193
    distal limb weakness and, 189t, 189–190
    generalized weakness and, 193

Habit spasm, 297–299
Hallervorden-Spatz disease, chorea and, 288–289
Hallucination, definition of, 43
    hypnagogic, 24–25
Haloperidol, overdose of, 66
Hands, weakness in. See *Limb weakness.*
Hartnup disease, acute ataxia and, 232–233
    chronic ataxia and, 245
Head, abnormal shape of, *373*, 373–375, 374t
    acrocephalosyndactyly and, 375
    craniostenosis and, 373–374
    Crouzon disease and, 374–375
    extracranial forces and, 373–374
    intracranial forces and, 373
    circumference of, in newborn, 91
    measurement of, 359
    normal growth of, *360*
    decreased size of. See *Microcephaly.*
    elevation of, for increased intracranial pressure,
    94–95
    increased size of. See *Macrocephaly.*
    injury to, closed, altered states of consciousness
    and, 68t, 68–69, *69*
    convergence palsy and, 315
    headache and, 83
    migraine and, 75
    mild, altered states of consciousness and, 67
    open, altered states of consciousness and, 69
    severe, altered states of consciousness and,
    67–70
    trauma to, 5
    facial weakness and, 345
    intracranial hemorrhage and, 101–102
    seizures and, 9
    vertigo and, 356–357
Headache, 73–88. See also *Migraine.*
    approach to, 73–75, 74t
    benign, exercise and, 82
    cluster, 77–78
        lithium carbonate for, 80
        methysergide maleate for, 80
        prednisone for, 80
        treatment of, 80
    connective tissue disorders and, 83
    diagnostic features of, 74, 74t
    dialysis and, 82
    encephalitis and, 83
    evaluation of, 75
    exertional, benign, 82

Headache (Continued)
eyestrain and, 84
hemispheric astrocytoma and, 97
hypersensitivity vasculitis and, 83
in cryptococcal meningitis, 113
intracranial pressure increase and, 91–92
mixed connective tissue disease and, 83
pain of, descriptions of, 74t, 74–75
psychogenic, 85–86
seizure, 86–87
sinusitis and, 84
sources of, 73t, 73–74
supratentorial malformation and, 106–107
systemic lupus erythematosus and, 83
tension, 83–84
chronic, 85–86
TMJ syndrome and, 84–85
vascular, nonmigrainous, 80t, 80–83
vasculitis and, 83
vasodilative, 80t, 80–83
alcohol and, 81
caffeine withdrawal and, 81
drugs and, 81
fever and, 81
food additives and, 81–82
hypertension and, 82
marijuana and, 81
orgasmic, 82
posttraumatic, 82–83
whiplash injury and, 84
Hearing, anatomic considerations in, 346
impairment of, 346–352. See also Deafness.
acquired, 350–352, 351t
acoustic neuroma and, 352, 352
drugs and, 350
genetic neurologic disorders and, 350
infectious diseases and, 350–351
metabolic disorders and, 350–351
pontobulbar palsy and, 350
skeletal disorders and, 351, 351t
trauma and, 351
tumor and, 352
assessment of, 347
brainstem auditory evoked response in, 347–
348, 348, 348t
central, 346
conductive, 346
diplacusis in, 347
hyperacusis and, 346–347
pure tone audiometry in, 347
recruitment in, 347
retinitis pigmentosa and, 350
Rinne test in, 347
sensorineural, 346
speech tests in, 347
symptoms of, 346–347
tests of, 347–349
tinnitus and, 346
Weber test in, 347
Hearing loss, language delay and, 119–120
Heart disease, congenital, acute hemiplegia and, 253–254
rheumatic, acute hemiplegia and, 254
Heart rate, apnea and, 4
Hemangioblastoma, cerebellar, chronic ataxia and, 237–238
Hematoma, epidural, 68–69, 69
spinal, paraplegia and, 275
subdural, 68–69

Hemiconvulsions-hemiplegia syndrome, 258
Hemidystonia, 294
Hemifacial spasm, 295–296
Hemiparesis, transitory, seizures and, 258
Hemiplegia, 248–262
acute, 248–260
absence status and, 258–259
arterial abscess and, 253–254
arterial embolism and, 253–254
arteriovenous malformations and, 257
L-asparaginase-induced thrombosis and, 256
cancer and, 256–257
carotid artery infection and, 252–253
carotid artery trauma and, 252
cerebral abscess and, 253–254
cerebrovascular disease and, 248–257
cervical infections and, 252–253
congenital heart disease and, 253–254
diabetes mellitus and, 259–260
differential diagnosis of, 248t
disseminated intravascular coagulation and, 256
epilepsy and, 258–259
fibromuscular dysplasia and, 253
hemiconvulsions and, 258
hemiparetic seizures and, 258
Henoch-Schönlein purpura, 255–256
hypersensitivity vasculitis and, 255–256
idiopathic capsular stroke and, 250–251
idiopathic cerebral artery infarction and, 251
infections and, 260
intracerebral hemorrhage and, 257
lipoprotein disorders and, 256
metastatic neuroblastoma and, 257
methotrexate-induced infarction and, 256–257
migraine and, 259
mitochondrial encephalopathy, lactic acidosis, and stroke-like syndrome and, 256
mitral valve prolapse and, 254
moyamoya disease and, 251–252
neck trauma and, 252
neonatal hemorrhage and, 257
neonatal infarction and, 249, 249t, 249–250
rheumatic heart disease and, 254
sickle cell anemia and, 254, 254–255
systemic lupus erythematosus and, 255
Takayasu arteritis and, 255
trauma and, 260
tumors and, 260
venous sinus thrombosis and, 253
venous thrombosis and, 257
vertebral artery trauma and, 252
chronic, 260
double, 277
progressive, chronic, 260, 260t
Hemolytic disease, neonatal, kernicterus with, 15
Hemorrhage, cerebellar, acute ataxia and, 233
intracerebral, acute hemiplegia and, 257
differential diagnosis of, 250t
focal clonic seizure and, 2
head injury and, 69
intracranial, increased intracranial pressure and, 101–107, 102
neonatal, 9
intraventricular, grades of, 103t
hydrocephalus and, 103
of newborn, 102, 102–105, 103t
of prematures, 103t, 103–104

Hemorrhage *(Continued)*
  intraventricular, of term infants, 104–105
    pathophysiology of, *102*
    phenobarbital and, 104
    vitamin E for, 104
  neonatal, acute hemiplegia and, 257
  subarachnoid, arterial aneurysm and, 105
    neonatal seizures and, 9
  subdural, neonatal seizures and, 9
Henoch-Schönlein purpura, acute hemiplegia and, 255–256
Heparin, maternal use of, embryopathy with, 349
Hepatolenticular degeneration, chorea and, 293–294
Hereditary motor sensory neuropathy, distal limb weakness and, 185–186
  type I, 185
  type II, 185–186
  type III, 186
  type IV, 186
Hereditary recurrent pressure palsy, monoplegia and, 284–285
Hereditary sensory and autonomic neuropathy, type I, 214–215
  type II, 215–216
  type III, 216
  type IV, 216–217
  with spastic paraplegia, 217
Hereditary sensory neuropathy, X-linked, 217
Hereditary sensory radiculoneuropathy, 214–215
Herniation, cerebellar, increased intracranial pressure and, 93t, 94
  falx, increased intracranial pressure and, 93
  of lumbar disk, sensory disturbance and, 219
  transtentorial, bilateral, increased intracranial pressure and, 93t, 94
    unilateral, increased intracranial pressure and, 93t, 93–94
Herniation syndromes, increased intracranial pressure and, 93t, 93–94
Heroin, neonatal withdrawal from, 14
Herpes simplex encephalitis, 49–50
  EEG in, 50, *51*
  neonatal seizures and, 13–14
Herpes zoster oticus, facial weakness and, 344
Heterophoria, 302
Heterotopia, 372
Hexosaminidase A, deficiency of, proximal limb weakness and, 174
Histidinemia, language delay and, 120
Histiocytosis, sea-blue, chronic ataxia and, 244–245
  DAF syndrome variant of, 315
Histoplasmosis, 115
Holoprosencephaly, hydranencephaly and, 367
  primary microcephaly and, 371
Homocystinuria, metabolic disturbance of, *126*
  progressive encephalopathy in, *126*, 126–127
Hopkins syndrome, 281
Horizontal suspension, infantile hypotension and, 149
Horn cell, anterior, degeneration of, incontinentia pigmentia and, 158
  infection of, 281
Horner syndrome, 335
Humerus, proximal, osteomyelitis of, monoplegia and, 280–281
Hunter syndrome, progressive encephalopathy and, 139

Huntington disease, progressive encephalopathy and, 142
Hurler syndrome, progressive encephalopathy and, 128, 128t
Hydranencephaly, holoprosencephaly and, 367
  porencephaly and, 367
Hydrocephalus, causes of, 360t
  communicating, achondroplasia and, 361
    benign subarachnoid space enlargement and, 361–362, *362*
    macrocephaly and, 361–363, *362, 363*
    meningeal malignancy and, 362–363, *363*
    tuberculous meningitis and, 110
  increased intracranial pressure and, 96
  intraventricular hemorrhage and, 103
  myelomeningocele and, 265
  noncommunicating, aqueductal stenosis and, 363–364, *364*
    congenital brain tumor and, 365
    Dandy-Walker malformation and, *364*, 364–365
    Klippel-Feil syndrome and, 365
    vein of Galen malformation and, 365–366
    Warburg syndrome and, 366–367
  posthemorrhagic, acetazolamide for, 104
    external ventricular drainage for, 104
    serial lumbar puncture in, 104
  progressive, infantile, 138
Hyperactivity, phenobarbital and, 37
Hyperacusis, 346–347
Hyperammonemia, encephalopathy and, 63
  neonatal seizures and, *12*, 12–13, 13t
Hypercalcemia, altered states of consciousness and, 63
  uremic encephalopathy and, 59
Hyperglycemia, altered states of consciousness and, 61–62
Hyperglycinemia, ketotic, neonatal seizures and, 11–12
Hypernatremia, altered states of consciousness and, 61
Hyperparathyroidism, altered states of consciousness and, 63
  facial weakness and, 345
  uremic encephalopathy and, 59
Hyperphenylalaninemia, differential diagnosis of, 125t
Hypersensitivity vasculitis, acute hemiplegia and, 255–256
  headache and, 83
Hypertension, encephalopathy and, 59–60, 70
  facial weakness and, 343
  headache and, 82
  intracranial, benign, 115t, 115–116
Hyperthermia, malignant, muscle stiffness and, 209–210
Hyperthyroidism, altered states of consciousness and, 63
  chorea and, 290
Hyperventilation, for increased intracranial pressure, 95
Hyperventilation syndrome, in children, 24
Hypoadrenalism, abnormal muscle activity and, 204
Hypobetalipoproteinemia, chronic ataxia and, 243–244
Hypocalcemia, abnormal muscle activity and, 203–204
  neonatal, seizures and, 10

Hypodipsia-hyponatremia syndrome, 331
Hypoglycemia, acute blindness and, 328
  altered states of consciousness and, 62–63
  neonatal, causes of, 10t
    seizures and, 9–10, 10t
Hypomagnesemia, encephalopathy and, 63
Hypomelanosis of Ito, megalencephaly and, 368
Hyponatremia, altered states of consciousness
    and, 62
Hypoparathyroidism, proximal limb weakness
    and, 183
Hypoplasia, cerebellar, chronic ataxia and, 238
Hypotension, infantile, horizontal suspension in,
    149
  vertical suspension in, 149
Hypothalamus, glioma of, progressive vision loss
    and, 331–332, *332*
Hypothermia, for increased intracranial pressure,
    95
Hypothyroidism, acquired, altered states of con-
    sciousness and, 63
  congenital, progressive encephalopathy and,
    124
  facial weakness and, 345
  hearing impairment and, 351
Hypotonia, appearance of, 147–148, *148*
  cerebral, 147
    diagnosis of, clues to, 149–150
    differential diagnosis of, 148t
    spinal cord injury and, 154–155
    with motor unit disorder, 149t
  congenital, benign, 153–154
  infantile, 147–169
    breech presentation injuries and, 154
    cerebral, 150–155, 151t
      benign, 153
      cerebrohepatorenal syndrome and, 152
      chromosome disorders and, 150–151
      chronic nonprogressive encephalopathy
        and, 151
      Cohen syndrome and, 153
      familial dysautonomia and, 153
      Lowe syndrome and, 153
      neonatal adrenoleukodystrophy and, 152
      oculocerebrorenal syndrome and, 153
      peroxisomal disorders and, 152
      Prader-Willi syndrome and, 151, 151t
    cervical presentation and, 154–155
    diagnostic approach to, 149t, 149–150
    fisting and, 150
    motor unit disorders and, 155–168
      leukodystrophy and, 186
    motor unit disorders with. See also *Motor
      unit, disorders of.*
      acid maltase deficiency and, 166
      botulism and, 160
      carnitine deficiency and, 167
      central core disease and, 163–164
      centronuclear myopathy and, 162–163
      cerebro-ocular dysplasia and, 165
      chronic inflammatory demyelinating poly-
        neuropathy in, 159
      congenital fiber type disproportion myopa-
        thy and, 162
      congenital hypomyelinating neuropathy in,
        159
      creatine kinase in, 155
      cytochrome-*c*-oxidase deficiency and, 166–
        167

Hypotonia *(Continued)*
  infantile, motor unit disorders with, electrodi-
      agnosis in, 155
    familial infantile myasthenia and, 161
    fiber type disproportion myopathies and,
        161–164, *162*, *163*
    juvenile myasthenia and, 160
    metabolic myopathy and, 166–168
    muscle biopsy in, 156
    muscular dystrophies and, *164*, 164–166
    myotonic dystrophy and, 165–166
    myotubular myopathy and, 162–163
    nemaline myopathy and, 163, *163*
    nerve biopsy in, 156
    neuromuscular transmission disorders in,
        160–161
    neuronal degeneration and, 158
    phosphofructokinase deficiency and, 167
    phosphorylase deficiency and, 167–168
    polyneuropathy in, 158–159, 159t
    Pompe disease and, 166
    rod myopathy and, 163, *163*
    spinal muscular atrophy and, 156–158,
        157
    Tensilon test in, 156
    transitory neonatal myasthenia and, 161
  myositis and, 168
  neurogenic arthrogryposis and, 158
  postural reflexes in, 150
  scissoring and, 150
  traction response in, 148–149, *149*
  plagiocephaly and, 373
Hypoxanthine guanine-phosphoribosyltransferase,
    deficiency of, 135
Hypoxia, 46–48
  high altitude and, 47
  prolonged, 46–47
Hypoxic-ischemic encephalopathy, neonatal, 6–9,
    8, 8t
Hypsarrhythmia, in infantile spasms, 21
Hysteria, acute blindness and, 329–330

I-cell disease, progressive encephalopathy and,
    128–129, *129*
Idiopathic nerve palsy, ophthalmoplegia and, 306
α-L-Iduronidase, deficiency of, 128
Immunization, encephalopathy with, 57–58
Incontinentia pigmenti, anterior horn cell degener-
    ation and, 158
  infantile seizures and, 20t
  neonatal seizures and, 15–16
Incontinentia pigmenti achromians, 368
Infantile bilateral striatal necrosis, chorea and, 288
Infarction, cerebral, evaluation of, 249t
    focal clonic seizure and, 2
    hemiplegia and, *249*, 249t, 249–250
  cerebral artery, idiopathic, acute hemiplegia
    and, 251
  neonatal, acute hemiplegia and, *249*, 249t,
    249–250
Infection, acute hemiplegia and, 260
  altered states of consciousness and, 48–55
  bacterial, vertigo and, 354–355
  enterovirus, generalized weakness and, 192–
    193
  facial weakness and, 343

Infection (Continued)
  fungal, increased intracranial pressure and, 112t, 112–115, 113t
  increased intracranial pressure and, 107t, 107–115, 108t, 109t, *111*
  intrauterine, developmental delay and, 122–123
    secondary microcephaly and, 372–373
  progressive encephalopathy and, 144
  viral, nerve palsy with, ophthalmoplegia and, 306
  vertigo and, 353
Internuclear ophthalmoplegia, 314
Intracranial pressure, increased, 89–117
  anterior fontanelle tension and, 91
  arterial aneurysms and, 105
  arteriovenous malformations and, 105–107
  bacterial meningitis and, 107t, 107–112, 108t, 109t, *111*
  benign intracranial hypertension and, 115t, 115–116
  bilateral transtentorial herniation and, 93t, 94
  brain abscess and, *111*, 111–112
  brain tumor and, 96–101, 97t
  candidal meningoencephalitis and, 114–115
  cerebellar herniation and, 93t, 94
  cerebral blood flow and, 90
  cerebral edema and, 90
  cerebrospinal fluid and, 89–90
  choroid plexus papilloma and, 100–101
  coccidioidomycosis and, 113–114
  diplopia and, 92
  ependymoma and, 99
  epidural empyema and, 112
  falx herniation and, 93
  fungal infections and, 112t, 112–115, 113t
  head circumference and, 91
  head elevation for, 94–95
  headache and, 91–92
  hemispheric astrocytomas and, 97–88, *98*
  herniation syndromes and, 93t, 93–94
  hydrocephalus and, 96
  hyperventilation for, 95
  hypothermia for, 95
  in children, 91–93, *92*, 92t, *93*, 93t
  in infant, 91
  infectious disorders and, 107t, 107–115, 108t, 109t, *111*
  intracranial arachnoid cysts and, 101
  intracranial hemorrhage and, 101–107, *102*
  intraventricular hemorrhage and, *102*, 102–105, 103t
  mass lesions and, 90
  medical treatment for, 94–96, 95t, *96*
  midline malformations and, 106
  osmotic diuretics for, 95
  papilledema and, 92
  pathophysiology of, 89–90
  pentobarbital coma for, 95–96, *96*
  pineal region tumors and, 100
  presenting features of, 89t
  primitive neuroectodermal tumor and, 99–100
  pseudotumor cerebri and, 115t, 115–116
  strabismus and, 92
  subdural empyema and, 112
  symptoms of, 90–94, *92*, 92t, *93*, 93t
  tuberculous meningitis and, 110

Intracranial pressure (Continued)
  increased, unilateral transtentorial herniation and, 93t, 93–94
  monitoring of, 94
Intrauterine infection, developmental delay and, 122–123
Intraventricular hemorrhage. See Hemorrhage, intraventricular.
Iris, hypoplasia of, 335
Isaacs syndrome, abnormal muscle activity and, 202
  hereditary form of, 202
Ischemia, 46–48
Ischemic exercise test, *205*, 205–206, *206*, 206t
Isometheptene, for migraine, 79
Isoniazid, neuropathy with, 188
Isovaleric acidemia, neonatal seizures and, 11, *11*
Isovaleryl-CoA dehyrogenase, *11*
Ito, hypomelanosis of, megalencephaly and, 368

Janz syndrome, 28–29
Japanese B encephalitis, 53
Jerk nystagmus, 317
Jitteriness, in newborn, 1, 5
Joubert syndrome, 238

Kawasaki disease, acute ataxia and, 234
Kayser-Fleischer ring, in Wilson disease, 293
Kernicterus, neonatal, seizures and, 15
Kernig sign, in bacterial meningitis, 109
Ketoacid dehydrogenase, *11*
  deficiency of, 127
Ketoacidosis, diabetic, 61–62
  cerebral edema and, 61
Kidney failure, encephalopathy with, 59–60
Kinky hair disease, progressive encephalopathy and, 134
Klippel-Feil syndrome, noncommunicating hydrocephalus and, 365
  paraplegia and, 268
Klonopin. See Clonazepam.
Krabbe disease, distal limb weakness and, 187
  progressive encephalopathy and, 131, 140–141
Kveim skin test, 344

Labyrinthitis, 355
Lactate, resting level of, myopathy and, 205
Lactate dehydrogenase, deficiency of, muscle abnormalities and, 207
Lafora disease, 29
Lance-Adams syndrome, 297
Landau-Kleffner syndrome, 31–32
Language delay, 118–120
  hearing loss and, 119–120
  histadinemia and, 120
  in infantile autism, 120
Lateral rectus palsy, transient, 311
Laughter, paroxysmal, in newborn, 2
Laurence-Moon-Biedl syndrome, progressive vision loss and, 334
Leber congenital amaurosis, congenital blindness and, 324

Leber optic neuropathy, progressive vision loss
and, 330
Legs, weakness in. See *Limb weakness.*
Leigh disease, progressive encephalopathy and,
133
Lennox-Gastaut syndrome, 23
Lens, abnormalities of, 323t
Lesch-Nyhan disease, progressive encephalopathy
and, 135
Lethargy, 42t
causes of, 44t
diagnostic approach to, 44, 46
patient history in, 44
physical examination in, 44, 46
Leukodystrophy, globoid, distal limb weakness
and, 187
late-onset, progressive encephalopathy and,
140
progressive encephalopathy and, 131
infantile hypotonia and, 165
metachromatic, distal limb weakness and, 186–
187
progressive encephalopathy and, 131–132,
141
Leukokoria, retinoblastoma and, 333
Leukomalacia, periventricular, intraventricular
hemorrhage and, 102
Limb weakness, distal, 183–192, 184t, 189t
causes of, 184t
Charcot-Marie-Tooth disease and, 185–186
Cockayne's syndrome and, 187
Déjérine-Sottas disease and, 186
diagnosis of, 183–184
drug effects and, 188
Emery-Dreifuss muscular dystrophy and,
191–192
globoid cell leukodystrophy and, 187
hereditary amyloid neuropathy and, 187
hereditary distal myopathy and, 191
hereditary motor sensory neuropathy and,
185–186
idiopathic, 189–190
isoniazid and, 188
Krabbe disease and, 187
metachromatic leukodystrophy and, 186–
187
myopathies and, 190–191
myotonic dystrophy and, 190–191
nitrofurantoin and, 188
pyruvate metabolism disorders and, 187
Refsum's disease and, 186
scapulo(humeral)peroneal syndromes and,
191–192
scapulohumeral syndrome and, 192
spinal muscular atrophy and, 191–192
causes of, 184–185
sulfatide lipidosis and, 186–187
systemic vasculitis and, 189
toxins and, 188
uremia and, 188–189
vasculopathy and, 189
vincristine and, 188
generalized, acute, 192–196
acute intermittent porphyria and, 196
botulism and, 194
enterovirus infections and, 192–193
familial hyperkalemic periodic paralysis
and, 195–196
familial hypokalemic periodic paralysis and,
195

Limb weakness *(Continued)*
generalized, acute, familial normokalemic periodic paralysis and, 196
Guillain-Barré syndrome and, 193
infectious disease and, 192–193
infectious myositis and, 194
myasthenia gravis and, 194
neuromuscular blockade and, 194
periodic paralysis and, 195–196
tick paralysis and, 194
lumbar plexitis and, 280
physical findings in, *171,* 171t, 171–172
presenting complaint of, 170–171, 171t
proximal, 172–183
Becker muscular dystrophy and, 175–178
clinical features of, 172t
debrancher enzyme deficiency and, 182
dermatomyositis and, 179–180, *180*
Duchenne muscular dystrophy and, 175–
178, *176, 177*
endocrine myopathies and, 183
facioscapulohumeral syndrome and, 178–
179
GM$_2$ gangliosidosis and, 174–175
inflammatory myopathies and, 179t, 179–
181, *180*
juvenile acid maltase deficiency and, 181–
182
limb-girdle muscular dystrophy and, 178, *178*
limb-girdle myasthenia and, 174–175
McArdle disease and, 182
metabolic myopathies and, 181–183
mitochondrial fatty acid oxidation disturbance
and, 182
mitochondrial myopathy and, 182–183, *183*
muscle carnitine deficiency and, 182
muscular dystrophies and, 175–178, *176,*
177
polymyositis and, 181
spinal muscular atrophies and, 172–175
signs of, 170–171, *171,* 171t
symptoms of, 170–172, *171,* 171t
Limb-girdle muscular dystrophy, vs. Becker muscular dystrophy, 178
Limb-girdle myasthenia, proximal limb weakness
and, 174–175
Linear nevus sebaceous syndrome, infantile seizures and, 20t
megalencephaly and, 368–369
Lipid(s), metabolic disorder of, progressive vision
loss and, 333
muscle storage of, proximal limb weakness and,
182
utilization of, defects of, decreased muscle energy and, 207–208
Lipidosis, glucosylceramide, progressive encephalopathy and, 130–131, 140
sphingomyelin, progressive encephalopathy
and, 140
sulfatide, distal limb weakness and, 186–187
juvenile, chronic ataxia and, 244
progressive encephalopathy and, 141
progressive encephalopathy and, 131–132
Lipofuscinosis, ceroid, juvenile type, progressive
encephalopathy and, 142
late infantile type of, progressive encephalopathy and, 141–142
neuronal, progressive encephalopathy and,
137
progressive encephalopathy and, 141

Lipoprotein, disorders of, acute hemiplegia and, 256
Lissencephaly, 372
Lithium carbonate, for cluster headache, 80
Liver failure, encephalopathy and, 60–61
Lobectomy, temporal, for complex partial seizures, 28
Locked-in syndrome, 42
Lowe syndrome, cerebral hypotonia and, 153
Lumbar disk, herniation of, sensory disturbance and, 219
Lumbar plexus, postnatal injury to, monoplegia and, 283
Lumbar puncture, in arterial aneurysm, 105
  in bacterial meningitis, 109
  serial, in intraventricular hemorrhage, 104
Lupus erythematosus, acute ataxia and, 233–234
  systemic, acute hemiplegia and, 255
    chorea and, 290
Lyme disease, 49
Lysosomal enzymes, disorders of, progressive childhood encephalopathy and, 139–141
    progressive encephalopathy and, 127–133, 128t, *129*, *130*, 130t

Machado-Joseph disease, chronic ataxia and, 240
Macrocephaly, 359–369, 360t
  achondroplasia and, 361
  anatomic megalencephaly and, 367–369
  aqueductal stenosis and, 363–364, *364*
  communicating hydrocephalus and, 361–363, *362*, *363*
  congenital brain tumors and, 365
  Dandy-Walker malformation and, *364*, 364–365
  genetic megalencephaly and, 367
  holoprosencephaly and, 367
  hydranencephaly and, 367
  hypomelanosis of Ito and, 368
  Klippel-Feil sydnrome and, 365
  linear nevus sebaceous syndrome and, 368–369
  megalencephaly and, gigantism with, 368
    neurologic disorders with, 367–368
  meningeal malignancy and, 362–363, *363*
  metabolic megalencephaly and, 369
  neurocutaneous disorders and, 368–369
  noncommunicating hydrocephalus and, 363–367, *364*, *366*
  porencephaly and, 367
  subarachnoid space enlargement and, 361–362, *362*
  vein of Galen malformation and, 365–366
  Warburg syndrome and, 366–367
Malignant hyperthermia, muscle stiffness and, 209–210
Mannosidosis, type II, progressive encephalopathy and, 140
Maple syrup urine disease, chronic ataxia and, 245
  intermittent, acute ataxia and, 232
  mild, progressive encephalopathy and, *126*, 127
  neonatal, seizures and, 10–11
Marijuana, abuse of, 66
  vascular headache and, 81
Marinesco-Sjögren syndrome, chronic ataxia and, 242–243

McArdle disease, muscle energy decrease and, 206–207
  proximal limb weakness and, 182
Measles, retinitis with, acute blindness and, 329
Measles encephalitis, 50–52
Medial longitudinal fasciculus, lesions of, ophthalmoplegia and, 314
Medulloblastoma, chronic ataxia and, *236*, 236–237
  noncommunicating hydrocephalus and, 365
Megalencephaly, 360t
  anatomic, 367–369
  genetic, 367
  gigantism and, 368
  hypomelanosis of Ito and, 368
  linear nevus sebaceous syndrome and, 368–369
  metabolic, 369
  neurocutaneous disorders and, 368–369
  neurologic disorder and, 367–368
Melkerrson syndrome, facial weakness and, 343
Meniere disease, hearing impairment and, 351
  vertigo and, 355–356
Meninges, malignancy of, communicating hydrocephalus and, 362–363, *363*
Meningismus, 49
Meningitis, aseptic, 49–55
  bacterial, 49
    cerebrospinal fluid analysis in, 108
    in children, 108–110, 109t
    in infant, 108–110, 109t
    in newborn, 107–108, 108t
    increased intracranial pressure and, 107t, 107–112, 108t, 109t, *111*
    lumbar puncture in, 109
    treatment of, in infants, 109, 109t
      in newborns, 108, 108t
  cryptococcal, increased intracranial pressure and, 112–113, 113t
  febrile seizures and, 19
  tuberculous, 110
Meningoencephalitis, candidal, increased intracranial pressure and, 114–115
Menkes syndrome, progressive encephalopathy and, 134
Menstrual cycle, migraine and, 76
Metabolism, inborn errors of, encephalopathy and, 58t, 58–59
  neonatal seizures and, 6, 6t
Metachromatic leukodystrophy, distal limb weakness and, 186–187
  progressive encephalopathy and, 131–132, 141
Methotrexate, infarction induced by, acute hemiplegia and, 256
Methsuximide, for seizures, 36
Methymalonyl-CoA mutase, *11*
Methymalonyl-CoA racemase, *11*
Methysergide maleate, for cluster headache, 80
Microcephaly, 369t, 369–373
  primary, 370–372
    anencephaly and, 370–371
    chromosome disorders and, 370
    corpus callosum agenesis and, 372
    defective cellular migration and, 372
    defective neurolation and, 370–371
    defective prosencephalization and, 371–372
    encephalocele and, 371
    holoprosencephaly and, 371
  secondary, 372–373
    intrauterine disorders and, 372

Microcephaly *(Continued)*
  secondary, perinatal brain injury and, 372
    postnatal systemic disease and, 373
    vascular aplasia and, 372
Microcephaly vera, 370
Midrin. See *Isometheptene.*
Migraine, 75–78, 76t
  acute ataxia and, 229–231, *230*
  acute hemiplegia and, 259
  Alice-in-Wonderland syndrome of, 77
  allergy and, 76
  altered states of consciousness and, 63–64
  aseptic meningitis and, 49
  basilar, acute ataxia and, 229–231, *230*
    EEG in, *230*
  calcium channel blocking agent prophylaxis for, 79
  cerebral, transient, migraine and, 75
  classic, 76–77
    visual aberrations in, 76–77
  clinical syndromes of, 76t, 76–78
  common, 77
  complicated, 77
  confusional, acute, 64
  cyproheptadine prophylaxis for, 80
  diagnosis of, 78
  diet and, 76
  electroencephalography for, 78
  epilepsy and, 25–26
  exercise and, 75
  head injury and, 75
  hemiplegic, familial, 64, 259
  in children, 25–26
  in infants, 23
  menstrual cycle and, 76
  ophthalmoplegic, 306
    vs. Tolosa-Hunt syndrome, 310
  prophylaxis for, 79
  propranolol prophylaxis for, 79
  retinal, acute blindness and, 326–327
  stress and, 75
  transient cerebral blindness and, 75
  transient posttraumatic cerebral blindness in, 328
  treatment of, 78–80, 79t
    chlorpromazine for, 79
    ergotamine for, 79
    isometheptene for, 79
  triggering factors in, 75–76
  vertigo and, 356
Migraine coma, 64
Miller Fisher syndrome, acute ataxia and, 226
  gaze palsy and, 314
Minocycline, vertigo and, 354
Mitochondrial disease, progressive vision loss and, 330
Mitochondrial encephalomyopathy, 142–143
Mitochondrial encephalopathy, lactic acidosis, and stroke-like syndrome, acute hemiplegia and, 256
Mitochondrial myopathy, decreased muscle energy and, 208–209, *209*
Mitral valve prolapse, acute hemiplegia and, 254
Mixed connective tissue disease, headache and, 83
Moebius syndrome, 304
  facial weakness and, 339–340
Mogadon. See *Nitrazepam.*
Monocular nystagmus, 319

Mononeuropathy, monoplegia and, 284–285
Monoplegia, 279–285
  acute, causes of, 280t
  acute idiopathic plexitis and, 279–280
  approach to, 279, 280t
  asthmatic amyotrophy and, 281
  brachial plexitis and, 279–280
  brachial plexus injury and, 283
  hereditary brachial plexopathy and, 281–282
  hereditary recurrent pressure palsy and, 284–285
  lumbar plexitis and, 280
  lumbar plexus injury and, 283
  mononeuropathies and, 284–285
  neonatal brachial neuropathy and, 282–283
  osteomyelitis-neuritis and, 280–281
  peroneal neuropathy and, 284
  plexopathies and, 279–284
  plexus tumors and, 283
  postnatal injuries and, 283
  radial neuropathy and, 284
  ulnar neuropathy and, 284
Monosodium glutamate (MSG), vascular headache and, 81–82
Monosomy, 12 p, 121t
  5 p, 121t
Morning glory disk, congenital blindness and, 324
Moro reflex, 132, 150
Morquio syndrome, paraplegia and, 268
Motion sickness, 356
Motor development, delayed, 120
Motor neuron, disorders of, 148t
Motor unit, 147
  continuous activity of, 200t, 200–202, 201t
  disorders of, cerebral hypotonia and, 149t
    creatine kinase and, 155
    diagnosis of, clues to, 150, 150t
    electrodiagnosis in, 155
    evaluation of, 155t, 155–156
    facial weakness and, 338–339
    infantile hypotonia and, 155–168
    muscle biopsy in, 156
    nerve biopsy in, 156
    perinatal respiratory distress and, 149t
Movement disorders, 286–301. See also *Chorea.*
  approach to, 286
  dystonia and, 291t, 291–295, 294t
  hemifacial spasm and, 295–296
  myoclonus and, 296–297
  tic syndromes and, 297–299
  tremor and, 299–300
Moyamoya disease, acute hemiplegia and, 251–252
MSG. See *Monosodium glutamate.*
Mucolipidosis, type II, progressive encephalopathy and, 128–129, *129*
  type IV, progressive encephalopathy and, 129
Mucopolysaccharidosis, evaluation of, *129*
  progressive encephalopathy and, 138–139
  type I, progressive encephalopathy and, 128, 128t
  type II, progressive encephalopathy and, 139
  type III, progressive encephalopathy and, 128
  type IV, paraplegia and, 268
  type VII, progressive encephalopathy and, 139
Multiple sclerosis, acute ataxia and, 227–228, *228*
Muscle(s), abnormal activity of, 200t, 200–204, 201t
  diseases with, 199t

Muscle(s) *(Continued)*
  abnormal activity of, hypoadrenalism and, 204
    hypocalcemia and, 203–204
    Isaacs syndrome and, 202
    myotonia congenita and, 202–203
    neuromyotonia and, 201
    Schwartz-Jampel syndrome and, 202
    Stiffman syndrome and, 200–201, 201t
    systemic disorders and, 203–204
    tetany and, 203–204
    thyroid disease and, 203
    uremia and, 203
  activity of, carbohydrate metabolism and, *204*
  biopsy of, creatine kinase level and, 205
    in infantile hypotonia, 156
  cramps of, 209–212
    Brody disease and, 211–212
    evaluation of, *206*
    tubular aggregates and, 211, *211*
  decreased activity of, 204–209
    ischemic exercise in, *205*, 205–206, *206*,
      206t
  decreased energy of, carbohydrate utilization
    defects and, 206–207
    carnitine palmityltransferase deficiency and,
      207–208
    diseases with, 200t
    lactate dehydrogenase deficiency and, 207
    lipid utilization defects and, 207–208
    mitochondrial myopathy and, 208–209
    myoadenylate deaminase deficiency and, 209
    phosphofructokinase deficiency and, 207
    phosphoglycerate kinase deficiency and, 207
    phosphoglycerate mutase deficiency and, 207
    respiratory chain abnormalities and, 208–
      209, *209*
  extraocular, 303t
    fibrosis of, 304
  stiffness of, 199, 209–212
    electromyography in, 200t
    malignant hyperthermia and, 209–210
    neuroleptic malignant syndrome and, 210
    rigid spine syndrome and, 210
    trilaminar myopathy and, 210
Muscular dystrophy, 148t
  Becker, 175–178
  clinical features of, 179t
  congenital, Fukuyama type, 164–165
    infantile hypotonia and, *164*, 164–165
  Duchenne, 175–178, *176*, *177*
    carrier status in, 177
    diagnosis of, 176
    treatment of, 176–177
  Emery-Dreifuss, distal limb weakness and, 191–
    192
  infantile hypotonia and, *164*, 164–166
  limb-girdle, 178, *178*
    vs. Becker muscular dystrophy, 178
  oculopharyngeal, facial weakness and, 342–343
  proximal limb weakness and, 175–179, *176*,
    177
Myasthenia, limb-girdle, familial, 174–175
  proximal limb weakness and, 174–175
  sporadic, 175
Myasthenia gravis, congenital, 304
  generalized weakness and, 194
  infantile, familial, hypotonia and, 161
  juvenile, hypotonia and, 160

Myasthenia gravis *(Continued)*
  neonatal, transitory, hypotonia and, 161
  ocular, 306–308
  progressive facial diplegia and, 342
  treatment of, 308
  unilateral ophthalmoplegia and, 306–308
Myasthenic crisis, 307
Myelitis, transverse, spinal paraplegia and, 270–
  271
Myelomeningocele, paraplegia and, 264–266
  treatment of, 266
Myoadenylate deaminase, deficiency of, decreased muscle energy and, 209
  muscle biopsy and, 206
  metabolic pathway of, *205*
Myoclonus, 296t, 296–297
  absence, in children, 28
  action, postanoxic, 47
  benign, in infants, 22
  essential, 296–297
  etiologic classification of, 296t
  focal, 297
  juvenile, 28–29
  nocturnal, benign, in newborn, 5
  palatal, 297
  posthypoxic, 297
  progressive, 29t, 29–30
  segmental, 297
  symptomatic, 297
Myoedema, 203
Myokymia, 200t
Myopathy, 147
  carbohydrate, proximal limb weakness and, 182
  centronuclear, infantile hypotonia and, 162–
    163
  disproportion, fiber type, 148t
    congenital, infantile hypotonia and, 162
    infantile hypotonia and, 161–164, *162*,
      163
  distal, hereditary, 191
    adult onset, 191
    infant onset, 191
  distal limb weakness and, 190–191
  endocrine, proximal limb weakness and, 183
  inflammatory, proximal limb weakness and,
    179t, 179–181, *180*
  lipid, proximal limb weakness and, 182
  metabolic, 148t
    infantile hypotonia and, 166–168
    proximal limb weakness and, 181–183
  mitochondrial, chronic ataxia and, 240
    decreased muscle energy and, 208–209
    proximal limb weakness and, 182–183, *183*
  myotubular, acute, infantile hypotonia and,
    162–163
    chronic, infantile hypotonia and, 163
    infantile hypotonia and, 162–163
  nemaline, infantile hypotonia and, 163, *163*
  rod, infantile hypotonia and, 163, *163*
  trilaminar, muscle stiffness and, 210
Myophosphorylase, deficiency of, muscle energy
  decrease and, 206–207
  proximal weakness and, 207
Myositis, infantile, hypotonia and, 168
  infectious, generalized weakness and, 194
  orbital, 310
Myotonia congenita, abnormal muscle activity
  and, 202–203

Myotonic discharge, 200t
Myotonic dystrophy, distal limb weakness and, 190–191
Mysoline. See *Primidone.*

Narcolepsy-cataplexy, in children, 24–25
Narcotics, neonatal withdrawal from, 14
Neck, injury to, headache and, 84
  trauma to, acute hemiplegia and, 252
Neck reflex, 150
Necrosis, striatal, bilateral, infantile, chorea and, 288
Neocortical death, 48
Nerve, biopsy of, in infantile hypotonia, 156
Nerve palsy, idiopathic, ophthalmoplegia and, 306
Neural crest syndrome, 216t
Neuritis, brachial, monoplegia and, 279–280
  sensory disturbances and, 218–219
  optic, 334
   idiopathic, acute blindness and, 326
Neuroaxonal dystrophy, infantile, progressive encephalopathy and, 136
Neuroblastoma, metastatic, acute hemiplegia and, 256
  myoclonic encephalopathy and, 227
  spinal paraplegia and, 269–270
Neurocutaneous disorders, megalencephaly and, 368–369
Neurocutaneous syndromes, progressive encephalopathy and, 135–136
Neuroectodermal tumor, primitive, increased intracranial pressure and, 99–100
Neurofibromatosis, infantile seizures and, 20t
  progressive encephalopathy and, 135–136
Neurolation, defective, primary microcephaly and, 370–371
Neuroleptic malignant syndrome, muscle stiffness and, 210
Neuroma, acoustic, acquired hearing impairment and, 352, *352*
Neuromuscular blockade, generalized weakness and, 194
Neuromuscular disese. See *Limb weakness.*
Neuromuscular transmission, disorders of, 148t
  infantile hypotonia and, 160–161
Neuromyelitis optica, spinal paraplegia and, 270–271
Neuromyotonia, 200t
  abnormal muscle activity and, 201
Neuron, defective migration of, primary microcephaly and, 372
Neuronal degeneration, infantile hyptonia and, 158
Neuronopathy, 147, 184
Neuropathy, 147. See also *Hereditary sensory and autonomic neuropathy.*
  amyloid, hereditary, distal limb weakness and, 187
  axonal, chronic, distal limb weakness and, 190
   giant, 190
  brachial, neonatal, monoplegia and, 282–283
  cranial, recurrent, causes of, 339t
  demyelinating, chronic, distal limb weakness and, 189t, 189–190
  diagnosis of, 183–184
  drugs and, 188
  electrodiagnosis in, 84t

Neuropathy *(Continued)*
  genetic, distal limb weakness and, 186–187
  hypomyelinating, congenital, hypotonia and, 159
  idiopathic, distal limb weakness and, 189–190
  motor sensory, hereditary, distal limb weakness and, 185–186
  optic, compressive, progressive vision loss and, 331–333, *332*
   demyelinating, acute blindness and, 325–326
   dominant, progressive vision loss and, 330–331
   indirect, acute blindness and, 328
   ischemic, acute blindness, 326–327
   Leber, chronic ataxia and, 245
    progressive vision loss and, 33
   toxic, acute blindness and, 328–329
  peroneal, monoplegia and, 284
  radial, monoplegia and, 284
  toxins and, 188
  ulnar, monoplegia and, 284
  uremia and, 188–189
Neuroretinitis, 326, *326*
Neuroretinopathy, progressive vision loss and, 330
Neurovascular reflex dystrophy, 218–219
Niemann-Pick disease, DAF syndrome variant of, 315
  progressive encephalopathy and, 140
  type A, progressive encephalopathy and, 130
Night terrors, 25
Nitrazepam, for seizures, 36
Nitrofurantoin, neuropathy with, 188
Nocturnal myoclonus, benign, in newborn, 5
Null point, ocular, 317
Nylen-Hallpike technique, 354
Nystagmus, 316t, 316–319
  acquired, 317–319
   divergence, 319
   downbeat, 318–319
   drug-induced, 318
   ictal, 318
   jerk, 317
   monocular, 319
   pendular, 317
   see-saw, 319
   upbeat, 318
   vestibular, 318
  congenital, 316–317
  optokinetic, 322
  visual acuity and, 316

Obscurations, 321
Obsessive-compulsive state, Tourette syndrome and, 298
Obtundation, 42t
Ocular bobbing, 316, 316t
Ocular dysmetria, 316, 316t
Ocular flutter, 316, 316t
Ocular motility, disorders of, 302–320
Ocular motor apraxia, congenital, 313–314
  vertical, congenital, 315
Oculocerebrorenal syndrome, cerebral hypotonia and, 153
Oculomotor nerve palsy, congenital, 303
Olivopontocerebellar degeneration, chronic ataxia and, 240

Ondine's curse, 46
Ophthalmoplegia, 303–313
    bilateral, acute, 312, 312t
        botulism and, 312, 312t
        drug intoxication and, 312, 312t
    chronic, 312–313, 313t
        thyrotoxicosis and, 313
    congenital, 303–305
        abducens nerve palsy and, 304
        Brown syndrome and, 304–305
        congenital ptosis and, 305
        extraocular muscle fibrosis and, 304
        myasthenia gravis and, 304
        oculomotor nerve palsy and, 303
        trochlear nerve palsy and, 303–304
    internuclear, 314
    unilateral, acute, 305–311, 306t
        aneurysm and, 309
        brainstem glioma and, *309*, 309–310
        brainstem stroke and, 310
        cavernous sinus fistula and, 311
        cavernous sinus thrombosis and, 311
        Gradenigo syndrome and, 308–309
        idiopathic nerve palsy and, 306
        migraine and, 306
        myasthenia gravis and, 306–308
        orbital pseudotumor and, 310
        orbital tumors and, 308
        Tolosa-Hunt syndrome and, 310
        trauma and, 311
Opisthotonos, 3, 46
Opsoclonus, 316, 316t
Optic atrophy, hereditary, vision loss and, 330–334
Optic disk, swollen, intracranial pressure and, *92*, 92t, 92–93, *93*, 93t
Optic nerve, glioma of, progressive vision loss and, 331–332, *332*
    hypoplasia of, congenital, blindness and, 323–324, *324*
    infarction of, acute blindness and, 326
Optic neuritis, idiopathic, acute blindness and, 326
    progressive, 334
Optic neuropathy, compressive, progressive vision loss and, 331–333, *332*
    demyelinating, acute blindness and, 325–326
    dominant, progressive vision loss and, 330–331
    indirect, acute blindness and, 328
    Leber, chronic ataxia and, 245
        progressive vision loss and, 330
    toxic, acute blindness and, 328–329
Optokinetic nystagmus, 322
Orbital pseudotumor, unilateral ophthalmoplegia and, 310
Orbital tumor, unilateral ophthalmoplegia and, 308
Organoid nevus syndrome, megalencephaly and, 368–369
Orgasm, headache and, 82
Ornithine, metabolic disorder of, progressive vision loss and, 333
Ornithine transcarbamylase, deficiency of, neonatal seizures and, *12*, 12–13, 13t
Osmolality, disorders of, altered states of consciousness and, 61–63
Osteomyelitis, tuberculous, paraplegia and, 273
Osteomyelitis-neuritis, monoplegia and, 280–281
Osteopetrosis, facial weakness and, 345

Otitis media, hearing impairment and, 350–353
Oxycephaly, 373t

Pachygyria, 372
Pain, congenital insensitivity to, hereditary sensory and autonomic neuropathy II and, 216
    hereditary sensory and autonomic neuropathy IV and, 216
    sensory disturbances and, 221–222
    headache, sources of, 73t, 73–74
Pallid syncope, in infants, 18
Palsy, Bell, facial weakness and, 341
    vs. herpes zoster oticus, 344
    bulbar, progressive, juvenile, 344–345
    cerebral, 276t, 276–277
    convergence, 315
    cranial, recurrent, causes of, 339t
    facial, recurrent, 343
    gaze, 313t, 313–315
        horizontal, 315
        vertical, 314–315
    pontobulbar, acquired hearing impairment and, 350
    pressure, recurrent, hereditary, 284–285
    pseudobulbar, facial weakness and, 338
Pancuronium, newborn paralysis with, seizures and, 1
Panencephalitis, rubella, progressive, 144
    sclerosing, subacute, 144
Panic disorder, altered states of consciousness and, 65
Papilledema, hemispheric astrocytoma and, 97
    intracranial pressure increase and, 92–93
    vs. drusen, 93, *93*
Papilloma, of choroid plexus, increased intracranial pressure and, 100–101
    noncommunicating hydrocephalus and, 365
Paraldehyde, for neonatal seizures, 17
Paralysis, periodic, generalized weakness and, 195–196
    hyperkalemic, familial, 195–196
    hypokalemic, familial, 195
    normokalemic, familial, 196
    tick, generalized weakness and, 194
    Todd, 258
Paramyotonia congenita, 195
Parapharyngeal space, infection of, acute hemiplegia and, 253
Paraplegia, approach to, 263
    cerebral, 276t, 276–277
        spastic, 276–277
    spastic, familial, 275–276
        autosomal dominant inheritance of, 275
        autosomal recessive inheritance of, 275
        hereditary sensory and autonomic neuropathy with, 217
    spinal, 263–276, 264t
        Adamkiewitz's artery embolization and, 273
        adrenoleukodystrophy and, 270–271
        arteriovenous malformation and, 267–268
        astrocytoma and, 269, *269*
        atlanto-axial dislocation and, 268
        causes of, 264t
        childhood trauma and, 273–275, *275*
        compressed vertebral body fracture and, 274
        congenital malformations and, 264–268
        Devic disease and, 270–271

Paraplegia *(Continued)*
spinal, diffuse encephalomyelitis and, 271
dysraphia and, 264–267
ependymoma and, 269–270
epidural abscess and, 272–273
epidural hematoma and, 275
fracture dislocation and, 274–275, *275*
infections and, 271–273, *272*
Klippel-Feil syndrome and, 268
Morquio syndrome and, 268
mucopolysaccharidosis IV and, 268
myelomeningocele and, 264–266
neuroblastoma and, 269–270
neuromyelitis optica and, 270–271
newborn trauma and, 273
signs of, 263–264
spinal cord concussion and, 274
spinal cord transection and, 274–275, *275*
spinal cord tumors and, 268–270, *269*
symptoms of, 263–264
tethered spinal cord and, 266–267, *267*
transverse myelitis and, 270–271
tuberculous osteomyelitis and, 273
Parathyroid gland, disorders of, altered states of
consciousness and, 63
Parinaud's syndrome, 100
Paroxysmal choreoathetosis, familial, 25
Paroxysmal disorders, 1–41. See also specific disorders, e.g., *Seizure(s).*
in children, 23–39, *27*, 29t, *31*, 32t
in newborns, 1–17, 2t, *3*, *4*, 5t, 6t, *8*, 10t, *11*,
12, 13t
of infants, 17t, 17–23, 20t, 21t
Paroxysmal laughter, in newborn, 2
Pelizaeus-Merzbacher disease, progressive encephalopathy and, 137–138
Pendred syndrome, congenital deafness and, 349
Pendular nystagmus, 316, 317
Pentobarbital coma, for increased incranial pres-
sure, 95–96, *96*
Periodic breathing, in newborn, 4
Periodic lateralizing epilepiform discharge, cerebral
necrosis and, *51*
Periodic paralysis, generalized weakness and,
195–196
hyperkalemic, familial, 195–196
hypokalemic, familial, 195
normokalemic, familial, 196
Peroneal nerve, injury to, monoplegia and, 284
Peroxisomes, disorders of, cerebral hypotonia
and, 152
Pertussis vaccine, encephalopathy with, 57–58
Phasic tone, 147
Phenacemide, for complex partial seizures, 28
for seizures, 36
Phenobarbital, for neonatal seizures, 16
for seizures, 37
intraventricular hemorrhage and, 104
Phenothiazine, overdose of, 66
Phenurone. See *Phenacemide.*
Phenylalanine, metabolism of, *125*
Phenylketonuria, progressive encephalopathy and,
125, 125t, 125–126
Phenytoin, for neonatal seizures, 16–17
for seizures, 36–37
Phosphofructokinase, deficiency of, infantile hypo-
tonia and, 167
muscle abnormalities and, 207

Phosphoglycerate kinase, deficiency of, muscle
abnormalities and, 207
Phosphoglycerate mutase, deficiency of, muscle
abnormalities and, 207
Phosphorylase, deficiency of, infantile hypotonia
and, 167–168
Photopsias, 321
Pineal region, tumors of, increased intracranial
pressure and, 100
Pituitary, adenoma of, progressive vision loss and,
332–333
infarction of, acute blindness and, 329
Plagiocephaly, 373t
Plexitis, brachial, monoplegia and, 279–280
idiopathic, acute, monoplegia and, 279–280
lumbar, monoplegia and, 280
Plexopathy, brachial, hereditary, monoplegia and,
281–281
monoplegia and, 279–284
Pneumonia, mycoplasmal, acute hemiplegia and,
252
Poisoning, 67. See also specific substances and
Drug(s).
facial weakness and, 345
neuropathy with, 188
Poliodystrophy, infantile, progressive, 133–134
Poliovirus, infection with, generalized weakness
and, 192–193
Polymyositis, proximal limb weakness and, 181
Polyneuropathy, amyloid, familial, sensory disturbances and, 218
cranial, idiopathic, facial weakness and, 341–
342
demyelinating, inflammatory, chronic, hypotonia and, 159
dysimmune, relapsing, 189
infantile hypotonia and, 158–159, 159t
Polyradiculoneuropathy, acute, generalized weakness and, 193
demyelinating, inflammatory, 189
Pompe disease, infantile hypotonia and, 166
Pontobulbar palsy, acquired hearing impairment
and, 350
Porencephaly, hydranencephaly and, 367
midline, congenital, 367
Porphyria, intermittent, acute, generalized weak-
ness and, 196
Post-traumatic sympathetic dystrophy, 218–219
Postconcussion syndrome, acute ataxia and, 228–
229
Postural reflexes, 150
Postural tone, 147
Posturing, abnormal. See *Dystonia.*
decerebrate, 3
Prader-Willi syndrome, cerebral hypotonia and,
151, 151t
Pregnancy, chorea and, 290
Primidone, for seizures, 37
Primitive neuroectodermal tumor, increased intra-
cranial pressure and, 99–100
Propionyl-CoA carboxylase, *11*
Propranolol, for migraine prophylaxis, 79
Proptosis, differential diagnosis of, 308
Prosencephalization, defective, primary micro-
cephaly and, 371–372
Pseudoataxia, 234
Pseudobulbar palsy, facial weakness and, 338
Pseudoseizures, 33

Pseudotumor, orbital, unilateral ophthalmoplegia and, 310
Pseudotumor cerebri, increased intracranial pressure and, 115t, 115–116
Psychomotor retardation, 118–123. See also *Developmental delay.*
Ptosis, congenital, 305
Pupil, aniridia of, 335
  Argyll Robertson, 335
  constriction of, 46
  dilated, fixed, 334–335
  dilation of, 46
  disorders of, 334–335
  essential anisocoria of, 334
  Horner syndrome of, 335
  tonic, 334
Pupillary light reflex, 46
Pure tone audiometry, 347
Pyridoxine, deficiency of, neonatal seizures and, 15
  for infantile spasms, 21–22
Pyruvate, metabolic defects of, distal limb weakness and, 187
  neonatal, 14
  progressive encephalopathy and, 133–134
Pyruvate decarboxylase, deficiency of, acute ataxia and, 231

Quadriplegia. See also *Paraplegia.*
  cerebral, 276t, 276–277
  spastic, 277
  spinal, 263–276, 264t

Radial nerve, injury to, monoplegia and, 284
Ramsay Hunt syndrome, 241–242
  facial weakness and, 344
  variants of, chronic ataxia and, 240–241
Rasmussen syndrome, 32
Recruitment test, 347
Reflex, Moro, 132, 150
  neck, 150
  postural, infantile hypotonia and, 150
  sucking, 337
  swallowing, 337
  tendon, 150
Reflex sympathetic dystrophy, sensory disturbances and, 218–219
Refsum disease, chronic ataxia and, 245
  distal limb weakness and, 186
  hearing impairment and, 350
Regression, psychomotor, 118–146. See also *Encephalopathy, progressive.*
Renal failure, encephalopathy with, 59
Respiratory chain abnormalities, decreased muscle energy and, 208–209, *209*
Respiratory distress, perinatal, motor unit disorders in, 149t
Retardation, psychomotor, 118–123. See also *Developmental delay.*
Retina, injury to, acute blindness and, 328
Retinal artery, obstruction of, acute blindness and, 327
Retinitis, measles, acute blindness and, 329
Retinitis pigmentosa, hearing impairment and, 350

Retinoblastoma, progressive vision loss and, 333
Rett syndrome, progressive encephalopathy and, 136–137
Reye syndrome, encephalopathy in, 54–55
Rhabdomyosarcoma, 101
Rheumatic chorea, 290
Rigid spine syndrome, muscle stiffness and, 210
Rigidity, decerebrate, 46
  decorticate, 46
  in newborn, 201t
Riley-Day syndrome, 216
  cerebral hypotonia and, 153
Ring lesion, 111, *111*
Rinne test, 347
Rolandic epilepsy, 30, *31*
Rosenthal fibers, 137
Roussy-Lévy syndrome, 185
Rubella, congenital, 144
Rubella embryopathy, developmental delay and, 123
Rubella panencephalitis, progressive, 144
Rubeola encephalitis, 50–52

Salicylates, ototoxicity of, 350
  Reye syndrome and, 54–55
Sandhoff disease, progressive encephalopathy and, 132–133
Sandifer syndrome, 295
Santavuori, neuronal ceroid lipofuscinosis and, 137
Sarcoidosis, facial weakness and, 344
Sarcoma, osteogenic, 101
Sarcoplasmic reticulum, calcium-activated ATP deficiency in, muscle crampls and, 211–212
  tubular aggregates of, muscle cramps and, 211, *211*
Scaphocephaly, 373, 373t
Scapulo(humeral)peroneal syndrome, distal limb weakness and, 191–192
Scapulohumeral syndrome, dementia and, distal limb weakness with, 192
Schilder's disease, 143
Schizophrenia, altered states of consciousness and, 65
Schwartz-Jampel syndrome, abnormal muscle activity and, 202
Scissoring, infantile hypotonia and, 150
Scoliosis, in syringomyelia, 220
Scotoma, 321
Sea-blue histiocytosis, chronic ataxia and, 244–245
  DAF syndrome variant of, 315
See-saw nystagmus, 319
Seizure(s), absence, in children, 26–27, *27*
  Lennox-Gastaut syndrome and, 23
  adversive, 315
  anticonvulsant drug therapy for, 33–38
    acetazolamide in, 35
    adverse reaction of, 34–35
    blood concentrations of, 34
    carbamazepine in, 35
    clonazepam in, 35–36
    clorazepate in, 36
    discontinuation of, 34
    ethosuximide in, 36
    indications for, 33

Seizure(s) *(Continued)*
 anticonvulsant drug therapy for, methsuximide
  in, 36
  nitrazepam in, 36
  phenacemide in, 36
  phenobarbital in, 37
  phenytoin in, 36–37
  primidone in, 37
  principles of, 34
  trimethadione in, 37
  valproic acid in, 38
 aphasia and, 31
 basilar migraine and, 229
 benign, 30, *31*
 clonic, focal, in newborn, 2
  multifocal, familial, 16
   in newborn, 2
 continual, 32, 251
 febrile, epilepsy and, 19
  in infants, 18–19
  meningitis and, 19
  pertussis vaccine and, 57
  treatment guidelines for, 19
  vs. myoclonic epilepsy, 22
 headache and, 86
 hemiparetic, 258
 hemispheric astrocytoma and, 97
 hysterical, 33
 in bacterial meningitis, 108
 in cherry-red spot–myoclonus syndrome, 29–
  30
 in Lafora disease, 29
 in Landau-Kleffner syndrome, 31–32
 in Rett syndrome, 137
 in Unverricht-Lundborg syndrome, 29
 mild head injury and, 67
 myoclonic, EEG appearance of, 21t
  in children, 28–30, 29t
  in newborns, 3
 neonatal, 1–17
  aminoacidopathies and, 10–13, *11, 12,* 13t
  anticonvulsant drugs for, 8t
  benign, 16
  etiology of, onset time and, 5t, 5–6
  glycine encephalopathy and, 11
  herpes simplex encephalitis and, 13–14
  hypocalcemia and, 10
  hypoglycemia and, 9–10, 10t
  hypoxic-ischemic encephalopathy and, 6–9,
   8, 8t
  incontinentia pigmenti and, 15–16
  isovaleric acidemia and, 11, *11*
  kernicterus and, 15
  ketotic hyperglycinemia and, 11–12
  mitochondrial disorders and, 14
  paraldehyde for, 17
  patterns of, 1–3, 2t, *3*
  phenobarbital for, 16
  phenytoin for, 16–17
  pyridoxine dependency and, 15
  subarachnoid hemorrhage and, 9
  subdural hemorrhage and, 9
  treatment of, 16–17
   duration of, 17
  urea cycle disturbances of, *12,* 12–13, 13t
 neurocutaneous cases of, in infants, 20t
 nonfebrile, in infants, 19–20
 nystagmus and, 318
 pancuronium and, 1

Seizure(s) *(Continued)*
 partial, complex, glioma and, 28
  in children, 27–28
  in children, 30–32, *31*
 patterns of, in newborn, 1–3, 2t, *3*
 posttraumatic, 69–70
 pseudo-, 33
 simulation of, 23–25
 subtle, in newborn, 1–2, *2,* 2t
 supratentorial malformation and, 106–107
 tonic, in newborn, 3
 tonic-clonic, absence seizures and, 26
  generalized, 32t, 32–33
 transient posttraumatic cerebral blindness in,
  328
Sensation, disturbances of, 214–222. *See also*
  *Hereditary sensory and autonomic neurop-
  athy.*
 brachial neuritis and, 218–219
 congenital pain insensitivity and, 221–222
 Déjérine-Roussy syndrome and, 221
 familial amyloid polyneuropathy and, 218
 hereditary sensory and autonomic neuropathy in, 214–218, 215t, 216t
 lumbar disk herniation and, 219
 reflex sympathetic dystrophy and, 218–219
 symptoms of, 214, 214t
 syringomyelia and, 219–220, *220*
 thalamic pain syndrome of Déjérine-Roussy
  and, 221
Sepsis, bacterial, 55–56
 gram-negative, 55
Shaking, injuries from, altered states of consciousness and, 67–68
Shock, hemorrhagic, encephalopathy and, 56
 septic, 55–56
Shoulder, osteomyelitis, monoplegia and, 280–
  281
SIADH. *See Syndrome of inappropriate antidiuretic hormone.*
Sialidosis, type II, progressive encephalopathy
  and, 129–130, 130t
Sickle cell anemia, acute hemiplegia and, 254–
  155
Sinusitis, headache and, 84
Skeletal disorders, hearing impairment and, 351,
  351t
Skull, fractures of, 69
Sleep paralysis, in children, 24
Sodium, loss of, altered states of consciousness
  and, 62
Sotos syndrome, 368
Spasms, 199
 habit. *See Tic.*
 hemifacial, 295–296
 infantile, 20t, 20–22
  ACTH for, 21
  diagnosis of, 21
  EEG appearance of, 21t
  pyridoxine for, 21–22
  treatment of, 21–22
Spasmus nutans, 317
Speech, disturbance of, dialysis dementia syn-
  drome and, 60
Speech discrimination test, 347
Speech reception threshold test, 347
Spielmeyer-Vogt-Sjögren disease, progressive en-
  cephalopathy and, 142
Spina bifida cystica, 265

Spina bifida occulta, 266
Spinal cord, imaging of, 264t
    infarction of, in newborn, 273
    injury to, infantile hypotonia and, 154–155
    tethered, paraplegia and, 266–267, 267
    transection of, paraplegia and, 274–275
    tumors of, paraplegia and, 268–270, 269
Spinal muscular atrophy, autosomal dominant
        type, 173–174
    autosomal recessive type, 173
    distal limb weakness and, 184–185, 191–192
    infantile, acute, 156–157, 157
        chronic, 157–158
    proximal limb weakness and, 172–174
Spine, concussion of, paraplegia and, 274
    dermal sinus of, 266
    diastematomyelia of, 266
    rigidity of, 210
    tuberculosis of, paraplegia and, 273
Spongy degeneration of infancy, progressive en-
        cephalopathy and, 138
SSPE, 144
St. Louis encephalitis, 52
Staphylococcus aureus, diskitis from, 271–272,
        272
    toxic shock syndrome and, 55
Staring spells, 26–28, 27
Status epilepticus, complex, partial, 28
    treatment of, 38–39
Stenosis, aqueductal, noncommunicating hydro-
        cephalus and, 363–364, 364
Steppage gait, 170, 223
Stiffman syndrome, abnormal muscle activity and,
        200–201, 201t
    genetic form of, 200–201, 201t
    sporadic form of, 201
Stiffness, in newborn, 201t
    myopathic, 209–212
Strabismus, intracranial pressure increase and, 92
    nonparalytic, 302–303
    paralytic, 303–313
Streptococcus pneumoniae, hearing loss and, 351
Streptomycin, vertigo and, 354
Stress, migraine and, 75
Striatal necrosis, bilateral, chorea and, 288
Stroke. See Cerebrovascular disease.
    brainstem, unilateral ophthalmoplegia and, 310
    capsular, idiopathic, acute hemiplegia and,
        250–251
Stupor, 42t
Sturge-Weber syndrome, infantile seizures and,
        20t
Subacute necrotizing encephalomyelopathy, 133
Subacute sclerosing panencephalitis, 144
Subarachnoid screw, for intracranial pressure
        monitoring, 94
Subarachnoid space, benign enlargement of, com-
        municating hydrocephalus and, 361–362,
        362
Subdural cup catheter, for intracranial pressure
        monitoring, 94
Subdural tap, in shaking injury, 68
Subthalamic nucleus, atrophy of, 240
Sucking reflex, 337
Sudeck atrophy, 218–219
Sulfatide lipidosis, distal limb weakness and, 187
    juvenile, chronic ataxia and, 244
        progressive encephalopathy and, 141
    progressive encephalopathy and, 131–132

Superior oblique palsy, unilateral ophthalmoplegia
        and, 311
Suspension, horizontal, in infantile hypotension,
        149
    vertical, in infantile hypotension, 149
Swallowing reflex, 337
Sydenham chorea, 290
Syncope, cyanotic, in infants, 18
    in children, 23–24
    in infants, 17–18
    pallid, in infants, 18
Syndrome of inappropriate antidiuretic hormone
        (SIADH), altered states of consciousness and,
        62
Syringobulbia, 219
    facial weakness and, 345
Syringomyelia, sensory disturbance and, 219–
        220, 220
Syrinx, formation of, 219
Systemic lupus erythematosus, acute hemiplegia
        and, 255
    chorea and, 290
    headache and, 83

Takayasu arteritis, acute hemiplegia and, 255
Tapetoretinal degeneration, progressive vision loss
        and, 333–334
Taps, subdural, in shaking injury, 68
Tardive dyskinesia, 287
Tay-Sachs disease, progressive encephalopathy
        and, 132
Telangiectasias, ataxia and, 242
Temporomandibular joint (TMJ) syndrome, head-
        ache and, 84–85
Tendon reflexes, 150
Tensilon test, 307
    in infantile hypotonia, 156
Tension headache, 83–84
Tentorial notch, herniation of, increased intracra-
        nial pressure and, 93t, 93–94
Teratoma, 100
    noncommunicating hydrocephalus and, 365
Tetany, 203–204
Tetrahydrobiopterin, deficiency of, 126
Thalamus, pain syndrome of, sensory disturbance
        and, 221
Thromboembolism, in homocystinuria, 126
Thrombosis, of cavernous sinus, unilateral
        ophthalmoplegia and, 311
    venous, acute hemiplegia and, 256
    venous sinus, acute hemiplegia and, 253
Thryoid disease, abnormal muscle activity and,
        203
Thyroid gland, disorders of, altered states of con-
        sciousness and, 63
Thyrotoxicosis, bilateral ophthalmoplegia and, 313
Thyroxine synthesis, defect of, congenital deafness
        and, 349
Tic, 297–299
    motor, simple, 297
Tick paralysis, generalized weakness and, 194
Tinnitus, 346
Titubation, 223
TMJ syndrome. See Temporomandibular joint
        syndrome.
Todd paralysis, 258
Toe-walking, 170

Tolosa-Hunt syndrome, facial weakness and, 342
  unilateral ophthalmoplegia and, 310
Tone, phasic, 147
  postural, 147
Tonic pupil syndrome, 334
Torticollis, 294t, 294–295
  paroxysmal, benign, 295
Tourette syndrome, 297–298, 297–299
  treatment of, 298–299
Toxic shock syndrome, 55
Toxin. See also *Drug(s)*.
  facial weakness and, 345
  neuropathy with, 188
Toxoplasmosis, developmental delay and, 122
Traction response, 148–149, *149*
Transferase deficiency, progressive encephalopathy and, 134–135
Transient global amnesia, 64
Transverse myelitis, spinal paraplegia and, 270–271
Tranxene. See *Clorazepate*.
Trauma, acute ataxia and, 228–229
  acute hemiplegia and, 260
  altered states of consciousness and, 67–70
  head, facial weakness and, 345
    vertigo and, 356–357
  hearing impairment and, 351
  unilateral ophthalmoplegia and, 311
Tremor, 299–300
  action, 299
  essential, 299–300
  familial, 299–300
  physiologic, 299
Tremulousness, in newborn, 5
Tricyclic antidepressants, overdose of, 65–66
Tridione. See *Trimethadione*.
Trigonocephaly, 373t
Trilaminar myopathy, muscle stiffness and, 210
Trimethadione, for seizures, 37–38
Trisomy, 10 p, 121t
  18, 121t
  21, 121t
Trochlear nerve palsy, congenital, 303–304
Tuberculosis, meningitis with, 110
  vertebral, paraplegia and, 273
Tuberous sclerosis, infantile seizures and, 20t
  progressive encephalopathy and, 135–136
Tubular aggregates, muscle cramps and, 211, *211*
Tumor. See also specific tumors, e.g., *Astrocytoma*.
  acute hemiplegia and, 260
  brain, acute ataxia and, 234
    noncommunicating hydrocephalus and, 365
  facial weakness and, 345
  hearing impairment and, 352
  intraocular, progressive vision loss and, 333
  meningeal, communicating hydrocephalus and, 362–363, *363*
  orbital, unilateral ophthalmoplegia and, 308
Tyrosinemia, transitory, 126

Ulcer, foot, hereditary sensory and autonomic neuropathy I and, 215
Ulnar nerve, injury to, monoplegia and, 284
Unverricht-Lundborg syndrome, 29
Upbeat nystagmus, 318

Urea cycle, disturbances of, neonatal seizures and, *12*, 12–13, 13t
Uremia, abnormal muscle activity and, 203
  neuropathy with, 188–189
Uremic encephalopathy, acute, 59
  chronic, 59
Usher syndrome, congenital deafness and, 349–350
Uveoparotitis, sarcoidosis and, 344

Vaccines, postimmunization encephalopathy with, 57–58
Valproic acid, for seizures, 38
  toxicity of, 19
Vascular disorders, acute ataxia and, 233–234
Vascular headache, nonmigrainous, 80t, 80–83
Vasculitis, headache and, 83
  hypersensitivity, acute hemiplegia and, 255–256
    headache and, 83
  systemic, neuropathy and, 189
Vasculopathy, 189
Vegetative state, persistent, 48
Vein of Galen malformation, increased intracranial pressure and, 106
  noncommunicating hydrocephalus and, 365–366
Venous sinus thrombosis, acute hemiplegia and, 253
Ventriculostomy, for intracranial pressure monitoring, 94
Vermis, aplasia of, chronic ataxia and, 238–239
Vertebra, compressed fracture of, paraplegia and, 274
  fracture dislocation of, paraplegia and, 274–275, *275*
Vertebral artery, trauma to, acute hemiplegia and, 252
Vertebrobasilar arteries, trauma to, acute ataxia and, 229
Vertical suspension, infantile hypotension and, 149
Vertigo, 352–357, 353t
  aminoglycosides and, 354
  anatomic considerations in, 352–353
  antibiotics and, 354
  approach to, 353–354
  bacterial infection and, 354–355
  caloric testing in, 353–354
  causes of, 353t
  central, vs. peripheral, 353t
  cholesteatoma and, 355
  drug effects and, 354
  electronystagmography in, 354
  epilepsy and, 354
  gentamicin and, 354
  history in, 353
  labyrinthitis and, 355
  Meniere disease and, 355–356
  migraine and, 23, 356
  minocycline and, 354
  motion sickness and, 356
  Nylen-Hallpike technique in, 354
  paroxysmal, benign, acute ataxia and, 230–231
  peripheral, vs. central, 353t
  physical examination in, 353

Vertigo *(Continued)*
  positional, paroxysmal, 357
  recurrent, benign, 356
  special tests for, 353–354
  streptomycin and, 354
  trauma and, 356–357
  vestibular concussion and, 356–357
  viral infections and, 355
  whiplash injury and, 357
Vestibular nystagmus, 318
Vesticular concussion, vertigo and, 356–357
Vincristine, neuropathy with, 188
Viral encephalitis, 48–49
Vision, aberrations of, classic migraine and, 76–77
  loss of. See also *Blindness.*
    progressive, 330–334
      aminoacidopathies and, 333
      causes of, 325t
      Cockayne syndrome and, 333
      compressive optic neuropathy and, 331–333, *332*
      craniopharyngioma and, 331
      dominant optic neuropathy and, 330–331
      hypothalamic glioma and, 331–332, *332*
      intraocular tumors and, 333
      juvenile diabetes mellitus and, 331
      Laurence-Moon-Biedel syndrome and, 334
      Leber optic neuropathy and, 330
      mitochondrial disease and, 330
      neuroretinopathy and, 330
      optic glioma and, 331–332, *332*
      pituitary adenoma and, 332–333
      progressive optic neuritis and, 334
      tapetoretinal degenerations and, 333–334
Visual acuity, assessment of, 321t, 321–322
  nystagmus and, 316t, 316–319
Visual evoked response, 322

Visual system, disorders of, 321–335. See also *Blindness; Vision, loss of.*
Vitamin E, for intraventricular hemorrhage, 104
Von Hippel–Lindau disease, chronic ataxia and, 237–238

Warburg syndrome, noncommunicating hydrocephalus and, 366–367
Weakness. See *Limb weakness.*
  facial. See *Facial weakness.*
Weber test, 347
West syndrome, 20
Western equine encephalitis, 52
Whiplash injury, headache and, 84
  vertigo and, 357
White matter, diseases of, progressive encephalopathy and, 143–144
  genetic disorders of, progressive encephalopathy and, 137–138
Wilson disease, chorea and, 293–294
Wohlfart-Kugelberg-Welander disease, 172–174
Writer's cramp, 295

X-linked hereditary sensory neuropathy, 217
Xanthomatosis, cerebrotendinous, progressive encephalopathy and, 143–144
Xeroderma pigmentosum, progressive encephalopathy and, 143

Zarontin. See *Ethosuximide.*